Looking Forward to the Future of Heparin: New Sources, Developments and Applications

Special Issue Editors

Giangiacomo Torri
Jawed Fareed

MDPI • Basel • Beijing • Wuhan • Barcelona • Belgrade

MDPI

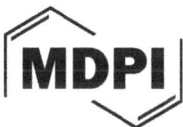

Special Issue Editors
Giangiacomo Torri
Ronzoni Institute
Italy

Jawed Fareed
Loyola University Medical Center
USA

Editorial Office
MDPI
St. Alban-Anlage 66
Basel, Switzerland

This edition is a reprint of the Special Issue published online in the open access journal *Molecules* (ISSN 1420-3049) from 2017–2018 (available at: http://www.mdpi.com/journal/molecules/special_issues/heparin).

For citation purposes, cite each article independently as indicated on the article page online and as indicated below:

Lastname, F.M.; Lastname, F.M. Article title. *Journal Name* **Year**, *Article number*, page range.

First Edition 2018

ISBN 978-3-03842-949-4 (Pbk)
ISBN 978-3-03842-950-0 (PDF)

Table of Contents

About the Special Issue Editors

Giangiacomo Torri, Dr., studied bioorganic chemistry at the University of Pavia. He joined the research group of Prof. B. Casu at the 'G. Ronzoni' Institute in 1973. He was a Harold Hibbert Fellow (1979–1980) at the "Department of Chemistry", of the McGill University of Montreal (Canada), as a guest of Prof. A.S. Perlin as a visiting scientist. From 2000 to 2015 Dr. Torri was the Director of the Ronzoni Research Institute. He is an expert in chemistry and biochemistry of bioactive carbohydrate polymers. He is especially involved in studies dealing with structural elucidation and modulation of sequences of glycosaminoglycans (GAGs), aimed at establishing structure–activity relationships. He contributed to the development of advanced approaches (especially by NMR spectroscopy and mass spectrometry) to the characterization of the structure, binding properties and complex formations of GAGs. He also contributed to the determination of the three-dimensional structure of GAG sequences both in the absence, and in the presence of binding proteins. He has wide experience in the coordination of interdisciplinary national and international research projects. He has over 250 scientific publications and patents. Since 2003, he has been President of the "Consortium for NMR research in Biotechnology and Material Science". From 2007 to 2016 he was an expert for the working party on Nuclear Magnetic Resonance Spectrometry of EU Pharmacopoeia Commission (EDQM). Since 2012, he has been the President of the "Centro Alta Tecnologia—Istituto G Ronzoni".

Jawed Fareed is a Professor of Pathology and Pharmacology and Director of the Hemostasis and Thrombosis Research Laboratories at Loyola University Medical Center, Chicago, IL. Dr. Fareed's main research interest is the development of glycosaminoglycan-derived drugs, such as heparins and novel anticoagulant and antithrombotic drugs. He is recognized for his role in the preclinical development and for initiating the first clinical trials of low-molecular-weight heparin and antithrombin agents in various vascular indications. He received his initial graduate training at the Imperial College, University of London in England, and at the University of Guelph in Ontario, Canada. In 1974, he completed his doctorate degree at Loyola University Chicago in the areas of pharmacology and experimental therapeutics. In 1996, he received the degree of Doctor Honoris Causa in hematology from the University of Bordeaux in France. He is the author or co-author of over 600 publications in the area of the diagnostic and therapeutic management of thrombotic disorders. In addition, he has authored several textbooks and has published extensively in the area of hemostasis and thrombosis. He also serves on the editorial boards of several leading journals in his area of expertise, including International Angiology and Journal of Clinical and Applied Thrombosis and Hemostasis where he serves as an Associate Editor. Dr. Fareed's professional affiliations include membership on the expert panel on biologicals for the World Health Organization, and fellowships of the American Heart Association, the American College of Angiology, and the Indian College of Interventional Cardiology. He is the founding director and vice president of the North American Thrombosis Forum. Currently he is the Chair of the scientific committee of the International Union of Angiology. He has received numerous awards from various national and international organizations, including the Lifetime Achievement award from the Association of Practicing Pathologists, India, in 2012, and the Mauro Bartolo Lifetime Achievement Award in 2017. Dr. Fareed views the current and past developments in heparin research as the foundation of thrombosis and hemostasis which also prompted progress made in the introduction of newer drugs to control thrombosis. He and his group is extensively involved in medical school and graduate education and research in vascular sciences.

molecules

MDPI

Editorial

Looking Forward to the Future of Heparin: New Sources, Developments and Applications

Giangiacomo Torri * and Giuseppe Cassinelli

Carbohydrate Sciences Department of Istituto di Ricerche Chimiche e Biochimiche "G. Ronzoni", 20133 Milan, Italy; ronzoni@ronzoni.it
* Correspondence: torri@ronzoni.it; Tel.: +39-02-70641621

Received: 26 January 2018; Accepted: 27 January 2018; Published: 31 January 2018

The seven reviews and the eleven articles in this special issue provide an updated survey of recent research and developments in the ever-growing field of heparin, along with low molecular weight heparins (LMWHs) and glycosaminoglycans (GAGs). The complex biosynthetic process, and the variability of tissues and animal species, has led to heparin chains heterogeneous in size and both N- and O-sulfation and N-acetylation patterns. Its low concentration in crude extracts, containing other heterogeneous GAGs, leads to a purification process that is very complex, and which is well-guarded by manufacturing companies. Van der Meer et al. [1], through a careful inspection of the academic and patent literature, provide a worthy overview of the multiple steps and variations in purification processes leading to active pharmaceutical ingredient (API)-grade heparin.

As a consequence of the "heparin crisis" in late 2007, an updating of heparin pharmacopeia monographies in the USA and the EU with new NMR and HPLC tests increased the quality control capabilities for crude and API porcine heparins, with some limitations in detecting the addition of non-porcine crude heparins or other GAG-like contaminants. An improvement to this process (Mauri L. et al.) [2] resulted from a collaborative study between the G. Ronzoni Institute and the Division of Pharmaceutical Analysis of Food and Drug Administration (FDA) in the USA. Analyzing 88 samples of commercial crude heparin through an orthogonal approach based on NMR chemometrics along with strong anionic exchange (SAX)—HPLC, they could be differentiated with regard to purity, as well as the mono- and disaccharide composition specific to each GAG family. Furthermore, heparin/heparan sulfate (HS) from different tissues and animal species, as well as from different manufacturing processes, can be characterized, and impurities such as dermatan- and chondroitin-sulfates quantified by the heteronuclear single-quantum correlation (HSQC) NMR approach and multivariate analysis (PCA).

Lima M. et al. [3] reviewed the newer applications of heparins and its analogs, as well as GAGs including marine organisms. The wide range of pharmacological activity of heparin can be attributed to its chemical features, which include heparan sulfate (HS), a widely occurring cell surface-bound polysaccharide, which participates in cell-cell signaling. Most of its potential applications seem to be partially associated with its anti-inflammatory effects, as well as to interactions with a multitude of proteins and inhibition of enzymes involved in pathologic processes, such as heparanase and metalloproteases. Additionally, the role of such mediators as selectins and galectins in cancer and metastasis, cathepsin-d and BACE-1, respectively, in Parkinson's and Alzheimer's diseases, human and microbial elastases in cystic fibrosis, and proteases and cytoadherence in parasite infections such as Leishmaniosis are elucidated. The ability to protect from viral infection through enveloped glycoproteins can open other potential applications for heparins and GAGs.

Two Italian teams (Poli M. et al.) [4] review their studies and recent findings with regard to the role of bone morphogenic proteins (BMPs, members of the TGF-β superfamily heparin/HS binding proteins) in activating the expression of hepcidin, the iron inflammation peptide hormone, which regulates systemic iron hemostasis, and can be deregulated by heparin. An in vivo screening allows the identification of non-anticoagulant glycol-split heparin, delivered by osmotic pumps, and supersulfated LMWH given orally as heparin antagonists and potential candidates for the treatment of anemias in chronic and genetic diseases.

The interactions and binding sites of heparin/HS with BMPs and cytokines of the TGF-β superfamily are reviewed by Rider C. and Mulloy B. [5]. The activity of TGF-β-cytokines in controlling proliferation, differentiation on survival in several cell types are also regulated by a number of secreted BMP antagonist proteins, the majority of which can also bind heparin. In conclusion, potential therapeutic applications of TGF-β cytokines on their own and those with BMP interactions with heparins/HS are described.

In a collaborative study of 6 laboratories in the USA, Europe and India (Bertini S. et al.) [6] the average MW of 20 lots of bovine mucosal heparin (BMH) were determined with the USP monograph method in comparison with porcine mucosal heparin (PMH) and bovine lung heparin (BLH) samples. Even with a wider variation, the average MW of BMH was found to be comparable to that of PMH, while BLH samples had a lower average MW. An alternative method using a polymer-based column with light scattering detection provided results that were in good agreement for all samples investigated in the study.

An article (Kim H. et al.) [7] reports a study exploring, in different bioreactor conditions, the yield, structure and activity of heparin/HS obtained by expressing serglycin in mammalian cells as an alternative source of these anticoagulant drugs, as well as of new bioengineered analogs.

Three Italian groups (Truzzi E. et al.) [8] explored the possibility of an intestinal lymphatic uptake of an orally formulated heparin. Self-assembled lipid nanoparticles were used to stabilize the heparin-coated iron-oxide nanoparticles. Then, the formulation was characterized with respect to its physical-chemical properties, encapsulation efficacy, in vitro stability, heparin leaking cytotoxicity and indirect indication of lymphatic up-take in $CaCo_2$ cells.

A collaborative study by an Israeli and Italian team (Vismara E. et al.) [9] led to the design and identification of a synthetic strategy for obtaining new theranostic super paramagnetic iron-oxide nanoparticle (SPION) systems decorating a magnetic iron-oxide core with an optimized ratio of bioorganic layer and of serum albumin and hyaluronic acid, which was selected to finally include paclitaxel and improve its efficacy. The TD-NMR experiments suggest their suitability for development as contrast agents in MRI.

The review by authors from the Departments of Neurosurgery at two US Universities (Hayman E. et al.) [10] suggests the therapeutic potential of heparins and derivatives for improving outcomes in aneurysm-associated subarachnoid hemorrhage (a-SAH). Retrospective analysis of preliminary clinical studies and experimental works suggest that the pleiotropic effects of heparins can be of benefit in blood-brain barrier dysfunctions, vasospasm, delayed cerebral ischemia and neuroinflammation preventing leukocyte extravasation, modulation of phagocyte activation, and inhibition of oxidative stress, all of which are involved in the complex a-SAH frame.

A Belgian team (Minet V.) [11] reviewed all of the current developed and evaluated functional assays for diagnosis in patients suspected of heparin-induced thrombocytopenia. Drawbacks in some assays, such as platelet activation and Hit antibody detection, are identified as being due to interlaboratory variability, lack of standardization and data control and interpretation.

Compositional analysis of both LMWH Dalteparin (Bisio et al.) [12] and Danaparoid (Gardini C. et al.) [13] and their enzymatically digested oligosaccharides have been determined at the G. Ronzoni Institute, by a combination of the more advanced LC/MS and NMR analytical methods. The API batch-to-batch variability of Dalteparin can also be assessed profiling octa- and deca-saccharides, and fractions endowed with different antithrombin affinity. Chromatographic fractionation and selected enzymatic digestion, as well as NMR analyses of Danaparoid, a GAG complex mixture extracted from porcine intestinal mucosa, allowed the characterization and quantification of the main component as LMW HS, and the minor ones dermatan and chondroitin sulfate, and identified oxidized glucosamine and uronic acid at the reducing ends.

The interactions of Tinzaparin, a LMWH used as antithrombotic prophylaxis in clinical oncology with *cis*-Pt, have been studied "in vitro" and in xenograft models (Mueller T. et al.) [14]. In vitro LMWH can reverse the *cis*-Pt resistance in a cancer-resistant cell line. In vitro preliminary studies show that Tinzaparin has no effect on *cis*-Pt accumulation in *cis*-Pt-resistant xenografts but strongly increases the Pt content in non-*cis*-Pt-resistant ones.

Component fractionation of Semuloparin, an ultra LMWH obtained by a depolymerization process preserving the AT binding region, has allowed a team at Sanofi (Mourier P. et al.) [15] to isolate five octadecasaccharides, each incorporating at least two AT-binding pentasaccharides. Full sequencing and "in vitro" testing of anti-FXa and anti-FIIa activities reveal the peculiarity of the pentasaccharide position within the octadecasaccharides for inhibition potency, which can differ up to twenty-fold in magnitude.

An extended physico-chemical characterization of Fondaparinux, the synthetic α-methyl glycoside of the AT binding pentasaccharide, and the active ingredient of the anticoagulant drug Arixtra®, have also been defined on the basis of a determination of single-crystal X-ray conformation. Quantitative NMR were also used, confirming that this method shows intrinsic robustness for content determination (de Wildt et al.) [16].

A team from Heidelberg University (Rappold M. et al.) [17] has synthesized and characterized a more sensitive probe (PDI-1) for the detection of dermatan sulfate by a mix-and-read assay in blood plasma in a clinically relevant concentration range (quantification limit in aqueous matrix 1 ng/mL).

Authors from the Trondheim University (Norway) (Arlov Ø. and Skjåk-Bræk G.) [18] review the synthesis and physico-chemical properties of sulfated alginates used as both a drug delivery system and a biomaterial component. Their superior biocompatibility, mild gelling conditions and structural versatility can open the way for new biomedical applications in fields next to those of GAGs.

Conflicts of Interest: The authors declare no conflict of interest.

References

1. Van der Meer, J.-Y.; Kellenbach, E.; van den Bos, L.J. From Farm to Pharma: An Overview of Industrial Heparin Manufacturing Methods. *Molecules* **2017**, *22*, 1025. [CrossRef] [PubMed]
2. Mauri, L.; Marinozzi, M.; Mazzini, G.; Kolinski, R.E.; Karfunkle, M.; Keire, D.A.; Guerrini, M. Combining NMR Spectroscopy and Chemometrics to Monitor Structural Features of Crude Heparin. *Molecules* **2017**, *22*, 1146. [CrossRef] [PubMed]
3. Lima, M.; Rudd, T.; Yates, E. New Applications of Heparin and Other Glycosaminoglycans. *Molecules* **2017**, *22*, 749. [CrossRef] [PubMed]
4. Poli, M.; Asperti, M.; Ruzzenenti, P.; Naggi, A.; Arosio, P. Non-Anticoagulant Heparins Are Hepcidin Antagonists for the Treatment of Anemia. *Molecules* **2017**, *22*, 598. [CrossRef] [PubMed]
5. Rider, C.C.; Mulloy, B. Heparin, Heparan Sulphate and the TGF-β Cytokine Superfamily. *Molecules* **2017**, *22*, 713. [CrossRef] [PubMed]
6. Bertini, S.; Risi, G.; Guerrini, M.; Carrick, K.; Szajek, A.Y.; Mulloy, B. Molecular Weights of Bovine and Porcine Heparin Samples: Comparison of Chromatographic Methods and Results of a Collaborative Survey. *Molecules* **2017**, *22*, 1214. [CrossRef] [PubMed]
7. Kim, H.N.; Whitelock, J.M.; Lord, M.S. Structure-Activity Relationships of Bioengineered Heparin/Heparan Sulfates Produced in Different Bioreactors. *Molecules* **2017**, *22*, 806. [CrossRef] [PubMed]
8. Truzzi, E.; Bongio, C.; Sacchetti, F.; Maretti, E.; Montanari, M.; Iannuccelli, V.; Vismara, E.; Leo, E. Self-Assembled Lipid Nanoparticles for Oral Delivery of Heparin-Coated Iron Oxide Nanoparticles for Theranostic Purposes. *Molecules* **2017**, *22*, 963. [CrossRef] [PubMed]
9. Vismara, E.; Bongio, C.; Coletti, A.; Edelman, R.; Serafini, A.; Mauri, M.; Simonutti, R.; Bertini, S.; Urso, E.; Assaraf, Y.G.; et al. Albumin and Hyaluronic Acid-Coated Superparamagnetic Iron Oxide Nanoparticles Loaded with Paclitaxel for Biomedical Applications. *Molecules* **2017**, *22*, 1030. [CrossRef] [PubMed]

10. Hayman, E.G.; Patel, A.P.; James, R.F.; Simard, J.M. Heparin and Heparin-Derivatives in Post-Subarachnoid Hemorrhage Brain Injury: A Multimodal Therapy for a Multimodal Disease. *Molecules* **2017**, *22*, 724. [CrossRef] [PubMed]

11. Minet, V.; Dogné, J.-M.; Mullier, F. Functional Assays in the Diagnosis of Heparin-Induced Thrombocytopenia: A Review. *Molecules* **2017**, *22*, 617. [CrossRef] [PubMed]

12. Bisio, A.; Urso, E.; Guerrini, M.; de Wit, P.; Torri, G.; Naggi, A. Structural Characterization of the Low-Molecular-Weight Heparin Dalteparin by Combining Different Analytical Strategies. *Molecules* **2017**, *22*, 1051. [CrossRef] [PubMed]

13. Gardini, C.; Urso, E.; Guerrini, M.; van Herpen, R.; de Wit, P.; Naggi, A. Characterization of Danaparoid Complex Extractive Drug by an Orthogonal Analytical Approach. *Molecules* **2017**, *22*, 1116. [CrossRef] [PubMed]

14. Mueller, T.; Pfankuchen, D.B.; Wantoch von Rekowski, K.; Schlesinger, M.; Reipsch, F.; Bendas, G. The Impact of the Low Molecular Weight Heparin Tinzaparin on the Sensitization of Cisplatin-Resistant Ovarian Cancers—Preclinical In Vivo Evaluation in Xenograft Tumor Models. *Molecules* **2017**, *22*, 728. [CrossRef] [PubMed]

15. Mourier, P.A.J.; Guichard, O.Y.; Herman, F.; Sizun, P.; Viskov, C. New Insights in Thrombin Inhibition Structure–Activity Relationships by Characterization of Octadecasaccharides from Low Molecular Weight Heparin. *Molecules* **2017**, *22*, 428. [CrossRef] [PubMed]

16. Wildt, W.; Kooijman, H.; Funke, C.; Üstün, B.; Leika, A.; Lunenburg, M.; Kaspersen, F.; Kellenbach, E. Extended Physicochemical Characterization of the Synthetic Anticoagulant Pentasaccharide Fondaparinux Sodium by Quantitative NMR and Single Crystal X-ray Analysis. *Molecules* **2017**, *22*, 1362. [CrossRef] [PubMed]

17. Rappold, M.; Warttinger, U.; Krämer, R. A Fluorescent Probe for Glycosaminoglycans Applied to the Detection of Dermatan Sulfate by a Mix-and-Read Assay. *Molecules* **2017**, *22*, 768. [CrossRef] [PubMed]

18. Arlov, Ø.; Skjåk-Bræk, G. Sulfated Alginates as Heparin Analogues: A Review of Chemical and Functional Properties. *Molecules* **2017**, *22*, 778. [CrossRef] [PubMed]

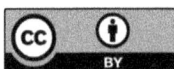

molecules

MDPI

Editorial

Remembering Professor Benito Casu (1927–2016)

Giangiacomo Torri * and Giuseppe Cassinelli

Carbohydrate Sciences Department of Istituto di Ricerche Chimiche e Biochimiche "G. Ronzoni", 20133 Milan, Italy; ronzoni@ronzoni.it
* Correspondence: torri@ronzoni.it; Tel.: +39-02-70641621

Received: 25 January 2018; Accepted: 26 January 2018; Published: 31 January 2018

Heparin and related drugs have contributed in so many different ways to the drug discovery process, and have provided a platform to understand the pathophysiology of vascular and inflammatory diseases for nearly 100 years. Despite its discovery in 1917 by Jay McLean, then a medical student, the scientific and clinical progress in the understanding of heparin and related drugs has continued to expand. This Special Issue of *Molecules* was developed in commemoration of the 100-year Anniversary of the discovery of Heparin. It would have been appropriate to have the lead article in this issue be by Professor Benito Casu, one of the lead pioneers who laid the foundation for the understanding of the heparin structure and function. Unfortunately, professor Casu unexpectedly and regrettably passed away on 11 November 2016. His legacy as a teacher, scientist, leader and a visionary who led a group of scientists at Ronzoni to advance the science of glycosaminoglycans will live for years to come. His diverse interest in this area is well represented in the manuscripts in this Special Issue.

At the G. Ronzoni Institute in Milan (Italy), he contributed over the last sixty years to the advancement of the knowledge of polysaccharide chemistry and biochemistry, especially both heparin and glycosaminoglycan (GAG) derivatives, analogs and mimetics. Several of these resulted from translational networks fruitfully set up by Professor Casu, who had the merit of sharing intuitions and projects with scientists, academic institutions, and industry. He had a unique attitude towards *"friendly competition"*, regardless of potential competitors, and used to cite a phrase of the Nobel Prize winner Rita Levi Montalcini: *"Research is a tool of knowledge and not a matter of power and competition"*.

In 1951, he started his scientific career with brilliant research on starch and cyclodextrins at the G. Ronzoni Institute. In 1969, he was first introduced to heparin during a sabbatical year at McGill University, Montreal (Canada), joining the group of Professor Arthur Perlin. The pioneer NMR studies on the structure and conformational flexibility of heparin provided him an international notoriety [1–3]. For over forty years, under his research coordination and operative direction, the Institute, through interdisciplinary and international networks and collaborations, significantly contributed to the development of both new analytical methodologies and novel heparin derivatives. This area of research provided a unique platform for research and education. This was the result of national and international exchange of students and senior scientists, all having the opportunity of sharing time and talent to advance the glycosciences. He promoted and organized, with his colleague Job Harenberg (Heidelberg-Mannheim University), the "1st Symposium on Glycosaminoglycans" at the Villa Vigoni, Loveno, Lake of Como (Italy) in 1991. The following twenty-four yearly symposia were always the preferred platform for pioneers, scholars and young investigators to present the more advanced research and multidisciplinary studies in the field. The 25th-Anniversary Symposium, in September 2017, was dedicated to Professor Casu.

In the framework of this preface, it is not possible to assess the content and richness of ideas, publications, reviews and patents of Prof. Casu. As a result of translational collaborations with academic institutions and/or industrial partners, the following highlights can be underscored:

- Structural characterization studies of heparin pentasaccharide sequence binding to antithrombin, fundamental for anticoagulant activity [4].
- Bioactive biotechnological heparins obtained by chemo-enzymatic modification of a biosynthetic precursor of bacterial origin [5].
- An honorary doctorate of the Uppsala University (Sweden), awarded in 1998 for outstanding contribution to heparin and GAGs knowledge and development.
- More recently, as a result of an international collaboration among G. Ronzoni Institute, Alabama University, USA (Prof. Sanderson), and Technion University, Haifa (Israel), granted by NCI, USA, the identification of a new class of non-anticoagulant heparins endowed with antineoplastic activity through the inhibition of heparanase [6,7], currently a lead compound under ongoing clinical trials.

The traditional interdisciplinary and international network of the Ronzoni Institute, under the guidance of Professor Casu and his group, is well expressed by the contributions of this special issue covering some of the translational steps "from bench to bedside".

Conflicts of Interest: The authors declare no conflict of interest.

References

1. Perlin, A.S.; Casu, B. Carbon-13 and proton magnetic resonance spectra of D-glucose-^{13}C. *Tetrahedron Lett.* **1969**, *10*, 2921–2924. [CrossRef]
2. Perlin, A.S.; Casu, B.; Sanderson, G.R.; Tse, J. Methyl α-and β-D-idopyranosiduronic acids synthesis and conformational analysis. *Carbohydr. Res.* **1972**, *21*, 123–132. [CrossRef]
3. Gatti, G.; Casu, B.; Perlin, A.S. Conformations of the major residues in heparin. ^{1}H-NMR spectroscopic studies. *Biochem. Biophys. Res. Commun.* **1978**, *85*, 14–20. [CrossRef]
4. Casu, B.; Oreste, P.; Torri, G.; Zoppetti, G.; Choay, J.; Lormeau, J.C.; Petitou, M.; Sinay, P. The structure of heparin oligosaccharide fragments with high anti-(factor Xa) activity containing the minimal antithrombin III-binding sequence. Chemical and ^{13}C nuclear-magnetic-resonance studies. *Biochem. J.* **1981**, *197*, 599–609. [CrossRef] [PubMed]
5. Casu, B.; Grazioli, G.; Razi, N.; Guerrini, M.; Naggi, A.; Torri, G.; Oreste, P.; Tursi, F.; Zoppetti, G.; Lindahl, U. Heparin-like compounds prepared by chemical modification of capsular polysaccharide from *E. coli* K5. *Carbohydr. Res.* **1994**, *263*, 271–284. [CrossRef]
6. Naggi, A.; Casu, B.; Perez, M.; Torri, G.; Cassinelli, G.; Penco, S.; Pisano, C.; Giannini, G.; Ishai-Michaeli, R.; Vlodavsky, I. Modulation of the heparanase-inhibiting activity of heparin through selective desulfation, graded N-acetylation, and glycol splitting. *J. Biol. Chem.* **2005**, *280*, 12103–12113. [CrossRef] [PubMed]
7. Ritchie, J.P.; Ramani, V.C.; Ren, Y.; Naggi, A.; Torri, G.; Casu, B.; Penco, S.; Pisano, C.; Carminati, P.; Tortoreto, M.; et al. SST0001, a chemically modified heparin, inhibits myeloma growth and angiogenesis via disruption of the heparanase/syndecan-1 axis. *Clin. Cancer Res.* **2011**, *17*, 1382–1393. [CrossRef] [PubMed]

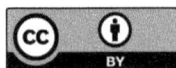

molecules

MDPI

Review

From Farm to Pharma: An Overview of Industrial Heparin Manufacturing Methods

Jan-Ytzen van der Meer *, Edwin Kellenbach and Leendert J. van den Bos

Development and Technical Support Aspen Oss, Kloosterstraat 6, P.O. Box 98, 5340 AB Oss, The Netherlands; ekellenbach@nl.aspenpharma.com (E.K.); lvandenbos@nl.aspenpharma.com (L.J.v.d.B.)
* Correspondence: jvandermeer@nl.aspenpharma.com; Tel.: +31-(0)88-277-9191

Academic Editors: Giangiacomo Torri and Jawed Fareed
Received: 19 May 2017; Accepted: 18 June 2017; Published: 21 June 2017

Abstract: The purification of heparin from offal is an old industrial process for which commercial recipes date back to 1922. Although chemical, chemoenzymatic, and biotechnological alternatives for this production method have been published in the academic literature, animal-tissue is still the sole source for commercial heparin production in industry. Heparin purification methods are closely guarded industrial secrets which are not available to the general (scientific) public. However by reviewing the academic and patent literature, we aim to provide a comprehensive overview of the general methods used in industry for the extraction of heparin from animal tissue.

Keywords: heparin; heparin process; manufacturing methods; industrial

---

1. Introduction

Heparin is a strongly charged polysaccharide anticoagulant which has been used and produced for nearly a century [1,2]. The heparin manufacturing methods used rely strongly on the unique molecular properties of heparin, including its acidity, high charge density and stability. These characteristics enable the purification of heparin despite the low concentration present in the starting material (~160–260 mg/kg). Therefore a short summary of the old and current views on structure and biosynthesis of heparin is given below, for more elaborate reviews on these topics see references [2–5]. Discussions on the structure of heparin date back to the 1920s. By the 1940s it was concluded that heparin consisted of uronic acids and amino sugars with a high content of ester sulfates and that the amino groups were (partly) acetylated [6]. Further biochemical characterization studies indicated that desulphonation resulted in loss of heparin activity [7]. Additionally, fractional precipitation of active material suggested that heparin consisted of a mixture of closely related structures instead of a single structure. [6,8] More recent studies have shown that these observations and conclusions were correct. We now know that heparin is indeed a highly sulfated polysaccharide consisting of alternating glucosamine and uronic acid units. In the biosynthetic pathway towards heparin, these monosaccharides (i.e., *N*-acetyl-D-glucosamine (GlcNAc) and D-glucuronic acid (GlcA)) are added to a tetrasaccharide linkage region (GlcA-Gal-Gal-Xyl-) which is attached to proteins containing Ser-Gly repeats. After this elongation step, heparin chains of up to 100 kDa are generated. During and after the elongation, several modifications can occur which include: epimerization of GlcA leading to L-iduronic acid (IdoA), *N*-deacetylation, *N*-sulfation, 2-*O*-sulfation, 6-*O*-sulfation, and more rarely 3-*O*-sulfation of the glucosamine [4]. The most prevalent disaccharide present in heparin is depicted below in Figure 1.

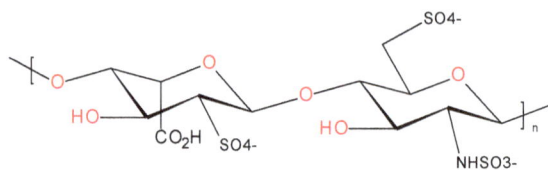

Figure 1. Major disaccharide found in heparin: (-4)-α-L-IdoA2S-(1-4)-α-D-GlcNS6S-(1-) [5].

The complete biosynthesis takes place in the Golgi compartment of mainly mast cells. These are a type of an immune cells containing heparin-rich granules. As a result of this biosynthesis and subsequent modifications, there are 32 theoretically possible disaccharides which make up heparin, making heparin more complex than other biopolymers such as proteins and nucleic acids [9]. Moreover, in contrast to proteins and nucleic acids, heparin is synthesized in a non-template directed fashion which results is a high degree of heterogeneity for all structural properties.

The anticoagulant activity of heparin is the result of its potentiating action on antithrombin (ATIII) which is an anti-coagulation factor. Potentiated ATIII, subsequently inhibits the action of pro-coagulation factors IIa (i.e., thrombin) and Xa by covalent binding, finally resulting in reduced coagulation. The molecular mechanism by which heparin potentiates ATIII differs for these two factors [5,10]. The potentiation of ATIII towards factor Xa mainly depends on an allosteric activation of ATIII by a specific pentasaccharide sequence in heparin. This pentasaccharide, which contains a unique 3-*O*-sulfate glucosamine triggers a conformational change in ATIII upon binding, which results in a ~1000-fold increasedaffinity of ATIII for Xa leading to increased inhibition of factor Xa [10]. The pentasaccharide sequence is sufficient for the Xa inhibition activity of heparin. For the inhibition of IIa, however, a heparin chain forms a bridge between ATIII and factor IIa by electrostatic interactions resulting in a stable ternary complex [10]. To enable this 'bridge' a heparin chain should be at least 15–16 saccharide units in length [11]. Besides chain length, also the overall charge (i.e., high sulfate to carboxylate ratio or S/C ratio) of a heparin chain is important for this mechanism since it enables strong interactions between heparin and ATIII and heparin and factor IIa.

The objective of the heparin manufacturing process is, therefore, to maximize the yield of highly charged, high molecular weight heparin chains present in the starting material without affecting the material by degradation (e.g., depolymerization and/or desulfation) caused by the applied process conditions. Typical industrial processes can be divided into five distinctive sections (Figure 2). Each of these section will be discussed in this review.

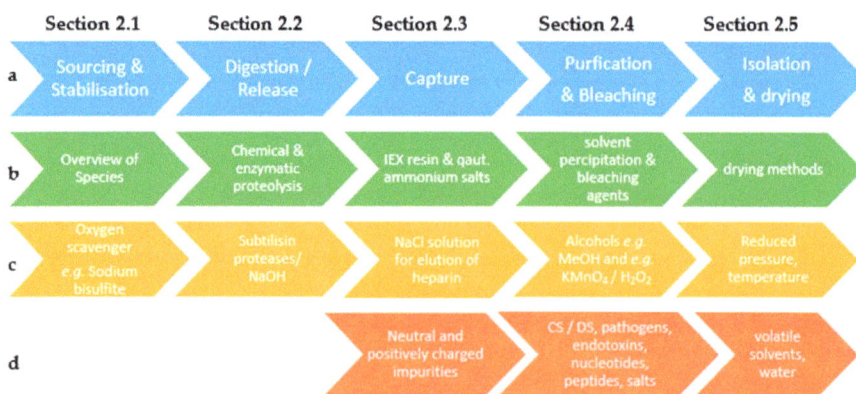

Figure 2. (**a**), Schematic representation of an industrial heparin purification process; (**b**) Discussed topics per section; (**c**) General process conditions and reagents; (**d**) Removed impurities per section.

1.1. Collection and Stabilization Starting Material

1.1.1. Regulatory Aspects Related to Sourcing

The biological material used for heparin production (i.e., mucosa or bovine lungs) should be derived from animals which meet the requirements for health suitable for human consumption [12]. This ensures the slaughtered animals are healthy and free of medication such as antibiotics. To guarantee this, several heparin producers provide full traceability of their starting material to the slaughterhouses and farms. Additionally, a polymerase chain reaction (PCR) or an immunochemical analysis is suggested by the FDA and European Pharmacopoeia to demonstrate the absence of any ruminant material in the starting material to mitigate the risk for contamination with BSE [12,13]. Moreover, from 2013 onwards, the complete supply chain of heparin, starting with the collection of the starting material, falls under EudraLex volume 4, annex 2 of the EU guidelines for "GMP for medicinal products for human and veterinary use" [14]. This indicates that the entire process falls under GMP control, albeit at different levels depending on the stage of the manufacturing process.

1.1.2. Sources: Porcine and Bovine

The first heparin production protocols used canine or bovine livers as a source. Later, mainly porcine mucosa and bovine lungs were used [15]. However, since porcine intestinal mucosa was found to be a much 'cleaner' source which required less degradation compared to bovine lungs and also as a result of the outbreak of bovine spongiform encephalopathy in the 1990s [3,16], heparin production from bovine material has decreased significantly. In fact, the only FDA-approved source of heparin is currently porcine mucosa [13,16]. However, several countries, including Brazil, Argentina and India, still allow bovine-derived heparin. Bovine heparin is preferred by some for religious reasons. Heparin is second only to insulin in application as a biological. To meet the annual heparin need, the offal of about 1.10^9 pigs are required, therefore there is a substantial risk for future heparin shortages. To prevent these potential shortages there is currently a strong debate ongoing to re-introduce bovine heparin in the USA [15]. Because strong drop of BSE prevalence in cows, the strongly increased knowledge on the disease and the prion reduction during the heparin purification process [17] the risks with respect to patient safety are now better understood [15]. This may facilitate the re-introduction of bovine heparin to the US market. There are however significant differences between porcine and bovine heparin. For instance, bovine heparin has substantially lower activity compared to porcine heparin [18] (see Table 1). A large amount of scientific literature is available describing structural differences between porcine and bovine derived heparin which might explain the difference in activity [15,17,19].

1.1.3. Other Mammalian Sources

Besides bovine and porcine heparin, sheep (ovine) intestines have been used in the past to produce pharmaceutical heparin. Ovine heparin is currently still available from chemical manufacturers for research purposes. An elaborate overview of physiochemical characteristics of commercially available ovine heparin compared to both porcine and bovine heparin has been given by Li Fu et al. [16]. Ovine heparin resembles porcine heparin more closely then bovine heparin based on the disaccharide composition, antithrombin affinity and M_W. Because of this resemblance, it was mentioned that programs to manufacture fractionated heparin from ovine sources have been initiated [20]. There are no religious restrictions on using sheep as a heparin-source however, a transmissible prion disease (scrapie) does occur in sheep. Although scrapie is not transmissible to humans, infected sheep are typically not used for consumption.

Dromedary (*Camelus dromedaries*) has been suggested as a heparin source since it is free of any religious and health reason concerns. To investigate this source heparin was isolated from dromedary intestines [21]. The disaccharide analysis in this study indicated that non- and monosulfated disaccharides were more abundant in dromedary heparin compared to porcine heparin. Consistent with this low degree of overall sulfation, dromedary raw heparin had a specific aXa activity of

~50–60 IU/mg which is approximately half of the activity of porcine heparin which was purified as a reference in that same study (see Table 1).

Table 1. Overview of characteristic of heparin derived from different sources.

Source	aXa Activity (IU/mg)	aPTT Activity	Average Mol. Weight (kDa)	S/C Ratio	Yield (mg/kg)	Refs
Porcine	148–219	168–277	15.0–19.0 [a]	2.31–2.57	160–260	[15,16,18,22]
Bovine [b]	123–156	103–181	16.2–16.5	2.29–2.40	n.d.	[16,18,19]
Ovine	142	150	22.9	3.66	n.d.	[16]
Dromedary	50–60	n.d.	24.0	2.0	400	[21]
Chicken	111	133	n.d.	2.26	n.d.	[18]
Turkey	16.6	n.d.	n.d.	n.d.	300	[23]
Salmon	110–137	n.d.	<8.0 [c]	2.20	n.d.	[24]
Shrimp	95–100	n.d.	8.5	n.d.	32	[25]
Clam	317	347	14.9	n.d.	2100	[26]

[a] Pharmacopoeial specification; [b] intestinal mucosa; [c] 96% was ≤8.0 Da.

1.1.4. Non-Mammalian Sources

By-products of the poultry industry might seem an obvious source for heparin production because of the high global chicken and turkey meat production. Active heparin can be derived from chicken intestines with a specific aXa activity of 111 IU/mg and slightly lower degree of sulfation compared to porcine heparin produced according to the same method (S/C ratio resp.: 2.26 and 2.40) [18]. In this study, however no yields have been reported. Heparin derived from chicken intestines appears to approach porcine-derived heparin based on disaccharide composition and aXa activity (111 IU/mg) [18]. The specific aXa activity of heparin derived from turkey intestines was extremely low (16.6 IU/mg) [23]. Although based on this information, chicken might be a potential source of biologically active heparin, to the best of our knowledge there is currently no heparin production on an (semi-) industrial scale using poultry-derived starting material. The obtained GAGs from turkey tissue mainly consisted of heparan sulfate. Differences between mammalian and avian immunological mechanisms might be an explanation for the absence of active heparin species in turkey [23].

A relatively recent report on heparin purification from salmon (*Salmo salar*) gills and intestines describes a partial purification where heparin was obtained with a low molecular weight (96% ≤ 8000 Da). The aXa activity of the salmon-derived heparin was in the range of clinically approved fractionated heparin (LMWH) [24].

Shrimp (*Penaeus brasiliensis*) heads can also be used as a source of natural LMWH with a yield of 32 mg/kg starting material [25]. This shrimp-derived heparin had a molecular weight of 8500 Da and an aXa activity of 95 IU/mg which is also comparable (on the low end) to LMWH. Nonetheless, in vivo experiments indicated that shrimp heparin had a slightly lower antithrombotic activity compared to pharmaceutical grade LMWH.

Heparin derived from clams (*Tapes phylippinarum*) was found to have substantially better aXa activity (317 IU/mg) compared to typical porcine heparin and an average molecular weight (Mw) of 14,900 Da, which is comparable to unfractionated heparin [26]. The yield of the clamp derived heparin was ~2.1 g/kg dry tissue which is a high yield. However, since the whole animal is used here, there is a strong competition with the food industry, which explains the high price of the starting material. To the best of our knowledge, there is currently no commercial heparin production from any of these sources.

1.1.5. Obtaining and Stabilizing Source Material

This section focusses on porcine intestinal mucosa, since this is the major source of the globally produced heparin. However, the processing steps also apply to bovine heparin. The mucosa production is highly linked to the production of casings for the sausage industry. A typical procedure starts with the removal of the content from the intestine and subsequent soaking of the intestine in a salt solution. After soaking, the mucosa is scraped from the intestines, yielding approximately 0.8 kg of mucosa per pig [22]. The emptied intestines are further processed as casings for the sausage industry and the mucosa is collected for further processing to heparin. Besides mucosa, whole porcine intestines can be used for heparin production and are referred to as "hashed porcine guts" [27,28]. It is known that chemical and/or enzymatic desulfation occurs after prolonged storage (mainly glucosamine 6-*O*-desulfation) resulting in decreased activity [18], therefore some sort of stabilization or preservation of the material is required. Typically, mucosa is preserved using an oxygen scavenger such as sodium bisulphite e.g., 1.5–2.5% *w*/*w* until further processing to limit microbiological growth [29]. Other preservatives which can be added to the mucosa include calcium propionate or phenol [22].

1.1.6. Heparin on Resin

To circumvent the transport of large volumes of mucosa and to reduce the risk of degradation during transport, a method was described [26] where the mucosa is hydrolyzed at the slaughterhouses and the resulting heparin subsequently loaded on an anion exchange resin. For this procedure, 3000–4000 L of intestinal mucosa (daily yield of a typical pig slaughterhouse) was enzymatically hydrolyzed using a subtilisin alkaline protease at 50–55 °C and at alkaline pH. After 3–4 h or when the viscosity was sufficiently reduced (threshold of 14.8 mPa·s) the enzyme was heat-inactivated and the hydrolysate was filtered. To this filtrate 24–30 kg of anion-exchange resin was added (examples described in the patent include Amberlite, Dowex, Duolite and Lewatit) and mixed for 10–13 h. The loaded resin was sieved off, dried and transferred to a container. As a preservative, 50 g/L of sodium bisulphite was added, and the container was shipped to a specialized chemical plant for further processing. Using this method the yield could be improved from 30,000 units per kg of mucosa to 48,000 units per kg mucosa, possibly because of the short processing times. Therefore, this approach can be highly advantageous, especially when sourcing mucosa at distant slaughterhouses. However, it does require more complex equipment, logistics and technical expertise at the slaughterhouses.

1.2. Digestion and Release of Heparin from Proteoglycans

The early heparin production procedures already included (e.g., [8]) a digestion step aiming to liberate the heparin from the (mast-) cells and proteoglycans. This digestion step can be done by autolysis, addition of pancreas extract, saliva, proteolytic enzymes or by chemical means. Chemical hydrolysis can be performed under acidic or alkaline conditions at high temperatures. This might affect the structure of the heparin. For instance, alkaline proteolysis at pH 11 leads to slight 2-*O*-desulfation of the uronic acids through base-catalyzed epoxide formation. [18] For an enzymatic digestion, a wide range of proteolytic enzymes (i.e., proteases) can be applied including trypsin, chymotrypsin [30], papaine [23] or subtilisin-type enzymes such as Alcalase® or Maxatase® [26,29,31]. For this enzymatic digestion, multiple tons of mucosa should be heated until the optimal temperature of the used enzyme (e.g., 50–60 °C for alcalase). Subsequently the pH should be set (e.g., 8.6 for subtilisins) [26,29] and the enzyme can be added at a typical enzyme:substrate ratio is 0.2–2 g/kg mucosa [31]. The reaction mixture is incubated for 4–16 h to ensure heparin is fully released from the proteoglycans.

1.3. Capture of the Heparin

Prior to the capture step, the heparin concentration in the digested starting material is extremely low (~0.01% *w*/*w*). Therefore, the aim of this step is to enrich the heparin content to enable further purification, at a higher concertation later in the process. Initial heparin extraction protocols describe the precipitation of heparin from autolyzed starting material by applying a low pH (2–2.5) and a high concentration of ammonium sulfate [7,8]. This step, most likely, precipitated mainly protein-bound heparins instead of free heparin, as the proteolytic (trypsin) digestion was conducted after this acid precipitation. The heparin crude obtained after this step still contained high amounts of protein [32]. Moreover, it was realized that this acid precipitation did not 'drop out all of the heparin' [33]. This is probably because heparin itself does not precipitate under these conditions. Therefore, in that latter patent a method was described using hydrophobic primary amines (such as hexylamine) which can form an insoluble complex with heparin under slightly acidic conditions due to their positive charge. This neutral heparin-amine complex was subsequently collected as a precipitate on the interface between the aqueous phase and an organic phase (e.g., methyl isobutyl ketone).

The principle of using ammonium cations such as in the example above is currently still the most widely used method for capturing heparin from digestion mixtures according to (patent-) literature. However, currently the quaternary ammonium cations are usually either immobilized on a resin (i.e., anion exchange resin) [29,31] or designed in such a way that they selectively form insoluble complexes with heparin (quaternary ammonium salts) [34,35]. Both methods exploit the polymeric nature and uniquely high charge density of heparin (~3.7 negative charges/disaccharide), distinguishing heparin from other biopolymers such as chondroitin sulfate (CS) (S/C ratio of ~1), dermatan sulfate (DS) (S/C ratio of ~1) or DNA/RNA (1 negative charge per disaccharide) present in the digestion mixture [36]. This allows a strong charge-based cooperative binding.

1.3.1. Precipitation with Quaternary Ammonium Salts

Several patents from the 1960s describe the precipitation of heparin with quaternary ammonium salts [34,35]. The general formula of such a salt is depicted below (Figure 3a) where the X represents any anion that does not render the salt water-insoluble, (e.g., chloride) and the ^{1}R and ^{2}R group represents an aliphatic hydrocarbon chain of at least eight carbons optionally interrupted by: aromatic rings, double bounds, oxygen- or nitrogen atoms and ^{2}R–^{4}R are groups consisting of 1–7 carbon atoms [35]. After incubation of the digestion mixture with such a salt, a water-insoluble complex is formed with the heparin chains. These insoluble complexes can be obtained as solids. One example of an applicable quaternary ammonium salt is Hyamine® 1622 (see Figure 3b) [34]. This patent describes a method were Hyamine 1622 is added to digested ground lungs, subsequently the precipitated Hyamine-heparin salt was filtered off and suspended in an organic solvent. This suspension was extracted with an aqueous solution, and from this solution the potassium salt of heparin precipitated by increasing the potassium acetate concentration to 30% (*w/v*). Approximately 0.6 g of crude material was obtained with an activity of 110 IU/mg from 2 kg of ground lungs using this method. Alternatively, the precipitated Hyamine-heparin complex can be extracted using a concentrated NaCl solution (i.e., 2M) to replace the heparin and subsequently precipitated with MeOH to obtain the heparin sodium salt [30]. Neither patents describe an extensive characterization on the obtained heparin, therefore there is no data on the amount of impurities such as nucleic acids and CS/DS.

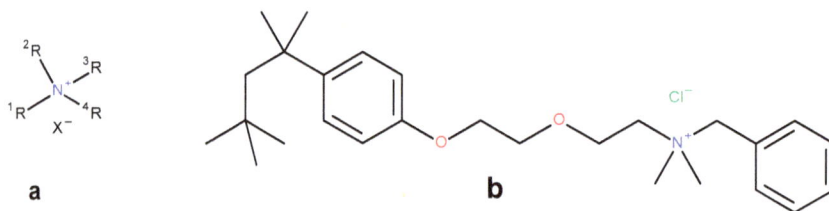

Figure 3. Structures of quaternary ammonium salts used for heparin capture by precipitation. (**a**) General structure of an applicable salt; (**b**) Structure of benzethonium chloride (Hyamine® 1622).

1.3.2. Ion Exchange Resins

Like Hyamine, the ion exchange resin can be added directly to the digestion mixture. Typical amounts of anion exchange resin include 2–4 L per 100 kg of mucosa [31]. Adsorption is typically done over several hours during which temperature, pH and salt concentration are critical parameters. Deviations on any of these parameters might result in increased binding of unwanted contaminants such as nucleic acids or other GAGs. After binding, the loaded resin has to be separated from the now heparin-free digestion mixture by sieving. To enable this sieving the anion exchanger (see Table 1, for functional groups) should be immobilized on a matrix which allows to be sieved. Examples thereof include crosslinked acrylic or polystyrene beads. After sieving the resulting waste stream (peptone) could be used as a fertilizer for farmlands, animal feed of for medical formulations for enteral or parental nutrition [37]. The loaded resin may be washed with water or a solution with a relatively low ionic strength (e.g., 5.8% NaCl m/v) to eliminate unbound material and to reduce less tightly bound compounds such as nucleic acids and other less charged GAGs [38]. This step can also be used to increase the activity of heparin (*vide infra*) by removing heparin with a low affinity to the resin. Subsequent elution with a high salt concentration (i.e., >14%) released the heparin from the column and enables further processing. There are several suitable anion exchange resins available on the market (Table 2). These resins might be the same type as the ones used for water treatment.

Table 2. Selected examples of functional groups used on anion exchange resins for heparin capture.

Resin Name	Functional Group	References
Amberlite IR-120, FPA98/, IRA900/CG-45		[24,29,31,36]
Dowex 22CL		[23]
Lewatitt CA9249		[26,31]
		[39]
DEAE		[39,40]

1.3.3. Resins or Fractional Elution for Activity Increase

Heparin's affinity to anion exchange resin depends both on its overall charge and its charge density. These are both closely related to degree of sulfation and chain length which are also important for its heparin activity. As a result, the binding affinity of heparin to anion exchange resin correlates with its activity. Therefore fractional elution or a washing step with a relatively low ionic strength (<3.5% NaCl) help to enrich highly active heparin chains [39–41]. Loaded resin (*N-N*-diethyl-2-hydroxypropyl ammonium functionalized cellulose) was washed with a ~2.3% NaCl solution. Subsequent fractional elution with a gradient from 2.3% to 8.2% NaCl enabled the inventors to obtain heparin fractions with a 2.5–5 fold increase of specific activity relative to the starting material yielding heparin with up to 500 IU/mg aXa activity and up to 400 IU/mg aIIa activity. Although for this invention purified heparin was fractionated instead of the more crude form of heparin which is bound to anion exchange resin, this patent illustrates the potential of applying the anion exchanger step to improve the activity, however at the expense of yield since low activity heparin still added to the initial yield. Other resin which can be used to improve heparin activity on lab scale include antithrombin-sepharose [42] and gel filtration columns. The first of these two selects heparin chains based on anti-thrombin affinity which is largely determined by the presence of the "high affinity pentasaccharide" and the second type separates heparin chains based on chain length. Both methods are highly useful analytical tools but due to scaling issues and considerable costs of the column material not practical for industrial scale heparin production.

1.4. Purification and Bleaching

At this stage of the production process, we have a heparin crude solution which is relatively pure. The main remaining contaminants at this stage are nucleic acids and non-heparin GAGs, such as chondroitin sulfate (CS) and dermatan sulfate (DS), which like heparin are biopolymers have a relatively high negative charge-density and therefore also adsorb to the anion exchange resin or precipitate with the quaternary ammonium salt. Moreover a variety of pathogens, including: viruses, bacteria and in the case of bovine starting material bovine spongiform encephalopathy (BSE) related prions may not have been adequately reduced to ensure patient safety. Therefore, the following steps are designed to reduce the inactive material such as DNA/RNA and to sufficiently reduce the infectious agents listed above.

1.4.1. (Fractional) Precipitation

Precipitation is both conducted to isolate the heparin or heparin crude from a solution and to remove impurities such as non-heparin GAGs and nucleic acids. It also serves to remove metal ions and small and/or less polar molecules such as peptide fragments generated during digestion and residues of chemicals used in processing: these will remain in the supernatant. For this step, different organic solvents such as methanol, ethanol, propanol, or acetone can be used [36,43]. As a result of decreasing polarity by addition of the antisolvent, the highly charged heparin chains precipitate. Most protocols in the literature apply either methanol or ethanol for this step with a percentage of ~50% (v/v). The concentration of the organic solvent is paramount at this stage as well as NaCl concentration and temperature. This was demonstrated by Volpi [36] who performed a fractional precipitation on a mixture of heparin, CS and DS with methanol, ethanol and propanol. Here it was observed that the order of precipitation of these compounds reflects their charge density (i.e., S/C ratios of resp. 2.4, 1.1 and 0.98). Using a relative volume of 1 methanol (i.e., ~50% v/v) precipitated nearly all the heparin from the mixture whereas a substantial concentration of CS and DS was still present in the supernatant (see Figure 4).

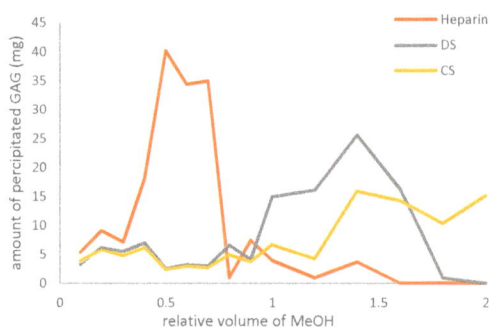

Figure 4. Fractional precipitation of heparin, DS and CS at different concentrations of methanol. Data derived from Volpi et al. [36].

1.4.2. Bleaching

The last step in most heparin processes usually includes an oxidation/bleaching step meant to remove/reduce color, endotoxins (depyrogenization), bacteria, mold, viruses and prions, followed by solvent precipitation sequence and a 0.22 µ sterile filtration to remove microbes and drying [43–47].

The oxidation is performed using e.g., potassium permanganate ($KMnO_4$) hydrogen peroxide (H_2O_2), peracetic acid (CH_3CO_3H), sodium hypochlorite (NaClO) or ozone (O_3) [48]. Prion reduction by hydrogen peroxide oxidation has been used by the FDA as a justification for the re-introduction of bovine heparin [15]. The term 'oxidation' is misleading here and 'bleaching' is more appropriate since the aim of the step is not to affect the heparin molecule by oxidation but rather to purify the heparin. However, this step can still result in the inadvertent modification of the heparin chains. This can result in damage to the heparin chain and/or a reduced biological activity [46,49,50]. In the wake of the 2008 contaminated heparin crisis, 1D ^{1}H-NMR was introduced as a pharmacopoeial release test. 1D ^{1}H-NMR had proved successful in detecting the contaminant oversulfated chondroitin sulfate which has a distinctive signal due to the glucosamine *N*-acetyl group [51–53]. This resulted in close inspection to heparin 1D ^{1}H-NMR spectra for unknown signals in specific spectral areas. Potassium permanganate oxidation has been shown to oxidize the reducing end hydroxyl of *N*-acetyl glucosamine to yield a carboxylate group resulting in a 2.10 ppm signal from the *N*-acetyl function in the NMR spectrum of potassium permanganate bleached heparin (see Figure 5, [54–57]).

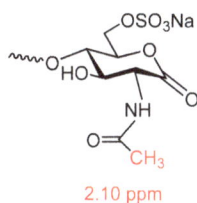

2.10 ppm

Figure 5. Reducing end oxidized *N*-acetylglucosamine heparin modification as a result of potassium permanganate bleaching.

Potassium permanganate oxidation also results in the reduction of the residual (glycol) serine at the reducing end of the heparin chain [50]. Oxidation by potassium permanganate results in an increase in carboxylate groups in heparin and concomitant chain breaks [50]. This should be taken into account when using the sulfate/carboxylate ratio which is commonly used as a measure for heparin sulfation [57]. Oxidation by peracetic acid results in the formation of 3-acetyluronic acid which displays a signal at 2.18 ppm in the ^{1}H-NMR spectrum of peracetic acid bleached heparin (Figure 6 [58]).

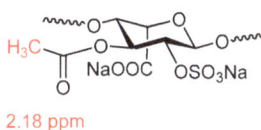

2.18 ppm

Figure 6. 3-Acetyluronic acid heparin modification as a result of peracetic acid bleaching.

Oxidation by other oxidation agents such as hydrogen peroxide and hypochlorite bleached heparin have not been reported to have a distinctive signals in its ^{1}H-NMR spectrum. Thus, these 'process signatures' allow to discriminate between oxidation methods used based on the ^{1}H-NMR spectroscopy [59]. Other products due to oxidation have been described in the literature [50]. Oxidation as purification step is only feasible because of the high intrinsic stability of the heparin molecule which is evident from a number of studies. [28,60,61] Less stable (bio-) molecules such as proteins would be degraded by these strongly oxidizing conditions, hence the strong virus/prion reductions achieved in this step [3,15]. The high stability of the heparin molecule together with its charged polymeric nature [60] enable it to be isolated in spite of being present at relatively low levels in the complex starting material [27].

1.5. Isolation and Drying

After this bleaching step, most properties of the heparin including: molecular composition, impurity profiles, microbial safety and color are determined. Therefore these steps are optimized to reach maximal yields and a minimum of residual solvents. There are several methods possible to isolate the heparin. Some of these methods include a precipitation step using a high percentage of methanol or ethanol ensuring that all heparin is precipitated. The precipitate is then collected and dried under vacuum at elevated temperatures (e.g., 40–75 °C) [62]. Alternatively, the heparin can be directly isolated from the solution by spray drying [63] or barrel drying [62].

2. Concluding Remark

Sourcing, isolation and purification of this 100 year old drug is still evolving for optimal efficacy and patient safety as well as production efficiency. The strict GMP regulations and pharmacopoeial criteria on the complete supply chain from farm to pharma will continue to assure the safety and efficacy of this WHO essential drug [64].

Acknowledgments: We thank Gijs van Dedem for critical reading of the paper and for his constructive comments.

Author Contributions: J.-Y.v.d.M., E.K. and L.J.v.d.B. constructed the idea for the manuscript, all authors contributed to the writing of the paper.

Conflicts of Interest: All authors hold positions in an enterprise which commercially manufactures heparin.

References

1.   Torri, G.; Naggi, A. Heparin centenary—An ever-young life-saving drug. *Int. J. Cardiol.* **2016**, *212*, S1–S4. [CrossRef]

2.   Yates, E.A; Rudd, T.R. Recent innovations in the structural analysis of heparin. *Int. J. Cardiol.* **2016**, *212*, S5–S9. [CrossRef]

3.   Barrowcliffe, T.W. History of heparin. In *Heparin-A Century of Progress*; Lever, R., Mulloy, B., Page, C.P., Eds.; Springer: Berlin/Heidelberg, Germany, 2012; pp. 3–22.

4.   Carlsson, P.; Kjellén, L. Heparin biosynthesis. In *Heparin—A Century of Progress*; Lever, R., Mulloy, B., Page, C.P., Eds.; Springer: Berlin/Heidelberg, Germany, 2012; pp. 23–41.

5.   Mulloy, B.; Hogwood, J.; Gray, E.; Lever, R.; Page, C.P. Pharmacology of heparin and related drugs. *Pharmacol. Rev.* **2016**, *68*, 76–141. [CrossRef] [PubMed]

6.   Jorpes, E. On the chemistry of heparin. *Biochem. J.* **1942**, *36*, 203–213. [CrossRef] [PubMed]

7.   Charles, A.F.; Scott, D.A. Studies on heparin: Observations on the chemistry of heparin. *Biochem. J.* **1936**, *30*, 1927–1933. [CrossRef] [PubMed]

8.   Kruizenga, M.H.; Spaulding, L.B. The preparation of highly active barium salt of heparin and its fractionation into two chemically and biologically different constituents. *J. Biol. Chem.* **1943**, *148*, 641–647.

9.   Shriver, Z.; Raman, R.; Venkataraman, G.; Drummond, K.; Turnbull, J.; Toida, T.; Linhardt, R.; Biemann, K.; Sasisekharan, R. Sequencing of 3-*O* sulfate containing heparin decasaccharides with a partial antithrombin III binding site. *Proc. Natl. Acad. Sci. USA* **2000**, *97*, 10359–10364. [CrossRef] [PubMed]

10. Olson, S.T.; Richard, B.; Izaguirre, G.; Schedin-Weiss, S.; Gettins, P.G. Molecular mechanisms of antithrombin-heparin regulation of blood clotting proteinases. A paradigm for understanding proteinase regulation by serpin family protein proteinase inhibitors. *Biochimie* **2010**, *92*, 1587–1596. [CrossRef] [PubMed]

11. Petitou, M.; Hérault, J.P.; Bernat, A.; Driguez, P.A.; Duchaussoy, P.; Lormeau, J.C.; Herbert, J.M. Synthesis of thrombin-inhibiting heparin mimetics without side effects. *Nature* **1999**, *398*, 417–422. [CrossRef] [PubMed]

12. European Pharmacopeia. *Monograph for Heparin Sodium Heparinum Natricum*, 9th ed.; 01/2017:0333; Council of Europe: Strasbourg, France, 2017.

13. Guidance for Industry-Heparin for Drug and Medical Device Use: Monitoring Crude Heparin for Quality. Available online: https://www.fda.gov/downloads/Drugs/GuidanceComplianceRegulatoryInformation/Guidances/UCM291390.pdf (accessed on 19 April 2017).

14. EudraLex. The Rules Governing Medicinal Products in the European Union, Volume 4: EU Guidelines for Good Manufacturing Practice for Medicinal Products for Human Van Veterinary Use, Annex 2 Manufacture of Biological Active Substances and Medicinal Products for Human Use. Ref. Ares(2012)118531-28/06/2012. Available online: https://ec.europa.eu/health/sites/health/files/files/eudralex/vol-4/vol4-an2_2012-06_en.pdf (accessed on 16 June 2017).

15. Keire, D.; Mulloy, B.; Chase, C.; Al-Hakim, A.; Cairatti, D.; Gray, E.; Hogwood, J.; Morris, T.; Mourão, P.A.S.; da Luz Carvalho Soares, M.; et al. Diversifying the Global Heparin Supply Chain: Reintroduction of Bovine Heparin in the United States? *Pharm. Technol.* **2015**, *28*, 36.

16. Fu, L.; Li, G.; Yang, B.; Onishi, A.; Li, L.; Sun, P.; Zhang, F.; Linhardt, R.J. Structural Characterization of Pharmaceutical Heparins Prepared from Different Animal Tissues. *J. Pharm. Sci.* **2013**, *102*, 1447–1457. [CrossRef] [PubMed]

17. Bett, C.; Grgac, K.; Long, D.; Karfunkle, M.; Keire, D.A.; Asher, D.M.; Gregori, L. A Heparin Purification Process Removes Spiked Transmissible Spongiform Encephalopathy Agent. *AAPS J.* **2017**, 1–7. [CrossRef] [PubMed]

18. Bianchini, P.; Liverani, L.; Mascellani, G.; Parma, B. Heterogeneity of unfractionated heparins studied in connection with species, source, and production processes. *Semin. Thromb. Hemost.* **1997**, *23*, 3–10. [CrossRef] [PubMed]

19. St. Ange, K.; Onishi, A.; Fu, L.; Sun, X.; Lin, L.; Mori, D.; Zhang, F.; Dordick, J.S.; Fareed, J.; Hoppensteadt, D.; et al. Analysis of heparins derived from bovine tissues and comparison to porcine intestinal heparins. *Clin. Appl. Thromb. Hemost.* **2016**, *22*, 520–527. [CrossRef] [PubMed]

20. Hoppensteadt, D.; Maia, P.; Silva, A.; Kumar, E.; Guler, N.; Jeske, W.; Kahn, D.; Walenga, J.M.; Coyne, E.; Fareed, J. Resourcing of Heparin and Low Molecular Weight Heparins from Bovine, Ovine, and Porcine Origin. Studies to Demonstrate the Biosimilarities. *Blood* **2015**, *126*, 4733. [CrossRef]

21. Warda, M.; Gouda, E.M.; Toida, T.; Chi, L.; Linhardt, R.J. Isolation and characterization of raw heparin from dromedary intestine: Evaluation of a new source of pharmaceutical heparin. *Comp. Biochem. Physiol. C Toxicol. Pharmacol.* **2003**, *136*, 357–365. [CrossRef] [PubMed]

22. Vreeburg, J.W.; Baauw, A. Method for Preparation of Heparin from Mucosa. Patent No. WO2010/110654 A1, 24 March 2009.

23. Warda, M.; Mao, W.; Toida, T.; Linhardt, R.J. Turkey intestine as a commercial source of heparin? Comparative structural studies of intestinal avian and mammalian glycosaminoglycans. *Comp. Biochem. Physiol. B Biochem. Mol. Biol.* **2003**, *134*, 189–197. [CrossRef]

24. Flengsrud, R.; Larsen, M.L.; Ødegaard, O.R. Purification, characterization and in vivo studies of salmon heparin. *Thromb. Res.* **2010**, *126*, e409–e417. [CrossRef] [PubMed]

25. Dietrich, C.P.; Paiva, J.F.; Castro, R.A.; Chavante, S.F.; Jeske, W.; Fareed, J.; Gorin, P.A.; Mendes, A.; Nader, H.B. Structural features and anticoagulant activities of a novel natural low molecular weight heparin from the shrimp *Penaeus brasiliensis. Biochim. Biophys. Acta* **1999**, *1428*, 273–283. [CrossRef]

26. Cesaretti, M.; Luppi, E.; Maccari, F.; Volpi, N. Isolation and characterization of a heparin with high anticoagulant activity from the clam *Tapes phylippinarum*: Evidence for the presence of a high content of antithrombin III binding site. *Glycobiology* **2004**, *14*, 1275–1284. [CrossRef] [PubMed]

27. Liu, H.; Zhang, Z.; Linhardt, R.J. Lessons learned from the contamination of heparin. *Nat. Prod. Rep.* **2009**, *26*, 313–321. [CrossRef] [PubMed]

28. Linhardt, R.J.; Gunay, N.S. Production and chemical processing of low molecular weight heparins. *Semin. Thromb. Hemost.* **1999**, *25*, 3–10.

29. Griffin, C.C.; Linhardt, R.J.; van Gorp, C.L.; Toida, T.; Hileman, R.E.; Schubert, R.L.; Brown, S.E. Isolation and characterization of heparan sulfate from crude porcine intestinal mucosal peptidoglycan heparin. *Carbohydr. Res.* **1995**, *276*, 183–197. [CrossRef]

30. Vidic, H.J. Process for Preparation of Heparin. U.S. Patent 4,283,530 A, 12 November 1976.

31. Van Houdenhoven, F.A.E.; Sanders, A.L.M.; van zuthpen, P.J.J. Process for the Purification of Heparin. U.S. Patent 6,232,093, 3 January 2000.

32. Homan, J.D.H.; Lens, J. A simple method for the purification of heparin. *Biochim. Acta* **1948**, *2*, 333–337. [CrossRef]

33. Bush, J.A.; Freeman, S.; Hagerty, E.B. Process for Preparing Heparin. U.S. Patent 2,884,358, 22 April 1957.

34. Nomine, G.; Pierre, B. Process of Purifying Heparin, and Product Produced Therefrom. U.S. Patent 2,989,438, 20 June 1961.
35. Mozen, M.M.; Evans, T.D. Process for Purifying Heparin. U.S. Patent 3,058,884, 14 September 1959.
36. Volpi, N. Purification of heparin, dermatan sulfate and chondroitin sulfate from mixtures by sequential precipitation with various organic solvents. *J. Chromatogr. B Biomed. Sci. Appl.* **1996**, *685*, 27–34. [CrossRef]
37. Van Gorp, C.L.; Vosburgh, F.; Schubert, R.L. Protein Hydrolysate from Mucosal Tissue. U.S. Patent 5,607,840, 30 November 1992.
38. Yamamoto, R.; Bellomo, E.G.; Kim, Y.; Rachana, V.Y.A.S. Method for Enhanced Heparin Quality. Patent No. WO2016/137471 A1, 26 February 2015.
39. Sache, E.; Maman, M.; Bertrand, H. New Heparin fractions Having Increased Anticoagulant Activities. Patent No. GB 2,051,103 A, 10 April 1980.
40. Toccaceli, N. Chromatographic Purification of Heparin. U.S. Patent 3,099,600, 30 July 1963.
41. Green, J.P. Fractionation of heparin on an anion exchanger. *Nature* **1960**, *186*, 472. [CrossRef] [PubMed]
42. Höök, M.; Björk, I.; Hopwood, J.; Lindahl, U. anticoagulant activity of heparin: Separation of high-activity and low-activity heparin species by affinity chromatography on immobilized antithrombin. *FEBS Lett.* **1976**, *66*, 90–93. [CrossRef]
43. Volpi, N. Fractionation of heparin, dermatan sulfate, and chondroitin sulfate by sequential precipitation: A method to purify a single glycosaminoglycan species from a mixture. *Anal. Biochem.* **1994**, *218*, 382–391. [CrossRef] [PubMed]
44. Arthur, B.E.; Ernest, H.J.; William, R.L. Process of Removing Colored Impurities from Heparin. U.S. Patent 2,830,931, 28 June 1954.
45. Bush, J.A.; Freeman, L.D.; Hagerty, E.B. Method for Purifying Sulfated Carbohydrates with Oxidizing Agents. U.S. Patent 31,356,660 A, 9 November 1956.
46. Ewards, F.R.; Horner, A.A. Purification of Heparin. U.S. Patent 3,179,566 A, 16 May 1963.
47. Celsus Website. Available online: https://www.heparin.com/manufacture_controls.php (accessed on 14 April 2017).
48. Coyne, E. Heparin—Past, present and future. In *Chemistry and Biology of Heparin*; Lundblad, R.L., Virgil Brow, W., Mann, K.G., Roberts, H.R., Eds.; Elsevier/North-Holland: Amsterdam, The Netherlands, 1981; pp. 9–17.
49. Yongjun, G. Refining Optimization Technology for Crude Heparin Sodium. Patent No. CN105,001,353 A, 17 August 2015.
50. Mourier, P.; Viskov, C. Process for Oxidizing Unfractionated Heparins and Detecting Presence or Absence of Glycoserine in Heparin and Heparin Products. Patent No. WO2005090411 A1, 24 March 2004.
51. Guerrini, M.; Beccati, D.; Shriver, Z.; Naggi, A.; Viswanathan, K.; Bisio, A.; Capila, I.; Lansing, J.C.; Guglieri, S.; Fraser, B.; et al. Oversulfated chondroitin sulfate is a contaminant in heparin associated with adverse clinical events. *Nat. Biotechnol.* **2008**, *26*, 669–675. [CrossRef] [PubMed]
52. Szajek, A.Y.; Chess, E.; Johansen, K.; Gratzl, G.; Gray, E.; Keire, D.; Linhardt, R.J.; Liu, J.; Morris, T.; Mulloy, B.; et al. The US regulatory and pharmacopeia response to the global heparin contamination crisis. *Nat. Biotechnol.* **2016**, *34*, 625–630. [CrossRef] [PubMed]
53. Szajek, A.Y.; Morris, T.S.; Koch, W.F.; Abernethy, D.R.; Williams, R.L. Inside USP: Heparin Monographs Further Revised. *Pharm. Technol.* **2009**, *33*, 136–137.
54. Beccati, D.; Roy, S.; Yu, F.; Gunay, N.S.; Capila, I.; Lech, M.; Linhardt, R.J.; Venkataraman, G. Identification of a novel structure in heparin generated by potassium permanganate oxidation. *Carbohydr. Polym.* **2010**, *82*, 699–705. [CrossRef] [PubMed]
55. Kellenbach, E.; Sanders, K.; Michiels, P.J.A.; Girard, F.C. 1H NMR signal at 2.10 ppm in the spectrum of KMnO4-bleached heparin sodium: Identification of the chemical origin using an NMR-only approach. *Anal. Bioanal. Chem.* **2011**, *399*, 621–628. [CrossRef] [PubMed]
56. Mourier, P.A.; Guichard, O.Y.; Herman, F.; Viskov, C. Heparin sodium compliance to the new proposed USP monograph: Elucidation of a minor structural modification responsible for a process dependent 2.10 ppm NMR signal. *J. Pharm. Biomed. Anal.* **2011**, *54*, 337–344. [CrossRef] [PubMed]
57. Casu, B.; Gennaro, U. A conductimetric method for the determination of sulphate and carboxyl groups in heparin and other mucopolysaccharides. *Carbohydr. Res.* **1975**, *39*, 168–176. [CrossRef]

58. Mourier, P.A.; Guichard, O.Y.; Herman, F.; Viskov, C. Heparin sodium compliance to USP monograph: Structural elucidation of an atypical 2.18 ppm NMR signal. *J. Pharm. Biomed. Anal.* **2012**, *67*, 169–174. [CrossRef] [PubMed]

59. Lee, S.E.; Chess, E.K.; Rabinow, B.; Ray, G.J.; Szabo, C.M.; Melnick, B.; Miller, R.L.; Nair, L.M.; Moore, E.G. NMR of heparin API: Investigation of unidentified signals in the USP-specified range of 2.12–3.00 ppm. *Anal. Bioanal. Chem.* **2011**, *399*, 651–662. [CrossRef] [PubMed]

60. Jandik, K.A; Kruep, D.; Cartier, M.; Linhardt, R.J. Accelerated stability studies of heparin. *J. Pharm. Sci.* **1996**, *85*, 45–51. [CrossRef] [PubMed]

61. Liu, L.; Linhardt, R.J.; Zhang, Z. Quantitative analysis of anions in glycosaminoglycans and application in heparin stability studies. *Carbohydr. Polym.* **2014**, *106*, 343–350. [CrossRef] [PubMed]

62. Huang, L.; Tang, J.; Wang, Z.; Zhou, J.; Yan, H. Method for Drying Heparin by Atomization. Patent No. CN1,218,058, 26 November 1997.

63. Raghavan, R.; Jett, J.L. Method to Produce a Solid Form of Heparin, U.S. Patent 2004/0176581, 27 February 2004.

64. WHO Model Lists of Essential Medicines. Available online: http://www.who.int/medicines/publications/essentialmedicines/EML_2015_FINAL_amended_NOV2015.pdf?ua=1 (accessed on 8 May 2017).

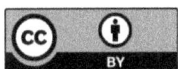

molecules

MDPI

Article

Combining NMR Spectroscopy and Chemometrics to Monitor Structural Features of Crude Heparin

Lucio Mauri [1], Maria Marinozzi [1], Giulia Mazzini [1], Richard E. Kolinski [2], Michael Karfunkle [2], David A. Keire [2] and Marco Guerrini [1,*]

[1] Institute for Chemical and Biochemical Research G. Ronzoni, via G. Colombo 81, 20133 Milan, Italy; mauri@ronzoni.it (L.M.); maria.marinozzi90@gmail.com (M.M.); giulia.mazzini@gmail.com (G.M.)

[2] Division of Pharmaceutical Analysis, Office of Testing and Research, Center for Drug Evaluation and Research, U.S. Food and Drug Administration, 645 S. Newstead Ave., St. Louis, MO 63110, USA; Richard.kolinski@fda.hhs.gov (R.E.K.); michael.karfunkle@fda.hhs.gov (M.K.); David.Keire@fda.hhs.gov (D.A.K.)

* Correspondence: guerrini@ronzoni.it; Tel.: +39-02-70641621

Received: 6 June 2017; Accepted: 5 July 2017; Published: 8 July 2017

Abstract: Because of the complexity and global nature of the heparin supply chain, the control of heparin quality during manufacturing steps is essential to ensure the safety of the final active pharmaceutical ingredient (API). For this reason, there is a need to develop consistent analytical methods able to assess the quality of heparin early in production (i.e., as the crude heparin before it is purified to API under cGMP conditions). Although a number of analytical techniques have been applied to characterize heparin APIs, few of them have been applied for crude heparin structure and composition analyses. Here, to address this issue, NMR spectroscopy and chemometrics were applied to characterize 88 crude heparin samples. The samples were also analyzed by strong anion exchange HPLC (SAX-HPLC) as an orthogonal check of the purity levels of the crudes analyzed by NMR. The HPLC data showed that the chemometric analysis of the NMR data differentiated the samples based on their purity. These orthogonal approaches differentiated samples according their glycosaminoglycan (GAG) composition and their mono and disaccharide composition and structure for each GAG family (e.g., heparin/heparan, dermatan sulfate, and chondroitin sulfate A). Moreover, quantitative HSQC and multivariate analysis (PCA) were used to distinguish between crude heparin of different animal and tissue sources.

Keywords: heparin; crude heparin; NMR; quantitative NMR; PCA; chemometric; HSQC

1. Introduction

In spite of its 100 year history, heparin and its lower molecular weight versions remain the most used anticoagulant and antithrombotic drug [1]. Heparin is a sulfated polysaccharide composed of alternating disaccharide sequences of uronic acid (either D-glucuronic or L-iduronic acid) and glucosamine. The glucosamine residue can be *N*-acetylated or *N*-sulfated in position 2, while both uronic acid and glucosamine can be sulfated in position 2 and 6, respectively. More rarely, the glucosamine residue can be sulfated in position 3, and found in the pentasaccharide sequence GlcNS/Ac-GlcA-GlcNS,3S,6S/OH-IdoA2S-GlcNS,6S, corresponding to the heparin binding site for antithrombin (AT). The degree of sulfation and distribution within the heparin chains depends on the animal or organ source; however, the detailed monosaccharide sequence is still largely undisclosed [2].

Until the late 1980s and early 1990s, when cases of bovine spongiform encephalopathy (BSE) were reported in United Kingdom and other countries, bovine heparin products were widely used together with those extracted from porcine intestine. As a result of BSE, bovine heparin was withdrawn from both the U.S. and European markets and entirely replaced by porcine mucosa heparin, limiting bovine heparin use to South America and some Islamic countries. The removal of bovine heparin from the market increased the market demand for porcine heparin. As a result, at present more than 50% of worldwide heparin production originates from China [3]. In addition, a shortage in the heparin supply (due also to a pig disease outbreak) was presumably the reason for the heparin contamination with the semisynthetic over-sulfated chondroitin sulfate (OSCS), an inexpensive adulterant with anticoagulant activity, which occurred in late 2007 in the US and Europe [4]. This so called heparin crisis, in addition to causing many deaths and severe side effects, demonstrated the vulnerability of the global heparin supply chain. Fortunately, the subsequent introduction of new tests (e.g., NMR and HPLC tests) to the heparin monographs of several pharmacopoeias around the world increased the degree of quality control of this drug, decreasing the risk of product adulteration [3]. However, the complexity of the heparin supply chain provides other opportunities for intentional adulteration, such as contamination with foreign substances or the addition of non-porcine sources of crude heparin (i.e., bovine or ovine heparin), which might not be detected by the current monograph test methods.

Heparin is produced from tissues of food animals, and for medical use the drug has been primarily obtained from pig or beef intestine, and can be sourced from sheep as well. Typically, the pig intestine is collected and processed in slaughterhouses approved by regulatory authorities and then transported to crude heparin processing facilities. In these facilities, the intestinal mucosa is removed and the dissociated mucosa is treated with proteolytic enzymes under alkaline conditions. After multiple steps, the highly anionic glycosaminoglycans (GAGs) can be adsorbed onto an anion exchange resin, which is washed. Then, the partially purified heparin is eluted, filtered, precipitated, and vacuum dried to form a substance known as crude heparin, where the glycosaminoglycan (GAG) fraction is concentrated. Crude heparin is then further purified at the level of active pharmaceutical ingredient (API) to remove impurities such as dermatan and chondroitins, nucleic acids, residual proteins, metal ions, and unwanted counterions. In addition, the purification involves oxidation ($KMnO_4$ or H_2O_2) and alkaline treatments to remove color and inactivate endotoxins and viruses that might be present in the product [5,6].

Whereas the purification of crude heparin to heparin sodium API is always conducted under cGMP conditions, only a few manufacturers can establish traceability back to the living animals. Many companies buy crude heparins from third parties, which have collected mucosa at multiple small slaughterhouses. These multiple sites increase the risk of un-intended or intentional contamination. Although it is impossible to eliminate all possible risks, reinforcing of appropriate requirements, controls, and best practices at the level of crude heparin as a key intermediate might help ensure the quality of the final pharmaceutical grade product.

A first step to define crude heparin as an intermediate in the production process of the API requires the specification of a normal range of composition found in heparin currently on the market. Different intermediates may exist and be qualified for use in the manufacture of heparin, such as resin bound heparin (early intermediates), a brown powder containing a large amount of RNA/DNA and galactosaminoglycans (mainly dermatan sulfate (DS) and chondroitin sulfate A (CSA)), or partly purified crude heparin, a light yellow powder containing only a small amount of dermatan sulfate [7]. Although different techniques have been used to identify and quantify OSCS in crude heparin, to our knowledge, these studies did not fully characterize the average composition of crudes produced in the global marketplace [8,9].

In the present study, 88 crude heparins collected from 2010 to 2015, representing 13 different manufacturers, have been characterized by NMR spectroscopy and strong anion exchange HPLC (SAX-HPLC). Particularly, a multivariate analysis (principal component analysis (PCA)) of one-dimensional (1D) proton NMR spectra was used to differentiate the crudes on the basis of their structural features and animal/organ of origin. Moreover, the quantitative composition of crude samples was performed using an adapted version of the HSQC method recently described in [10].

2. Results

2.1. Protocol for Sample Preparation

Crude heparin samples are often not completely soluble in water. Therefore, to avoid the presence of insoluble material in the NMR tube, a protocol of sample separation by centrifugation was developed. Three parameters of the separation protocol were evaluated for their effect on the supernatant content, including: the amount of insoluble material present, crude concentration, and the method of solution equilibration (with or without stirring). Each of the eight combinations of the parameters was tested. Moreover, three separations were performed for a single parameter set to evaluate the precision of the data, giving a total of ten separations. For each separation, two parameters were measured after lyophilization of the supernatant or the pellet: the total weight loss and the amount of precipitate, both expressed as a percentage of the original weight (Table 1).

Table 1. Recovering of soluble and insoluble material obtained by two crude heparin samples. Weightings before and after the separation and lyophilization procedure are shown.

Sample	Crude (mg/mL)	Stirring	Supernatant (mg)	Precipitate (mg)	Weight loss % (%w)	Precipitate (%w)
G9709	40.4	No	35.3	1.2	9.7	3.3
G9709	40.8	No	35.4	1.0	10.8	2.7
G9709	38.9	No	33.7	1.2	10.3	3.4
G9709	39.0	Yes	34.0	1.1	10.0	3.1
G9709	79.7	No	60.4	10.0	11.7	14.2
G9709	81.4	Yes	62.4	9.4	11.8	13.1
G9710	39.0	No	33.8	2.7	6.4	7.4
G9710	39.3	Yes	33.2	2.1	10.2	5.9
G9710	79.5	No	56.8	13.8	11.2	19.5
G9710	80.5	Yes	59.3	13.0	10.2	18.0

With the exclusion of one result, the loss of water due to lyophilization was around 10%, regardless of sample concentration. While the stirring procedure during solution equilibration did not affect the yield on a percentage basis, the amount of precipitate was related to the sample concentration, showing that the precipitate still contains soluble material. To verify that the procedure does not result in the selective separation of glycosaminoglycan species, a precipitate obtained at a higher concentration (80 mg/mL) was re-suspended in 1 mL of D_2O, centrifuged, and the spectrum of the supernatant compared with that obtained after the first solubilization. While no differences in the glycosamonoglycan pattern were found, higher non-GAG signals in the re-suspended precipitate were observed (Figure S1). Based on these results, to collect enough soluble material for the NMR characterization, an aliquot of 60 mg of crude heparin was determined to be sufficient for analysis in 1.5 mL of D_2O. The average weights of the 88 crude samples are shown in Table S1.

The proton chemical shifts of heparin are affected both by the pH and concentration of the solution [11,12]. Crude heparin does not contain only heparin, but also other GAGs (heparan, dermatan, and chondroitin sulfate), as well as non-GAG material, mainly DNA and RNA, some proteinaceous material, and a variable amount of water and salts. For these reasons, the proton spectra of crude heparins in D_2O were not fully reproducible, and a shift of signals, particularly those of anomeric glucosamine and iduronic acid residues, was often observed (Figure S2). The maximum shift of both peaks observed was about 10–12 Hz (0.015–0.020 ppm), presumably due to the different concentration of GAG components in the samples, which affect the pH of the solution. These spectra cannot be easily compared, particularly when they are analysed by multivariate analysis (e.g., PCA). To remove the effect of pH variability, the samples were solubilized in 0.15 M of phosphate buffer at pH 7.1, containing 3 mM of perdeuterated EDTA. The complexation of bivalent or paramagnetic ions induced by the addition of perdeuterated EDTA provides narrower lines and improved resolution. A comparison of crude proton spectra recorded in water and the buffer solution is shown in Figure S2.

2.2. One-Dimensional (1D) Spectra Library and PCA

The proton spectra of eighty-eight crude heparin samples were registered by the NMR analysis protocol indicated in the experimental section. The spectra show very high variability of composition, both in terms of non-GAGs components (broad signals at both aromatic and aliphatic regions due to DNA/RNA and other impurities, Figure S1) and galactosaminoglycans components, mainly dermatan and chondroitin sulfate (Figure 1).

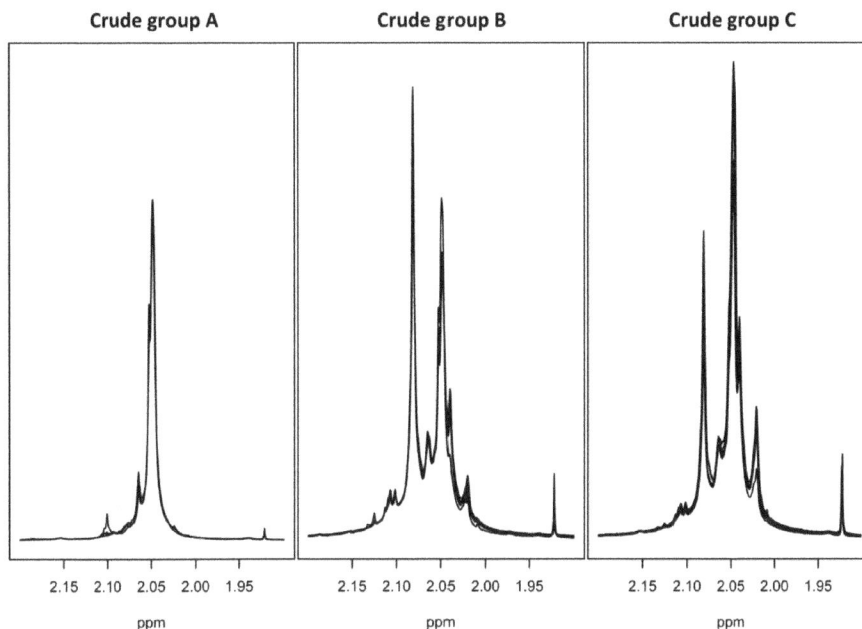

Figure 1. ^{1}H-NMR spectra. Acetyl region of proton spectra of samples of group A, group B, and group C (see Figure 2) registered at 600 MHz, showing methyl signals of Dermatan (2.08 ppm), Heparin (2.05 ppm), and Chondoritin (2.02 ppm) components.

Due to this variability and the difficulties in establishing quantitative ratios among diagnostic signals, the spectral complexity was reduced to the basic elements which best define the crucial differences between samples by employing chemometric techniques.

One of the most common tools used to explore a complex dataset is principal component analysis (PCA). Typically, this tool takes a large number of correlated variables and transforms the data into a smaller number of uncorrelated variables (principal components), while extracting the maximal amount of variation, thus making it easier to analyse the data and make predictions [13].

The score plot of the first two components, generated by the PCA of 88 ^{1}H-NMR spectra of the crude samples, is shown in Figure 2. The graph, displaying the variance accounted for by the principal components, shows that only two components are necessary to account for more than 80% of the total variance, indicating that the differences among the samples are mainly distributed along the components **1** and **2**.

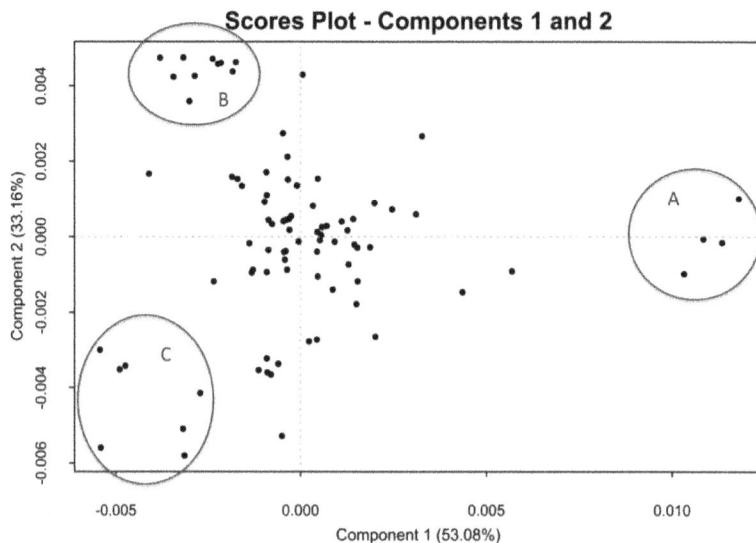

Figure 2. Score plot of the first two components generated by principal component analysis (PCA) of the GAGs signals region of the ^{1}H-NMR spectrum. Most of the samples are centered in the PCA, while there are 21 more peripheral samples: highlighted as A, B, and C.

In the loading plot of the first principal component, the negative signal of the acetyl protons of dermatan sulfate was observed (Figure 3). By contrast, in the loading of the second principal component, signals belonging to the trisulfated disaccharide (corresponding to the most abundant dissaccharide of heparin chains) are positive, while the other heparin and chondroitin acetyl signals are negative. The analysis of the loading plots suggested that samples having a positive score in component 1 (Figure 2, group A) contain a low amount of dermatan sulfate, while those having negative score in component 2 (Figure 2, group C) contain highly acetylated heparin with a larger amount of chondroitin. The samples contained within the group B have instead a higher degree of sulfation, together with a large amount of dermatan. The proton spectra of the samples belonging to these groups confirm what was observed by PCA, showing that the spectra of samples belonging to the group A, in the absence of dermatan and chondroitin acetyl signals, match with those of purified heparin (Figure 1).

Since the major differences among the crude samples defined by PCA are due to the content of galactosaminoglycan and the acetylation degree of the heparin component, the PCA was performed also on part of the anomeric region of the proton spectra (5.75–4.94 ppm). In this region, with the exclusion of the weak H1 of I2S of dermatan sulfate (5.18 ppm), no signals belonging to dermatan and chondroitin are present. Before the PCA analysis, the selected region of the proton spectra was aligned with a custom algorithm (Table S14 and Figure S9), because without alignment the shift effect was dominant in the loading plot of the first principal component. After the alignment, PCA differentiates samples on the basis of the sulfation pattern of the heparin/heparan sulfate components. The score plot generated by the PCA of this spectral region is shown in Figure 4. No evident clusters are visible, and the loading plot of the first principal component (Figure S3) can be interpreted in terms of the degree of sulfation of the samples, where the samples positioned in the negative score of the first principal component are more highly sulfated. Although the loading plot of the second component is difficult to interpret, the negative signals corresponding to the H1 of GlcNS,6OH and I2S linked to GlcNS,6OH indicate that the samples with lower 6-O-sulfation are located in the negative score of the second principal component (Figure S3).

Loadings Plots - Components 1, 2

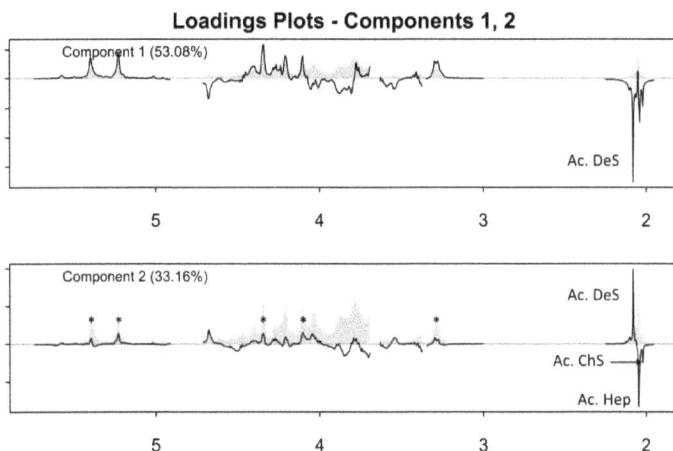

Figure 3. Loading plot of the first two components of the PCA of the GAGs signals region. In the loading plot of component 1, a negative signal corresponding to the N-acetyl residue of dermatan is observed. Positive signals corresponding to the trisulfated disaccharide (*) (-I2S-GlcNS,6S-) and negative signals corresponding to the N-acetyl residue of glucosamine (Hep) and galatosamine (ChS) are observed in the loading plot of component 2.

Scores Plot - Components 1 and 2

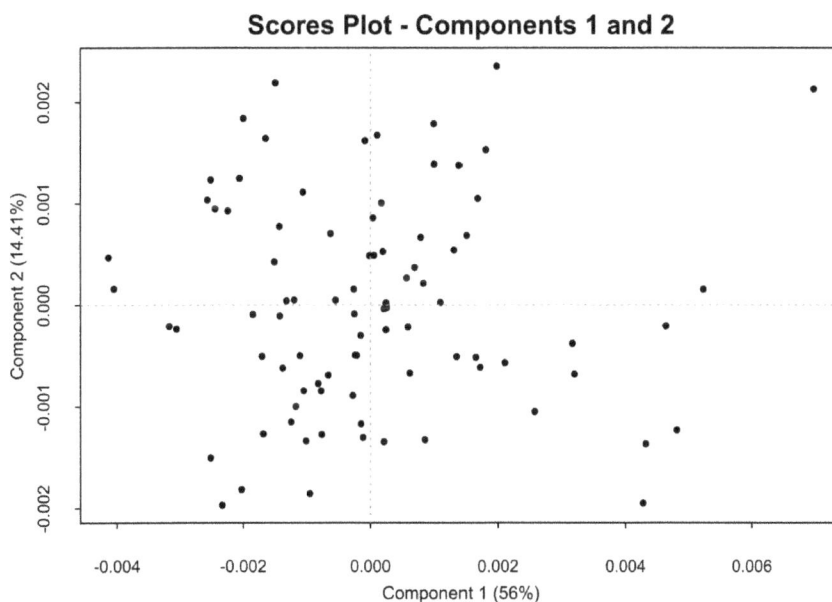

Figure 4. Score plot of the first two components generated by PCA of part of anomeric signals region. No clusters are defined. Only one sample appears isolated in the upper-right of the figure.

2.3. SAX-HPLC Analysis

To confirm the results of the NMR chemometric analysis data, the purity of the crude heparin samples was analyzed with a lower resolution method; SAX-HPLC. The SAX-HPLC method applied here separates heparin (~2.5 sulfates per disaccharide) from less sulfated (e.g., ~1 sulfate per disaccharide,

DS/CSA/heparan) or more sulfated (e.g., 4 sulfates per disaccharide, over sulfated chondroitin sulfate (OSCS)) GAGs based on negative charge [9,14]. As shown in Figure 5, the crude heparins in group A were the most pure, with the majority of the signal eluting at ~20.5 min consistent with heparin sodium API. For group B, two major peaks (17.0 and 20.4 min) of similar intensity were observed and attributed to primarily DeS and heparin, respectively. For group C, three major peaks were observed (14.5, 16.6, and 20.5 min), with the intensity of the 14.5 and the 16.6 peaks being much higher than the heparin peak at 20.5 min. These group C peaks are attributed to DNA/RNA, heparan/CSA, DeS, and heparin sulfate. Thus, group C samples contain DNA/RNA impurities as well as more less sulfated GAGs (i.e., CSA/heparan/DeS) than the group B or group A samples (Figure S4). Overall, the chemometric analysis of the NMR data and the visual examination of the SAX-HPLC chromatograms of the crude heparin samples can be used to order the crudes from highest (A) to lowest purity (C) as A, B, and C, respectively.

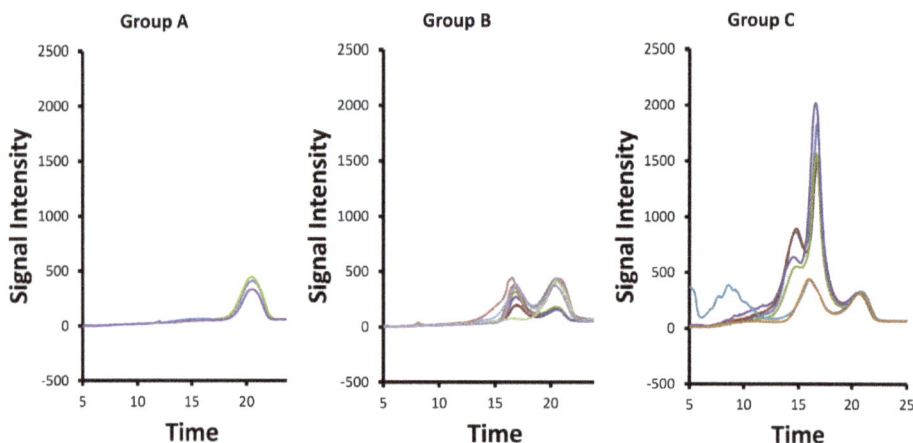

Figure 5. The 5 min to 25 min portion of the strong anion exchange HPLC (SAX-HPLC) chromatograms with UV detection at 215 nm of crudes differentiated into groups A, B, and C by NMR data as shown in Figure 2. Generally, the lower resolution HPLC method shows these groups have increasing levels of different impurities, going from group A to B to C, respectively.

2.4. HSQC Analysis

Quantitative HSQC was recently applied to heparin and low molecular weight heparins (LMWHs). The ^{1}H,^{13}C-HSQC data acquired on heparin APIs were used for calculating the percentage of mono- and disaccharides by normalizing volumes with reference to the sum of volumes of signals corresponding to each monosaccharide type (glucosamines or uronic acids) and the same carbon-proton pair type (e.g., anomeric or C2 position pairs) [10,15–17]. In the HSQC spectra collected here, signals belonging to high molecular weight species, mainly DNA and RNA, were not detected, presumably due to the increased linewidths associated with these slower tumbling larger molecules.

The HSQC spectrum of crude heparin also contains signals belonging to galactosaminoglycan components (DS and CSA), which partially overlap with those of the heparin/heparan sulfate (HS) components. By contrast, in the H2/C2 region, signals belonging to *N* acetyl glucosamine were completely separated from those of the *N*-acetyl-galactosamine residues (3.90 ppm/56.0–56.6 ppm and 4.02 ppm/53.8–54.6 ppm, respectively; Figure S5). Thus, the percentage of glucosamine and galactosamino residues could be calculated by the integration of the corresponding residues (Table 2). In addition, the uronic acid components of the galactosaminoglycans were well separated in the anomeric region of the crude heparins (Figure 6). Beside the major IdoA-GalNAc,4S sequences, DeS contains about 10% of disulfated disaccharide sequences, mostly consisting of IdoA2S-GalNAc,4S [18]. The anomeric signals of IdoA and IdoA2S of dermatan sulfate, at 4.88/106.1 ppm and 5.18/103.4 ppm, respectively, could be integrated to determine the IdoA2S/IdoA ratio. Similarly, the anomeric signal of the glucuronic acid of the chondroitin presents distinct chemical shift values on the basis of the position of the sulfate group of the following *N*-Acetyl-galactosamine residue (Figure 6) (4.47/106.6 ppm and 4.50/107.1 ppm for the ChS4S or ChS6S, respectively) [19], allowing the evaluation of the GalNAc,6S/GalNAc,4S ratio. Unfortunately, the anomeric signals of the DeS and ChS *N*-acetyl-galactosamine residues partially overlap with the anomeric signal of heparin glucuronic acid. In particular, if chondroitin is present, the amount of glucuronic acid linked to trisulfated glucosamine (G-$A_{NS,3S,6X}$) could be overestimated.

Table 2. Molar average composition of 88 crude heparin samples. PMHC = pig mucosa heparin crude; Hep = Heparin; DeS = Dermatan sulfate; ChS = Chondroitin sulfate; A = Glucosamine; I = Iduronic acid; G = Glucuronic acid; X = SO_3^- or H; SDEG = Heparin disaccharide degree of sulfation.

PMHC	Hep	DeS	ChS	ANH26X	ANAc6X	ANS3S6X	A6S	G2OH	G2S	I2OH	I2S	SDEG
average	89.3	8.6	2.4	1.8	16.3	4.5	73.3	18.0	0.01	10.5	71.5	2.31
median	89.2	8.7	2.1	1.9	16.3	4.4	73.7	17.9	0.00	10.6	71.4	2.32
st.dev.	4.1	3.1	1.9	0.7	2.0	0.7	3.4	1.9	0.09	0.9	2.5	0.08
min	79.9	0.0	0.0	0.0	11.6	3.1	63.3	14.0	0.00	8.2	65.4	2.13
max	100.0	16.6	7.7	3.0	21.1	5.9	79.8	22.4	0.75	12.4	76.8	2.46

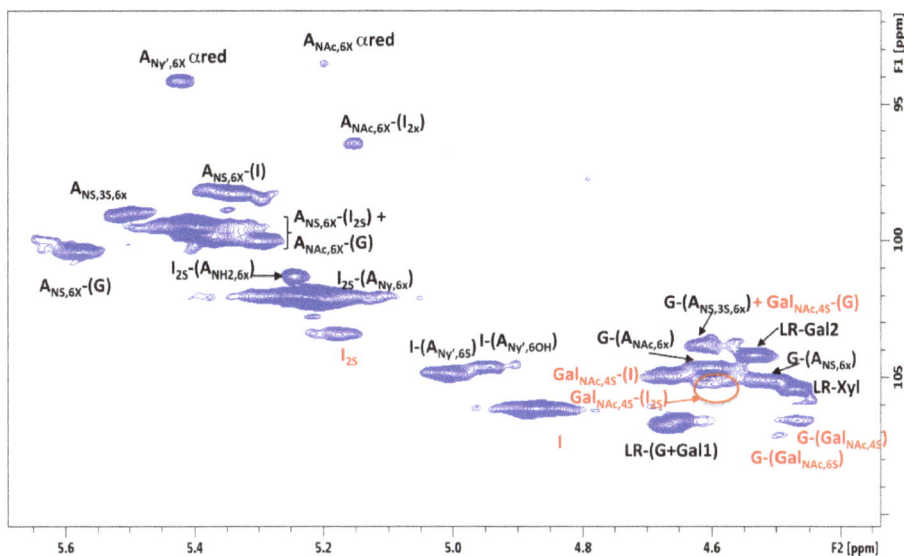

Figure 6. Anomeric region of a crude heparin HSQC spectrum. Signal assignments of heparin and DeS/ChS components are in black and red, respectively.

Finally, the composition of the heparin fraction was obtained as for the API product [10]. Tables S2 and S3 show the signals assignment and the detailed formulas for the calculations. The precision of the method was evaluated using a crude sample positioned close to the origin (0) of the PCA scores plot of Figure 2, therefore having an average composition in DeS/ChS comparable with the whole library of 88 samples. The intermediate precision was determined combining two operators and two spectrometers operating at 500 and 600 MHz (Tables S7–S9). Using a reasonable experimental time (6 h at 600 MHz and 8 h at 500 MHz) it was possible to quantify with sufficient precision all of the fragments above 3%, compared to 2% for API heparin with 2 h at 600 MHz and $3\frac{1}{2}$ h at 500 MHz [10]. This was considered a good result also in view of the fact that the concentration in the NMR tube was limited to 20 mg/0.6 mL compared to 35 mg/0.6 mL for API heparin. Clearly, the limit of quantification (LOQ) of heparin fragments might change according to the dermatan and chondroitin content. It was verified that a reliable estimation of the LOQ is given by the formula

$$\text{LOQ} = 2000 \times \text{VOL}/(\text{VOL\_SUM} \times \text{SNR}) \tag{1}$$

where VOL_SUM is the sum of all heparin anomeric signals, while VOL and SNR are the volume and signal to noise ratio of the anomeric signal of $\text{I-(A}_{NY',6S})$ or $\text{I-(A}_{NY',6OH})$ (Figure 6; both residues give comparable values for LOQ). If the LOQ is too high, the spectrum can be acquired again with more scans (NS) for better SNR, as the SNR term is proportional to the square root of NS. The robustness of the method was also evaluated by identifying the most critical parameters of the analytical method: pH of buffer, sample concentration, acquisition temperature, and spectrum phasing. These four parameters where studied at two levels in a Plucket–Burman design (Tables S4–S6). The heparin fragment quantification showed good robustness with respect to all of the parameters. The GAGs content was sensitive to variations of temperature, probably due to the different mobility of the heparin, DeS, and ChS chains.

A summary and the details of the obtained composition of a series of 75 out of 88 crude heparin samples are shown in Table 2 and Tables S10–S13, respectively.

As already observed in the PCA, crude heparin samples are characterized by a large variation in galactosaminoglycan content (0–20%), while the heparin component varies in N-acetylation, 6-O-sulfation, and nonsulfated uronic acid content (11–21%, 63–79%, and 23–35% respectively). Notably, the serine of the linkage region is almost exclusively present in its intact form (CHα at 4.00/57.4 ppm; Figure S5). However, the oxidized form of serine [20] was detected in the samples of group A by the reduction or absence of the CHα signal and the presence of the anomeric signal of xylose linked to oxidized serine residue (4.48/105.5 ppm; Figure S6). The presence of the oxidized forms in the linkage region suggests that crude heparin has been subject to an oxidizing process; usually, such a step is applied during the purification of crude to API heparin. In fact, the monosaccharide composition of the samples present in group A of the PCA results is compatible with a semi purified product. In addition to showing serine in the oxidized form, their spectra do not contain signals belonging to galactosaminoglycan or DNA/RNA impurities, making the whole spectral profile similar to that of an API product (Figure S6).

2.5. Crude of Different Origin

As porcine, bovine, and ovine API heparins differ in many aspects of their structure and activity [21–25], it is important to verify if their structural differences can be observed in the corresponding crude. Six heparin crude samples from bovine intestinal mucosa (BMHC), two from bovine lung (BLHC) and three from ovine intestinal mucosa (OMHC) were characterized by proton and HSQC analysis. The PCA of the GAGs signals region of proton spectra of these samples against the library of porcine crude heparin was not able to differentiate samples according their origin (Figure S7). In spite of the structural differences between the heparins in these crudes, the galactosaminoglycan content mostly contributes to the samples' separation in component 1 (Figure 3). By contrast, PCA performed exclusively on the anomeric region was able to group samples on the basis of their origin, separating them in function of their sulfation pattern in component 1 and of the 6-O-sulfation in component 3 (Figure 7 and Figure S8). Indeed, BMHC and PMHC are not fully separated in components 1 and 2 because of their similar degree of sulfation, while in component 3 BMHC are fully distinguished from other crude heparin (Figure 7).

3D Score Plot - Components 1, 2 and 3

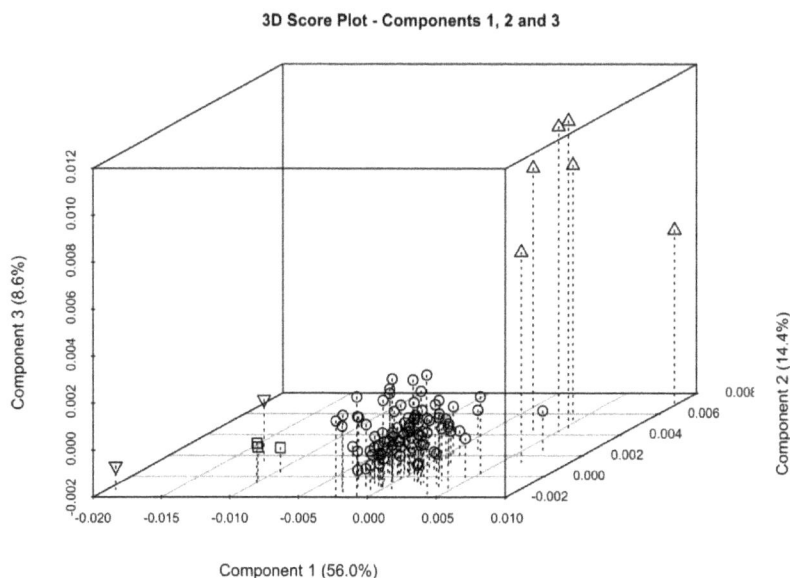

Figure 7. Three-dimensional (3D) Score plot generated by PCA of part of the anomeric signals region. Sample clusters corresponding to the different families of crude heparin are defined. BMHC (above pointing triangles), OMHC (squares) and BLHC (below pointing triangles), against the library of PMHC (circles).

The monosaccharide composition of each crude family was determined by HSQC analysis (Tables 2 and 3). The bovine lung crude shows the highest degree of sulfation and lowest content of acetylation and nonsulfated uronic acid. The lower 6-*O*-sulfation of the bovine mucosa crude agree with those observed in the corresponding API [25], while the degree of sulfation and amount of *N*-acetylation measured for the ovine crude samples is intermediate to that of bovine lung and porcine mucosa heparin, as also observed by the integration of C13 spectra of the purified heparin samples [24]. The greater structural detail obtained applying the HSQC method allows the detection of minor residues in crude heparin, such as G2S, that is more abundant in BMHC compared to ovine or porcine heparins [25].

Table 3. Molar average composition of crude heparin of different species/organ.

BMHC	Hep	DeS	ChS	ANH26X	ANAc6X	ANS3S6X	A6S	G2OH	G2S	I2OH	I2S	SDEG
average	94.7	4.2	0.4	1.5	10.6	2.0	51.7	14.1	1.5	6.8	77.1	2.20
median	98.1	1.1	0.0	1.9	9.6	1.8	52.4	13.8	2.0	6.3	76.9	2.19
st.dev.	5.9	5.8	0.9	3.3	3.3	0.7	4.0	2.0	1.2	1.2	2.8	0.07
min	85.3	0.0	0.0	0.0	8.2	1.3	47.1	11.9	0.0	6.0	73.4	2.12
max	98.8	12.5	2.1	2.6	17.2	3.5	57.2	17.4	2.5	9.2	81.0	2.31
BLHC	**Hep**	**DeS**	**ChS**	**ANH26X**	**ANAc6X**	**ANS3S6X**	**A6S**	**G2OH**	**G2S**	**I2OH**	**I2S**	**SDEG**
Sample 1	94.7	4.2	0.4	1.9	6.6	2.8	85.8	7.8	0.0	4.6	87.6	2.68
Sample 2	98.1	1.1	0.0	0.0	1.6	2.5	90.2	2.3	0.5	2.8	93.4	2.85
OMHC	**Hep**	**DeS**	**ChS**	**ANH26X**	**ANAc6X**	**ANS3S6X**	**A6S**	**G2OH**	**G2S**	**I2OH**	**I2S**	**SDEG**
Sample 1	98.9	1.1	0.0	1.5	8.8	5.0	80.5	10.2	0.0	7.0	82.8	2.58
Sample 2	97.7	2.3	0.0	1.8	8.8	4.7	82.2	10.5	0.0	7.2	82.3	2.59
Sample 3	98.7	1.3	0.0	1.6	7.8	5.3	82.2	9.7	0.0	7.0	83.4	2.61

3. Discussion

The major goals in the analysis of a large number of porcine crude heparins and a range of crude heparin from different animal or tissue sources were: (1) to establish reliable test methods to differentiate them at the crude stage of manufacturing; and (2) to propose a definition for crude heparins as a key intermediate in drug manufacturing. Similar tests can be used to assure the quality of the porcine heparin or bovine heparin API used clinically. Importantly, by checking heparin quality earlier in the supply chain, contaminated material can be prevented from reaching the active pharmaceutical ingredient purification processes, which are often performed under cGMP in U.S. based plants. Because the supply chain for heparin is complex and a global one, controlling the quality of this widely used drug, its intermediates, and starting materials (at least as early as the crude heparin warehouse) solely through cGMP inspection is insufficient and often impractical, in part due to the limited resources that the regulatory authorities have. Thus, there is a need to develop strong analytics and appropriate specifications for crude heparin to ensure the consistent high quality of the final heparin drug substance. For this reason, the tests and the data obtained by applying them will help assure the quality of heparin sodium and LMWH drug products by improving the quality of the entire global heparin supply chain.

In this work, strong anion exchange HPLC (SAX-HPLC) and NMR spectroscopy coupled with chemometrics was demonstrated to be a feasible strategy to characterize crude heparin samples. The proton NMR and HPLC data clearly show that crude heparins vary in terms of glycosaminoglycan composition, amount of DNA/RNA, and other impurities. Proton spectra, when the samples were properly prepared, could be analyzed by PCA, grouping samples based on their composition (relative amount of dermatan, chondroitin, and heparin) or structural properties (degree of sulfation). The presence in the library of some samples that were almost free from galactosaminoglycans and DNA/RNA components suggests that some batches have undergone different levels of purification treatments consistent with the known differences in the way heparins are manufactured by different companies. Quantitative HSQC analysis, recently applied to determine the mono- and disaccharide composition of heparin and LMWH [10], can be extended to crude heparin, allowing an in-depth study of the structural features of samples. Particularly, the degree of sulfation can vary starting from 2.1 to 2.4, the latter value is typical of the purified porcine heparin. Notably, the group of samples that lacked dermatan and chondroitin also contained oxidized serine, suggesting that the products were treated with oxidizing agents, such as those typically used during the production of API. Overall, PCA and HSQC analyses were able to distinguish between crude heparins of different animal and organ sources and manufactured by different processes.

4. Methods

4.1. Reagents and Starting Material

Deuterium oxide 99.9%, sodium dihydrogenphosphate hydrate (NaH2PO4 H2O), disodium hydrogen phosphate dihydrate ($Na_2HPO_4 \cdot H_2O_2$), and 3-(trimethylsilyl)propionic-2,2,3,3-d4 acid sodium salt (TSP) were purchased from Sigma-Aldrich (Milan, Italy). Deuterated EDTA d-16 98% was obtained from Product Cambridge Isotope Laboratories, Inc.

The crude heparin samples were dissolved in phosphate buffer solution, which was prepared as follows: 49.7 mg of sodium dihydrogenphosphate hydrate (0.36 mmol), 202.9 mg of disodium hydrogen phosphate dihydrate (1.14 mmol), and 9.2 mg deuterated EDTA d-16 (0.03 mmol) were dissolved in 10 mL of water. The pH was checked at 7.1. The solution was distributed into 1.3 mL aliquots and then lyophilized. Each aliquot was dissolved in 0.2 mL of D_2O and lyophilized again. Finally, the buffer was dissolved in 1.3 mL deuterium oxide with 0.002% TSP (12 mM).

4.2. Strong Anion Exchange HPLC:

Solutions of crude heparin were prepared as described in Keire et al. [9]. SAX-HPLC separations were performed on a Dionex IonPac® AS11-HC (250 mm × 4 mm) column (Dionex, Sunnyvale, CA, USA). The AS11-HC column's characteristics are: a bead diameter of 9 m with a 2000 Å pore size, particles made of a divinylbenzene/ethylvinylbenzene polymer cross-linked at 55%, coated with microporous latex (DVB/EVB 6% cross-linked) 70 nm particles with hydroxyalkyl quaternary ammonium functional groups, and capacity of 290 equiv./4 mm × 250 mm column. A column temperature of 35 °C was used. The mobile phase was MilliQ water (buffer A) and 2.5 M NaCl with 20 mM TRIS adjusted to pH 3.0 by addition of phosphoric acid (buffer B). The gradient was 0–2 min at 95% A with 5% B, followed by a linear gradient to 100% B at 26 min, a hold at 100% B until 31 min, a linear gradient to 95% A with 5% B at 32 min, and a hold until end of run at 40 min. The flow rate was constant at 0.8 mL/min. The UV detector was set at 215 nm. A 40 L injection volume was used. The liquid chromatography system consisted of Agilent HPLC with a G1314A variable wavelength detector, G1322A degasser, G1311A quaternary pump, column thermostat, and G1313A autosampler.

4.3. Sample Preparation

A 60 mg aliquot of each sample was dissolved in 1.5 mL of D_2O. After two hours, the samples were centrifuged for 4′ at 12,000 rpm, and the supernatant was separated from the precipitated pellet. The supernatant and precipitated pellet were lyophilized. A 20 mg aliquot of the lyophilized supernatant powder was dissolved in 0.6 mL of phosphate buffer solution and transferred to a 5 mm NMR tube.

4.4. ^{1}H-NMR

NMR spectra were measured on a Bruker AVANCE III 600 MHz spectrometer (Karlsruhe, Germany) equipped with TCI 5 mm cryogenic probe. The experiments were acquired with a constant presaturation power of 7 Hz at 298 K, and the following acquisition parameters were used: number scan 32, dummy scan 8, relaxation delay 12 s, spectra width 18 ppm, transmitter offset 4.7 ppm. After exponential multiplication (line broadening of 0.3 Hz), the spectra were Fourier transformed, phased, baseline corrected, and calibrated on the TSP signal.

4.5. HSQC-NMR

The 2D-^{1}H,^{13}C-HSQC spectra were measured on a Bruker AVANCE III 600 MHz spectrometer or on a Bruker AVANCE III HD 500 MHz spectrometer (Karlsruhe, Germany), equipped with TCI 5 mm cryogenic probes, using the Bruker library hsqcetgpsisp2.2 pulse sequence.

The experiments were recorded at 298 K using the following acquisition parameters: number of scan 24 (600 MHz) or 40 (500MHz), dummy scan 16, relaxation delay 2.5 s (600 MHz) or 2 s (500 MHz), spectral width 8 ppm (F2) and 80 ppm (F1), transmitter offset 4.7 ppm (F2) and 80 ppm (F1), 1JC-H = 150 Hz. The chosen processing parameters are: zero filling to 4k in F2; linear prediction to 640 points and zero filling to 1k in F1; and apodization by a 90° shifted squared sine bell function in both dimensions. The spectra were processed and integrated using Topsin software version 3.5 (Bruker BioSpin, Rheinstetten, Germany).

4.6. PCA

Proton NMR spectra were imported into R (R Core Team (2016). R: A language and environment for statistical computing. R Foundation for Statistical Computing, Vienna, Austria. URL https://www.R-project.org/) (R version 3.3.1) and cut according to the chosen spectral region (GAGs signals region: 1.95–2.25, 3.0–3.345, 3.37–3.63, 3.69–4.714, and 4.912–5.75 ppm regions, or part of the anomeric signals region: 4.938–5.75 ppm region). Bucketing was then applied (16 points for GAGs region and 8 points for Heparin/HS region). Spectra were normalized for total area, in the Heparin/HS region case aligned (details in Table S14 and Figure S9), and mean centered. Principal Components Analysis (PCA) was performed using the prcomp function from the R stats package.

Supplementary Materials: Figures S1–S9 and Tables S1–S14 are available online

Acknowledgments: In part this study was supported by the FDA Critical Path Program and Ronzoni Foundation funds.

Author Contributions: M.G. and D.A.K. drew up the study plan and discussed it with L.M. R.E.K. and M.K. L.M., M.M. and G.M. performed NMR experiments; L.M. performed chemometric studies and organized NMR results; R.E.K. and M.K. performed HPLC study. M.G., D.A.K. and L.M. wrote the paper and revised the manuscript.

Conflicts of Interest: The authors declare no conflict of interest. FDA Disclaimer: This publication reflects the views of the author and should not be construed to represent the FDA's views or policies.

References

1. Lever, R.; Mulloy, B.; Page, C.P. (Eds.) *Heparin—A Century of Progress*, 1st ed.; Springer: Berlin/Heidelberg, Germany, 2012.
2. Casu, B. Structure and active domains of heparin. In *Chemistry and Biology of Heparin and Heparan Sulphate*, 1st ed.; Garg, H.G., Linhardt, R.J., Hales, C.A., Eds.; Elsevier Ltd: Oxford, UK, 2005; pp. 1–28.
3. Keire, D.; Mulloy, B.; Chase, C.; Al-Hakim, A.; Cairatti, D.; Gray, E.; Hogwood, J.; Morris, T.; Mourão, P.; Da Luz Carvalho Soares, M.; et al. Diversifying the Global Heparin Supply Chain: Reintroduction of Bovine Heparin in the United States? *Pharm. Technol.* **2015**, *11*, 2–9.
4. Guerrini, M.; Beccati, D.; Shriver, Z.; Naggi, A.; Viswanathan, K.; Bisio, A.; Capila, I.; Lansing, J.C.; Guglieri, S.; Fraser, B.; et al. Oversulfated chondroitinsulfate is a contaminant in heparin associated with adverse clinical events. *Nat. Biotechnol.* **2008**, *26*, 669–675. [CrossRef] [PubMed]
5. Liu, H.; Zhanga, Z.; Linhardt, R.J. Lessons learned from the contamination of heparin. *Nat. Prod. Rep.* **2008**, *26*, 313–321. [CrossRef] [PubMed]
6. Linhardt, R.J.; Gunay, N.S. Production and chemical processing of low molecular weight heparins. *Semin. Thromb. Hemost.* **1999**, *25*, 5–16. [PubMed]
7. U.S. Department of Health and Human Services. Food and Drug Administration. *Guidance for Industry: Heparin for Drug and Medical Device Use: Monitoring Crude Heparin for Quality*; FDA: Silver Spring, MD, USA, 2013. Available online: https://www.fda.gov/downloads/Drugs/GuidanceComplianceRegulatoryInformation/Guidances/UCM291390.png (accessed on 24 April 2017).
8. Sommers, C.D.; Mans, D.J.; Mecker, L.C.; Keire, D.A. Sensitive detection of oversulfated chondroitin sulfate in heparin sodium or crude heparin with a colorimetric microplate based assay. *Anal. Chem.* **2011**, *83*, 3422–3430. [CrossRef] [PubMed]
9. Keire, D.A.; Trehy, M.L.; Reepmeyer, J.C.; Kolinski, R.E.; Ye, W.; Dunn, J.; Westenberger, B.J.; Buhse, L.F. Analysis of crude heparin by ^{1}H-NMR, capillary electrophoresis, and strong-anion-exchange-HPLC for contamination by over sulfated chondroitin sulfate. *J. Pharm. Biomed. Anal.* **2010**, *11*, 921–926. [CrossRef] [PubMed]
10. Mauri, L.; Boccardi, G.; Torri, G.; Karfunkle, M.; Macchi, E.; Muzi, L.; Keire, D.; Guerrini, M. Qualification of HSQC methods for quantitative composition of heparin and low molecular weight heparins. *J. Pharm. Biomed. Anal.* **2017**, *136*, 92–105. [CrossRef] [PubMed]
11. Gatti, G.; Casu, B.; Hamer, G.K.; Perlin, A.S. Studies on the conformation of heparin by ^{1}H and ^{13}C NMR spectroscopy. *Macromolecules* **1979**, *12*, 1001–1007. [CrossRef]
12. Nguyen, K.; Rabenstein, D.L. Determination of the primary structure and carboxyl pKAs of heparin-derived oligosaccharides by band-selective homonuclear-decoupled two-dimensional ^{1}H-NMR. *Anal. Bioanal. Chem.* **2011**, *399*, 663–671. [CrossRef] [PubMed]
13. Jolliffe, I.T. *Principal Component Analysis*, 2nd ed.; Bickel, P., Diggle, P., Fienberg, S., Krickeberg, K., Olkin, I., Wermuth, N., Zeger, S., Eds.; Springer: New York, NY, USA, 2002.
14. Keire, D.A.; Mans, D.J.; Ye, H.; Kolinski, R.E.; Buhse, L.F. Assay of possible economically motivated additives or native impurities levels in heparin by ^{1}H-NMR, SAX-HPLC, and anticoagulation time approaches. *J. Pharm. Biomed. Anal.* **2010**, *52*, 656–664. [CrossRef] [PubMed]

15. Guerrini, M.; Naggi, A.; Guglieri, S.; Santarsiero, R.; Torri, G. Complex glycosaminoglycans: Profiling substitution patterns by two dimensional NMR spectroscopy. *Anal. Biochem.* **2005**, *337*, 35–47. [CrossRef] [PubMed]

16. Guerrini, M.; Guglieri, S.; Naggi, A.; Torri, G. LMWHs: Structural differentiation by bidimensional NMR spectroscopy. *Semin. Thromb. Hemost.* **2007**, *33*, 478–487. [CrossRef] [PubMed]

17. Keire, D.; Buhse, L.F.; al-Hakim, A. Characterization of currently marketed heparin products: Composition analysis by 2D-NMR. *Anal. Methods* **2013**, *5*, 2984–2994. [CrossRef]

18. Mascellani, G.; Liverani, L.; Prete, A.; Bergonzini, G.; Bianchini, P.; Torri, G.; Guerrini, M.; Casu, B. Quantitation of dermatan sulfate active site for the heparin cofactor II by ^{1}H Nuclear Magnetic Resonance spectroscopy. *Anal. Biochem.* **1994**, *223*, 135–141. [CrossRef] [PubMed]

19. Mucci, A.; Schenetti, L.; Volpi, N. ^{1}H and ^{13}C nuclear magnetic resonance identification and characterization of components of chondroitin sulfates of various origin. *Carbohydr. Polym.* **2000**, *41*, 37–45. [CrossRef]

20. Mourier, P.; Anger, P.; Martinez, C.; Herman, F.; Viskov, C. Quantitative compositional analysis of heparin using exhaustive heparinase digestion and strong anion exchange chromatography. *Anal. Chem. Res.* **2015**, *3*, 46–53. [CrossRef]

21. Casu, B.; Guerrini, M.; Naggi, A.; Torri, G.; De-Ambrosi, L.; Boveri, G.; Gonella, S. Differentiation of beef and pig mucosal heparins by NMR spectroscopy. *Thromb. Haemost.* **1995**, *74*, 1205. [PubMed]

22. Watt, D.K.; Yorke, S.C.; Slimb, G.C. Comparison of ovine, bovine and porcine mucosal heparins and low molecular weight heparins by disaccharide analyses and ^{13}C NMR. *Carbohydr. Polym.* **1997**, *33*, 5–11. [CrossRef]

23. Tovar, A.M.F.; Teixeira, A.C.; Rembold, S.M.; Leite, M., Jr.; Lugon, J.R.; Mourão, P.A.S. Bovine and porcine heparins: Different drugs with similar effects on human haemodialysis. *BMC Res. Notes* **2013**, *6*, 230–237. [CrossRef] [PubMed]

24. Fu, L.; Li, G.; Yang, B.; Onishi, A.; Li, L.; Sun, P.; Zhang, F.; Linhardt, R.J. Structural Characterization of Pharmaceutical Heparins Prepared from Different Animal Tissues. *J. Pharm. Sci.* **2013**, *102*, 1447–1457. [CrossRef] [PubMed]

25. Naggi, A.; Gardini, C.; Pedrinola, P.; Mauri, L.; Urso, E.; Alekseeva, A.; Casu, B.; Cassinelli, G.; Guerrini, M.; Iacomini, M.; et al. Structural peculiarity andantithrombin binding region profile of mucosal bovine and porcine heparins. *J. Pharm. Bioanal. Anal.* **2016**, *118*, 52–63. [CrossRef] [PubMed]

Sample Availability: Samples of the compounds are not available from the authors.

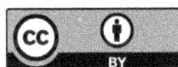

molecules

Article

Molecular Weights of Bovine and Porcine Heparin Samples: Comparison of Chromatographic Methods and Results of a Collaborative Survey

Sabrina Bertini [1] , Giulia Risi [1,2], Marco Guerrini [1], Kevin Carrick [3], Anita Y. Szajek [3,4] and Barbara Mulloy [5,*]

[1]   Istituto di Ricerche Chimiche e Biochimiche "G. Ronzoni" via G. Colombo 81, 20133 Milano, Italy; bertini@ronzoni.it (S.B.); giulia.risi02@universitadipavia.it (G.R.); guerrini@ronzoni.it (M.G.)
[2]   Department of Chemistry, University of Pavia, viale Taramelli 12, 27100 Pavia, Italy
[3]   U.S. Pharmacopeial Convention (USP), 12601 Twinbrook Parkway, Rockville, MD 20852, USA; klc@usp.org (K.C.); anita.szajek@nih.gov (A.Y.S.)
[4]   Center for Scientific Review (CSR), National Institutes of Health, 6701 Rockledge Dr. Rm. 4187, Bethesda, MD 20892, USA
[5]   Institute of Pharmaceutical Science, Franklin Wilkins Building, King's College London, 150 Stamford St., London SE1 9NH, UK
*   Correspondence: barbara.mulloy@kcl.ac.uk; Tel.: +44-207-848-4295

Received: 24 May 2017; Accepted: 15 July 2017; Published: 19 July 2017

Abstract: In a collaborative study involving six laboratories in the USA, Europe, and India the molecular weight distributions of a panel of heparin sodium samples were determined, in order to compare heparin sodium of bovine intestinal origin with that of bovine lung and porcine intestinal origin. Porcine samples met the current criteria as laid out in the USP Heparin Sodium monograph. Bovine lung heparin samples had consistently lower average molecular weights. Bovine intestinal heparin was variable in molecular weight; some samples fell below the USP limits, some fell within these limits and others fell above the upper limits. These data will inform the establishment of pharmacopeial acceptance criteria for heparin sodium derived from bovine intestinal mucosa. The method for MW determination as described in the USP monograph uses a single, broad standard calibrant to characterize the chromatographic profile of heparin sodium on high-resolution silica-based GPC columns. These columns may be short-lived in some laboratories. Using the panel of samples described above, methods based on the use of robust polymer-based columns have been developed. In addition to the use of the USP's broad standard calibrant for heparin sodium with these columns, a set of conditions have been devised that allow light-scattering detected molecular weight characterization of heparin sodium, giving results that agree well with the monograph method. These findings may facilitate the validation of variant chromatographic methods with some practical advantages over the USP monograph method.

Keywords: bovine heparin; porcine heparin; molecular weight; size exclusion chromatography; pharmacopeia

---

1. Introduction

Heparin preparations for medical use are polydisperse polymers derived from mast cell containing tissues, with molecular weights determined by both the tissue of origin and the processes involved in heparin manufacture [1]. Measurement of the molecular weight distribution of heparin samples usually involves size exclusion chromatography (SEC) with some form of light scattering detection, as this technique does not depend on calibrant reference materials [2,3]. A chromatographic method was developed for inclusion as an identification method in the USP monograph for heparin sodium [4], using a sample of porcine mucosal heparin as a broad standard calibrant, characterized in a collaborative study involving eight laboratories. Though all these laboratories were expert in light scattering detection, reproducibility of results between laboratories was not strong. However, it was possible to combine the experimental results of this study to give a characteristic molecular weight distribution for the calibrant material, expressed as a slice table allowing the use of the calibrant as a broad standard (the USP Heparin Sodium Molecular Weight Calibrant (Reference Standard) RS) [5].

Only heparin from porcine intestinal mucosa (porcine mucosal heparin) is currently approved for use in the USA, but the US Food and Drugs Administration (FDA) is investigating the possibility of introduction of heparin sodium from bovine intestinal mucosa (bovine mucosal heparin) into the US market [6]. Bovine mucosal heparin is licensed for use in several countries in the world. As porcine and bovine heparin differ in many aspects of their structure and activity [7–10], data have been collected on the potency and physicochemical characteristics of bovine heparin lots in current use in these countries. The USP will use the collected data to generate proposed acceptance criteria for potency and identification assays including molecular weight average and distributional parameters.

A multi-laboratory collaborative study has therefore been organized by the USP to obtain consensus molecular weight data using the USP Heparin Sodium monograph method [4,5] for a panel of bovine heparin samples in comparison with standard samples of porcine mucosal heparin. In addition to its data-gathering role for specification setting, this set of samples provides an opportunity to investigate further the discrepancies between light scattering methods and the USP calibrant-based method, and to determine whether alternative column types, as compared with those referred to in the USP Heparin Sodium monograph, might have acceptable chromatographic properties for heparin sodium MW determination either using light scattering detection or with the use of the USP Heparin Sodium Molecular Weight Calibrant RS.

Summary and Aims of the Study

Phase 1: Molecular weight parameters as described in the USP Heparin Sodium monograph [4] were measured in six laboratories using the method described in the USP Heparin Sodium monograph [4] for 20 lots of bovine mucosal heparin, 2 lots of bovine lung heparin, and 2 standard samples of porcine mucosal heparin. The data collected in this phase of the study will contribute to the establishment of suitable acceptance criteria for the molecular weight distribution of bovine mucosal heparin sodium.

Phase 2: Using the same heparin samples as Phase 1, a single laboratory assessed results from 12 distinct chromatographic methods, varying in column type, mobile phase, and calibration method. The aim of this phase of the study was to identify alternative chromatographic methods giving similar molecular weight values to those obtained using the USP Heparin Sodium monograph method, avoiding some practical disadvantages of the USP method.

2. Results and Discussion

2.1. Phase 1: Collaborative Survey of Bovine and Porcine Heparin Samples

Results for 10 heparin samples were obtained from six participating laboratories, and for a further 14 samples from five laboratories. The sample codes are listed in Table S1 (Supplementary Materials), with species and tissue of origin; there were 20 samples of heparin manufactured from bovine intestinal mucosa (bovine mucosal heparin), two samples of bovine lung heparin, and two samples of heparin manufactured from porcine intestinal mucosa (porcine mucosal heparin). System suitability requirements described in Materials and Methods (below) were met for each laboratory on each day of the study.

An earlier study of heparin samples from porcine intestinal mucosa, currently the only acceptable source for heparin sodium in the USA, was used to derive appropriate acceptance criteria for molecular weight distribution by setting limits to the weight-average molecular weight M_w (15,000 to 19,000 g/mol), $M_{24,000}$ (no more than 20%) and the ratio $M_{8000-16,000}/M_{16,000-24,000}$ (no less than 1.0) [5].

These molecular weight characteristics for all 24 heparin samples, as determined in the participating laboratories, are listed in Table S2A (M_w), Table S2B ($M_{24,000}$) and Table S2C ($M_{8000-16,000}/M_{16,000-24,000}$) (Supplementary Materials) and summarized in Figure 1.

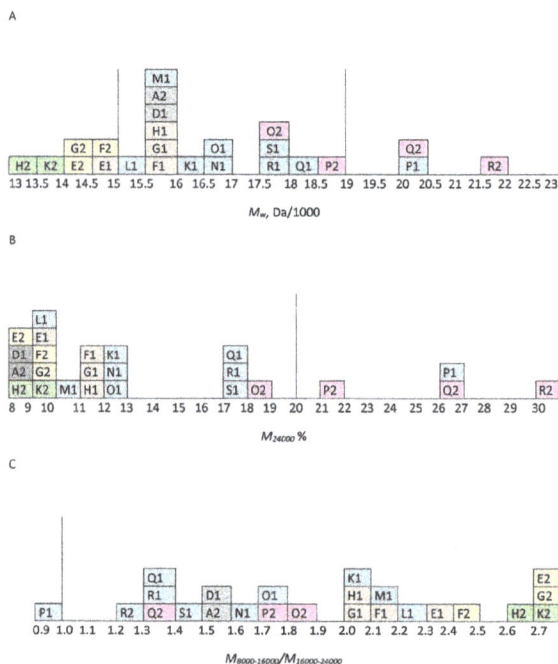

A

		M1						
		A2						
		D1						
		H1				O2		
	G2 F2	G1		O1		S1		Q2
H2 K2	E2 E1 L1	F1	K1 N1		R1 Q1 P2		P1	R2

13 13.5 14 14.5 15 15.5 16 16.5 17 17.5 18 18.5 19 19.5 20 20.5 21 21.5 22 22.5 23

M_w, Da/1000

B

L1						
E2 E1						
D1 F2	F1 K1		Q1			
A2 G2	G1 N1		R1		P1	
H2 K2 M1 H1 O1		S1 O2	P2	Q2	R2

8 9 10 11 12 13 14 15 16 17 18 19 20 21 22 23 24 25 26 27 28 29 30

M_{24000} %

C

	Q1			K1		E2
	R1	D1	O1	H1 M1		G2
P1	R2 Q2 S1 A2 N1 P2 O2	G1 F1 L1 E1 F2	H2 K2

0.9 1.0 1.1 1.2 1.3 1.4 1.5 1.6 1.7 1.8 1.9 2.0 2.1 2.2 2.3 2.4 2.5 2.6 2.7

$M_{8000-16000}/M_{16000-24000}$

Figure 1. Histogram plots of Phase 1 summary results for 24 heparin samples (see Table S1) (**A**) M_w, (**B**) $M_{24,000}$ and (**C**) $M_{8000-16,000}/M_{16,000-24,000}$ for bovine lung heparin (green), porcine mucosal heparin (grey), and bovine mucosal heparin from sample donors 1 (orange), 3 (blue), 4 (pink), and 6 (yellow). Values recorded are the mean values from five or six laboratories (see Table S2A–C) The vertical lines indicate upper and lower limit acceptance criteria in the USP monograph for heparin sodium.

The two porcine mucosal heparins A-3 and D-1 have M_w near 16,000 Da, a typical value for heparin sodium as previously determined [5] and close to the characteristic value of 16,000 Da for the USP Heparin Sodium Identification RS. They have $M_{24,000}$ of about 9%, and the ratio $M_{8000-16,000}/M_{16,000-24,000}$ is about 1.5. Two bovine lung heparins H-2 and K-2 have lower M_w, outside the acceptable range for heparin sodium at about 13,500 Da. This is consistent with values determined for bovine lung heparins dating from the 1950s to the 1990s [11].

For the 20 bovine mucosal heparins, variability between individual samples is similar to that for porcine heparin before introduction of molecular weight acceptance criteria, as determined previously [5]. Three samples out of 23 (P-1, Q-2, and R-2) have M_w higher than the top limit of 19,000 Da, and the same three samples have more than the limit of $M_{24,000}$ (20%). One of these samples also has a low value for the ratio $M_{8000-16,000}/M_{16,000-24,000}$, though the mean value from five laboratories rounds up to 1.0, the lower limit for this value. Figure 1 is shaded to indicate the donor numbers of each sample, and systematic differences can be seen in the molecular weight profiles of samples from each source. These differences are likely to originate from variant manufacturing protocols, though variations in the source tissues due to climate, nutrition, etc. are also possible.

Figure 2 illustrates RI-detected chromatograms of the two bovine heparin samples with the lowest (E-2) and highest (R-2) values of M_w. Though there is considerable overlap between the two samples, it is clear that sample E-2 contains a major amount of low molecular weight material, with longer retention time, compared with sample R-2. At higher molecular weights (short retention time), sample R-2 has about 30% material over 24,000 Da (well outside the USP's acceptable range for porcine heparin sodium) whereas sample E-2 only has about 8% (values of $M_{24,000}$ from Table S2B). Values for $M_{8000-16,000}/M_{16,000-24,000}$ reflect the molecular weight distribution in the mid-range; this ratio varies from 2.70 for sample E-2 to 1.28 for sample R-2 (Table S2C).

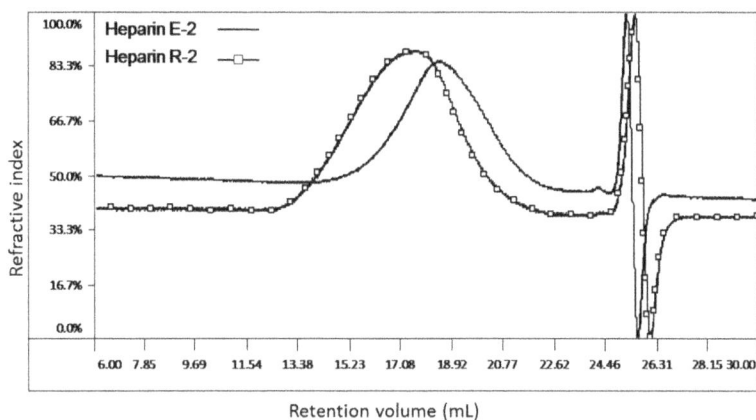

Figure 2. Phase 1: Molecular weight distributions for the samples of bovine mucosal heparin with highest (R-2) and lowest (E-2) molecular weights as measured by the USP Heparin Sodium monograph method. Chromatographic profiles refer to Method 1.

2.2. Phase 2: Comparison of Different Chromatographic Methods

20 Samples of bovine mucosal heparin, two samples of bovine lung heparin, two samples of porcine mucosal heparin and one USP Heparin Sodium Identification RS were analyzed in different chromatographic conditions (see Table S5) by one laboratory involved in the project, with the purpose of comparing the conventional USP calibration method to a light-scattering method; furthermore, an evaluation of silica (two column sets, called A and B) and polymeric columns (two column sets, called C and D) chromatographic performances was done to determine whether polymeric columns might have acceptable chromatographic properties for heparin sodium MW determination (method details are reported below and in the Supplementary Material). Actually, most of the pharmacopeia chromatographic assays for the molecular weight distributions of heparin use silica columns, for which the great advantage of high resolution is countered by very short life time and many problems of compatibility with samples (interactions, pH, and so on).

After first analysis with silica columns sets A and B (respectively Methods 1 and 2), samples were analyzed with polymer column set C (Methods from 3 to 7) and finally with polymer column set D (Methods from 8 to 12). The chromatographic profiles overlay of the USP Heparin Sodium Identification RS is reported in Figure 3. As can be observed, the elution peak is well separated from the mobile phase peak, so all chromatographic conditions tested are suitable for the analysis of this sample. Same results were obtained for the analysis of the other samples (chromatograms not reported). After acquisition, data were elaborated using suitable GPC software, as described in Supplementary Material section. Results for weight-average molecular weight M_w of the heparin samples, percent proportion of material $M_{24,000}$ and the ratio $M_{8000-16,000}/M_{16,000-24,000}$ are reported in Table S3A–C of the Supplementary Material section; results obtained for the analysis of the USP Heparin Sodium Identification RS are reported in Table 1.

Table 1. Phase 2: Weight-average molecular weight (M_w, Da), percent proportion of material above 24,000 Da ($M_{24,000}$) and the ratio $M_{8000–16,000}/M_{16,000–24,000}$ (Ratio) of USP Heparin Sodium Identification RS, as measured using 12 distinct chromatographic methods. Results refer to the mean values of duplicate injections. Values were rounded to the nearest 100 Da.

Value	Chromatographic Methods (see Text and Table S5)											
	1	2	3	4	5	6	7	8	9	10	11	12
M_w (kDa)	15.8	17.7	15.7	15.2	16.7	16.1	17.0	15.8	15.7	16.0	16.2	16.4
$M_{24,000}$	8.8	16.86	8.93	8.17	13.39	9.12	14.79	8.96	8.47	7.93	6.20	8.32
Ratio	1.89	0.99	1.82	1.97	1.49	1.64	1.48	1.72	1.82	1.37	1.24	1.15

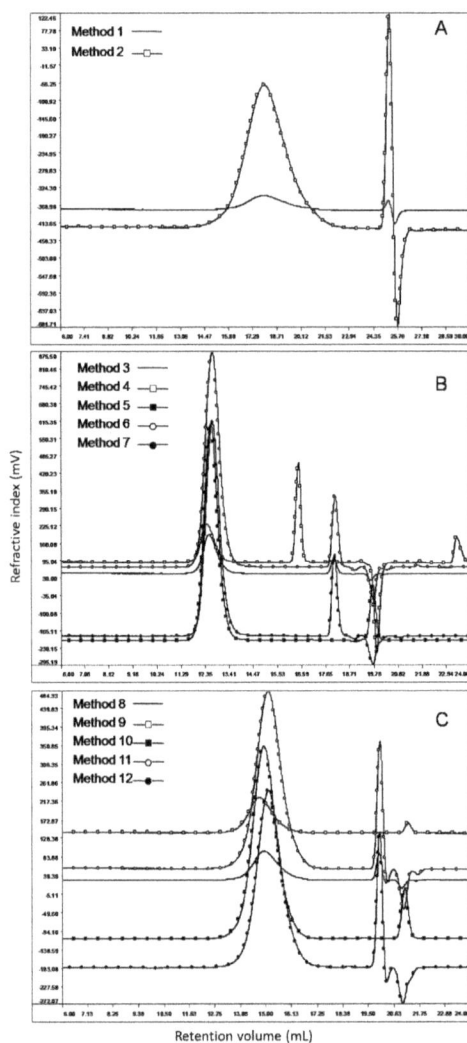

Figure 3. Phase 2: Overlay view of USP Heparin Sodium Identification RS chromatographic profiles in 12 distinct chromatographic systems. Panels: (**A**) Methods 1 and 2; (**B**) Methods 3–7; (**C**) Methods 8–12.

The weight-average molecular weight M_w range calculated for the USP Heparin Sodium Identification RS, as measured to assess system suitability (see Methods section), is between 15,200 and 17,700 Da, with an average value of 16,200 Da. Acceptance criteria for the system suitability test indicate that M_w for this sample should lie within +/−500 Da of the established value of 16,000 Da (see Methods for the full set of system suitability requirements). Results for Methods 2, 4, 5 and 7, respectively 17,700, 15,200, 16,700 and 17,000 Da are out of the USP acceptance criteria, but considering all 12 methods M_w results, the RSD% calculated is 4.17%, an acceptable value taking into account the instrument sensitivity and the different chromatographic conditions tested. One of the most critical points in the analysis with light-scattering detector is the use of the correct dn/dc value, a parameter that is a function not only of the sample but also of the chromatographic conditions, and this is the base of the differences observed in molecular weight distribution results [5]. The values used in this work were experimentally calculated for a heparin sodium sample by the laboratory involved in the comparison of chromatographic methods.

More in detail: Methods 5 and 7 were acquired at 40 °C with same columns and both gave high molecular weight and of course higher $M_{24,000}$ in comparison with Method 1 (official USP method for the analysis of heparin sodium molecular weight distribution); instead Methods 3, 4 and 6, acquired at 30 °C with the same columns but different calibration, gave lower molecular weight in comparison to 5 and 7 (although Methods 3 and 6 respects USP acceptance criteria). So, it is clear that column set C does not completely have the acceptable chromatographic properties required. The main reason of these differences could be the different particle size between columns sets C and A (both columns of the set C have a particle size of 7 μm, while columns set A have a particle size of 5 and 8 μm). Regarding to the columns set B, both molecular weight and ratio $M_{8000–16,000}/M_{16,000–24,000}$ are out of the acceptance criteria; again, the main problem could be the particle size of the columns set (5 μm). As a conclusion for this first part, it seems that with a chromatographic system in which the particle size is the same for each column used in series, the correct resolution required is not reached, with the only exception of Method 3 chromatographic conditions, very similar to the USP official method. Looking at Methods 8 to 12, each of these chromatographic conditions results are within the acceptance criteria; the fact that column set D particle sizes are different (respectively 10 μm for the TSKG4000SWXL and 7 μm TSKG3000PWXL) could be a confirmation that having a single particle size in a column set cannot reach the right resolution required. Particularly remarkable is that the use of a light-scattering detector allows us to reach results comparable with the official USP method for the analysis of heparin sodium.

Taking into account results from the whole set of 24 heparin samples, values for M_w (Table S3A) and $M_{24,000}$ (Table S3B) can be used to compare methods for use over a wide range of heparin samples (Figure 4). Methods 3, 8 and 9 give results in especially good agreement with Method 1 over the entire range; few values for M_w are more than 500 Da away from the Method 1 value, and few values for $M_{24,000}$ are outside +/−10% of the Method 1 value.

Methods 10 and 11 use the same column set as Methods 8 and 9, but use the Broad Standard calibrant (The USP Heparin Sodium Molecular Weight Calibrant RS). This calibrant was characterized for use with the L59 silica columns specified in the monograph. The calibrant information for a broad standard is a slice table of mass fraction vs. molecular weight (for example Table S4), which is a property of the calibrant material, theoretically independent of the chromatographic system used. In principle therefore, the broad standard calibrant should be transferable to any SEC column for which the sample is fully included. Methods 10 and 11 give reasonable agreement with Method 1 across most of the range of heparin samples in the panel, but less good agreement than do light-scattering Methods 8 and 9. Transference of this calibration method to column types other than those specified in the monograph cannot be guaranteed, and is particularly poor for column set C in this study (see Figure 4, Methods 5, 6 and 7), but appears to work best when used for heparin samples with molecular weight distributions within the current USP acceptance criteria (Table S3A,B).

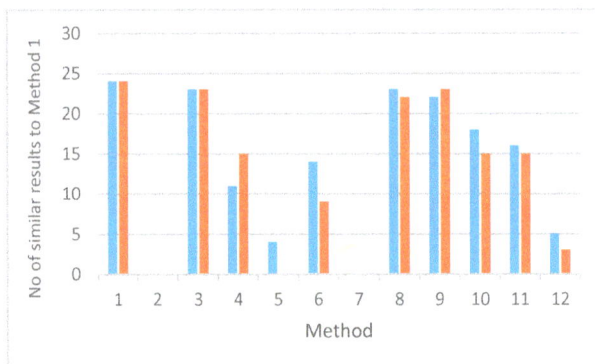

Figure 4. Phase 2: Column chart indicating similarity in molecular weight results for 24 heparin samples, between the USP Heparin Sodium monograph method (Method 1) and 11 other distinct chromatographic methods (Table S5). Blue columns plot M_w data and orange columns plot $M_{24,000}$. Data are taken from Table S3A,B; similarity criteria are for M_w, values differ from Method 1 by less than 500 Da; for $M_{24,000}$ values differ from Method 1 by less than 10%.

3. Materials and Methods

3.1. Materials

USP Heparin Sodium Molecular Weight Calibrant and USP Heparin Sodium Identification RS were provided by USP. Twenty heparin sodium samples from bovine intestinal mucosa, and two from bovine lung were donated by four manufacturers of heparin; two standard samples from porcine intestinal mucosa were from USP and NIBSC. Sample codes are listed in Table S1.

3.2. Phase 1: The Collaborative Study

For the collaborative study, participants followed protocols based on the USP Heparin Sodium Monograph Identification Test D: Molecular weight determinations [4]. Briefly, the samples were analyzed by SEC on silica-based size exclusion columns USP code L59 (for example, a TSK G4000 SWXL (7.8 mm × 30 cm) and a TSK G3000 SWXL column (7.8 mm × 30 cm) in series, preceded by a TSK SWXL guard column; Tosoh Bioscience) using 0.1 M ammonium acetate (with 0.02% sodium azide preservative) as a mobile phase at a flow rate of 0.6 mL/min. Detection was by refractive index (RI) increment; the columns and detector were maintained at 30 °C. The calibrant, system suitability sample, and all heparin samples were taken up at 5 mg/mL in mobile phase; injection volume was 20 µL. Duplicate determinations were performed for each heparin sample in each laboratory, and results were reported to the USP.

Analysis of the Chromatographic Data

Broad standard calibration was performed using a chromatogram of the USP Heparin Sodium Molecular Weight Calibrant RS, baseline corrected and integrated; the cumulative area at each point under the heparin peak was calculated. Using the broad standard table (Table S4), points in the chromatogram were identified for which the percent cumulative area was closest to the percent fractions listed in the table; the molecular weight (MW) in the table was then assigned to the corresponding retention time (RT) in the chromatogram. For the set of retention times and molecular weights identified, log(MW) vs. RT was fitted to a third-order polynomial function. For each injection of the heparin samples and the system suitability sample, the weight average molecular weight M_w was calculated according to the formula

$$\overline{M}_w = \frac{\sum_i RI_i M_i}{\sum_i RI_i} \tag{1}$$

where RI_i is detector response at each point i and M_i is molecular weight at each point i.

Proportions of material within specific molecular weight ranges were calculated as follows: the percentage of heparin with molecular weight in the range 8000 to 16,000 Da, $M_{8000-16,000}$, the percentage of heparin with molecular weight in the range 16,000 to 24,000 Da, $M_{16,000-24,000}$, and the percentage of heparin with molecular weight greater than 24,000 Da, $M_{24,000}$.

System suitability criteria were as follows, taken from the USP Heparin Sodium monograph: in the chromatogram of the system suitability sample (the USP Heparin Sodium Identification RS), there is a baseline resolution between the heparin and salt peaks. The linear regression coefficient of the calibration curve fitted to the broad standard table values must be not less than 0.990 in magnitude, using a third order polynomial equation. The mean of the calculated M_w from the duplicate injections of system suitability solution rounded up to the nearest 100 Da is within 500 Da of the assigned value of 16,000. The peak molecular weights (M_p) of the duplicate injections of system suitability solution do not differ by more than 5% of the upper value.

3.3. Phase 2: Comparison of Different Chromatographic Methods

In Phase 2 of the study 12 different GPC methods were compared in a single laboratory. Details of the chromatographic conditions used in each of the 12 methods are given in the text of the Supplementary Materials, and in Table S5. The heparin samples characterized in Phase 2 were the same set as for Phase 1 of the study.

Analysis of the Chromatographic Data

Two methods for derivation of molecular weights from chromatograms were employed. For methods 1 (the USP monograph method), 5, 6, 7, 10, 11 and 12, in which only the refractive index detector is involved , a broad standard calibration was performed using a chromatogram of the USP Heparin Sodium Molecular Weight Calibrant RS, as described for Phase 1. Methods 2, 3, 8 and 9 used both RI and Right Angle Laser Light Scattering (RALLS) detection, for which no calibrant reference standard is needed. The relationship between refractive index increment and concentration of the analyte, known as the dn/dc parameter, changed as a function of the mobile phase used, as described in Supplementary Material section. As for the Phase 1 study, the weight-average molecular weight M_w, the percentage of heparin with molecular weight in the ranges 8000 to 16,000, $M_{8000-16,000}$, and 16,000 to 24,000, $M_{16,000-24,000}$, and the percentage of heparin with molecular weight greater than 24,000, $M_{24,000}$ were evaluated.

Acceptance criteria were as for Phase 1: The chromatographic system is suitable if the chromatographic profile of samples does not overlap the mobile phase peak; secondly, the M_w value determined for USP Heparin Sodium Identification RS (the system suitability sample) has to be within 500 Da of the assigned value of 16,000 Da [4].

4. Conclusions

A panel of 20 lots of bovine mucosal heparin had average molecular weights similar to those of porcine mucosal heparin samples, but with a wider variation from sample to sample, probably reflecting differences in manufacturing methods for heparin from a single species and tissue source. Some molecular weight values fall outside current USP acceptance criteria for heparin sodium.

Bovine lung heparin samples were lower in average molecular weight than mucosal heparin, as has been reported in the past.

Alternative SEC methods for molecular weight analysis of heparin sodium give varying degrees of comparability with the USP monograph method. Use of the USP Heparin Sodium Molecular Weight Calibrant RS with long-lived polymer based columns gave comparable results with the USP monograph method for samples within the current acceptable range of heparin sodium samples; some methods using polymer-based columns with light scattering detection gave good agreement throughout the full range of heparin samples investigated in this study.

Supplementary Materials: Supplementary Materials are available online. 1. Table S1: Heparin sample codes and origin; 2. Table S2A–C: Molecular weight measurements from the Phase 1 study; 3. Further details of materials and methods; 4. Table S3A–C: Molecular weight measurements for the Phase 2 study; 5. Table S4: Broad standard table for the USP Heparin Sodium Molecular Weight Calibrant RS; 6. Table S5: Summary of methods used for Phase 2.

Acknowledgments: We gratefully acknowledge the contributions of the participants in the collaborative study, and the donors of the materials. Participants: C.S. Venkatesan, V.N.S.M.V.G Raju, A. Vijaya, A. Kishore, N. Swapna, and S. Kanaka Durga—Gland Pharma, India; Elaine Gray and John Hogwood—National Institute for Biological Standard and Control, UK; Robert J. Linhardt—Rensellaer Polytechnic Institute, USA; Marco Guerrini, Sabrina Bertini, and Giulia Risi—Istituto Ronzoni, Italy; Christian Viskov and Julie Cegarra—Sanofi Chimie, France; David Keire, Michael Karfunkle, and Hongping Ye—USFDA. Donors of material: Bioiberica S.A., Spain; Extrasul, Brasil; Gland Pharma, India; Kin Master Produtos Quimicas, Brasil; National Institute for Biological Standards and Control, UK; Syntex S.A. Argentina; United States Pharmacopeia. We also thank all the members of the United States Pharmacopeia's Expert Panel on Bovine Heparin for their discussions and insights.

Author Contributions: A.J.Z. and B.M. conceived, designed and organized the Phase 1 collaborative study; A.J.Z., K.C. and B.M. collated and interpreted the collaborative study results; M.G. and S.B. conceived and designed the Phase 2 comparison of chromatographic methods; S.B. and G.R. performed the comparison of chromatographic methods; all authors co-wrote the paper.

Conflicts of Interest: The authors declare no conflict of interest.

Disclaimer: This article was prepared while Anita Szajek was employed with the United States Pharmacopeial Convention. The opinions expressed in this article are the author's own and do not reflect the view of the National Institutes of Health, the Department of Health and Human Services, or the United States government.

References

1. Mulloy, B.; Hogwood, J.; Gray, E.; Lever, R.; Page, C.P. Pharmacology of Heparin and Related Drugs. *Pharmacol. Rev.* **2016**, *68*, 76–141. [CrossRef] [PubMed]
2. Bertini, S.; Bisio, A.; Torri, G.; Bensi, D.; Terbojevich, M. Molecular weight determination of heparin and dermatan sulfate by size exclusion chromatography with a triple detector array. *Biomacromolecules* **2005**, *6*, 168–173. [CrossRef] [PubMed]
3. Sommers, C.D.; Ye, H.; Kolinski, R.E.; Nasr, M.; Buhse, L.F.; Al-Hakim, A.; Keire, D.A. Characterization of currently marketed heparin products: Analysis of molecular weight and heparinase-I digest patterns. *Anal. Bioanal. Chem.* **2011**, *401*, 2445–2454. [CrossRef] [PubMed]
4. United States Pharmacopeial Convention. Heparin Sodium. In *United States Pharmacopeia USP40-NF35*; United States Pharmacopeial Convention: Rockville, MD, USA, 2017; pp. 4475–4480.
5. Mulloy, B.; Heath, A.; Shriver, Z.; Jameison, F.; Al-Hakim, A.; Morris, T.S.; Szajek, A.Y. USP compendial methods for analysis of heparin: Chromatographic determination of molecular weight distributions for heparin sodium. *Anal. Bioanal. Chem.* **2014**, *406*, 4815–4823. [CrossRef] [PubMed]
6. Keire, D.; Mulloy, B.; Chase, C.; Al-Hakim, A.; Cairatti, D.; Gray, E.; Hogwood, J.; Morris, T.; Mourão, P.; Soares, M.; et al. Diversifying the Global Heparin Supply Chain: Reintroduction of Bovine Heparin in the United States? *Pharm. Technol.* **2015**, *39*, 28–35.
7. Santos, G.R.; Tovar, A.M.; Capille, N.V.; Pereira, M.S.; Pomin, V.H.; Mourao, P.A. Structural and functional analyses of bovine and porcine intestinal heparins confirm they are different drugs. *Drug Discov. Today* **2014**, *19*, 1801–1807. [CrossRef] [PubMed]
8. Tovar, A.M.; Santos, G.R.; Capille, N.V.; Piquet, A.A.; Glauser, B.F.; Pereira, M.S.; Vilanova, E.; Mourao, P.A. Structural and haemostatic features of pharmaceutical heparins from different animal sources: Challenges to define thresholds separating distinct drugs. *Sci. Rep.* **2016**, *6*, 35619. [CrossRef] [PubMed]

9. St Ange, K.; Onishi, A.; Fu, L.; Sun, X.; Lin, L.; Mori, D.; Zhang, F.; Dordick, J.S.; Fareed, J.; Hoppensteadt, D.; et al. Analysis of Heparins Derived from Bovine Tissues and Comparison to Porcine Intestinal Heparins. *Clin. Appl. Thromb. Hemost.* **2016**, *22*, 520–527. [CrossRef] [PubMed]

10. Fu, L.; Li, G.; Yang, B.; Onishi, A.; Li, L.; Sun, P.; Zhang, F.; Linhardt, R.J. Structural Characterization of Pharmaceutical Heparins Prepared from Different Animal Tissues. *J. Pharm. Sci.* **2013**, *102*, 1447–1457. [CrossRef] [PubMed]

11. Mulloy, B.; Gray, E.; Barrowcliffe, T.W. Characterization of unfractionated heparin: Comparison of materials from the last 50 years. *Thromb. Haemost.* **2000**, *84*, 1052–1056. [PubMed]

Sample Availability: Samples of the compounds are not available from the authors.

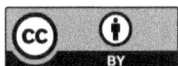

molecules

MDPI

Article

Structure-Activity Relationships of Bioengineered Heparin/Heparan Sulfates Produced in Different Bioreactors

Ha Na Kim, John M. Whitelock and Megan S. Lord *

Graduate School of Biomedical Engineering, University of New South Wales, Sydney, NSW 2052, Australia;
h.n.kim@unsw.edu.au (H.N.K.); j.whitelock@unsw.edu.au (J.M.W.)
* Correspondence: m.lord@unsw.edu.au; Tel.: +61-2-9385-3910

Academic Editors: Giangiacomo Torri and Jawed Fareed
Received: 3 May 2017; Accepted: 11 May 2017; Published: 15 May 2017

Abstract: Heparin and heparan sulfate are structurally-related carbohydrates with therapeutic applications in anticoagulation, drug delivery, and regenerative medicine. This study explored the effect of different bioreactor conditions on the production of heparin/heparan sulfate chains via the recombinant expression of serglycin in mammalian cells. Tissue culture flasks and continuously-stirred tank reactors promoted the production of serglycin decorated with heparin/heparan sulfate, as well as chondroitin sulfate, while the serglycin secreted by cells in the tissue culture flasks produced more highly-sulfated heparin/heparan sulfate chains. The serglycin produced in tissue culture flasks was effective in binding and signaling fibroblast growth factor 2, indicating the utility of this molecule in drug delivery and regenerative medicine applications in addition to its well-known anticoagulant activity.

Keywords: heparin; heparan sulfate; serglycin; proteoglycan; recombinant expression; bioreactor

---

1. Introduction

Heparin is used clinically as an anticoagulant due to its ability to bind anti-thrombin and modulate downstream events in the clotting cascade [1,2]. The large market for clinical heparin, including more than 300,000 doses used per day in the US [3,4], has also enabled researchers to explore its therapeutic application to reduce the thrombogenecity of materials and deliver growth factors for tissue repair [5]. Heparan sulfate is structurally similar to heparin with both being linear polysaccharides composed of repeating disaccharides of hexuronic acid and glucosamine. Heparin contains a higher degree of sulfation than heparan sulfate [6] with, on average, 2.7 sulfate groups per disaccharide, whereas heparan sulfate contains at least one sulfate group per disaccharide [7].

Heparin is only known to be expressed by mast cells in tissues that are in direct contact with the environment, including lung, skin, and intestine, and decorates the protein core of a single intracellular proteoglycan, serglycin [8–11]. Thus, the biological function of heparin is unlikely to be the prevention of blood coagulation. Heparan sulfate, however, is ubiquitous on the cell surface and in the extracellular matrix of tissues and decorates the protein core of many cell surface, including syndecans and glypicans, and extracellular matrix, including perlecan, agrin, and type XVIII collagen, proteoglycans and displays tissue-specific sulfation patterns [12,13]. These structural differences account for tissue-specific activities of heparan sulfates in modulating cellular interactions, as well as the binding and activity of enzymes, growth factors and extracellular matrix proteins [14,15]. Thus, there is growing interest in the therapeutic application of heparan sulfates for selective biological activities.

Both heparin and heparan sulfate isolated from tissues vary in composition and sequence between sources due to their synthesis via a non-template-driven process involving the timed activity of approximately twenty enzymes in the Golgi [16], although the regulators of the expression of these enzymes are not fully understood. These enzymes are involved in chain initiation, elongation, epimerization, and sulfation. While this structural heterogeneity provides an opportunity to fine-tune the biological activity for particular applications, the precise identification of structure-function relationships has been challenging [17]. However, certain structural features are known to be required for highly-specific interactions, such as a pentasaccharide structure containing an 3-*O*-sulfated glucosamine for binding to anti-thrombin III [18], whereas other structures are less specific, such as a contiguous string of highly-sulfated disaccharides for binding to fibroblast growth factor (FGF) and downstream growth factor activation [19].

Heparin is sourced predominantly from animal tissues, particularly porcine intestinal mucosa and, to a lesser extent, bovine lung tissues due to concerns over bovine spongiform encephalopathy contamination [20]. Commercially-available heparan sulfates are synthesized as byproducts of heparin production or by selective de-sulfation of heparin [21,22]. The production of heparan sulfate libraries from tissues is time consuming and technically challenging [23]. The growing demand for heparin and heparan sulfates for clinical applications has led researchers to explore alternative methods of production including chemoenzymatic synthesis [24], chemical synthesis [25], sulfation of polysaccharides [26], and metabolic engineering [27]. A bioengineered heparin-like heparan sulfate was recently reported by the authors by expressing serglycin in mammalian cells [1]. This recombinant serglycin was decorated with chondroitin/dermatan sulfate in addition to heparin/heparan sulfate chains [1,28] similar to serglycin isolated from natural sources where it has been shown to be decorated with multiple types of glycosaminoglycan chains covalently attached to its eight glycosaminoglycan attachment sites [8–11].

The aim of this study was to explore the effect of different bioreactor conditions on the yield, structure, and activity of heparin/heparan sulfates produced by expressing serglycin in mammalian cells. Bioreactors, including tissue culture flasks, continuously-stirred tank reactors (CSTR), and shaker flasks, were investigated as each of these have been used for commercial scale production of bioactives [29]. Different bioreactors and culture conditions were found to change the structure of the heparin/heparan sulfate chains produced by the cells with the serglycin produced being effective at binding and signaling FGF-2. This supports the use of these bioreactors and our approach to produce heparin/heparan sulfates for use in the clinic as an anticoagulant, as well as future uses in drug delivery and regenerative medicine applications.

2. Results

2.1. The Effect of Different Bioreactors on Serglycin Production

HEK-293 cells expressing serglycin were cultured for three days in different bioreactors, including batch culture in tissue culture flasks, CSTR, and shaker flasks (Figure 1A). The morphology of cells after three days in culture was analyzed by phase contrast microscopy (Figure 1B). Cells cultured in the tissue culture flasks formed a confluent monolayer of cells with the characteristic polygonal morphology of adherent cells (Figure 1B(i)). In contrast, aggregated spheroids of cells were found in both the CSTR and shaker flasks (Figure 1B(ii),(iii)). Cells cultured in the CSTR were stirred at 100 rpm, which produced aggregates in the size range 50–300 μm (Figure 1B(ii)). Cells cultured in the shaker flasks were subjected to constant agitation using an orbital shaker operated at 80 rpm, which induced the formation of uniform cell spheroids that ranged in size from 180–200 μm (Figure 1B(iii)).

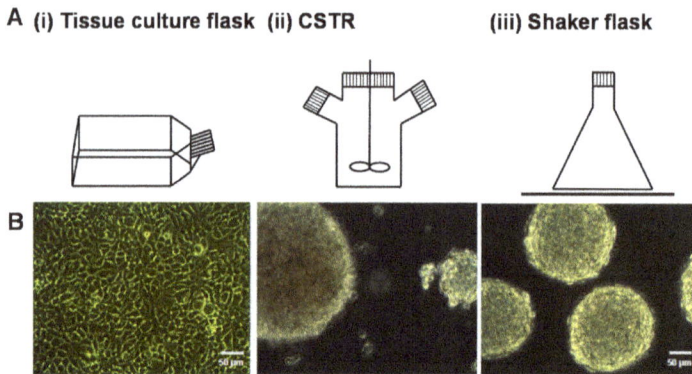

Figure 1. (**A**) Schematic of different bioreactors used to culture the HEK-293 cells expressing serglycin including (**i**) tissue culture flasks, (**ii**) continuously stirred tank reactors (CSTR), and (**iii**) shaker flasks; and (**B**) phase contrast images of cells after three days of culture in the different bioreactor conditions. The scale bar represents 50 μm.

The influence of the different bioreactors on cell proliferation was analyzed over three days (Figure 2). Cells cultured in the tissue culture flasks supported the highest level of cell proliferation. Both the CSTR and shaker flasks supported significantly reduced ($p < 0.05$) cell proliferation compared to the cultures in the tissue culture flasks. The CSTR and shaker flasks induced the formation of spheroid cultures that appeared to have reduced the proliferation of the cells.

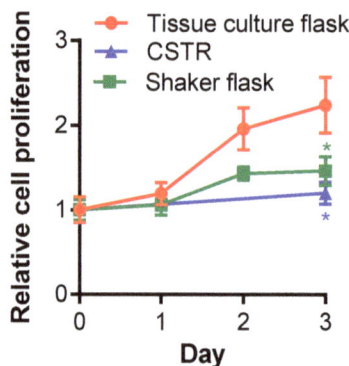

Figure 2. The relative number of cells measured over three days in the different bioreactors, including tissue culture flasks, CSTR, and shaker flasks. Data are presented as means ± standard deviation ($n = 3$). * indicates significant differences ($p < 0.05$) compared to tissue culture flasks at day 3 analyzed by one-way ANOVA.

The influence of the different bioreactors on the cells was also analyzed in terms of yield of proteins and glycosaminoglycans after enrichment of the conditioned medium by anion exchange chromatography for proteoglycans, of which the major proteoglycan produced by these cells was serglycin. The highest yield of proteins was obtained from the tissue culture flasks, followed by the CSTR, and then the shaker flasks, which demonstrated the lowest yield (Figure 3A). The highest yield of glycosaminoglycans was obtained from the CSTR and shaker flasks, and the lowest yield of glycosaminoglycans was obtained from the tissue culture flasks (Figure 3B). Analysis of the ratio of glycosaminoglycan to protein yields indicated that the CSTR and shaker flasks produced the highest amount, and the tissue culture flasks the least (Figure 3C). These data suggest that the spheroid cultures reduced cell proliferation and encouraged glycosaminoglycan decoration of the serglycin protein core to a greater extent than tissue culture flasks that encouraged cell proliferation and protein production.

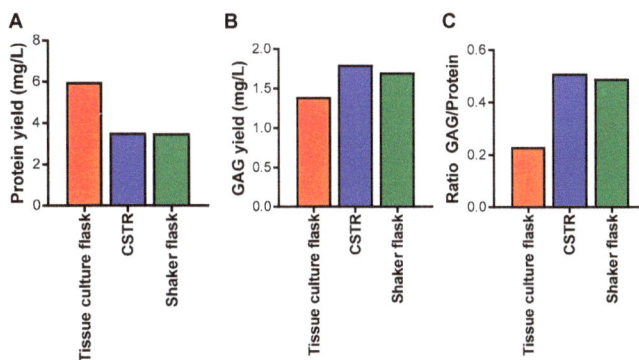

Figure 3. Yield of (**A**) protein; (**B**) glycosaminoglycan (GAG); and (**C**) the ratio of GAG to protein from HEK-293 cells expressing serglycin cultured in different bioreactors over three days and purified by anion exchange chromatography. Protein concentration was measured by Coomassie protein assay and GAG concentration was measured by Dimethylmethylene Blue (DMMB) assay.

The effect of bioreactors on serglycin production and glycosaminoglycan decoration was also explored. There was no difference on the level of serglycin produced by cells in each of the bioreactors (Figure 4A). Tissue culture flasks and the CSTR produced the same level of heparin/heparan sulfate chains as detected by the presence of the HS stub structure that is demonstrated following heparinase III (HepIII) digestion and recognized by the monoclonal antibody 3G10 (Figure 4B). In contrast, the shaker flasks significantly reduced ($p < 0.05$) the level of heparin/heparan sulfate chains (Figure 4B). Unlike heparin/heparan sulfate, which has one stub structure, chondroitin sulfate (CS) has multiple stub structures, following chondroitinase (C'ase) ABC digestion, including the 4- or 6-sulfated stub that can be detected with monoclonal antibodies 2B6 or 3B3, respectively (Figure 4C). While the level of chondroitin sulfate chains with 6-sulfated stub structures was not altered in any of the bioreactors analyzed, the level of 4-sulfated stub structures was significantly reduced in the shaker flasks compared to the tissue culture flask and CSTR (Figure 4C).

The effect of the different bioreactors was further assessed by analyzing the sub-structure of the heparan and chondroitin sulfate chains produced by ELISA (Figure 5). Interestingly, the CSTR promoted the production of heparan sulfate chains containing N-acetylated glucosamine resides, as detected using the heparan sulfate chain antibody, to a significantly greater ($p < 0.05$) extent than either the tissue culture flasks or the shaker flasks (Figure 5A). Together with the data presented in Figure 4B, this indicated that the tissue culture flasks promoted heparan sulfate/heparin chains with a different structure to the CSTR as they exhibited the same level of heparan sulfate/heparin chains. It is speculated that the tissue culture flasks promoted heparan sulfate/heparin chains with sulfated disaccharides, as observed previously [1]. The shaker flasks facilitated minimal heparan sulfate/heparin chain production with no detectable heparan sulfate chains using the heparan sulfate chain antibody (Figure 5A). Both the tissue culture flasks and the CSTR supported the production of chondroitin sulfate containing type A and C disaccharides, while the shaker flask did not support the production of this type of chondroitin sulfate chain (Figure 5B). These data align with the level of 4-sulfated chondroitin sulfate stub structures detected in each of the cultures (Figure 4C).

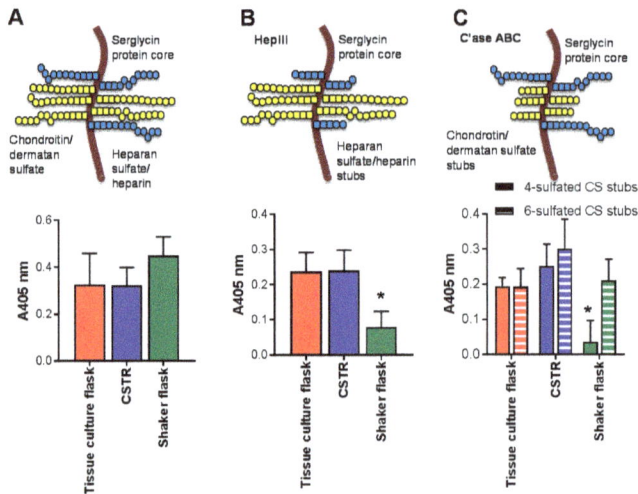

Figure 4. The effect of bioreactors on the production of serglycin, heparin/heparan sulfate and chondroitin sulfate. The schematic indicates the structure of serglycin with eight glycosaminoglycan attachment sites that can be decorated with either chondroitin/dermatan sulfate or heparin/heparan sulfate chains. The effect of glycosaminoglycan lyase digestion on the glycosaminoglycan chains are indicated in panels (**B,C**) with HepIII removing heparin/heparan sulfate chains to reveal a single stub structure and chondroitinase ABC (C'ase ABC) removing chondroitin/dermatan sulfate chains to reveal a stub structure. ELISA for the presence of (**A**) serglycin core protein; (**B**) heparin/heparan sulfate stubs detected using anti-heparan sulfate/heparin-stub antibody clone 3G10 following HepIII digestion, and (**C**) chondroitin sulfate stubs detected using anti-4-sulfated chondroitin sulfate stub antibody clone 2B6 and anti-6-sulfated chondroitin sulfate stub antibody clone 3B3 following C'ase ABC digestion. Data are presented as means $\pm$ standard deviation ($n = 3$). * indicates significant differences ($p < 0.05$) compared to tissue culture flasks analyzed by one-way ANOVA.

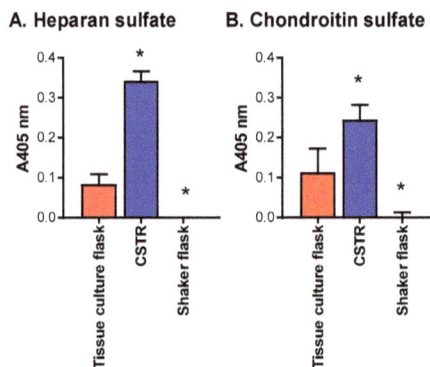

Figure 5. Effect of bioreactors on heparan and chondroitin sulfate structure. ELISA for the presence of (**A**) heparan sulfate chains detected using anti-heparan sulfate chain antibody clone 10E4 and (**B**) chondroitin sulfate chains detected using anti-chondroitin sulfate chain antibody clone CS-56. Data are presented as means $\pm$ standard deviation ($n = 3$). * indicates significant differences ($p < 0.05$) compared to batch cultures analyzed by one-way ANOVA.

2.2. The Effect of Different Culture Conditions on Serglycin Production

As the tissue culture flasks promoted the production of heparan sulfate/heparin, this type of bioreactor was explored further over a seven-day batch culture with HEK-293 cells expressing serglycin. Cells were cultured in three different glucose concentrations of 5.5, 25, and 50 mM as a previous study where the cultures that were passaged weekly and fed every three days indicated that the level of glucose in the medium affected heparin/heparan sulfate production [1]. The influence of glucose concentration on the cells was analyzed in terms of serglycin production and glycosaminoglycan decoration after enrichment of the conditioned medium by anion exchange chromatography for serglycin (Figure 6). Increasing the level of glucose in the medium increased the level of serglycin produced (Figure 6A). There was, however, no difference in the level of heparan sulfate/heparin stubs produced by cells in each of the conditions (Figure 6B) and only baseline levels of heparan sulfate chains containing *N*-acetylated glucosamine residues detected in each condition (Figure 6C). It is speculated that cells grown in tissue culture flasks for extended periods, regardless of glucose concentration, promoted heparan sulfate/heparin chains with sulfated disaccharides, as observed previously [1]. In contrast, cells cultured in medium containing 5.5 mM glucose produced significantly ($p < 0.05$) lower levels of chondroitin sulfate containing type A and C disaccharides compared to cells cultured in medium containing either 25 or 50 mM glucose (Figure 6D).

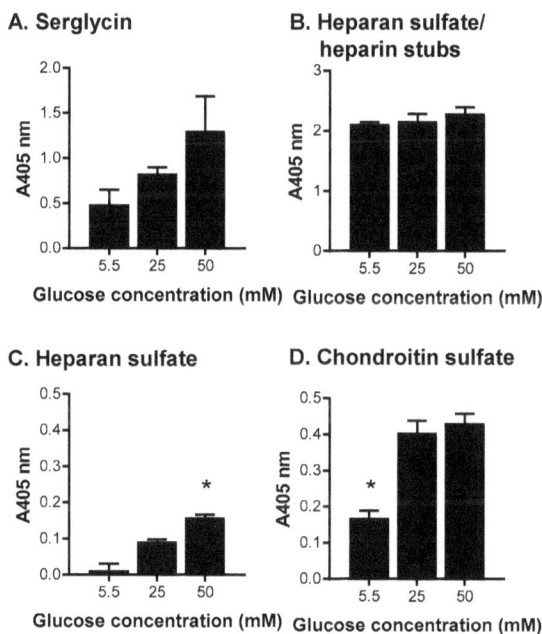

Figure 6. The effects of altering glucose concentrations in media for the production of serglycin, heparan sulfate/heparin and chondroitin sulfate. ELISA for the presence of (**A**) serglycin was detected using a polyclonal anti-serglycin antibody; (**B**) heparan sulfate/heparin stubs were detected using anti-heparan sulfate stub antibody clone 3G10 following HepIII digestion; (**C**) heparan sulfate chains were detected using anti-heparan sulfate antibody clone 10E4; and (**D**) chondroitin sulfate chains were detected using anti- chondroitin sulfate chain antibody clone CS-56. Data are presented as means ± standard deviation ($n = 3$). * indicates significant differences ($p < 0.05$) compared to 25 mM glucose analyzed by one-way ANOVA.

2.3. The Effect of Serglycin Glycosaminoglycan Decoration on Growth Factor Binding and Signaling

One of the major functions of the glycosaminoglycans, such as heparin/heparan sulfate, is to bind and signal growth factors. The production of proteoglycans capable of recapitulating this function in vivo is of therapeutic interest due to the relatively low abundance of naturally-occurring proteoglycans at sites of wound healing. Thus the binding and signaling of the mitogenic growth factor, FGF-2, was analyzed using the BaF32 cell assay. The BaF32 cells proliferate when biologically-active ternary complexes are formed between cell surface FGF receptors, FGF-2 and heparin/heparan sulfate. The positive control for the assay was the FGF receptor type 1c expressing cells exposed to heparin and FGF-2 as shown by the significant ($p < 0.05$) increase in absorbance compared to cells exposed to either heparin or FGF-2 (Figure 7). The addition of serglycin produced by cells cultured for seven days in medium containing 25 mM glucose, as this preparation contained both highly-sulfated heparan sulfate/heparin and chondroitin sulfate, bound and signaled FGF-2 as shown by the significant ($p < 0.05$) increase in cell proliferation compared to cells only exposed to serglycin. Digestion of the chondroitin sulfate chains that decorated serglycin resulted in significantly ($p < 0.05$) greater proliferation of the cells when exposed to FGF-2 compared to cells exposed to undigested serglycin and FGF-2. These data indicated that removal of the chondroitin sulfate chains increased the ability of the heparin/heparan sulfate chains that decorated serglycin to bind and signal FGF-2. Digestion of the heparin/heparan sulfate chains that decorated serglycin resulted in no significant difference in the proliferation of the cells when exposed to FGF-2 compared to cells exposed to undigested serglycin and FGF-2. Digestion of the heparin/heparan sulfate and chondroitin sulfate chains that decorated serglycin resulted in a significant ($p < 0.05$) increase in the proliferation of the cells when exposed to FGF-2 compared to cells exposed to undigested serglycin and FGF-2. Together these data suggested that the heparin/heparan sulfate chains released from the serglycin core protein by HepIII digestion were able to form active complexes with FGF-2 and FGF receptor type 1c.

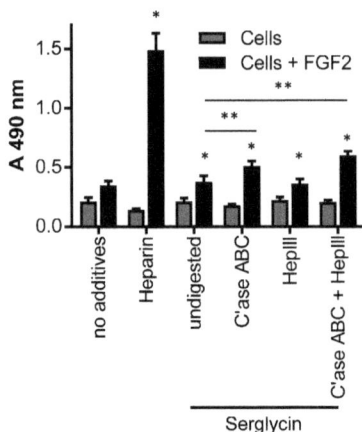

Figure 7. Activity of serglycin with heparin/heparan sulfate and chondroitin sulfate chains determined by the signaling of FGF receptor type 1c expressing BaF32 cells in the presence of FGF-2 as mesured by the MTS assay. Cells in the presence of FGF-2 and heparin were used as a control for the formation of active ternary complexes. Negative controls were cells in the presence of no additives, heparin, or FGF-2. Selected serglycin preparations were digested with either chondroitinase ABC, hepIII or both glycosaminoglycan lysases prior to the assay. Cell proliferation was measured after 72 h. * indicated significant differences ($p < 0.05$) within treatments for cells and FGF-2 compared to cells only as determined by a one-way ANOVA; ** indicated significant differences ($p < 0.05$) as determined by two-way ANOVA.

3. Discussion

This study explored the production of recombinant serglycin in different bioreactors including tissue culture flasks, CSTR, and shaker flasks. Bioreactors that maintain cells in a suspension culture are widely used in industry enabling scale-up of bioactive production [29]. The HEK-293 cells used in this study that had been transfected to stably express serglycin are an adherent cell line, so it was of interest to subject them to the CSTR and shaker flask bioreactors that did not provide conditions for cell adhesion and explore their ability to proliferate and express serglycin. Interestingly, the cells cultured in these bioreactors proliferated, albeit at reduced levels compared to the cells grown in tissue culture flasks. In addition, the cells in both the CSTR and shaker flasks formed spheroids similar to what can be achieved with packed bed bioreactors, however, without an adhesive bead matrix to support cell adhesion [30]. The cell spheroids formed in the CSTR and shaker flasks indicated that the cells under these conditions, formed stable cell-cell contacts providing a different microenvironment to cells grown in the tissue culture flasks.

The microenvironment of cells is known to affect the type and structure of glycosaminoglycans that decorate proteoglycans leading to tissue-specific sulfation patterns [12,13]. The authors recently reported that mast cells cultured in different microenvironments change the type of glycosaminoglycans that they produce [31]. Thus, it was not surprising to discover in this study that the type of bioreactor used to produce proteoglycans altered the production of heparin/heparan and chondroitin sulfate chains. Interestingly, while there were differences in the extent and type of glycosaminoglycans produced, there was no change in the level of serglycin produced in each of the bioreactors. It was interesting to note that while the CSTR and shaker flask bioreactors both induced cell spheroid cultures, albeit of different sized spheroids, the cells produced a similar level of glycosaminoglycan decoration of the protein cores, but with different structures. This finding further supports the concept that the microenvironment plays a key role in determining the type and structure of glycosaminoglycans.

The level of glucose in the culture medium has been reported to affect cell proliferation [32], as well as protein production and glycosylation [33–36]. A comparison of the results of this study and a previous study by the authors indicated that changes in the method of culture in tissue culture flasks is sufficient to alter both serglycin protein core production and the type of glycosaminoglycans [1]. Previously, the cells were cultured for seven days in tissue culture flasks in medium containing 5.5, 25, or 50 mM glucose, passaged weekly and fed every three days. These conditions indicated that the level of glucose in the medium affected both serglycin and heparin/heparan sulfate production [1]. In contrast, this study, cells were grown for three days in tissue culture flasks in medium containing 5.5, 25, or 50 mM glucose prior to passaging, demonstrated that the level of glucose in the medium also affected chondroitin sulfate production.

As the recombinant serglycin produced in this study was decorated with heparin/heparan sulfate chains, it was of interest to determine its ability to bind and signal growth factors. Heparin/heparan sulfate chains are known to bind FGF-2 involving regions of high sulfation called S-domains [19,37]. Thus the serglycin preparation containing sulfated heparan sulfate/heparin and chondroitin sulfate was explored for FGF-2 signaling. This study found that the serglycin bound and signaled FGF-2 through its heparin/heparan sulfate chains both when attached to the serglycin protein core and following HepIII digestion. HepIII depolymerizes heparan sulfate by elimination of hexuronic acids acting next to *N*-sulfated or *N*-acetated residues without sulfation, or with low levels of O-sulfation [38]. Thus HepIII has a limited ability to depolymerize heparin. The heparin/heparan sulfate chains attached to serglycin used in this assay were found to contain highly-sulfated disaccharides, thus, treatment with HepIII would have released heparin/highly-sulfated heparan sulfated oligomers accounting for the FGF-2 activity of the heparin/heparan sulfate chains in solution in addition to when presented on the protein core of serglycin. While chondroitin sulfate is not involved in FGF-2 signaling [39], removal of the chondroitin sulfate chains from serglycin in this study was able to enhance the binding and signaling of the heparin/heparan sulfate bound to serglycin. This is likely due to the close proximity of the eight glycosaminoglycan attachment sites within the central region of the serglycin protein core. Removal of the chondroitin sulfate chains from the protein core of serglycin is likely to have enabled increased flexibility of the heparin/heparan sulfate chains attached to serglycin. A similar phenomenon has been observed for perlecan decorated with both heparan and chondroitin sulfate [40].

In conclusion, this study demonstrated that different bioreactors, including tissue culture flasks, CSTRs, and shaker flasks, in addition to different levels of glucose in the media, produced unique microenvironments that differentially decorated serglycin with heparin/heparan sulfate, as well as chondroitin sulfate. The serglycin produced bound and signaled FGF 2 via its heparin/heparan sulfate chains both when presented as a proteoglycan or as isolated glycosaminoglycan chains. These data demonstrate that the recombinant expression of serglycin is a promising approach for the production of tailored glycosaminoglycan structures with broad applications in drug delivery and regenerative medicine.

4. Materials and Methods

4.1. Culture of Mammalian Cells Expressing Serglycin

Human embryonic kidney (HEK-293) cell were transfected to stably express serglycin, as previously described [1]. Cells were maintained with DMEM culture medium containing 25 mM glucose, 10% (*v/v*) fetal bovine serum (FBS) and 100 µg/mL penicillin and streptomycin at 37 °C, 5% CO_2 in a humidified incubator. Cells seeded at 2×10^5 cells/mL were cultured in standard T75 culture flasks (reactor volume of 10 mL), a continuously-stirred tank reactor (CSTR) operated at 100 rpm, or a conical shaker flask on an orbital shaker operated at 80 rpm, each with a reactor volume of 250 mL. The speed of rotation of the CSTR and shaker flasks was determined with reference to previous studies using suspension cells [31]. Each of the bioreactors was operated in batch mode over three days. Additionally, cells were cultured in DMEM culture medium containing 5.5, 25, or 50 mM glucose, 10% (*v/v*) FBS and 100 µg/mL penicillin and streptomycin at 37 °C, 5% CO_2 in a humidified incubator in standard T75 culture flasks in batch mode for seven days.

4.2. Cell Proliferation Assay

At each time point 50 µL of cell suspension was removed from the CSTR and shaker flasks and the number of viable cells analyzed using a hemocytometer and the trypan blue exclusion dye. For the tissue culture flasks, cell proliferation was analyzed by setting up parallel conditions in a 96 well tissue culture plate seeded with 2×10^5 cells/mL and the number of cells at each time point was analyzed by the MTS assay using Cell Titer 96 Aqueous One Solution Reagent (Promega, Madison, WI, USA) and absorbance was measured at 490 nm.

4.3. Isolation of Serglycin

Serglycin was isolated from the conditioned medium by anion exchange chromatography. The diethylaminoethyl (DEAE) column was equilibrated at 1 mL/min with running buffer (250 mM NaCl, 20 mM Tris, 10 mM EDTA, pH 7.5) before the addition of medium conditioned by cells and the baseline absorbance was re-established with running buffer. Serglycin was eluted using an eluting buffer (1 M NaCl, 20 mM Tris, 10 mM EDTA, pH 7.5) and concentrated. Serglycin-enriched fractions were subsequently concentrated and analyzed for protein concentration using a Coomassie Blue protein assay (Thermo Scientific, Scoresby, Australia). Glycosaminoglycan concentration was determined using the Dimethylmethylene Blue assay (DMMB) as previously described [41].

4.4. Glycosaminoglycan Digestion

Samples were digested with 50 mU/mL proteinase-free chondroitinase (C'ase) ABC (EC 4.2.2.4) purified from *Proteus vulgaris* in 0.1 M Tris acetate, pH 8 at 37 °C for 16 h to confirm the presence of CS/DS. Samples were digested with 10 mU/mL of heparinase (Hep) III (EC 4.2.2.8) purified from

Flavobacterium heparinum (Seikagaku Corp., Tokyo, Japan) diluted in 10 mM Tris-HCl, pH 7.4 at 37 °C for 16 h to determine the presence of heparin/HS.

4.5. ELISA

Serglycin-enriched samples (10 µg based on Coomassie protein assay) with and without glycosaminoglycan lyase digestion were coated onto high-binding 96-well ELISA plates (Greiner, Frickenhausen, Germany) for 2 h at 25 °C. Wells were rinsed twice with Dulbecco's phosphate-buffered saline, pH 7.4 (DPBS) followed by blocking with 0.1% (*w/v*) casein in DPBS for 1 h at 25 °C. Wells were rinsed twice with DPBS with 1% (*v/v*) Tween 20 (PBST) followed by incubation with primary antibodies diluted in 0.1% (*w/v*) casein in DPBS for 2 h at 25 °C. Primary antibodies used included a rabbit polyclonal anti-serglycin antibody (ascites 1:5000), mouse monoclonal anti-4-sulfated chondroitin sulfate stub antibody (clone 2B6, gift from Prof Bruce Caterson, Cardiff University, conditioned medium 1:1000), mouse monoclonal anti-6-sulfated chondroitin sulfate stub antibody (clone 3B3, gift from Prof Bruce Caterson, Cardiff University, conditioned medium 1:1000), mouse monoclonal anti-heparan sulfate stub antibody (clone 3G10, Seikagaku, 1 µg/mL), mouse monoclonal anti-chondroitin sulfate type A and C antibody (clone CS-56, ascites 1:2500), and mouse monoclonal anti-heparan sulfate antibody (clone 10E4, Seikagaku Corp., 1 µg/mL). Wells were rinsed twice with PBST, followed by incubation with biotinylated secondary antibodies (1:1000) diluted in 0.1% (*w/v*) casein in DPBS for 1 h at 25 °C, rinsed twice again with PBST, and then incubated with streptavidin-HRP (1:500) for 30 min at 25 °C. Binding of the antibodies to the samples was detected using the colorimetric substrate, 2,2-azinodi-(3-ethylbenzthiazoline sulfonic acid), and absorbance was measured at 405 nm.

4.6. Growth Factor Binding and Signaling of FGF-2

BaF32 cells were derived from an IL-3-dependent and heparan sulfate proteoglycan-deficient myeloid B cell line that has been stably transfected with fibroblast growth factor receptor (FGFR) 1c [42]. BaF32 cells represent a model system developed to identify heparin/heparan sulfate structures that interact with FGFs and their receptors. The readout of this assay is cell proliferation which indicated the formation of ternary complexes on the cell surface between heparin/heparan sulfate, FGF-2 and FGFR1c. BaF32 cells were maintained in RPMI 1640 medium containing 10% (*v/v*) FBS, 10% (*v/v*) WEHI-3BD conditioned medium, 100 µg/mL penicillin, and streptomycin. WEHI-3BD cells were maintained in RPMI 1640 medium supplemented with 2 g/L sodium bicarbonate, 10% (*v/v*) FBS, 100 µg/mL penicillin, and streptomycin, and the conditioned medium was collected three times per week and stored at −20 °C until it was required. For the mitogenic assays, the BaF32 cells were transferred into IL-3 depleted medium for 24 h prior to experimentation and seeded into 96-well plates at a density of 2×10^4 cells/well in the presence of medium only, 120 nM heparin, 0.5 µg/mL serglycin either in the presence or absence of 0.03 nM FGF-2. To analyze the role of the different glycosaminoglycans that decorated recombinant serglycin, serglycin was also treated with C'ase ABC and/or HepIII prior to use in the assay. Cells exposed to heparin and FGF-2 were used as a positive control for the assay, as this combination is known to induce cell proliferation, while cells exposed to each of the treatments in the absence of FGF-2 were used as a negative control. Background absorbance readings were also obtained for each of the treatments in the absence of cells. Cells were incubated for 72 h in 5% CO_2 at 37 °C, and the number of cells present was assessed using the MTS assay. The MTS reagent (Promega, Madison, WI, USA) was added to the cell cultures 6 h prior to measurement of the absorbance at 490 nm.

Acknowledgments: The authors thank Achilles Theocharis (University of Patras, Greece) for the rabbit polyclonal anti-serglycin antibody. The authors acknowledge Phoebe Lingat for technical assistance. The authors acknowledge grant support from the Australian Research Council Linkage Project Scheme.

Author Contributions: H.N.K., J.M.W., and M.S.L. conceived and designed the experiments, analyzed the data and wrote the paper; and H.N.K. performed the experiments.

Conflicts of Interest: The authors declare no conflict of interest.

References

1. Lord, M.S.; Cheng, B.; Tang, F.; Lyons, J.G.; Rnjak-Kovacina, J.; Whitelock, J.M. Bioengineered human heparin with anticoagulant activity. *Metab. Eng.* **2016**, *38*, 105–114. [CrossRef] [PubMed]
2. Lindahl, U.; Backstrom, G.; Hook, M.; Thunberg, L.; Fransson, L.A.; Linker, A. Structure of the antithrombin-binding site in heparin. *Proc. Natl. Acad. Sci. USA* **1979**, *76*, 3198–3202. [CrossRef] [PubMed]
3. Linhardt, R.J. 2003 Claude S. Hudson Award address in carbohydrate chemistry. Heparin: Structure and activity. *J. Med. Chem.* **2003**, *46*, 2551–2564. [CrossRef] [PubMed]
4. Bhaskar, U.; Sterner, E.; Hickey, A.M.; Onishi, A.; Zhang, F.; Dordick, J.S.; Linhardt, R.J. Engineering of routes to heparin and related polysaccharides. *Appl. Microbiol. Biotechnol.* **2012**, *93*, 1–16. [CrossRef] [PubMed]
5. Sakiyama-Elbert, S.E. Incorporation of heparin into biomaterials. *Acta Biomater.* **2014**, *10*, 1581–1587. [CrossRef] [PubMed]
6. Lever, R.; Page, C.P. Novel drug development opportunities for heparin. *Nat. Rev. Drug Discov.* **2002**, *1*, 140–148. [CrossRef] [PubMed]
7. Toida, T.; Yoshida, H.; Toyoda, H.; Koshiishi, I.; Imanari, T.; Hileman, R.E.; Fromm, J.R.; Linhardt, R.J. Structural differences and the presence of unsubstituted amino groups in heparan sulphates from different tissues and species. *Biochem. J.* **1997**, *322*, 499–506. [CrossRef] [PubMed]
8. Kolset, S.O.; Gallagher, J. Proteoglycans in haemopoietic cells. *Biochim. Biophys. Acta* **1990**, *1032*, 191–221. [CrossRef]
9. Kolset, S.O.; Mann, D.M.; Uhlin-Hansen, L.; Winberg, J.O.; Ruoslahti, E. Serglycin-binding proteins in activated macrophages and platelets. *J. Leukoc. Biol.* **1996**, *59*, 545–554. [PubMed]
10. Kolset, S.O.; Pejler, G. Serglycin: A structural and functional chameleon with wide impact on immune cells. *J. Immunol.* **2011**, *187*, 4927–4933. [CrossRef] [PubMed]
11. Kolset, S.O.; Tveit, H. Serglycin—Structure and biology. *Cell. Mol. Life Sci.* **2008**, *65*, 1073–1085. [CrossRef] [PubMed]
12. Kato, M.; Wang, H.; Bernfield, M.; Gallagher, J.T.; Turnbull, J.E. Cell surface syndecan-1 on distinct cell types differs in fine structure and ligand binding of its heparan sulfate chains. *J. Biol. Chem.* **1994**, *269*, 18881–18890. [PubMed]
13. Iozzo, R.V.; Schaefer, L. Proteoglycan form and function: A comprehensive nomenclature of proteoglycans. *Matrix Biol.* **2015**, *42*, 11–55. [CrossRef] [PubMed]
14. Bernfield, M.; Gotte, M.; Park, P.W.; Reizes, O.; Fitzgerald, M.L.; Lincecum, J.; Zako, M. Functions of cell surface heparan sulfate proteoglycans. *Annu. Rev. Biochem.* **1999**, *68*, 729–777. [CrossRef] [PubMed]
15. Lin, X. Fuctions of heparan sulfate proteoglycans in cell signaling during development. *Development* **2004**, *131*, 6009–6021. [CrossRef] [PubMed]
16. Salmivirta, M.; Lidholt, K.; Linhadl, U. Heparan sulfate: A piece of information. *FASEB J.* **1996**, *10*, 1270–1279. [PubMed]
17. Turnbull, J.E. Heparan sulfate glycomics: Towards systems biology strategies. *Biochem. Soc. Trans.* **2010**, *38*, 1356–1360. [CrossRef] [PubMed]
18. Rosenberg, R.D.; Shworak, N.W.; Liu, J.; Schwartz, J.J.; Zhang, L. Heparan sulfate proteoglycans of the cardiovascular system. Specific structures emerge but how is synthesis regulated? *J. Clin. Investig.* **1997**, *99*, 2062–2070. [CrossRef] [PubMed]
19. Kreuger, J.; Salmivirta, M.; Sturiale, L.; Gimenez-Gallego, G.; Lindahl, U. Sequence analysis of heparan sulfate epitopes with graded affinities for fibroblast growth factors 1 and 2. *J. Biol. Chem.* **2001**, *276*, 30744–30752. [CrossRef] [PubMed]
20. Linhardt, R.J.; Gunay, N.S. Production and chemical processing of low molecular weight heparins. *Semin. Thromb. Hemost.* **1999**, *25*, 5–16. [PubMed]
21. Ashikari-Hada, S.; Habuchi, H.; Kariya, Y.; Itoh, N.; Reddi, A.H.; Kimata, K. Characterization of growth factor-binding structures in heparin/heparan sulfate using an octasaccharide library. *J. Biol. Chem.* **2004**, *279*, 12346–12354. [CrossRef] [PubMed]
22. Yates, E.A.; Guimond, S.E.; Turnbull, J.E. Highly diverse heparan sulfate analogue libraries: Providing access to expanded areas of sequence space for bioactivity screening. *J. Med. Chem.* **2004**, *47*, 277–280. [CrossRef] [PubMed]
23. Powell, A.K.; Ahmed, Y.A.; Yates, E.A.; Turnbull, J.E. Generating heparan sulfate saccharide libraries for glycomics applications. *Nat. Protoc.* **2010**, *5*, 821–833. [CrossRef] [PubMed]

24. DeAngelis, P.L.; Liu, J.; Linhardt, R.J. Chemoenzymatic synthesis of glycosaminoglycans: Re-creating, re-modeling and re-designing nature's longest or most complex carbohydrate chains. *Glycobiology* **2013**, *23*, 764–777. [CrossRef] [PubMed]

25. Choay, J.; Petitou, M.; Lormeau, J.C.; Sinaÿ, P.; Casu, B.; Gatti, G. Structure-activity relationship in heparin: A synthetic pentasaccharide with high affinity for antithrombin III and eliciting high anti-factor Xa activity. *Biochem. Biophys. Res. Commun.* **1983**, *116*, 492–499. [CrossRef]

26. Farrugia, B.L.; Lord, M.S.; Melrose, J.; Whitelock, J.M. Can we produce heparin/heparan sulfate biomimetics using 'mother-nature' as the gold standard? *Molecules* **2015**, *20*, 4254–4276. [CrossRef] [PubMed]

27. Baik, J.Y.; Gasimli, L.; Yang, B.; Datta, P.; Zhang, F.; Glass, C.A.; Esko, J.D.; Linhardt, R.J.; Sharfstein, S.T. Metabolic engineering of Chinese hamster ovary cells: Towards a bioengineered heparin. *Metab. Eng.* **2012**, *14*, 81–90. [CrossRef] [PubMed]

28. Lord, M.S.; Cheng, B.; Farrugia, B.L.; McCarthy, S.; Whitelock, J.M. Platelet factor 4 binds to vascular proteoglycans and controls both growth factor activities and platelet activation. *J. Biol. Chem.* **2017**, *292*, 4054–4063. [CrossRef] [PubMed]

29. Eibl, R.; Kaiser, S.; Lombriser, R.; Eibl, D. Disposble bioreactors: The current state-of-the-art and recommended applications in biotechnology. *Appl. Microbiol. Biotechnol.* **2010**, *86*, 41–49. [CrossRef] [PubMed]

30. Meuwly, F.; Ruffieux, P.A.; Kadouri, A.; von Stockar, U. Packed-bed bioreactors for mammalian cell culture: Bioprocess and biomedical applications. *Biotechnol. Adv.* **2007**, *25*, 45–56. [CrossRef] [PubMed]

31. Lord, M.S.; Jung, M.; Whitelock, J.M. Optimization of bioengineered heparin/heparan sulfate production for therapeutic applications. *Bioengineered* **2017**, *10*, 1–4. [CrossRef] [PubMed]

32. Sugiura, T. Effects of glucose on the production of recombinant protein C in mammalian cell culture. *Biotechnol. Bioeng.* **1992**, *39*, 953–959. [CrossRef] [PubMed]

33. Whitford, W.G. Fed-batch mammalian cell culture in bioproduction. *BioProcess. Int.* **2006**, *4*, 30–40.

34. Cechowska-Pasko, M.; Bańkowski, E. Glucose deficiency inhibits glycosaminoglycans synthesis in fibroblast cultures. *Biochimie* **2010**, *92*, 806–813. [CrossRef] [PubMed]

35. Wang, A.; Midura, R.J.; Vasanji, A.; Wang, A.J.; Hascall, V.C. Hyperglycemia diverts dividing osteoblastic precursor cells to an adipogenic pathway and induces synthesis of a hyaluronan matrix that is adhesive for monocytes. *J. Biol. Chem.* **2014**, *289*, 11410–11420. [CrossRef] [PubMed]

36. Vogl-Willis, C.A.; Edwards, I.J. High-glucose-induced structural changes in the heparan sulfate proteoglycan, perlecan, of cultured human aortic endothelial cells. *Biochim. Biophys. Acta* **2004**, *1672*, 36–45. [CrossRef] [PubMed]

37. Gallagher, J.T. Heparan sulfate: Growth control with a restricted sequence menu. *J. Clin. Investig.* **2001**, *108*, 357–361. [CrossRef] [PubMed]

38. Wei, Z.; Lyon, M.; Gallagher, J.T. Distinct substrate specificities of bacterial heparinases against *N*-unsubstituted glucosamine residues in heparan sulfate. *J. Biol. Chem.* **2005**, *280*, 15742–15748. [CrossRef] [PubMed]

39. Chuang, C.Y.; Lord, M.S.; Melrose, J.; Rees, M.D.; Knox, S.M.; Freeman, C.; Iozzo, R.V.; Whitelock, J.M. Heparan sulfate dependent signaling of fibroblast growth factor (FGF) 18 by chondrocyte-derived perlecan. *Biochemistry* **2010**, *49*, 5524–5532. [CrossRef] [PubMed]

40. Smith, S.M.L.; West, L.A.; Govindraj, P.; Zhang, X.; Ornitz, D.M.; Hassell, J.R. Heparan and chondroitin sulfate on growth plate perlecan mediate binding and delivery of FGF-2 to FGF receptors. *Matrix Biol.* **2007**, *26*, 175–184. [CrossRef] [PubMed]

41. Davies, N.P.; Roubin, R.H.; Whitelock, J.M. Characterization and purification of glycosaminoglycans from crude biological samples. *J. Agric. Food Chem.* **2008**, *56*, 343–348. [CrossRef] [PubMed]

42. Ornitz, D.M.; Yayon, A.; Flanagan, J.G.; Svahn, C.M.; Levi, E.; Leder, P. Heparin is required for cell-free binding of basic fibroblast growth factor to a soluble receptor and for mitogenesis in whole cells. *Mol. Cell Biol.* **1992**, *12*, 240–247. [CrossRef] [PubMed]

Sample Availability: Samples of the compounds are available upon request from the authors.

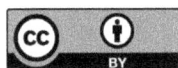

molecules

MDPI

Review

Sulfated Alginates as Heparin Analogues: A Review of Chemical and Functional Properties

Øystein Arlov [1] and Gudmund Skjåk-Bræk [2,*]

[1] Department of Biotechnology and Nanomedicine, SINTEF Materials and Chemistry,
Richard Birkelands vei 3B, 7034 Trondheim, Norway; oystein.arlov@sintef.no
[2] Department of Biotechnology, Norwegian University of Science and Technology, Sem Sælands vei 6/8, 7034 Trondheim, Norway
* Correspondence: gudmund.skjak.brak@ntnu.no; Tel.: +47-7359-3323

Academic Editor: Giangiacomo Torri
Received: 5 April 2017; Accepted: 5 May 2017; Published: 11 May 2017

Abstract: Heparin is widely recognized for its potent anticoagulating effects, but has an additional wide range of biological properties due to its high negative charge and heterogeneous molecular structure. This heterogeneity has been one of the factors in motivating the exploration of functional analogues with a more predictable modification pattern and monosaccharide sequence, that can aid in elucidating structure-function relationships and further be structurally customized to fine-tune physical and biological properties toward novel therapeutic applications and biomaterials. Alginates have been of great interest in biomedicine due to their inherent biocompatibility, gentle gelling conditions, and structural versatility from chemo-enzymatic engineering, but display limited interactions with cells and biomolecules that are characteristic of heparin and the other glycosaminoglycans (GAGs) of the extracellular environment. Here, we review the chemistry and physical and biological properties of sulfated alginates as structural and functional heparin analogues, and discuss how they may be utilized in applications where the use of heparin and other sulfated GAGs is challenging and limited.

Keywords: heparin; alginate; sulfated alginate; biomaterials

---

1. Introduction

Glycosaminoglycans (GAGs) are a group of negatively charged linear polysaccharides found in virtually all animal tissues. The majority of GAG subtypes are associated with the plasma membrane via a protein core, referred to as proteoglycans, and are key components of the extracellular matrix (ECM) in providing structural support and hydration. The sulfated GAGs have additional vital roles in the development, maintenance, and pathophysiology of mammalian tissues, and may serve as receptors, co-receptors, and reservoirs through electrostatic interaction with proteins. Heparin differs from other GAGs in that it is primarily produced by mast cells, and is released from storage granules into the extracellular space by exocytosis. Heparin is a potent anticoagulant, and is widely used in the clinic as an intravenously administered blood thinner and as a coating material for medical devices. While structurally related to heparan sulfate (HS), heparin undergoes a greater degree of enzymatic modification during synthesis, resulting in highly diverse biological activities. Heparin has the highest sulfation degree of the GAGs, and a higher charge density than any known biopolymer, thus associating with a plethora of proteins including coagulation factors, growth factors, cytokines, adhesion proteins, and pathogen-related proteins.

The use of heparin for other biomedical applications than anticoagulation is however limited, partly due to rapid turnover in biological systems and risks of excessive bleeding upon administration. Heparin has a high degree of heterogeneity in its monosaccharide sequence and modification pattern, depending on the source, and has few options for structural customizability. This complicates tuning of the drug's efficacy, as well as the characterization of biological activity and structure-function relationships required for exploring new potential applications. An additional aspect regarding widespread use of heparin is concerns regarding safety and sustainability in its production, as the most widely used derivatives of heparin are isolated from animal tissues [1]. For these reasons, over the last few decades numerous heparin derivatives and analogues from natural sources, chemical synthesis, and chemical and/or enzymatic functionalization of polysaccharides have been described [2–5]. Some of the heparin analogues described in the literature aim to emulate the anticoagulant properties of heparin, to provide more sustainable and safe drug manufacturing and/or allow greater control over pharmacokinetic and –dynamic properties. Others are directed toward novel pharmaceutical applications or as components in biomaterials, where the physicochemical properties and highly specific anticoagulating action of heparin pose limitations.

This review aims to present current knowledge and studies on sulfated alginates as novel heparin analogues, based on the authors' own work and the available recent literature. We further wish to discuss future directions of this research, as well as areas of application where sulfated alginates can potentially provide a viable alternative to heparin or other sulfated GAGs and derivatives.

1.1. Heparin Molecular Structure and Physical Properties

Heparin and heparan sulfate are synthesized as alternating copolymers of 1→4-linked N-acetylglucosamine (GlcNAc) and glucuronic acid (GlcA). During synthesis, the nascent chain is modified by a series of enzymes in the Golgi apparatus, namely N-deacetylase-N-sulfotransferases, C-5 epimerases, and 2-O, 3-O, and 6-O sulfotransferases [6]. Epimerization of GlcA into iduronic acid (IdoA) confers structural flexibility to the polysaccharide chains, in that IdoA can assume one of three stable conformations ($^4C_1$, $^1C_4$, or $^2S_0$) depending on the modification pattern and induced effects upon protein interaction [7]. The expression of tissue-specific isozymes [8,9] and varying combinations of modifications confer a high degree of structural complexity and variability to heparin and HS, requiring a great effort for their functional and structural characterization. Heparin has a higher degree of sulfation and epimerization compared to HS, where the trisulfated disaccharide IdoA2S-GlcNS6S (Figure 1) constitutes 60–85% of the heparin chain, depending on the source [10,11]. However, there are no repeating sequences in heparin as the trisulfated disaccharides are interspersed by undersulfated residues of varying lengths. Heparan sulfate exhibits long unmodified regions between heparin-like motifs with high sulfation and epimerization degrees [12]. Epimerization of GlcA to IdoA has been demonstrated in vitro, using Glucuronyl C5-epimerase isolated from bovine tissue and the K5 capsular polysaccharide (GlcA-GlcNAc) [13]. To the authors' knowledge, only one prokaryotic GlcA C5-epimerase has been identified and utilized for in vitro epimerization of K5. As the activity of the enzymes was relatively low, the results indicated that the native substrate differs from heparin and HS-like polysaccharides [14]. Of note, in vitro epimerization of GlcA is readily reversible, in contrast to the reaction in vivo due to subsequent O-sulfation following epimerization [13,15].

Commercial heparin is generally classified as unfractionated heparin (UFH, ~15 kDa), low molecular weight heparin (LMWH, ~6 kDa), or ultra-low molecular weight heparin (ULMWH, <2 kDa), where the most common ULMWHs are chemically synthesized oligosaccharides including the antithrombin (AT)-binding region [16]. Whereas chemical synthesis of heparin has had major limitations in terms of oligosaccharide length, recent advances have demonstrated production of up to 40-mers by iterative homologation of tetrasaccharides [17]. However, this approach generates repeating sequences, which are not found in native heparin.

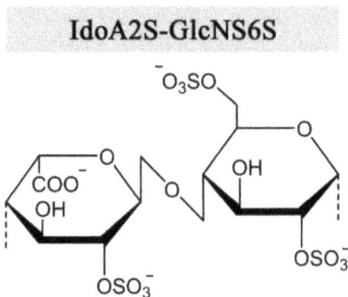

Figure 1. The prevalent disaccharide structure in heparin.

1.2. Biological Properties of Heparin and Structure-Function Relationships

Heparin has potent anticoagulating properties and has widespread use in the clinic as an intravenously administered drug and as a coating material on medical devices. Its anticoagulating effect is primarily mediated by highly specific binding and activation of antithrombin, which in turn inactivates several proteases of the coagulation cascade, namely thrombin and Factors X, IX, XI, and XII [18].

Furthermore, heparin has demonstrated anti-inflammatory effects, presumably by multiple functions due to its broad substrate affinity. For instance, heparin has long been known to bind complement factors, where its anti-coagulating effects can supplement this effect through cross talk between the complement and coagulation pathways [19,20], as well as pro-inflammatory cytokines [21]. Binding of heparin to these proteins can exert an inhibitory effect through preventing receptor interaction, conformational changes, or proteolytic cleavage. An additional postulated mechanism is the binding of heparin to P- and L-selectins, inhibiting interaction with endothelial proteoglycans and thus adhesion and extravasation of leukocytes [22]. Heparin has also been evaluated as a potential antiviral drug due to association with viral capsule proteins [23]. Heparan sulfate and other GAGs on the cell surface can be utilized as a receptor for pathogens initiating adhesion and eventual cell entry, where soluble heparin can serve as an antagonist [24].

Heparin has been demonstrated to bind a plethora of proteins with varying interaction strengths. Asides from the well characterized AT interaction, the selectivity of heparin-protein interactions, and whether specific sequences are "programmed" into the heparin chains, remains a controversial subject. For a more comprehensive discussion of the topic, the reader is referred to the works of Lindahl and associates [25,26]. As a relevant point to the present review, it is evident that variance in monosaccharide sequences and modification patterns can have a large impact on protein interaction strength, tied to optimal alignment for ionic interactions and van der Waals forces [7]. For example, Hu and co-workers generated a HS disaccharide library, demonstrating that only 4 out of 48 disaccharides bind fibroblast growth factor-1 (FGF-1) with high affinity [27]. The presence of IdoA has been demonstrated to be critical for the interaction strength to specific proteins, where a large degree of chain flexibility can contribute to improved alignment between heparin and the protein surface, compared to a more rigid polysaccharide with equivalent charge. For example, the $^1C_4$ conformation forms a kink in the heparin/HS chain which greatly enhances FGF interaction, but is not present in IdoA-containing dermatan sulfate due to the different interspersed monosaccharides and linkage patterns [28]. Studies have also shown the effect of various sulfation patterns in heparin on binding to P and L-selectins, revealing that 6-O-sulfation is critical for interaction with both selectins [29]. Furthermore, LMWH interacts less strongly with selectins compared with UFH, indicating an additional dependence of chain length, or that critical structural patterns are disrupted during fragmentation [30]. These examples emphasize that there are additional aspects beyond charge density that influence the biological activity of sulfated GAGs, which must be addressed in the design of functional analogues.

2. Sulfated Alginates

2.1. Properties of Alginate

Alginates, in contrast to GAGs, are produced in brown algae *(Pheaophyceae)*, where they serve as structural polysaccharides, or in certain genera of gram-negative bacteria (*Azotobacter* and *Pseudomonas* sp.) where alginates as exocellular polysaccharides confer different protective functions and virulence factors [31]. Still, they share some structural features with heparin and heparin sulfate besides all being linear uronans. Alginates are copolymers of 1→4-linked β-D-mannuronic acid (M) and α-L-guluronic acid (G) (Figure 2), which are C-5 epimers of each other, analogous to GlcA and IdoA in heparin/HS. Moreover, they are arranged in G-and M-blocks of various length interspaced with regions of alternating sequences (MG-block) akin to the sulfate-, IdoA-rich and undersulfated GlcA-rich regions(NS and NA domains, respectively) found in heparan sulfate [32]. Alginates form hydrogels through ionic cross-linking with divalent cations such as calcium, where the gel properties are largely influenced by the content and length of the G-blocks [33]. Alginate is synthetized as homopolymeric mannuronan, which in a post-polymerization step is converted into alginate by C-5 epimerization, similar to the GlcA→IdoA conversion in the biosynthesis of heparin and heparan sulfate. Due to the action of these post-polymerization epimerases, both GAGs and alginate possess non-random block sequential structures. Whereas the introduction of IdoA in heparin/HS provides conformational flexibility significant for protein interactions, the main effect of epimerization in alginates is the introduction of calcium binding G-blocks responsible for gel formation. The alginate-producing bacterium *Azotobacter vinelandii* expresses seven exocellular epimerases (AlgE1-7), which have been cloned and can be used to engineer alginates with compositionally homogeneous structures not found in nature [34].

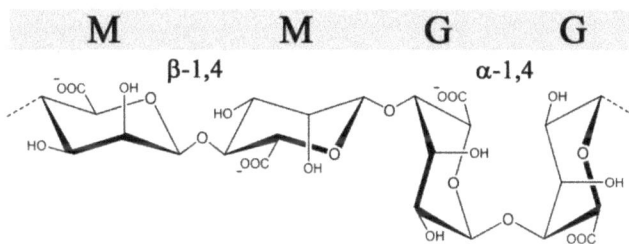

Figure 2. The structures and glycosidic bond conformations of β-D-mannuronic acid and α-L-guluronic acid in alginates.

Of note, the AlgE4 enzyme can be used to introduce an alternating sequence (poly-MG), similar to the basic backbone structure of heparin [35]. Enzymatic and chemical modifications of alginates have been extensively described in previous reviews, illustrating a great structural and functional versatility [36,37]. Alginate has been evaluated for numerous biomedical applications, primarily due to their gentle gelling conditions, including immunoisolation of cell transplants [38], slow-release systems [39], in vitro tissue engineering [40], and 3D-bioprinting [41]. Purified alginates are relatively inert toward cells and biomolecules, providing good biocompatibility but simultaneously discouraging favourable interactions with cell receptors and vital soluble factors that are characteristic of glycosaminoglycans in the extracellular matrix. Thus, great efforts have been made to functionalize alginates to provide a biomimetic environment, while maintaining their biocompatibility and gelling properties. One such strategy is by chemical sulfation, to emulate the structure of sulfated GAGs.

2.2. Synthesis and Characterization of Sulfated Alginates

Multiple strategies have been described for chemical sulfation of alginates (Figure 3). Huang and co-workers first employed chlorosulfonic acid (HClSO$_3$) in formamide, resulting in a reported degree of sulfation (DS) of approximately 1.2 sulfate groups per monosaccharide. As a means to reduce the adverse effects from over-sulfation, the sulfated alginates were conjugated with quaternary amine groups, allowing a controlled reduction of anti-coagulating properties [42]. We found that the sulfation degree could be reproducibly tuned by varying the chlorosulfonic acid concentration, but the DS was found to reach a plateau around DS = 1.0–1.2, depending on the monosaccharide sequence and their relative solubility in acid [43,44]. Sulfation of dextran has been performed using sulfur trioxide (SO$_3$) in pyridine, which was reported to result in a more homogeneous substitution compared with the HClSO$_3$/formamide method [45]. This approach was used for alginate by Mhanna and coworkers, using a tetrabutylammonium (TBA) salt of alginate to increase solubility in pyridine [46], but was found to have challenges related to reproducibility of the sulfation degree in following studies. An alternative strategy employs a carbodiimide-H$_2$SO$_4$ intermediate reacting directly with alginate [47], or via the TBA salt of alginate in DMF [48]. One challenge with the described methods is the strong acidic conditions used to obtain a high sulfation degree, resulting in partial depolymerization of high-molecular weight alginates [47], whereas the relatively low solubility of alginate in acid can reduce reaction reproducibility and throughput. Fan and co-workers reported a novel strategy for the sulfation of polysaccharides under non-acidic conditions, obtaining a DS of approximately 2 sulfates/monosaccharide at optimal conditions [49]. Although the authors of this review were not able to sulfate alginates using the method as described, the procedure could have a large potential for preventing depolymerization and allowing a DS approaching that of heparin, if successfully established.

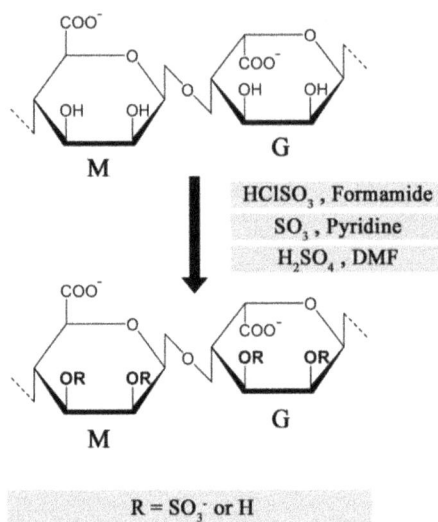

Figure 3. Published methods for chemical sulfation of alginate using different reagents [9,42,46,48].

The molecular structure of sulfated alginates has been characterized primarily by utilizing Fourier-transform infrared (FTIR) spectroscopy, Nuclear magnetic resonance (NMR), and Mass spectrometry (MS)-based methods. In the FTIR spectrum, sulfation of the hydroxyl groups in alginate results in the appearance of a distinct peak corresponding to the symmetric stretching of the S=O bond [42,48]. However, this method provides little qualitative data and cannot clearly distinguish substitution at C-2 from C-3, nor the M from G in alginate. NMR can provide detailed structural data, but generates highly complicated spectra due to the heterogeneity in the substitution patterns and monosaccharide sequences of sulfated alginates. We generated alginates with homogeneous sequences (poly-M, poly-G, and poly-MG) with three specific degrees of sulfation using HClSO$_3$, and employed various 2D NMR techniques to assign the 1D ^{13}C spectrum and identify the substitution pattern for the distinct alginate sequences [43,44]. Consistent with previous studies, the sulfation followed a random substitution pattern, indicated by the increase in spectrum heterogeneity at low sulfation degrees [43]. Based on the NMR data, no apparent selectivity was found for the substitution of M/G, or C-2/C-3. This was also found by Zhao and co-workers in an early study on low-molecular weight sulfated guluronate, by NMR characterization [50]. Following this presumption, the sulfate groups are evenly distributed along the polysaccharide chains and not organized in domains of varying density (e.g., following alginate block sequences), in contrast with heparan sulfate [51]. The degree of sulfation (DS) can thus be expressed as the average number of sulfates per monosaccharide, and determined by biochemical methods or mass spectrometry-based elemental analysis [44,52].

Chemical sulfation of alginates results in a less heterogeneous substitution pattern compared with natural heparin and heparan sulfate, as the sulfate groups are presumably equally distributed between C-2 and C-3 of the mannuronic acid and guluronic acid moieties. This provides as mentioned a relatively homogeneous charge distribution along the polysaccharide chain, which can contribute to the study of structure-function relationships while reducing batch-to-batch variability. The published methods demonstrate limitations in terms of sulfation degree, as the substitution is restricted to the free hydroxyl group, while di-sulfated monosaccharides are presumably discouraged from steric effects. The different substitution pattern and lower charge density of sulfated alginates can in turn lead to more transient protein interactions, or the utilization of alternative interaction sites compared with heparin/HS. Additional strategies for C-6 sulfation can therefore be explored to emulate highly sulfated moieties [53]. Furthermore, monosaccharide-specific sulfation of alginate would carry a substantial benefit, as sulfation of primarily mannuronic acid would allow unimpaired cross-linking of guluronic acid blocks and a vast improvement in sulfated alginate gel strength and stability. This is, however, yet to be demonstrated, as there are great challenges in discerning between the monosaccharides chemically.

2.3. Chemical and Physical Properties of Sulfated Alginates

Introduction of a charged and relatively bulky substituent notably alters the chemical structure of alginates, which is of great relevance to their inherent properties in solution and in ionically-crosslinked hydrogels. Steric hindrance reduces rotation around the glycosidic bond, conferring a more extended and rigid conformation in polysaccharides [54]. The sulfate groups can further promote intramolecular charge repulsion, although this effect is reduced by the presence of sodium counter ions similarly to the carboxyl groups of alginate and is presumably negligible compared with steric effects. The precise effect of sulfation on alginate conformation in solution remains to be elucidated, and can be approached utilizing homogeneous sequences of alginates that have previously been studied in terms of chain extension and bond rotation [55]. The stiffness of the polysaccharide chain can influence interaction strengths with proteins, and thus the biological properties of the polysaccharides.

Sulfation generally has a deteriorating effect on the gelling ability of alginates, where the resulting gels have a lower stiffness and increased rate of swelling and destabilization compared with unmodified alginate [46,56]. Negatively charged sulfate groups associate with divalent cations, but disrupt the long G-blocks that are responsible for the cooperative binding of ions and forming of cross-linking junction zones in the gel network, as described in the "egg-box" model [57]. In a recent study, we characterized gels made exclusively from sulfated alginates with varying sulfation degrees, as well as the effect of combining highly sulfated alginate (DS = 1) in unmodified alginate gels at various proportions. Sulfated alginate alone (150 kDa) was found to form stable gels with calcium up to a sulfation degree of approximately 0.4, whereas increasing the sulfation level required either the inclusion of unmodified alginate or utilization of gelling ions with a higher affinity for alginate (e.g., barium, strontium) [58]. An alternative strategy that has not yet been explored to the authors' knowledge is covalent cross-linking between sulfated alginates, or to unmodified alginates, which can be a feasible approach where a higher gel stiffness is required. As highly sulfated alginates presumably only form transient cross-links within the hydrogel matrix, they diffuse out in the surrounding medium upon swelling of the gels at a higher rate than unmodified alginate, particularly at low molecular weight. Interestingly, a low amount (20%) of S-Alg mixed with unmodified alginate consistently demonstrated decreased stiffness but a lower swelling potential in saline than the alginate control, potentially due to a higher charge density, retention of gelling ions slowing the exchange with Na^+, and osmotic influx of water [58].

The use of heparin analogues in hydrogels are of great interest for encapsulation of cells and proteins (e.g., in tissue engineering). Sulfated alginates demonstrate great potential with its inherent gelling capability and has, similarly to native alginate, a great versatility in properties and gelling conditions to allow the tuning of hydrogel characteristics toward specific applications. These include enzymatic engineering to increase gel strength [34], and the utilization of alternative cross-linking ions [59] and gelling techniques, for example, $CaCl_2$ for immediate gelling versus $CaCO_3$ and glucono-δ-lactone GDL for a gradual release of calcium in injectable solutions and in situ gelation [60].

2.4. Effects of Sulfated Alginates on the Coagulation Cascade

As heparin is most widely known and used due to its potent anticoagulating properties, it is of great interest to investigate whether similar effects can be achieved utilizing the structurally analogous sulfated alginates. Huang and co-workers studied the activated partial thrombosis time (APTT), thrombin time (TT), and prothrombin time (PT) in plasma, using sulfated algal alginates with an approximate DS of 1.0 sulfate per monosaccharide. Although heparin was not included as a control in the present study, sulfated alginates prolonged the APTT with increasing treatment concentrations while showing no significant effects on the TT and PT [42]. Conversely, Ma and co-workers showed a pronounced elevation of the TT increasing with the sulfation degree and concentration of sulfated alginate, whereas no comparison with heparin was made. The authors further demonstrated a procedure for coating a polyethersulfone membrane with sulfated alginate, resulting in prolonged coagulation compared with the non-coated membrane [47]. By hydrolysis and separation, Li and co-workers prepared low-molecular weight (6–7 kDa) alginates enriched in mannuronic acid or guluronic acid, and studied the anticoagulating effects of their sulfated derivatives. Similarly to the study by Huang, SA was found to increase the APTT compared to the saline control and the non-sulfated alginates, whereas a two- and eight-fold greater effect was observed for LMWH and heparin, respectively, at similar concentrations [61]. The results indicate that sulfated alginates may inhibit the extrinsic coagulation pathway through binding and sequestration and/or prevention of protease activity of upstream factors, but are unable to bind antithrombin selectively to inhibit tissue factor (TF)-mediated activation of Factor X, and thrombin. Lacking AT activation was also evident from the TT test where sulfated alginate was unable to prolong coagulation time in the presence of excess thrombin. Heparin does not deactivate TF directly in vivo, but induces secretion of an inhibitor (TFPI) from endothelial cells, resulting in a less pronounced effect on the PT in vitro [62]. To the authors' knowledge, the release of TF has not been demonstrated for sulfated alginates or similar heparin analogues in in vivo models.

The mechanism behind the observed anticoagulating effects of sulfated alginates are still not clear, whereas the presented research does not strongly support the specific antithrombin activation that is characteristic of heparin. Presumably, the sulfated alginates non-specifically bind multiple coagulation factors, having a partial antagonizing or deactivating effect on the proteases or indirectly through other regulatory proteins (Figure 4). Alternatively, interaction outside the active sites may lead to aggregation and sequestration of precursors such as fibrinogen, as proposed for other heparin mimetics [63]. As the sulfated alginates were postulated to have a greater influence on the intrinsic coagulation pathway [42], interaction studies with individual coagulation factors can help further elucidate their effect on the coagulation cascade, by indicating whether the interactions are largely non-specific or if there is a selectivity for certain factors. Furthermore, platelet aggregation and activation are vital steps within the coagulation cascade, and should be studied for hydrogels or surface coatings of sulfated alginates to evaluate if they exhibit effects similar to heparin and other well-characterized heparin analogues [5,64].

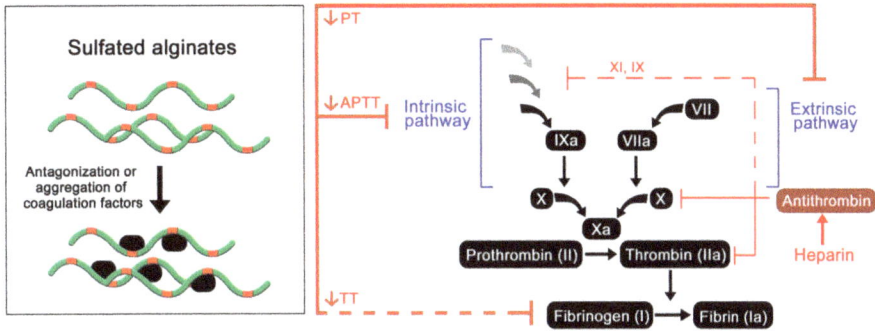

Figure 4. Postulated effect of sulfated alginates on the coagulation cascade resulting in prolonged coagulation time [42,47,49,50,61].

2.5. Immunological Effects of Sulfated Alginates

The mechanisms behind the anti-inflammatory properties of heparin and similar sulfated polysaccharides are still not fully understood. Several studies demonstrate interactions with cytokines, chemokines, growth factors, and signalling cascade factors, potentially resulting in altered protein half-life, sequestration of ligands from their receptors, and/or prevention of proteolytic cleavage or conformational changes in proteins. The cellular response to inflammation can also be affected more directly by heparin, through association with adhesion proteins that mediate extravasation of leukocytes across the endothelium [29].

To study the anti-inflammatory properties of sulfated alginates, we employed two different model systems, where multiple anti-inflammatory effects were observed (Figure 5). In the first study, sulfated alginates were incorporated in alginate microspheres either as a secondary coat on polycation-coated microcapsules or mixed with non-sulfated alginate in uncoated microspheres, followed by incubation in whole human blood anti-coagulated with lepirudin [65]. Microspheres with sulfated alginates were found to attenuate the inflammatory response, by lowering the expression of several inflammatory cytokines, including interleukin (IL)-1β, TNF, and IL-8. The sulfated alginate gels were found to inhibit the complement cascade in blood, as well as in plasma in soluble form [44], indicating direct interaction with complement factors as previously demonstrated for heparin [19,66]. Sequestration of complement factors prevents assembly of the convertases and terminal complement complex, whereas we additionally demonstrated interaction between sulfated alginates and complement inhibitory Factor H, which can contribute to suppression of the complement cascade on microsphere surfaces [65]. Lastly, there is significant cross talk between the coagulation and complement cascades [20,67], where the previously described anticoagulating activities of sulfated alginates can have an indirect influence on the inflammatory response. Sulfated alginates were further found to reduce integrin alpha M (ITGAM/CD11b) expression on leukocytes, which can be attributed to indirect effects from sequestration of cytokines and complement factors. In the second study, human chondrocytes were encapsulated in alginate or sulfated alginate gels, prior to inflammatory induction with IL-1β. Chondrocytes in sulfated alginate gels demonstrated lowered expression of inflammatory and catabolic markers, as well as reduced nuclear factor-kappa b NF-κB and p38-mitogen activated protein kinase (MAPK)-mediated signaling compared with the alginate controls. Sulfated alginate was found to bind IL-1β, presumably sequestering the cytokines in the gel matrix and preventing induction of the encapsulated cells [58]. Similarly, Freeman and co-workers demonstrated binding to IL-6, further indicating that sulfated alginates can regulate cytokine activity as well as their expression [48]. Inhibition of cytokine activity through binding can appear to contradict with the potentiating effect of binding growth factors, and will depend on whether the interaction sites between sulfated alginates and proteins interfere with receptor binding, or if there is a co-receptor functionality as previously established for heparan sulfate and FGF [68]. Heparin has previously been demonstrated to inhibit leukocyte activity through associating with L- and P-selectins [22], which has not yet been demonstrated for sulfated alginates, but can potentially reveal additional anti-inflammatory effects in alternative model systems. As a model for chronic inflammation, Zhao and co-workers studied granuloma formation in rats, and found that ingested sulfated guluronate reduced the size of the granuloma [50]. The mechanisms behind this effect are still unclear, and sulfated alginates may act on multiple levels such as inflammation and coagulation pathways, and adhesion molecules [69,70].

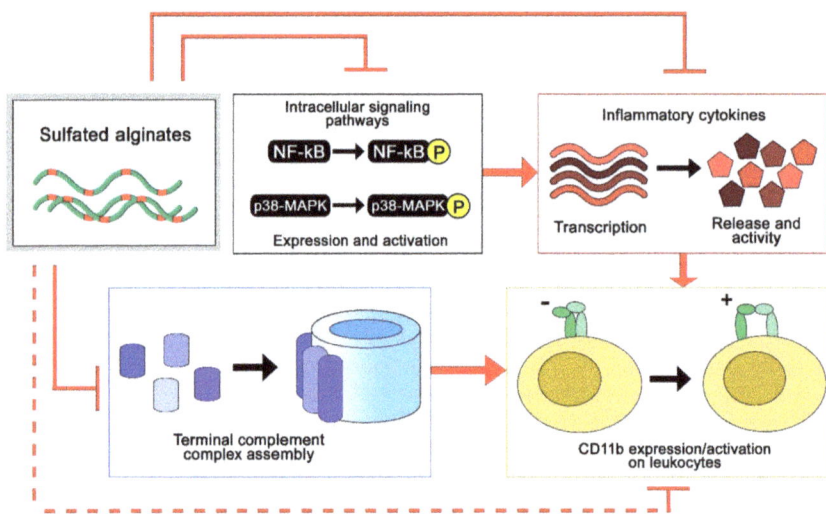

Figure 5. Anti-inflammatory effects of sulfated alginates from whole blood and cell culture models [58,65].

2.6. Sulfated Alginates in Tissue Engineering and Drug Delivery

The use of heparin and other GAGs in biomaterials intended for long-term implantation is limited partly due to their rapid turnover in vivo. The exploration of more stable analogues has therefore been encouraged for a range of applications in tissue engineering and encapsulation of therapeutics. Cohen and co-workers initially reported sulfated alginates to associate with multiple heparin-binding growth factors, highlighting their potential to serve as a reservoir and a slow-release system for growth factors toward tissue cultivation and drug delivery [48]. Sulfated alginate hydrogels loaded with growth factors were further found to promote angiogenesis and blood perfusion in animal tissues, and have been formulated as injectable solutions for gelation in situ [71,72]. In a separate study, heterogeneous hydrogels with layered organization of specific growth factors were found to support compartmentalized differentiation of mesenchymal stem cells into osteoblasts and chondrocytes [73]. In a recent study, Ruvinov and colleagues proposed a model where the multiple heparin-binding proteins and sulfated alginate chains spontaneously assemble into nanoparticles with a fiber-like structure and a net negative surface charge, which can subsequently be immobilized in injectable hydrogels such as unmodified alginates or various nanoparticle formulations [74]. This demonstrates a great potential and versatility for formulating hydrogel- and nanoparticle-based delivery of heparin-binding proteins, whereas modifications to the structure and sequence of the sulfated alginates can additionally contribute to the release rate by tuning the interaction strength with various proteins [43,44]. In addition to providing prolonged delivery of growth factors through their associative retention, the binding of sulfated alginate has been demonstrated to protect the proteins from proteolytic cleavage by trypsin [74], which is one of the postulated effects of heparin and other sulfated glycosaminoglycans in regulating cell signaling.

Zenobi-Wong and colleagues initially employed sulfated alginate hydrogels for the cultivation of cartilage, and found that the gels promoted proliferation and prolonged viability of the chondrocytes (Figure 6). Furthermore, the sulfated alginates were able to sustain the cartilaginous phenotype over long culture times, demonstrated by a high degree of collagen 2 expression and repressed collagen 1 expression [46]. The inductive effect on chondrocyte proliferation was attenuated by blocking beta1 integrins, indicating that the sulfated alginates interact (presumably indirectly) with integrins and potentially other adhesion proteins on the cell surface to support anchorage and migration. The chondrogenic effects were additionally related to a high degree of FGF retention in the hydrogels, where the sulfated alginates are proposed to act as a co-receptor to the cellular FGF receptor, analogous to heparan sulfate in vivo [56]. This was indicated by the ability of sulfated alginates to restore FGF-mediated proliferation of HS-deficient BaF3 cells [56], and was later reproduced by Li and co-workers utilizing additional growth factors and different sequences of sulfated alginate [61]. Due to their beneficial effects on chondrocyte proliferation and phenotype maintenance, sulfated alginates have further been evaluated as a component in bioinks for 3D-bioprinting, including nanocellulose fibers to retain the shape of printed structures prior to ionic crosslinking [75].

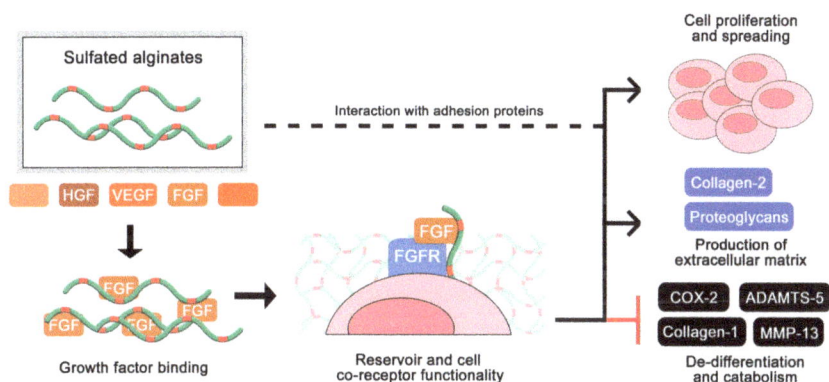

Figure 6. Sulfated alginates bind multiple growth factors [48], and have an inductive effect in chondrocyte cultivation [46,56,58].

Whereas the degradation of sulfated alginates has not yet been studied in vivo, alginates are not depolymerized by any known enzyme in mammals. Sulfated alginates may thus provide more stable hydrogels for long-term implants, where alteration of the sulfation degree, monosaccharide sequence, and gelling conditions can tune properties such as swelling and porosity, degradability, and retention of matrix-binding proteins. Despite a low inflammatory response from the innate immune system, in vivo experiments in certain rat models and primates have uncovered a fibrotic reaction to pure alginate implants, which will presumably occur in human subjects as well and impair the function of the hydrogels and encapsulated cells. As elaborated in the previous section, sulfated alginates show potent anti-inflammatory properties, which can reduce immunological rejection and fibrosis toward long-term implants and potentially overcome these challenges with alginate-based biomaterials. The encapsulation of cells in biomimetic matrices is a highly relevant approach for generating more advanced in vitro tissue models, and for clinical tissue engineering including matrix-assisted cell implantation and injectable matrices such as supporting scaffolds for tissue repair [76,77].

2.7. Structure-Function Relationships in Sulfated Alginates

The conformations of M and G are $^4C_1$ and $^1C_4$, respectively, with glycosidic bonds that are di-equatorial, di-axial, or equatorial-axial for MM, GG, and MG, resulting in varying orientations of the sulfated C2 and C3 hydroxyl groups (Figure 2). The sequences vary in their extension and rigidity, where the GG sequences have a more compact conformation with higher charge density per unit length compared with MM. The MG sequence was initially demonstrated by Smidsrød and colleagues to have a more flexible backbone compared with MM and GG [55], which is also supported by its higher solubility in water at low pH [78]. Similar to heparin, structural and conformational properties, alongside the negative charge density, can influence the interaction strength between sulfated alginates and proteins, emphasizing the importance of characterizing structure-function relationships.

Oligosaccharides of sulfated alginates have been utilized to study the minimal degree of polymerization (DP) required for binding to proteins. In one of our studies using a sulfated alternating alginate sequence (S-MG, DS~0.9), a minimum length of 8-mer was required for significant interaction with HGF, whereas 14-mers approached the interaction strength of poly-S-MG (DP = 80) and LMWH. For FGF-2, a low degree of interaction was observed for 6-mers of S-MG, whereas the 14-mers did not show the efficacy of poly-SMG. Overall, the S-MG samples showed a lower degree of interaction with FGF-2 compared with HGF, and did not approach the efficacy of heparin. Liu and co-workers prepared and sulfated (DS~1.5) M-rich oligosaccharides obtained from hydrolysis and separation of algal alginate, and studied the binding interaction to HIV envelope protein gp120, as a potential anti-HIV therapy. It was demonstrated that a minimal length of an 8-mer was required for interaction, whereas multivalent interactions were observed for >15–16 mers as well as a higher binding affinity compared with heparin [79]. As alginates can be reproducibly hydrolysed and separated into low-disperse fractions based on size and monosaccharide composition, optimizing the molecular weight of samples can potentially contribute to reducing adverse effects in therapeutic applications, similarly to the use of UFH/LMWH/ULMWH.

To assess the impact of the alginate monosaccharide sequence, we initially utilized homogeneous sequences (poly-M, poly-G, and poly-MG) of sulfated alginates with similar sulfation degrees and analysed the interaction with HGF [44]. Here, it was found that at high sulfation degrees (DS~1) the efficacy of the varying sequences was similar, whereas at intermediate sulfation degrees (DS~0.5) the interaction strength increased in the order of poly-M < poly-G < poly-MG. This points towards an influence of chain flexibility as the highly sulfated alginates are presumed to display a more rigid conformation, thus reducing the effect of backbone flexibility in the unmodified alginate sequences. To further investigate the effect of chain flexibility, we performed a periodate oxidation of sulfated poly-M alginates, causing hexuronic ring opening in non-sulfated monosaccharides and an introduction of flexible junction zones [43]. This resulted in increased interaction strength with HGF and FGF-2, correlated with the oxidation degree of the sulfated alginates. The importance of chain flexibility is expected to vary between proteins of different sizes and surface patterns of basic amino acid residues. It was discovered that sulfated poly-M alginates interacted more strongly to FGF-2 than the sulfated poly-MG alginates, while periodate oxidation had a smaller impact on interaction strength compared with that for HGF, indicating that the monosaccharide structure and charge orientation contributes to interaction strength alongside chain flexibility. This was again demonstrated by Li and co-workers, who found that sulfated G-rich oligosaccharides were more effective that M-rich oligosaccharides at prolonging coagulation time, and at mediating FGF-8 signalling in BaF3 cell cultures [61]. As over-sulfated alginates may exert a high degree of non-specific and potential adverse effects, chemo-enzymatic engineering of the backbone may provide a versatile tool to improve interaction strengths and potentially confer increased ligand selectivity compared to sulfation alone, similarly to the role of IdoA in heparin and heparan sulfate.

3. Conclusions and Future Directions

From the present status of knowledge, sulfated alginates show in particular promise for cell immobilization and tissue engineering applications, as presented through the works of Zenobi-Wong and Cohen with their respective groups. The sulfated alginates act as analogues of cell surface GAGs in mediating growth factor signalling, while creating a biomimetic physical environment for the proliferation and migration of cells, extracellular matrix deposition, and tissue maturation. Similarly, the sulfated alginate matrix may provide a reservoir for growth factors, where the affinity toward specific growth factors may be altered through chemo-enzymatic engineering of the alginate, for a tuned and sustained delivery to tissues. There have further been demonstrated anti-inflammatory properties in sulfated alginates, which can aid in matrix-assisted cell- and tissue transplantations by suppressing pro-catabolic and inflammatory responses from surrounding tissues and in encapsulated cells. However, additional in vivo studies to assess gel stability, immunological and fibrotic responses, and implant survival are required. Non-coagulating heparins have previously been evaluated for anti-inflammatory and anti-cancer therapeutics, highlighting an additional potential application for heparin analogues with customizable pharmacokinetic and -dynamic properties in treating acute and chronic inflammatory conditions.

Several studies on sulfated alginates have focused on their anti-coagulant properties. However, there are no clear indications of specific antithrombin activation, where substantially higher concentrations of sulfated alginates are required to approach the efficacy of heparin. While sequences of sulfated alginate with a higher affinity for antithrombin can potentially be generated through chemo-enzymatic engineering, emulation of the specific heparin pentasaccharide may prove challenging. As an intravenously administered drug with rapid onset, heparin benefits from a short half-life. Sulfated alginates are presumably eliminated through renal excretion alone, which is a slower mechanism compared to depolymerization, where extended activity may lead to a severe drop in blood pressure and additional adverse effects. The use of sulfated alginates as anticoagulants can therefore show greater promise as a coating for medical devices and biomaterials, where a high surface stability is desirable and the additional anti-inflammatory effects can potentially reduce fibrosis or immunological rejection of implanted devices or materials.

Chemical sulfation of alginates allows for the simple and reproducible synthesis of heparin-like molecules in large batches and at low cost. However, much work remains to explore novel strategies for milder and more selective syntheses, to further characterize and understand their interaction with heparin-binding proteins, and to evaluate the potential of sulfated alginates toward novel biomedical applications. Compared to GAGs and other heparin analogues, the utility of sulfated alginates is tied to their gelling capability and their structural customizability, allowing tuning of physical and biological properties, and bioavailability. The majority of studies have employed commercial algal alginates and have performed sulfation of C2 and C3, whereas exploring non-conventional sequence patterns (alternative sources, enzymatic engineering), novel sulfation strategies (M/G preference, C6-sulfation), and conjugation to other functional groups can provide new properties and potentially improved selectivity of protein interactions. Ideally, a sulfated alginate oligosaccharide library with defined modification patterns can be established and applied to gain a deeper understanding of their structure-function relationships. In conclusion, sulfated alginates have unique characteristics as heparin analogues, and while they are relatively unstudied, they demonstrate a wide range of biological properties and a structural versatility that can provide novel biomedical applications and a deeper understanding of the biological functions of sulfated glycosaminoglycans.

Acknowledgments: This work was supported by the Norwegian Research Council through the MARPOL project (grant no. 221576), and by SINTEF Materials and Chemistry, Trondheim, Norway.

Author Contributions: Ø.A. and G.S.-B. reviewed the literature and wrote the paper.

Conflicts of Interest: The authors declare no conflict of interest.

References

1. Liu, H.Y.; Zhang, Z.Q.; Linhardt, R.J. Lessons Learned from the Contamination of Heparin. *Nat. Prod. Rep.* **2009**, *26*, 313–321. [CrossRef] [PubMed]
2. Lindahl, U.; Li, J.P.; Kusche-Gullberg, M.; Salmivirta, M.; Alaranta, S.; Veromaa, T.; Emeis, J.; Roberts, I.; Taylor, C.; Oreste, P.; et al. Generation of "Neoheparin" from E Coli K5 Capsular Polysaccharide. *J. Med. Chem.* **2005**, *48*, 349–352. [CrossRef] [PubMed]
3. Codee, J.D.C.; Stubba, B.; Schiattarella, M.; Overkleeft, H.S.; van Boeckel, C.A.A.; van Boom, J.H.; van der Marel, G.A. A Modular Strategy toward the Synthesis of Heparin-Like Oligosaccharides Using Monomeric Building Blocks in a Sequential Glycosylation Strategy. *J. Am. Chem. Soc.* **2005**, *127*, 3767–3773. [CrossRef] [PubMed]
4. Jiao, G.L.; Yu, G.L.; Zhang, J.Z.; Ewart, H.S. Chemical Structures and Bioactivities of Sulfated Polysaccharides from Marine Algae. *Mar. Drugs* **2011**, *9*, 196–223. [CrossRef] [PubMed]
5. Deng, J.; Liu, X.Y.; Ma, L.; Cheng, C.; Shi, W.B.; Nie, C.X.; Zhao, C.S. Heparin-Mimicking Multilayer Coating on Polymeric Membrane Via Lbl Assembly of Cyclodextrin-Based Supramolecules. *ACS Appl. Mater. Interfaces* **2014**, *6*, 21603–21614. [CrossRef] [PubMed]
6. Sasisekharan, R.; Venkataraman, G. Heparin and Heparan Sulfate: Biosynthesis, Structure and Function. *Curr. Opin. Chem. Biol.* **2000**, *4*, 626–631. [CrossRef]
7. Raman, R.; Venkataraman, G.; Ernst, S.; Sasisekharan, V.; Sasisekharan, R. Structural Specificity of Heparin Binding in the Fibroblast Growth Factor Family of Proteins. *Proc. Natl. Acad. Sci. USA* **2003**, *100*, 2357–2362. [CrossRef] [PubMed]
8. Habuchi, H.; Tanaka, M.; Habuchi, O.; Yoshida, K.; Suzuki, H.; Ban, K.; Kimata, K. The Occurrence of Three Isoforms of Heparan Sulfate 6-*O*-Sulfotransferase Having Different Specificities for Hexuronic Acid Adjacent to the Targeted *N*-Sulfoglucosamine. *J. Biol. Chem.* **2000**, *275*, 2859–2868. [CrossRef] [PubMed]
9. Aikawa, J.; Grobe, K.; Tsujimoto, M.; Esko, J.D. Multiple Isozymes of Heparan Sulfate/Heparin Glcnac *N*-Deacetylase/Glcn *N*-Sulfotransferase-Structure and Activity of the Fourth Member, Ndst4. *J. Biol. Chem.* **2001**, *276*, 5876–5882. [CrossRef] [PubMed]
10. Sudo, M.; Sato, K.; Chaidedgumjorn, A.; Toyoda, H.; Toida, T.; Imanari, T. H-1 Nuclear Magnetic Resonance Spectroscopic Analysis for Determination of Glucuronic and Iduronic Acids in Dermatan Sulfate, Heparin, and Heparan Sulfate. *Anal. Biochem.* **2001**, *297*, 42–51. [CrossRef] [PubMed]
11. Guerrini, M.; Bisio, A.; Torri, G. Combined Quantitative H-1 and C-13 Nuclear Magnetic Resonance Spectroscopy for Characterization of Heparin Preparations. *Semin. Thromb. Hemost.* **2001**, *27*, 473–482. [CrossRef] [PubMed]
12. Maccarana, M.; Sakura, Y.; Tawada, A.; Yoshida, K.; Lindahl, U. Domain Structure of Heparan Sulfates from Bovine Organs. *J. Biol. Chem.* **1996**, *271*, 17804–17810. [CrossRef] [PubMed]
13. Hagner-McWhirter, A.; Lindahl, U.; Li, J.P. Biosynthesis of Heparin/Heparan Sulphate: Mechanism of Epimerization of Glucuronyl C-5. *Biochem. J.* **2000**, *347*, 69–75. [CrossRef] [PubMed]
14. Raedts, J.M.; Lundgren, M.; Kengen, S.W.M.; Li, J.P.; van der Oost, J. A Novel Bacterial Enzyme with D-Glucuronyl C5-Epimerase Activity. *J. Biol. Chem.* **2013**, *288*, 24332–24339. [CrossRef] [PubMed]
15. Lidholt, K.; Fjelstad, M.; Jann, K.; Lindahl, U. Biosynthesis of Heparin 25. Substrate Specificities of Glycosyltransferases Involved in Formation of Heparin Precursor and Escherichia-Coli K5 Capsular Polysaccharides. *Carbohydr. Res.* **1994**, *255*, 87–101. [CrossRef]
16. Lindahl, U.; Backstrom, G.; Hook, M.; Thunberg, L.; Fransson, L.A.; Linker, A. Structure of the Antithrombin-Binding Site in Heparin. *Proc. Natl. Acad. Sci. USA* **1979**, *76*, 3198–3202. [CrossRef] [PubMed]
17. Hansen, S.U.; Miller, G.J.; Cliff, M.J.; Jaysonc, G.C.; Gardiner, J.M. Making the Longest Sugars: A Chemical Synthesis of Heparin-Related [4](N) Oligosaccharides from 16-Mer to 40-Mer. *Chem. Sci.* **2015**, *6*, 6158–6164. [CrossRef]
18. Rosenberg, R.D. Actions and Interactions of Antithrombin and Heparin. *N. Engl. J. Med.* **1975**, *292*, 146–151. [PubMed]
19. Sahu, A.; Pangburn, M.K. Identification of Multiple Sites of Interaction between Heparin and the Complement-System. *Mol. Immunol.* **1993**, *30*, 679–684. [CrossRef]

20. Amara, U.; Flierl, M.A.; Rittirsch, D.; Klos, A.; Chen, H.; Acker, B.; Bruckner, U.B.; Nilsson, B.; Gebhard, F.; Lambris, J.D.; et al. Molecular Intercommunication between the Complement and Coagulation Systems. *J. Immunol.* **2010**, *185*, 5628–5636. [CrossRef] [PubMed]

21. Gandhi, N.S.; Mancera, R.L. The Structure of Glycosaminoglycans and Their Interactions with Proteins. *Chem. Biol. Drug Des.* **2008**, *72*, 455–482. [CrossRef] [PubMed]

22. Nelson, R.M.; Cecconi, O.; Roberts, W.G.; Aruffo, A.; Linhardt, R.J.; Bevilacqua, M.P. Heparin Oligosaccharides Bind L-Selectin and P-Selectin and Inhibit Acute-Inflammation. *Blood* **1993**, *82*, 3253–3258. [PubMed]

23. Joyce, J.G.; Tung, J.S.; Przysiecki, C.T.; Cook, J.C.; Lehman, E.D.; Sands, J.A.; Jansen, K.U.; Keller, P.M. The L1 Major Capsid Protein of Human Papillomavirus Type 11 Recombinant Virus-Like Particles Interacts with Heparin and Cell-Surface Glycosaminoglycans on Human Keratinocytes. *J. Biol. Chem.* **1999**, *274*, 5810–5822. [CrossRef] [PubMed]

24. Ascencio, F.; Fransson, L.A.; Wadstrom, T. Affinity of the Gastric Pathogen Helicobacter-Pylori for the N-Sulfated Glycosaminoglycan Heparan-Sulfate. *J. Med. Microbiol.* **1993**, *38*, 240–244. [CrossRef] [PubMed]

25. Spillmann, D.; Lindahl, U. Glycosaminoglycan Protein Interactions-a Question of Specificity. *Curr. Opin. Struct. Biol.* **1994**, *4*, 677–682. [CrossRef]

26. Lindahl, U. A Personal Voyage through the Proteoglycan Field. *Matrix Biol.* **2014**, *35*, 3–7. [CrossRef] [PubMed]

27. Hu, Y.P.; Zhong, Y.Q.; Chen, Z.G.; Chen, C.Y.; Shi, Z.; Zulueta, M.M.; Ku, C.C.; Lee, P.Y.; Wang, C.C.; Hung, S.C. Divergent Synthesis of 48 Heparan Sulfate-Based Disaccharides and Probing the Specific Sugar-Fibroblast Growth-Factor-1 Interaction. *J. Am. Chem. Soc.* **2012**, *134*, 20722–20727. [CrossRef] [PubMed]

28. Foxall, C.; Holme, K.R.; Liang, W.H.; Wei, Z. An Enzyme-Linked-Immunosorbent-Assay Using Biotinylated Heparan-Sulfate to Evaluate the Interactions of Heparin-Like Molecules and Basic Fibroblast Growth-Factor. *Anal. Biochem.* **1995**, *231*, 366–373. [CrossRef] [PubMed]

29. Wang, L.C.; Brown, J.R.; Varki, A.; Esko, J.D. Heparin's Anti-Inflammatory Effects Require Glucosamine 6-O-Sulfation and Are Mediated by Blockade of L- and P-Selectins. *J. Clin. Investig.* **2002**, *110*, 127–136. [CrossRef] [PubMed]

30. Koenig, A.; Norgard-Sumnicht, K.; Linhardt, R.; Varki, A. Differential Interactions of Heparin and Heparan Sulfate Glycosaminoglycans with the Selectins-Implications for the Use of Unfractionated and Low Molecular Weight Heparins as Therapeutic Agents. *J. Clin Investig.* **1998**, *101*, 877–889. [CrossRef] [PubMed]

31. Skjåk-Bræk, G.; Donari, I.; Paoletti, S. Alginate Hydrogels: Properties and Applications. In *Polysaccharide Hydrogels*; Matricardi, P., Alhaique, F., Coviello, T., Eds.; Pan Stanford: Boca Raton, FL, USA, 2015.

32. Sarrazin, S.; Lamanna, W.C.; Esko, J.D. Heparan Sulfate Proteoglycans. *Cold Spring Harbor Perspect. Biol.* **2011**, *3*, 1–33. [CrossRef] [PubMed]

33. Stokke, B.T.; Smidsrød, O.; Bruheim, P.; Skjåk-Bræk, G. Distribution of Uronate Residues in Alginate Chains in Relation to Alginate Gelling Properties. *Macromolecules* **1991**, *24*, 4637–4645. [CrossRef]

34. Mørch, Y.A.; Donati, I.; Strand, B.L.; Skjåk-Bræk, G. Molecular Engineering as an Approach to Design New Functional Properties of Alginate. *Biomacromolecules* **2007**, *8*, 2809–2814. [CrossRef] [PubMed]

35. Høidal, H.K.; Ertesvåg, H.; Skjåk-Bræk, G.; Stokke, B.T.; Valla, S. The Recombinant Azotobacter Vinelandii Mannuronan C-5-Epimerase Alge4 Epimerizes Alginate by a Nonrandom Attack Mechanism. *J. Biol. Chem.* **1999**, *274*, 12316–12322. [CrossRef] [PubMed]

36. Pawar, S.N.; Edgar, K.J. Alginate Derivatization: A Review of Chemistry, Properties and Applications. *Biomaterials* **2012**, *33*, 3279–3305. [CrossRef] [PubMed]

37. Ertesvåg, H. Alginate-Modifying Enzymes: Biological Roles and Biotechnological Uses. *Front. Microbiol.* **2015**, *6*, 1–10.

38. Jacobs-Tulleneers-Thevissen, D.; Chintinne, M.; Ling, Z.; Gillard, P.; Schoonjans, L.; Delvaux, G.; Strand, B.L.; Gorus, F.; Keymeulen, B.; Pipeleers, D.; et al. Sustained Function of Alginate-Encapsulated Human Islet Cell Implants in the Peritoneal Cavity of Mice Leading to a Pilot Study in a Type 1 Diabetic Patient. *Diabetologia* **2013**, *56*, 1605–1614. [CrossRef] [PubMed]

39. Zhang, J.; Wang, Q.; Wang, A. In Situ Generation of Sodium Alginate/Hydroxyapatite Nanocomposite Beads as Drug-Controlled Release Matrices. *Acta Biomate.* **2010**, *6*, 445–454. [CrossRef] [PubMed]

40. Sandvig, I.; Karstensen, K.; Rokstad, A.M.; Aachmann, F.L.; Formo, K.; Sandvig, A.; Skjåk-Bræk, G.; Strand, B.L. Rgd-Peptide Modified Alginate by a Chemoenzymatic Strategy for Tissue Engineering Applications. *J. Biomed. Mater. Res. Part A* **2015**, *103*, 896–906. [CrossRef] [PubMed]

41. Markstedt, K.; Mantas, A.; Tournier, I.; Martinez, H.; Hägg, D.; Gatenholm, P. 3D Bioprinting Human Chondrocytes with Nanocellulose-Alginate Bioink for Cartilage Tissue Engineering Applications. *Biomacromolecules* **2015**, *16*, 1489–1496. [CrossRef] [PubMed]

42. Huang, R.H.; Du, Y.M.; Yang, J.H. Preparation and in Vitro Anticoagulant Activities of Alginate Sulfate and Its Quaterized Derivatives. *Carbohydr. Polym.* **2003**, *52*, 19–24.

43. Arlov, Ø.; Aachmann, F.L.; Feyzi, E.; Sundan, A.; Skjåk-Bræk, G. The Impact of Chain Length and Flexibility in the Interaction between Sulfated Alginates and Hgf and Fgf-2. *Biomacromolecules* **2015**, *16*, 3417–3424. [CrossRef] [PubMed]

44. Arlov, Ø.; Aachmann, F.L.; Sundan, A.; Espevik, T.; Skjåk-Bræk, G. Heparin-Like Properties of Sulfated Alginates with Defined Sequences and Sulfation Degrees. *Biomacromolecules* **2014**, *15*, 2744–2750. [CrossRef] [PubMed]

45. Miyaji, H.; Misaki, A. Distribution of Sulfate Groups in the Partially Sulfated Dextrans. *J. Biochem.* **1973**, *74*, 1131–1139. [CrossRef] [PubMed]

46. Mhanna, R.; Kashyap, A.; Palazzolo, G.; Vallmajo-Martin, Q.; Becher, J.; Möller, S.; Schnabelrauch, M.; Zenobi-Wong, M. Chondrocyte Culture in Three Dimensional Alginate Sulfate Hydrogels Promotes Proliferation While Maintaining Expression of Chondrogenic Markers. *Tissue Engl. Part A* **2014**, *20*, 1454–1464. [CrossRef] [PubMed]

47. Ma, L.; Cheng, C.; Nie, C.X.; He, C.; Deng, J.; Wang, L.R.; Xia, Y.; Zhao, C.S. Anticoagulant Sodium Alginate Sulfates and Their Mussel-Inspired Heparin-Mimetic Coatings. *J. Mater. Chem. B* **2016**, *4*, 203–215. [CrossRef]

48. Freeman, I.; Kedem, A.; Cohen, S. The Effect of Sulfation of Alginate Hydrogels on the Specific Binding and Controlled Release of Heparin-Binding Proteins. *Biomaterials* **2008**, *29*, 3260–3268. [CrossRef] [PubMed]

49. Fan, L.H.; Jiang, L.; Xu, Y.M.; Zhou, Y.; Shen, Y.A.; Xie, W.G.; Long, Z.H.; Zhou, J.P. Synthesis and Anticoagulant Activity of Sodium Alginate Sulfates. *Carbohydr. Polym.* **2011**, *83*, 1797–1803. [CrossRef]

50. Zhao, X.; Yu, G.L.; Guan, H.S.; Yue, N.; Zhang, Z.Q.; Li, H.H. Preparation of Low-Molecular-Weight Polyguluronate Sulfate and Its Anticoagulant and Anti-Inflammatory Activities. *Carbohydr. Polym.* **2007**, *69*, 272–279. [CrossRef]

51. Lindahl, U.; Kusche-Gullberg, M.; Kjellen, L. Regulated Diversity of Heparan Sulfate. *J. Biol. Chem.* **1998**, *273*, 24979–24982. [CrossRef] [PubMed]

52. Dodgson, K.S.; Price, R.G. A Note on the Determination of the Ester Sulphate Content of Sulphated Polysaccharides. *Biochem. J.* **1962**, *84*, 106–110. [CrossRef] [PubMed]

53. Yang, J.H.; Du, Y.M.; Huang, R.H.; Wan, Y.Y.; Wen, Y. The Structure-Anticoagulant Activity Relationships of Sulfated Lacquer Polysaccharide—Effect of Carboxyl Group and Position of Sulfation. *Int. J. Biol. Macromol.* **2005**, *36*, 9–15. [CrossRef] [PubMed]

54. Heymann, B.; Grubmuller, H. Chair-Boat' Transitions and Side Groups Affect the Stiffness of Polysaccharides. *Chem. Phys. Lett.* **1999**, *305*, 202–208. [CrossRef]

55. Smidsrød, O.; Glover, R.M.; Whittington, S.G. The Relative Extension of Alginates Having Different Chemical Composition. *Carbohydr. Res.* **1973**, *27*, 107–118. [CrossRef]

56. Öztürk, E.; Arlov, Ø.; Aksel, S.; Li, L.; Ornitz, D.M.; Skjåk-Bræk, G.; Zenobi-Wong, M. Sulfated Hydrogel Matrices Direct Mitogenicity and Maintenance of Chondrocyte Phenotype through Activation of Fgf Signaling. *Adv. Funct. Mater.* **2016**, *26*, 3649–3662. [CrossRef]

57. Grant, G.T.; Morris, E.R.; Rees, D.A.; Smith, P.J.C.; Thom, D. Biological Interactions between Polysaccharides and Divalent Cations-Egg-Box Model. *Febs. Lett.* **1973**, *32*, 195–198. [CrossRef]

58. Arlov, Ø.; Steinwachs, M.; Skjåk-Bræk, G.; Zenobi-Wong, M. Biomimetic Sulphated Alginate Hydrogels Suppress Il-1beta-Induced Inflammatory Responses in Human Chondrocytes. *Eur. Cell. Mater.* **2017**, *33*, 76–89. [CrossRef] [PubMed]

59. Mørch, Ý.A.; Donati, I.; Strand, B.L.; Skjåk-Bræk, G. Effect of Ca^{2+}, Ba^{2+}, and Sr^{2+} on Alginate Microbeads. *Biomacromolecules* **2006**, *7*, 1471–1480. [CrossRef] [PubMed]

60. Draget, K.I.; Østgaard, K.; Smidsrød, O. Homogeneous Alginate Gels-a Technical Approach. *Carbohydr. Polym.* **1990**, *14*, 159–178. [CrossRef]

61. Li, Q.C.; Zeng, Y.Y.; Wang, L.L.; Guan, H.S.; Li, C.X.; Zhang, L.J. The Heparin-Like Activities of Negatively Charged Derivatives of Low-Molecular-Weight Polymannuronate and Polyguluronate. *Carbohydr. Polym.* **2017**, *155*, 313–320. [CrossRef] [PubMed]

62. Mousa, S.A.; Mohamed, S. Inhibition of Endothelial Cell Tube Formation by the Low Molecular Weight Heparin, Tinzaparin, Is Mediated by Tissue Factor Pathway Inhibitor. *Thromb. Haemost.* **2004**, *92*, 627–633. [CrossRef] [PubMed]

63. Ma, L.; Cheng, C.; He, C.; Nie, C.X.; Deng, J.; Sun, S.D.; Zhao, C.S. Substrate-Independent Robust and Heparin-Mimetic Hydrogel Thin Film Coating Via Combined Lbl Self-Assembly and Mussel-Inspired Post-Cross-Linking. *ACS Appl. Mater. Interfaces* **2015**, *7*, 26050–26062. [CrossRef] [PubMed]

64. Niimi, Y.; Ichinose, F.; Ishiguro, Y.; Terui, K.; Uezono, S.; Morita, S.; Yamane, S. The Effects of Heparin Coating of Oxygenator Fibers on Platelet Adhesion and Protein Adsorption. *Anesth. Analg.* **1999**, *89*, 573–579. [PubMed]

65. Arlov, Ø.; Skjåk-Bræk, G.; Rokstad, A.M. Sulfated Alginate Microspheres Associate with Factor H and Dampen the Inflammatory Cytokine Response. *Acta Biomater.* **2016**, *42*, 180–188. [CrossRef] [PubMed]

66. Weiler, J.M.; Edens, R.E.; Linhardt, R.J.; Kapelanski, D.P. Heparin and Modified Heparin Inhibit Complement Activation Invivo. *J. Immunol.* **1992**, *148*, 3210–3215. [PubMed]

67. Oikonomopoulou, K.; Ricklin, D.; Ward, P.A.; Lambris, J.D. Interactions between Coagulation and Complement-Their Role in Inflammation. *Semin. Immunopathol.* **2012**, *34*, 151–165. [CrossRef] [PubMed]

68. Spivak-Kroizman, T.; Lemmon, M.A.; Dikic, I.; Ladbury, J.E.; Pinchasi, D.; Huang, J.; Jaye, M.; Crumley, G.; Schlessinger, J.; Lax, I. Heparin-Induced Oligomerization of Fgf Molecules Is Responsible for Fgf Receptor Dimerization, Activation, and Cell-Proliferation. *Cell* **1994**, *79*, 1015–1024. [CrossRef]

69. Izaki, S.; Goldstein, S.M.; Fukuyama, K.; Epstein, W.L. Fibrin Deposition and Clearance in Chronic Granulomatous Inflammation: Correlation with T-Cell Function and Proteinase Inhibitor Activity in Tissue. *J. Investig. Dermatol.* **1979**, *73*, 561–565. [CrossRef] [PubMed]

70. Lukacs, N.W.; Chensue, S.W.; Strieter, R.M.; Warmington, K.; Kunkel, S.L. Inflammatory Granuloma-Formation Is Mediated by Tnf-Alpha-Inducible Intercellular-Adhesion Molecule-1. *J. Immunol.* **1994**, *152*, 5883–5889. [PubMed]

71. Ruvinov, E.; Leor, J.; Cohen, S. The Effects of Controlled Hgf Delivery from an Affinity-Binding Alginate Biomaterial on Angiogenesis and Blood Perfusion in a Hindlimb Ischemia Model. *Biomaterials* **2010**, *31*, 4573–4582. [CrossRef] [PubMed]

72. Freeman, I.; Cohen, S. The Influence of the Sequential Delivery of Angiogenic Factors from Affinity-Binding Alginate Scaffolds on Vascularization. *Biomaterials* **2009**, *30*, 2122–2131. [CrossRef] [PubMed]

73. Re'em, T.; Witte, F.; Willbold, E.; Ruvinov, E.; Cohen, S. Simultaneous Regeneration of Articular Cartilage and Subchondral Bone Induced by Spatially Presented Tgf-Beta and Bmp-4 in a Bilayer Affinity Binding System. *Acta Biomater.* **2012**, *8*, 3283–3293. [CrossRef] [PubMed]

74. Ruvinov, E.; Freeman, I.; Fredo, R.; Cohen, S. Spontaneous Coassembly of Biologically Active Nanoparticles Via Affinity Binding of Heparin-Binding Proteins to Alginate-Sulfate. *Nano Lett.* **2016**, *16*, 883–888. [CrossRef] [PubMed]

75. Müller, M.; Ece, Ö.; Øystein, A.; Paul, G.; Zenobi-Wong, M. Alginate Sulfate–Nanocellulose Bioinks for Cartilage Bioprinting Applications. *Annals Biomed. Eng.* **2016**, *45*, 210–223. [CrossRef] [PubMed]

76. Makris, E.A.; Gomoll, A.H.; Malizos, K.N.; Hu, J.C.; Athanasiou, K.A. Repair and Tissue Engineering Techniques for Articular Cartilage. *Nat. Rev. Rheumatol.* **2015**, *11*, 21–34. [CrossRef] [PubMed]

77. Duflo, S.; Thibeault, S.L.; Li, W.H.; Shu, X.Z.; Prestwich, G.D. Vocal Fold Tissue Repair in Vivo Using a Synthetic Extracellular Matrix. *Tissue Eng.* **2006**, *12*, 2171–2180. [CrossRef] [PubMed]

78. Hartmann, M.; Dentini, M.; Draget, K.I.; Skjåk-Bræk, G. Enzymatic Modification of Alginates with the Mannuronan C-5 Epimerase Alge4 Enhances Their Solubility at Low Ph. *Carbohydr. Poly.* **2006**, *63*, 257–262. [CrossRef]

79. Liu, H.Y.; Geng, M.Y.; Xin, X.L.; Li, F.C.; Zhang, Z.Q.; Li, J.; Ding, J. Multiple and Multivalent Interactions of Novel Anti-Aids Drug Candidates, Sulfated Polymannuronate (Spmg)-Derived Oligosaccharides, with Gp120 and Their Anti-Hiv Activities. *Glycobiology* **2005**, *15*, 501–510. [CrossRef] [PubMed]

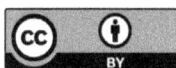

Article

Self-Assembled Lipid Nanoparticles for Oral Delivery of Heparin-Coated Iron Oxide Nanoparticles for Theranostic Purposes

Eleonora Truzzi [1], Chiara Bongio [2], Francesca Sacchetti [1], Eleonora Maretti [1], Monica Montanari [3], Valentina Iannuccelli [1], Elena Vismara [2,*] and Eliana Leo [1,*]

1. Department of Life Sciences, University of Modena and Reggio Emilia, via Campi 103, 41125 Modena, Italy; eleonora.truzzi@unimore.it (E.T.); francesca.sacchetti@unimore.it (F.S.); eleonora.maretti@unimore.it (E.M.); valentina.iannuccelli@unimore.it (V.I.)
2. Department of Chemistry, Materials and Chemical Engineering "G. Natta", via Mancinelli 7, Politecnico di Milano, 20131 Milano, Italy; chiara.bongio@polimi.it
3. Department of Life Sciences, University of Modena and Reggio Emilia, via Campi 287, 41125 Modena, Italy; monica.montanari@unimore.it
* Correspondence: elena.vismara@polimi.it (E.V.); eliana.leo@unimore.it (E.L.); Tel.: +39-02-2399-3098 (E.V.); +39-059-205-8558 (E.L.)

Academic Editors: Giangiacomo Torri and Jawed Fareed
Received: 12 May 2017; Accepted: 5 June 2017; Published: 9 June 2017

Abstract: Recently, solid lipid nanoparticles (SLNs) have attracted increasing attention owing to their potential as an oral delivery system, promoting intestinal absorption in the lymphatic circulation which plays a role in disseminating metastatic cancer cells and infectious agents throughout the body. SLN features can be exploited for the oral delivery of theranostics. Therefore, the aim of this work was to design and characterise self-assembled lipid nanoparticles (SALNs) to encapsulate and stabilise iron oxide nanoparticles non-covalently coated with heparin (Fe@hepa) as a model of a theranostic tool. SALNs were characterised for physico-chemical properties (particle size, surface charge, encapsulation efficiency, in vitro stability, and heparin leakage), as well as in vitro cytotoxicity by methyl thiazole tetrazolium (MTT) assay and cell internalisation in CaCo-2, a cell line model used as an indirect indication of intestinal lymphatic absorption. SALNs of about 180 nm, which are stable in suspension and have a high encapsulation efficiency (>90%) were obtained. SALNs were able to stabilise the heparin coating of Fe@hepa, which are typically unstable in physiological environments. Moreover, SALNs–Fe@hepa showed no cytotoxicity, although their ability to be internalised into CaCo-2 cells was highlighted by confocal microscopy analysis. Therefore, the results indicated that SALNs can be considered as a promising tool to orally deliver theranostic Fe@hepa into the lymphatic circulation, although further in vivo studies are needed to comprehend further potential applications.

Keywords: theranostics; solid lipid nanoparticles; iron oxide nanoparticles; heparin coating; intestinal lymphatic absorption

---

1. Introduction

Currently, oral delivery is the most accepted route of drug administration, even though it is associated with poor drug bioavailability. One of the most promising strategies to overcome these limitations is the use of nanomedicine or nano-drug delivery systems [1]. As an example, solid lipid nanoparticles (SLNs) have attracted increasing attention owing to their biocompatibility and biodegradability. SLNs are composed of lipids in a solid state at room temperature and surfactants. They are produced using hot or cold homogenisation without the employment of organic solvents and generally have low production costs. SLNs offer advantages such as good tolerability, high oral drug bioavailability and low acute and chronic toxicity [2,3]. Moreover, being composed of lipids, SLNs have shown good potential in achieving drug delivery into the systemic circulation through intestinal lymphatic absorption [4–6]. After oral administration, small and hydrophilic substances enter in the systemic circulation by a passive absorption mechanism through enterocytes. On the contrary, large and lipophilic compounds with a logP $\geq$ 5 (where P is the octanol/water partition coefficient), such as components of SLNs, are metabolically stable (in the intestinal lumen and within enterocytes) and can be considered good candidates for lymphatic transport to the systemic circulation [7]. Drug adsorption via the intestinal lymphatic system has several major advantages, including circumventing first-pass metabolism and targeting drugs to diseases that spread through the lymphatic system. For example, cancer cells use the lymph nodes as a reservoir to spread to the other areas of the body [8].

The main ways to deliver drugs to intestinal lymphatic vessels are through lymphatic capillaries, gut-associated lymphoid follicles that form Peyer's patch, and finally the intestinal walls via transcellular absorption. This last route is the lymphatic target of lipid-based nanoformulations because during transit across the enterocyte the lipids become associated with chylomicrons which are secreted into the mesenteric lymph duct [9–12].

SLNs have to satisfy certain requirements to achieve lymphatic delivery. It was observed that the uptake and fate of SLNs are influenced by particle size, surface hydrophobicity, type of lipids, and concentration of the emulsifier [1,6,13]. Also, the surface charge plays an important role: negatively-charged carriers have been reported to show higher lymphatic uptake than neutral or positively-charged particles [1,9,14]. SLNs promote lymphatic absorption and can also be exploited for theranostic purposes, which to the best of our knowledge, have not been extensively investigated [15]. Theranostics is the fusion of therapeutic and diagnostic approaches aiming to personalise and advance medicine. Magnetic nanoparticles (MNPs) represent a particularly appropriate tool based on their ability to be simultaneously functionalised and guided by external magnetic fields [16]. Some MNPs-based therapeutic applications include magnetic fluid hyperthermia (MFH), magnetic resonance imaging (MRI) and magnetic drug targeting [17,18]. In this field, iron oxide (Fe_3O_4) MNPs provide a unique nanoplatform with tunable sizes and surface chemistry studied extensively for MRI and MFH applications [19]. Without a coating, MNPs have hydrophobic surfaces with a high area to volume ratio and a propensity to agglomerate. An appropriate surface coating allows MNPs to be and remain homogenously dispersed for longer times. Several materials have been used to modify the surface of MNPs, such as organic polymers (dextran, chitosan, polyethylene glycol), organic surfactants (sodium oleate and dodecylamine), and metals [16]. Vismara et al. proposed the use of heparin as a non-covalent coating for iron oxide nanoparticles (Fe@hepa) [20]. Heparin, a natural polysaccharide with many bioactive properties, is a heterogeneous, polydispersed, highly sulphated glycosaminoglycan composed of 1 $\rightarrow$ 4 linked disaccharide repeating units. Each unit consists of an α-D-glucosamine and either a hexuronic acid, α-L-idruronic or β-D-glucoronicacid unit, with O-sulphate groups at different positions of the disaccharide. Various studies have demonstrated that heparin and low-molecular-weight heparins, in addition to having anticoagulant properties, are anti-angiogenic agents and can be used as vectors to reach tumour sites due to their ability to bind over-expressed proteins [21–23]. Thanks to these features, the heparin coating specifically directs iron oxide nanoparticles to tumour environments in order to accomplish the theranostic aim. Moreover, Vismara et al. demonstrated an increased stability in a water suspension of Fe@hepa nanoparticles with respect to naked iron oxide by conferring a negative charge due to the heparin coating [20]. However, the heparin surface shell is instable in physiologic environment where the presence of ions reduces the strength of the electrostatic bond between the positive iron oxide core and the negative heparin chain.

Therefore, the purpose of the present work was to design a nano-theranostic tool based on Fe@hepa nanoparticles for oral absorption through the lymphatic route. To the best of our knowledge, in the theranostic field poor attention has been addressed to the study of this promising approach. In order to stabilise the heparin coating in physiological environments, and at the same time promote oral absorption through the lymphatic route, Fe@hepa were encapsulated in a biocompatible solid lipid shell to obtain self-assembled lipid nanoparticles (SALNs). SALNs were obtained by self-emulsification process and were characterised with regard to their size, encapsulation efficiency, in vitro cytotoxicity and ability to be internalised into the CaCo-2 cell line (colon rectal adenocarcinoma cell line of human origin) used as a model for an indirect indication of lymphatic uptake.

2. Results

2.1. SALN Characterisation

By using the original self-emulsification process, two SALNs–Fe@hepa samples were developed using 1 or 5 mg of Fe@hepa (namely SALNs–Fe@hepa1 and SALNs–Fe@hepa5, respectively). The particle size, polydispersity index (PDI) and Z-potential values obtained with photon correlation spectroscopy (PCS) analysis are shown in Table 1. No differences in the particle size nor in the PDI values were observed, regardless of the amount of Fe@hepa used (all the samples were roughly of 180 nm with a PDI of 0.3), while the negative charge of the particle surface (Z-potential value) increased with the increase of the initial amount of Fe@hepa utilised in the preparation. The particle size was monitored for one month and no significant changes were observed (data not shown). The size and the Z-potential of naked Fe@hepa were previously reported [20] and were 92 nm and −61 mV, respectively.

Table 1. Size, polydispersity index (PDI) and Z-potential values of loaded and unloaded self-assembled lipid nanoparticles (SALNs). Fe@hepa1: iron oxide nanoparticles non-covalently coated with heparin (1 mg); Fe@hepa5: iron oxide nanoparticles non-covalently coated with heparin (5 mg).

Sample	Size (nm)	PDI	Z-Potential (mV)
Unloaded SALNs	182 ± 15	0.295 ± 0.015	−16.4 ± 4.7
SALNs–Fe@hepa1	183 ± 18	0.278 ± 0.008	−15.5 ± 5.8
SALNs–Fe@hepa5	186 ± 21	0.364 ± 0.013	−24.0 ± 5.5

2.2. Morphological Studies

Morphological characterisation of the samples was performed using the scanning electron microscopy analysis (SEM modality) to visualise the particles in solid form, while the scanning transmission electron microscopy analysis (STEM modality) was used to observe the samples as suspension. Both the analyses were performed in high-vacuum conditions. Figure 1A shows, as an example, the image of SALNs–Fe@hepa1 at high magnification (100,000×) using the SEM technique. Even if SALNs appear aggregated in clusters, each single particle can be clearly recognised as a distinct solid structure with a roughly spherical morphology.

By STEM modality (Figure 1B), unloaded SALNs in suspension are hardly detectable due to their intrinsically low electron density that limits the resolution. However, even if the particles appear as weak-contrast dark formations, their imperfectly spherical morphology is easily observable.

Figure 1C,D shows the STEM images of loaded particles (SALNs–Fe@hepa5). At low magnification (Figure 1C), SALNs–Fe@hepa5 appear irregular in the shape, as observed also for the unloaded particles, but with a darker inner structure. The high-contrast dark part in the core region of each particle can be assigned to the Fe@hepa clusters, while the clear part surrounding the core regions can be attributable to the lipid shell. At high magnification (Figure 1D) one single particle with a rough contour is observed. Within the particle, even if not perfectly in the centre, dark small dots, due to clusters of Fe@hepa nanoparticles, are clearly visible. The clusters appear surrounded by a weak-contrast dark part attributable to the lipid matrix, according to the images of the unloaded sample (Figure 1B). The particle sizes of SALNs–Fe@hepa5 as well as of the Fe@hepa nanoparticles are also consistent with PCS analysis results reported in Table 1 and in previous studies [20], respectively.

To confirm the composition of the particles observed by the electron microscopy analysis, the qualitative energy dispersive X-ray (EDX) analysis was performed by the single-point method. A single loaded nanoparticle, as observed in the image reported in Figure 1D, was analysed in comparison with an individual unloaded nanoparticle and the qualitative composition was reported in the EDX spectra representing the plots of X-ray counts vs. elements. In spectrum relating to SALNs–Fe@hepa, the peak of iron is clearly visible (Figure 2A), while it is absent in unloaded particles (Figure 2B), confirming the presence of Fe@hepa into the loaded SALNs. In the spectra, the presence of Al and Si are probably due to the support used for the analyses.

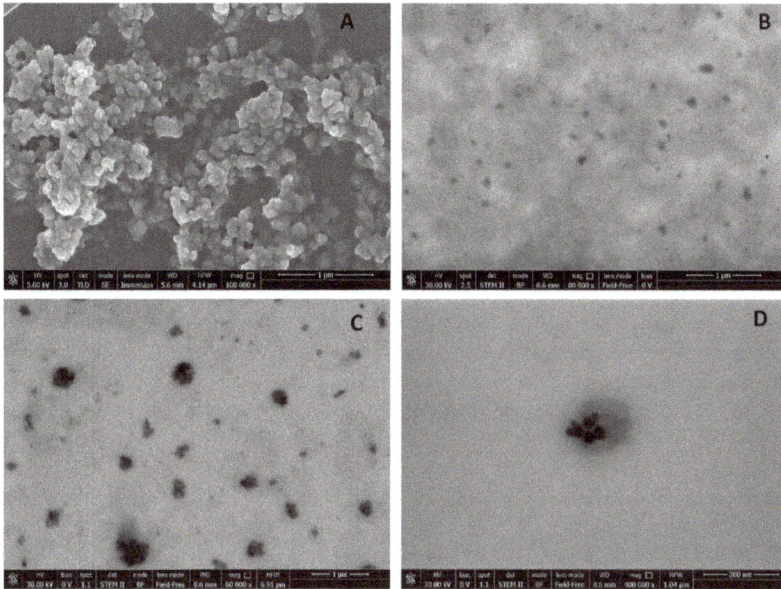

Figure 1. (**A**) SEM microphotograph of SALNs–Fe@hepa1 at high magnification (100,000×); (**B**) Representative scanning transmission electron microscopy (STEM) image of unloaded SALNs; (**C**) Representative STEM image of SALNs–Fe@hepa5 at low magnification (60,000×); (**D**) Representative STEM image of SALNs–Fe@hepa5 at high magnification (400,000×).

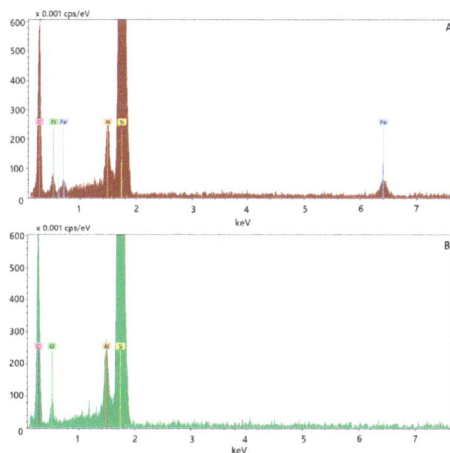

Figure 2. Energy dispersive X-ray (EDX) spectra referred to SALNs–Fe@hepa5 (**A**) and unloaded SALNs (**B**).

2.3. Drug Loading and Encapsulation Efficiency

The amount of Fe@hepa loaded inside SALNs was calculated by indirect method, i.e., analysing the non-encapsulated amount of Fe@hepa. No significant differences are observed in the encapsulation efficiency (EE%) between the samples ($p > 0.05$), while the drug loading (DL) increases five-fold in SALNs-Fe@hepa5 ($p < 0.001$) (Table 2).

Table 2. Encapsulation efficiency (EE%) and drug loading (DL) of SALNs–Fe@hepa.

Sample	EE%	DL (μg Fe@hepa/mg SALNs-Fe@hepa)
SALNs–Fe@hepa1	86.6 ± 2.76	5.14 ± 0.01
SALNs–Fe@hepa5	91.5 ± 3.09	26.38 ± 0.70

2.4. In Vitro SALNs-Fe@hepa Stability

In order to verify the retention of Fe@hepa in SALNs stored as suspension at 4 °C, the spontaneous Fe@hepa sedimentation from SALNs–Fe@hepa was monitored for both the samples for one month after the preparation (t_0). At predetermined time interval, the amount of Fe@hepa separated from the suspension was measured by spectrophotometric method. These data were subtracted from the initial Fe@hepa loading and the results are reported in the graph (Figure 3). The data indicate that SALNs–Fe@hepa5 are more stable compared to the SALNs–Fe@hepa1. Indeed, for this sample, after 4 days, the loss of the cargo was only 4% compared to the initial content, indicating a good stability of the system. Then, a very slow sedimentation rate of free Fe@hepa is observed in the remaining time until a total loss of 6%. On the contrary, SALNs–Fe@hepa1 appeared quite instable in suspension, showing a fast initial loss of cargo corresponding to about 11% in 4 days followed by a slower phase of Fe@hepa release up to a total loss of 20% in one month. Therefore, given the weak stability in suspension of SALNs–Fe@hepa1, this sample was not taken into account in the further experiments.

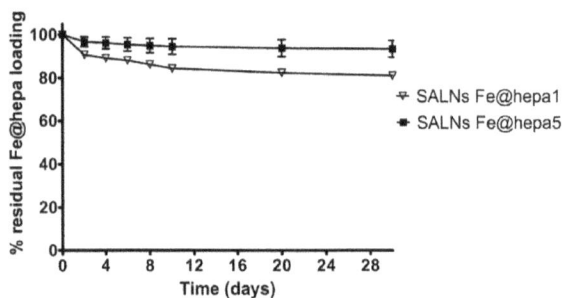

Figure 3. Percentage of Fe@hepa released from SALNs-Fe@hepa1 and SALNs–Fe@hepa5 stored as a suspension at 4 °C for one month, where 100% corresponds to initial SALNs–Fe@hepa drug loading. Error bars indicate standard deviation (SD); where not visible, error bars did not exceed symbol size.

2.5. Stabilisation of Heparin Coating

In order to evaluate if the encapsulation of the Fe@hepa into SALNs was able to stabilise the heparin coating, the leakage of heparin form both naked Fe@hepa and SALNs-Fe@hepa5 was measured in physiologic solution (NaCl 0.9%). Indeed, the heparin shell is stable in water [20] but in the presence of saline medium the interaction between heparin and iron oxide became weaker, resulting in the release of heparin and in the loss of stability of the colloidal suspension [24]. Therefore, to measure the stability of the coating, experimental conditions with minimal perturbation (saline solution) were considered and the amount of heparin released after only 1 h at room temperature was evaluated. As reported in Table 3, in the case of naked Fe@hepa, as expected, a leakage of about 70% of the initial amount of heparin occurred while in the case of the SALNs–Fe@hepa5 no release of heparin in solution was observed in the time period considered.

Table 3. Evaluation of the amount of heparin released in saline solution from SALNs–Fe@hepa5 and naked Fe@hepa.

Sample	Mass of Fe@hepa (µg)	Initial Amount of Heparin in Fe@hepa (µg)	% of Heparin Released in NaCl 0.9%
SALNs–Fe@hepa5	810	72.9	0
Fe@hepa	620	55.8	72

2.6. Cytotoxicity Assay

In order to determine the in vitro cytotoxicity of SALNs–Fe@hepa5 compared to naked Fe@hepa and unloaded SALNs, the methyl thiazole tetrazolium test (MTT) was performed on the intestinal CaCo-2 cell line after different incubation times (2, 4, and 6 h). For each time, various concentrations of SALNs (0.8, 1.2, 1.6, 2 mg/mL) and the respective amount of Fe@hepa (21, 32, 42, 53 µg/mL) were tested and the results are reported in Figure 4. The cytotoxicity of Fe@hepa is always higher than that of the other samples, but the cellular viability never dropped below 74%. Unloaded SALNs show a higher cell viability with respect to the control, while SALNs–Fe@hepa5 show a cell viability intermediate between the other two samples. However, significant differences are evident only within unloaded SALNs and the other two samples at the concentration of 2 mg/mL after 2 and 4 h of treatment.

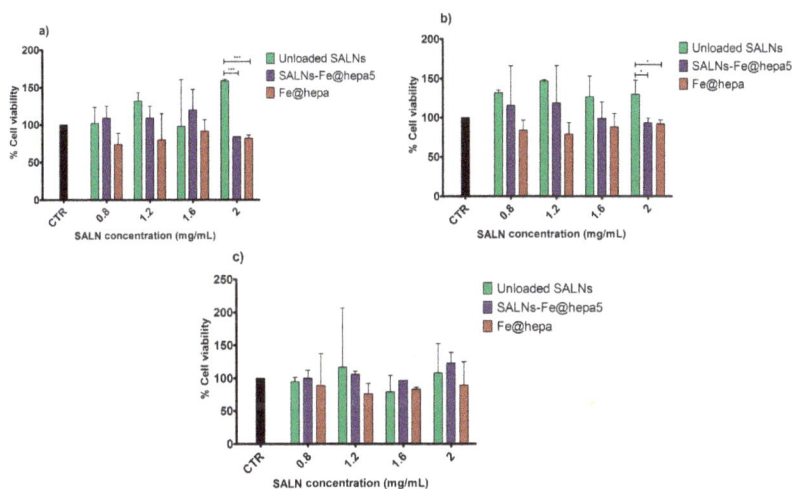

Figure 4. Analyses of cytotoxicity of the samples at different concentrations on CaCo-2 cells (colon rectal adenocarcinoma cell line of human origin) after 2 (**a**), 4 (**b**) and 6 h (**c**) of treatment, using methyl thiazole tetrazolium test (MTT) assay. SALN concentrations of 0.8, 1.2, 1.6, 2 mg/mL correspond to 21, 32, 42, 53 µg/mL of naked Fe@hepa, respectively. Comparison between samples was performed by ANOVA one-way test. Statistical significance levels were defined as: * ($p < 0.05$), *** ($p < 0.001$). Error bars indicate SD; where not visible, error bars did not exceed symbol size.

2.7. Quantification of SALNs–Fe@hepa in the CaCo-2 Cell Line

Considering the results obtained from the study of cytotoxicity, the concentration of SALNs equal to 2 mg/mL (corresponding to 53 µg/mL of Fe@hepa) is considered optimal to study the internalisation of the systems in the CaCo-2 cell line, a colorectal cell line adopted as a model for lymphatic absorption [10,25].

Cells were preventively incubated for 2, 4 and 6 h with naked Fe@hepa and SALNs–Fe@hepa5, washed with phosphate buffer saline (PBS) and then lysated.

The percentages of iron oxide found in the cell lysate respect to the amount used for the incubation are shown in Figure 5. After two hours of incubation, the percentage of iron oxide present into cell lysate was the same for both the samples (naked Fe@hepa and SALNs–Fe@hepa5). For the other incubation times, iron oxide in cell lysate resulted higher after the treatment with naked Fe@hepa. Moreover, a time-dependent correlation can be noticed: the amount of iron oxide increases with the increasing incubation time. Significant differences can be observed between the samples after 4 and 6 h of incubation ($p < 0.05$).

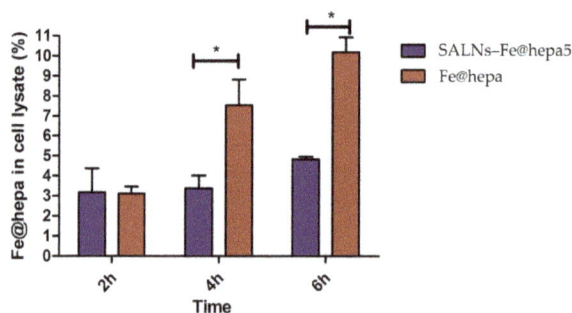

Figure 5. Quantification of iron oxide in CaCo-2 cells after 2, 4 and 6 h of treatment with SALNs–Fe@hepa5 at the concentration of 2 mg/mL (corresponding to 53 μg/mL of Fe@hepa) and naked Fe@hepa at the concentration of 53 μg/mL. A comparison between samples was performed by ANOVA one-way test. Statistical significance levels were defined as: * ($p < 0.05$).

In order to visualise the internalisation of the sample in the CaCo-2 cell model (Figure 6), confocal laser scanning microscopy analysis was performed. Cellular nuclei were stained in blue, SALNs were labelled in red, while Fe@hepa, owing to their density, were visible as black spots in white-light channel.

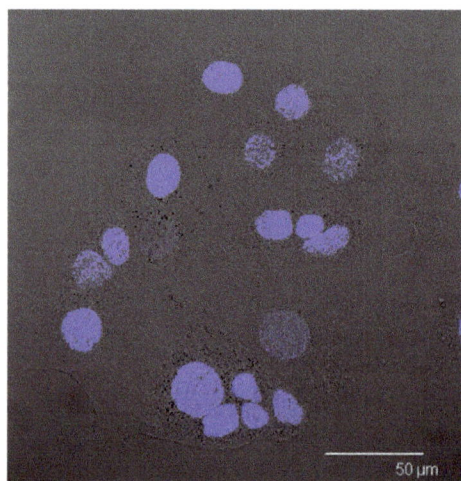

Figure 6. Confocal microscopy image of CaCo-2 cells after nuclei staining with Hoechst.

CaCo-2 cells were treated with Nile red-labelled unloaded SALNs, Nile red-labelled SALNs–Fe@hepa5 and naked Fe@hepa. Figure 7A shows CaCo-2 cells incubated with Fe@hepa. Black spots with different sizes, attributed to clusters of iron oxide nanoparticles, are visible near the cytoplasm but clearly in a different z-thickness compared to the nuclei.

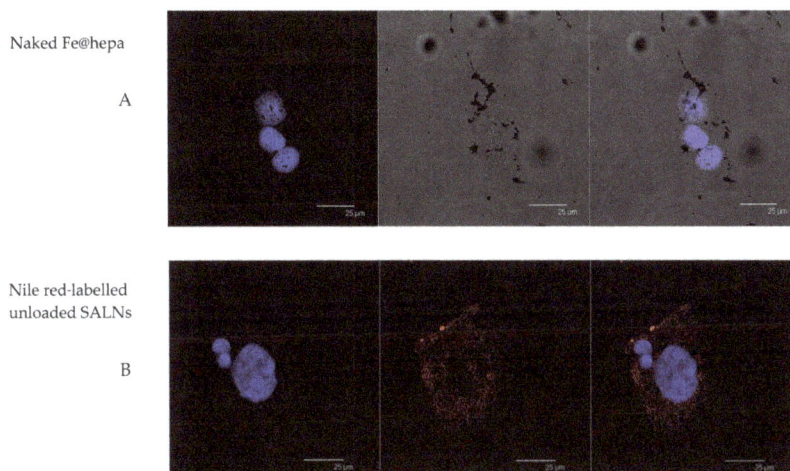

Figure 7. (**A**) Confocal microscopy images of CaCo-2 cells after nuclei staining and 4 h incubation with naked Fe@hepa. From left to right: blue channel (Hoechst), white-light channel and merged image. (**B**) Confocal microscopy images of CaCo-2 cells after nuclei staining and 4 h of incubation with Nile red-labelled unloaded SALNs. From left to right: blue channel (Hoechst), red channel (Nile red) and merged image.

After incubation with Nile red-labelled unloaded SALNs (Figure 7B), red fluorescence is noticeable around the nuclei of CaCo-2 cells. Red spots are attributable to Nile red-labelled SALNs because no red fluorescence is observed in untreated CaCo-2 cells (Figure 6). The image clearly indicates that SALNs are localised inside the cells because the red fluorescence is located in the area surrounding the nuclei correspondent to the cytoplasm.

After treatment with Nile red-labelled SALNs-Fe@hepa5 (Figure 8), in addition to red spots, it is possible to appreciate, in a white-light channel, a grey shading around the nuclei where also red fluorescence is located. Moreover, black spots attributable to Fe@hepa clusters are clearly visible externally to cells revealing the presence of non-encapsulated Fe@hepa, which have tendency to form clusters outside the cells.

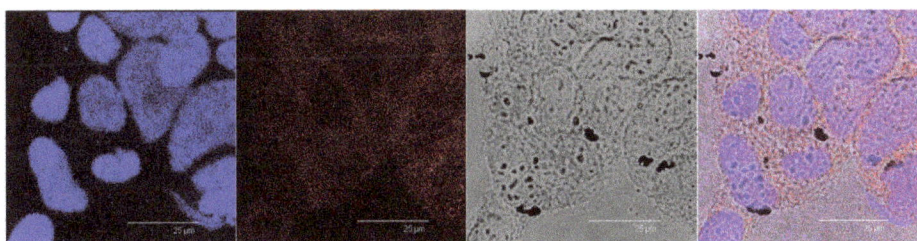

Figure 8. Confocal microscopy images of CaCo-2 cells after nuclei staining and 4 h of incubation with Nile red-labelled SALNs-Fe@hepa5. From left to right: blue channel (Hoechst), red channel (Nile red), white-light channel and merged image.

3. Discussion

Iron oxide nanoparticles have attracted considerable interest due to their superparamagnetic properties and their potential biomedical applications. The dimensions of these nanoparticles make them ideal candidates for nano-engineering of surfaces to develop non-toxic and biocompatible nanoparticles. Moreover, different coating materials can prevent their irreversible aggregation in aqueous or biological media [26]. Vismara et al. proposed heparin coating as an attractive strategy to achieve a theranostic aim exploiting anti-angiogenic activity of native heparin [20]. However, this coating is instable in physiological conditions. The goal of this work was to stabilise Fe@hepa by encapsulation in SALNs, envisaging an oral absorption through a lymphatic route.

SALNs are biocompatible, biodegradable, and can be used as controlled drug delivery and targeting system. Owing to their composition, SALNs possess a structure very similar to that of glyceride-rich chylomicrons which are believed to allow lymphatic transport of drugs into the intestinal lymphatic circulation [27].

It is known that lipid nanoparticles based on triglycerides with a high carbon chain length are less susceptible to intestinal lipase than those composed of a shorter carbon chain and are preferably transported into the intestinal lymphatic system [11,25,28]. For this reason, Geleol™ and Gelucire 50/13® high carbon chain length lipids, both generally recognised as safe and biocompatible materials (manufacturer's information), were selected as the lipid matrix for the SALN preparation. Moreover, these lipids have a low melting point, avoiding the risk of degradation of the drug during the preparation. Gelucire 50/13® is composed of mono-, di-, and triglycerides with mono- and di-fatty acid esters of polyethylene glycol (PEG). Owing to the composition, it exhibits surfactant and solubility enhancing properties that can be exploited to better incorporate lipophilic compounds and to stabilise the lipid nanosystem [29,30]. Moreover, it has been demonstrated that Gelucire® decreases P-glycoprotein efflux, making it a good candidate to gain lymphatic uptake [31,32].

After different formulation attempts, the preparation was optimised to achieve a reproducible and stable colloidal suspension without an observed particle dimensional change when Fe@hepa were encapsulated in the lipid matrix. The average diameter (around 180 nm) and the lipid nature of the particles make this system potentially suitable for intestinal lymphatic uptake associated with chylomicrons synthesised within enterocytes [1,6]. Alternatively, large molecular weight drug-carrier constructs may be selectively taken up intact via the lymphatic system because their large size favours uptake via the leakier structure of the lymphatic vessels, as compared to blood capillaries [33]. The size of the particles suitable for this pathway is a controversial matter [34]. However, it is recognised that the minute size of this formulation enables efficient uptake into the intestine, particularly via the lymphatic route, favoured by particles between 20 and 500 nm in diameter [9].

Regarding the zeta potential, unloaded SALNs measured slightly negative (−16 mV), and became progressively more negative with increasing amounts of Fe@hepa. Considering that Fe@hepa are strongly negative (about −61 mV) due to the presence of heparin coating, the more negative surface charge observed for SALNs–Fe@hepa with respect to unloaded SALNs can be attributable to a portion of Fe@hepa next to the SALN surface as observed in the STEM pictures (Figure 1C,D).

Morphological studies were performed to better understand the nanoparticle structure. The images obtained by SEM modality on the dried samples confirmed that the structure of the system is solid due to the lipid core made of solid components (Gelucire 50/13® and Geleol™), as can be seen in Figure 1A. However, the SEM modality does not allow the observation of particle contour due to the poor resolution under low-voltage operating conditions (5 kV). Thus, pictures of SALNs in suspension were obtained in STEM modality, highlighting a rough surface structure probably due to the presence of a mixture of the two lipids in the particle matrix. In Figure 1D, at high magnification, it is possible to observe black spots, attributable to Fe@hepa. The clusters of Fe@hepa appear surrounded by the lipid matrix and the presence of Fe@hepa nanoparticles located in a peripheral position in the SALNs are also visible (Figure 1C,D). The presence of Fe@hepa close to the surface of the particles might explain the negative Z-potential value noticed for SALNs–Fe@hepa5. In addition, this finding is in agreement with EDX analysis that shows the superficial elemental composition of the particles. Indeed, EDX study shows the clear presence of iron in the spectrum of SALNs-Fe@hepa (Figure 2A) while no iron signal is evident in the spectrum of unloaded SALNs. On the other hand, the incorporation of Fe@hepa into the lipid matrix, as observed by electronic microscopy, should lead to a stabilisation of the heparin coating. To confirm if this goal was achieved, the release of heparin from the system in physiologic solution was evaluated comparing naked Fe@hepa and SALNs–Fe@hepa. The results (Table 3) show that no heparin was released from the SALNs–Fe@hepa sample, indicating that the encapsulation of Fe@hepa inside SALNs is a good strategy to avoid the loss of heparin coating occurring for the naked Fe@hepa. Indeed, heparin, selected as an iron oxide coating for its antiangiogenic features in tumour environments [21–23], is linked to the particle surface by ionic bonds between the positive iron oxide core and its negative chain. Therefore, Fe@hepa are destabilised in biological isotonic fluid where the electrostatic interaction between iron oxide and heparin become weaker. On the other hand, when Fe@hepa are surrounded by lipid matrix, the interaction with the biological fluids is avoided and no leakage of heparin occurs.

To better understand the potential of Fe@hepa–loaded SALNs, the particles were prepared using two different dosages (1 or 5 mg). The analyses indicate that in both SALNs–Fe@hepa samples the percentage of Fe@hepa incorporated is around 90%. This means that, increasing the initial loading, the encapsulation efficiency remains stable, suggesting that using only 1 mg of Fe@hepa the loading capacity of the lipid system was far from saturation. As evidence of this, increasing the initial amount of drug by five-fold, the loading increases proportionally from 5.14 µg/mg to 26.4 µg/mg (Table 2). However, during storage it was possible to notice a progressive sediment of Fe@hepa, indicating a probable desorption of Fe@hepa nanoparticles from the system. For this reason, the stability of SALNs–Fe@hepa samples was monitored for one month after the preparation (Figure 3). The data indicated that during one month, the higher loaded sample (SALNs–Fe@hepa5) was by far more stable than the less loaded sample (SALNs–Fe@hepa1). It can be assumed that in both the cases, the initial rapid loss of cargo is probably due to Fe@hepa non-embedded inside the lipid matrix or highly dispersed in the suspension. Afterwards, a release of Fe@hepa with a slower rate was observed; this was attributed to a leakage of Fe@hepa owing to its high density and to the magnetic forces between iron oxide nanoparticles. The results indicate clearly that the loss of Fe@hepa was larger for the lower loaded sample (SALNs–Fe@hepa1). To explain this finding, it can be assumed that when high amounts of Fe@hepa are embedded in the lipid matrix, the forces of attraction within Fe@hepa clusters are prevalent, stabilising the cargo. On the contrary, when poor amounts of Fe@hepa are loaded, the forces of attraction of the clusters inside the particles are weaker in respect to the attraction of the non-embedded particles, leading to a progressive leakage of the cargo. For this reason, all subsequent studies on cells were conducted using only the most loaded and stable sample (SALNs–Fe@hepa5).

The MTT assay on CaCo-2 cells was performed after different times of exposure (2, 4, 6 h) to compare the cytotoxicity induced by unloaded SALNs, naked Fe@hepa, and SALNs–Fe@hepa5. The CaCo-2 cell line was used because it has been reported to be an indirect indication of intestinal lymphatic transport [10,25]. The results of the analyses indicated that the lipids used to develop SALNs are not toxic but, on the contrary, they seem to improve the cell viability as the percentage of cell vitality observed after the treatment with unloaded SALNs resulted equal to or higher than the control (Figure 4). Only a slight cytotoxicity was observed for naked Fe@hepa since cell viability, at the experimental conditions adopted, never dropped below 74% compared to the control. Cytotoxicity studies reported in the literature and conducted on naked iron oxide nanoparticles demonstrated that these systems induce a reduction of cell viability depending on their coating, time of exposure, concentrations and cell type evaluated [35–37]. Thus, the results obtained in this work demonstrated that the coating with heparin allows biocompatible and non-toxic nanoparticles to be obtained. The cytotoxicity of SALNs–Fe@hepa falls in the middle between that of unloaded SALNs and Fe@hepa at all concentrations and incubation times considered, probably because the partial negative effects of Fe@hepa are compensated by the positive effect of unloaded SALNs. Therefore, it is possible to conclude that all the samples, at all the concentrations tested, do not exhibit toxicity on CaCo-2 cell model and the results indicate that the cytotoxicity is neither time- nor concentration-dependent. For this reason, to carry out the studies regarding the ability of the particles to enter the CaCo2 cells, the highest concentration (cell viability more than 80%) has been selected and therefore all the experiments were conducted using the concentration of 2 mg/mL.

The ability of the particles to enter in CaCo-2 cells was evaluated by measuring the amount of iron transported in the cells by the two systems (Fe@hepa and SALNs-Fe@hepa5). The results (Figure 5) indicated that the amount of iron found in the cells was higher for the cells incubated with naked Fe@hepa respect to cells incubated with SALNs–Fe@hepa, especially for longer incubation times. These findings seem to be in contrary to expectations because in the literature SALNs resulted able to improve the internalisation of drugs thanks to their composition [4–6]. However, it is important to notice that the higher percentage of iron found in the cells treated with Fe@hepa might be due to the precipitation of naked iron oxide on the bottom of the wells, because of the loss of the heparin coating in biological fluids. Indeed, during the experiments, it was observed that in the case of cells treated with naked Fe@hepa, dark spots attributable to iron remained attached to the well bottom, even after the washing with PBS (see Section 4.11). On the contrary, in the case of cells incubated with SALNs–Fe@hepa5, the non-internalised particles were easily removed with washing owing to the low density of their lipid composition. As a result, in the case of cells treated with Fe@hepa an overestimation of Fe@hepa associated with the cells might have occurred.

In order to support this assumption, confocal laser scanning microscopy analysis was performed using Nile red as a probe to visualise SALNs in the red channel, while no probe was used for Fe@hepa since their clusters appeared as dark spots by observation in white-light channel. Observing the cells treated with Fe@hepa, the dark spots attributed to the Fe@hepa clusters seem to be localised in a different z-thickness compared to nuclei, indicating that they were not internalised by CaCo-2 cells (Figure 7A). This observation indicated that iron clusters had not entered the cells, giving evidence of the overestimation of Fe@hepa associated with the cells. On the contrary, both unloaded SALNs and SALNs–Fe@hepa5 seem to be internalised in the cells because a slight red fluorescence is noticeable around the nuclei, highlighting that the particles were localised in the cytoplasm. However, the iron particles embedded in the SALNs were not visible, probably owing to their small dimension even thought they could be considered responsible of the grey shading visible around the nuclei (Figure 8). On the other hand, regarding the black spots visible outside the cells in the image of cells incubated with SALNs–Fe@hepa, they could be attributable to Fe@hepa not embedded in the lipid matrix but only absorbed on the surface or highly dispersed in the suspension according to what was observed in the in vitro stability studies (Figure 7).

4. Materials and Methods

4.1. Chemicals

Geleol™ (Glycerol Monostearate 40–55, type I) and Gelucire 50/13® Pellets (Stearoyl Macrogol-32 Glycerides) were a kind gift from Gattefossè (Saint-Priest, France). Fe@hepa (containing 9% w/w of heparin) were provided by the laboratory of Prof. E. Vismara and synthesised as previously described [20]. Azure II and Nile red were purchased from Sigma-Aldrich Italia (Milan, Italy). Potassium thiocyanate was purchased from Carlo Erba Reagenti (Milan, Italy). Hoechst 33342 stain was purchased from ThermoFisher (Monza, Italy). Dulbecco's Modified Eagle's Medium with high glucose (DMEM), L-glutamine, fetal bovine serum (FBS), penicillin–streptomycin (P/S), phosphate buffer saline (PBS), sodium pyruvate and other culture reagents were purchased from EuroClone (Milan, Italy).

A MilliQ water system (Millipore; Bedford, MA, USA) provided high purity water (18.2 MΩ) for these experiments.

All other chemical reagents were obtained commercially as reagent-grade products.

4.2. SALN Formulation

SALNs were obtained by a self-assembling process using an original technique in which no organic solvents were employed (Figure 9). Briefly, a mixture of Geleol:Gelucire 1:1 *w/w* was melted at 65 °C after the addition of 50 μL of MilliQ water containing Fe@hepa (1 or 5 mg) and emulsified by ultrasound energy (Vibra-Cell, Sonic & Materials, Inc. 53 Church Hill Road, Newton, CT, USA) at 10 output Watt for 30 s. This water/oil (W/O) dispersion was rapidly solidified in ice bath and then added to 15 mL of MilliQ water, previously heated at 65 °C. To obtain the SALNs, the dispersion was homogenized for 3 min at 24,000 rpm by Ultra Turrax (T-25 basic IkaLabortecnik, Staufen, Germany) and then cooled in ice for about 10 min to allow the SALN solidification. SALNs–Fe@hepa were purified by centrifugation at 2000 rpm for 5 min at 20 °C (Rotina 380R, Hettich, Kirchlengern, Germany) to remove the non-encapsulated Fe@hepa. The purified suspensions of SALNs were stored at +4 °C. Unloaded SALNs were obtained omitting the addition of Fe@hepa in the 50 μL of MilliQ water, while labelled SALNs for cell internalisation studies were obtained by adding Nile red (0.01%) in the melted Geleol™.

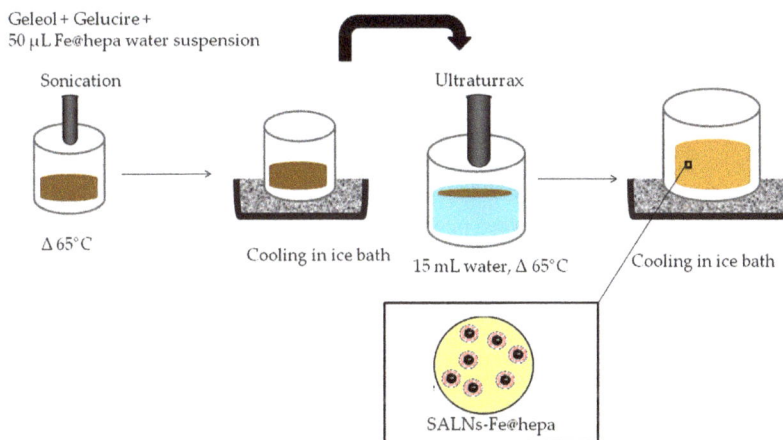

Figure 9. Scheme of self-assembling process used for SALN formulation.

4.3. SALN Characterisation

SALN size and polydispersity index (PDI) were determined by photon correlation spectroscopy (PCS) technique using a Zetasizer Nano ZS analyser system (Zetasizer version 6.12; Malvern Instruments, Worcs, UK). The results were expressed as the average of three different measurements.

Particle surface charge (Z-Potential value) was measured by using the same apparatus, equipped with a 4 mW He–Ne laser (633 nm) and DTS software (Version 5.0, Malvern Instruments, Worcs, UK). Measurements were performed in triplicate and each measurement was averaged over at least 12 runs.

4.4. Morphological Studies

SALN morphological features were analysed by field-emission gun scanning electron microscopy (SEM-FEG, Nova 11 NanoSEM 450, Fei, Eindhoven, The Netherlands) using both the SEM and the TEM mode. For the SEM mode, a few drops of the SALNs suspension were placed on an aluminum stub (TAAB Laboratories Equipment Ltd., Aldermaston, Berks, UK) covered by a double side sticky tab (TAAB Laboratories Equipment Ltd., Aldermaston, Berks, UK) and, after drying, vacuum coated with gold–palladium in an argon atmosphere for 60 s (Sputter Coater Emitech K550, Emitech LTD, Ashford, Kent, UK).

For the TEM mode a STEM detector characterised by a low voltage electron beam (30 kV) was employed. TEM 200 mesh Formvar/Carbor Coppergrids (TAAB Laboratories Equipment Ltd., Berks, UK) were immersed in SALNs diluted suspension (1:10 v/v in water) and dried at room conditions (25 °C, 760 mmHg) before the analysis.

Elemental composition of Fe@hepa loaded or unloaded SALNs was determined by energy disperse X-ray (EDX) analysis with X-EDS Bruker QUANTAX-200 (Bruker Nano GmbH, Berlin, Germany) coupled with SEM-FEG. Elements can be identified qualitatively and semi-quantitatively as a function of the X-ray energy emitted by their electrons transferring from a higher energy shell to a lower energy one. The X-ray emissions from the Kα or Lα levels were measured for the following atoms: oxygen (Kα = 0.525 keV), carbon (Kα = 0.277 keV), silicon (Kα = 1.740 keV), aluminium (Kα = 1.487 keV) and iron (Kα = 6.404 keV, Lα = 0.705 keV).

4.5. Drug Loading and Encapsulation Efficiency

The determination of Fe@hepa loaded in SALNs was performed by indirect method analysing the amount of non-encapsulated Fe@hepa by a spectrophotometric method based on the formation of highly-coloured complexes iron-thiocyanate ion.

Briefly, after obtaining SALNs, the separation of the non-encapsulated Fe@hepa (free Fe@hepa) was carried out by centrifugation (see Section 4.2). The pellet was re-suspended in 200 µL of milliQ water and digested in 1 mL of HCl 37% w/w for 2 h at 60 °C. Subsequently, 1.5 mL of 0.1 M solution of potassium thiocyanate (KSCN) was added to form the red-coloured [FeKSCN]$^{2+}$ iron complex. The amount of free Fe@hepa was determined by recording absorbance at 480 nm (Lambda 35 UV/VIS, Perkin-Elmer, Norwalk, CT, USA). The standard calibration curve for iron complex was performed under identical conditions with known amounts of naked Fe@hepa and using KSCN and HCl solution as blank [38].

The encapsulation efficiency (EE%) and drug loading (DL µg/mg) were calculated by using the following equations:

$$EE\% = \frac{\text{initial Fe@hepa(mg)} - \text{free Fe@hepa determined(mg)}}{\text{initial Fe@hepa(mg)}} \times 100$$

$$DL\left(\frac{\mu g}{mg}\right) = \frac{\text{encapsulated Fe@hepa(µg)}}{\text{total mass of SALNs composition(mg)(lipids and Fe@hepa)}}$$

where encapsulated Fe@hepa were calculated by subtracting the amount of free Fe@hepa determined from the initial amount added to the preparation. The experiments were conducted in triplicate and the results were expressed as average ± standard deviation (SD).

4.6. In Vitro SALNs-Fe@hepa Stability

In order to evaluate the in vitro stability of SALNs–Fe@hepa, the amount of Fe@hepa separated gradually at 4 °C for one month by spontaneous precipitation was quantified.

Practically at predetermined intervals (2, 4, 6, 8, 10, 20 and 30 days), the pellet deposited at the bottom of the vials of the SALNs-Fe@hepa suspension was determined. The pellet was recovered, re-suspended in 200 µL of milliQ water and digested in 1 mL of HCl 37% w/w for 2 h at 60 °C. After that, the solution was analysed to determine the amount of iron in accordance with the method described above. The analyses were performed in triplicate.

4.7. Stability of Heparin Coating

In order to analyse the stability of the heparin coating in Fe@hepa before and after the formation of SALNs, the amount of heparin released in saline solution from naked Fe@hepa and SALNs–Fe@hepa was evaluated.

Briefly, a known amount of sample was incubated under magnetic stirring in 0.9% NaCl water solution at 37 °C for 1 h. Then, the suspension was centrifuged for 25 min at 9500 rpm at room temperature (Rotina 380R) in order to separate nanoparticles (naked Fe@hepa or SALNs–Fe@hepa) from the supernatant. The amount of heparin released in the supernatant was determined by using a modified Azure II colorimetric method [39]. Typically, aliquots (500 µL) of aqueous solution were reacted with 4.5 mL of the Azure solution (0.01 mg/mL) and assayed at 654 nm by vis-spectroscopy (Lambda 35 UV/VIS). Quantification was achieved by comparing the absorbance of the samples to a regression curve determined from medium spiked with increasing amount of heparin. The experiments were conducted in triplicate.

4.8. In Vitro Nile Red Release

Nile red released from SALNs was evaluated during 24 h. Labelled SALNs (40 mg) were incubated at 37 °C in 40 mL of phosphate buffer (20 mM, pH 7.4) or DMEM added with serum, under magnetic stirring. One millilitre of SALNs suspension was withdrawn from the system at time intervals of 30 min and replaced with 1 ml of fresh solvent to maintain constant volume. The sample was centrifuged at 9500 rpm for 25 min and Nile red content was determined in the supernatant by vis-spectroscopy at 525 nm. The analysis was performed in triplicate.

4.9. Cell Culture

CaCo-2 cell line were cultured as a monolayer in Dulbecco's Modified Eagle's Medium with high glucose (DMEM) containing L-glutamine 2 mM, penicillin 100 UI/mL, streptomycin 100 µg/mL, sodium pyruvate and 10% of fetal bovine serum (FBS) at 37 °C in a humidified atmosphere (5% CO_2). Cells were sub-cultured when the confluence was $\geq$80%.

4.10. Cytotoxicity Assay

CaCo-2 cells were seeded at a density of 60,000 cells/well in 24-well plate in complete DMEM medium for 48 h. Cells were then treated with Fe@hepa, unloaded SALNs and SALNs–Fe@hepa samples at different concentrations (0.8, 1.2, 1.6 and 2 mg/mL for SALNs, and respective Fe@hepa concentrations) for 2, 4, and 6 h.

After incubation times the methyl thiazole tetrazolium test (MTT) was performed to assess cell viability. Optical densities were measured spectrophotometrically at 570 nm with a multiplate reader (TecanGenios Pro with Magellan 6 software). Cell viability was expressed as a percentage of cell survival respect to the control (untreated cells).

The experiment was performed in triplicate.

4.11. Quantification of SALNs–Fe@hepa on CaCo-2 Cell Model

The amount of Fe@hepa up-taken by the CaCo-2 cells after treatment with Fe@hepa and SALNs–Fe@hepa at different incubation times was quantified by adapting a method previously reported [40]. Cells were seeded in 6-well plate at density of 250,000 cells per well in complete DMEM medium for 48 h. Then, cells were incubated with 2 mg/mL of SALNs–Fe@hepa and a proportional amount of naked Fe@hepa (53 µg/mL) for 2, 4 and 6 h. At the end of the incubation time, cells were washed with PBS and the amount of iron associated to the cells was quantified using the method described in Section 4.5. The experiments were performed in triplicate. In order to compensate the matrix effect, the calibration curve for iron quantification was prepared incubating different known amounts of Fe@hepa in the presence of unloaded SALNs into CaCo-2 cells.

4.12. CLSM Studies of Monolayers

The confocal laser scanning microscopy (CLSM) of fixed cells was performed with a Leica DM IRE2 microscope (Mannheim, Germany) and a Leica Confocal System equipped with a scanner multiband 3-channel Leica TCS SP2 with AOBS, laser diode blue COH (405 nm/25 mW), laser Ar (458 nm/5 mW) (476 nm/5 mW) (488 nm/20 mW) (496 nm/5 mW) (514 nm/20 mW), laser HeNe (543 nm/1.2 mW), laser HeNe (594 nm) (orange) and laser HeNe (633 nm/102 mW). CaCo-2 cells, seeded at a density of 100,000 cells per well in a chambered coverglass (Lab-Tek®, Thermo-scientific, Milan, Italy), were incubated with naked Fe@hepa (53 µg/mL), Nile red-labelled unloaded SALNs (2 mg/mL), and Nile red-labelled SALN–Fe@hepa (2 mg/mL). After 4 h of incubation, the treated cells were washed twice with PBS, fixed in paraformaldehyde (3% *w/v*) for 20 min at room temperature, stained with 2 µg/mL Hoechst 33342 dye and analysed with CLSM.

4.13. Statistical Analysis

Statistical analysis was performed using the one-way analysis of variance (ANOVA). The data are represented as mean ± SD. Difference was considered statistically significant at *p*-values less than 0.05.

5. Conclusions

In this work it was demonstrated that SALNs are an efficient carrier for Fe@hepa, reducing their cytoxicity to CaCo-2 cells and overcoming the loss of heparin coating in biological fluids. SALNs–Fe@hepa resulted able to be efficiently internalised in CaCo-2 cells, and were demonstrated to be a promising tool for delivering the theranostic Fe@hepa to lymphatic circulation by the oral route, although further studies are needed to comprehend the potential in vivo applications. Moreover, it would be interesting in the future to replace native heparin with low-molecular-weight heparins, which showed a less anticoagulant activity while maintaining antiangiogenic activity, in order to reduce risks of bleeding.

Acknowledgments: The authors are grateful to Cassa di Vignola for its generous financial support. Thanks are also due to Miriam Hanuskova and to Federica Mazza for their valuable contribution to the work.

Author Contributions: Elena Vismara and Eliana Leo conceived and designed the experiments; Eleonora Truzzi and Chiara Bongio performed the experiments; Francesca Sacchetti and Eleonora Maretti analysed the data; Valentina Iannuccelli contributed to the in vitro characterisation of the particles; Monica Montanari contributed to the experiments on the CaCo-2 cell line.

Conflicts of Interest: The authors declare that there are no conflicts of interest.

References

1. Chaudhary, S.; Garg, T.; Murthy, R.S.R.; Rath, G.; Goyal, A.K. Recent approaches of lipid-based delivery system for lymphatic targeting via oral route. *J. Drug Target.* **2014**, *22*, 871–882. [CrossRef] [PubMed]
2. Wissing, S.A.; Kayser, O.; Müller, R.H. Solid lipid nanoparticles for parenteral drug delivery. *Adv. Drug Deliv. Rev.* **2004**, *56*, 1257–1272. [CrossRef] [PubMed]
3. Doktorovova, S.; Souto, E.B.; Silva, A.M. Nanotoxicology applied to solid lipid nanoparticles and nanostructured lipid carriers—A systematic review of in vitro data. *Eur. J. Pharm. Biopharm.* **2014**, *87*, 1–18. [CrossRef] [PubMed]
4. Singh, I.; Swami, R.; Khan, W.; Sistla, R. Lymphatic system: A prospective area for advanced targeting of particulate drug carriers. *Expert Opin. Drug Deliv.* **2014**, *11*, 211–229. [CrossRef] [PubMed]
5. Cho, H.J.; Park, J.W.; Yoon, I.S.; Kim, D.D. Surface-modified solid lipid nanoparticles for oral delivery of docetaxel: Enhanced intestinal absorption and lymphatic uptake. *Int. J. Nanomed.* **2014**, *9*, 495–504.
6. Aji Alex, M.R.; Chacko, A.J.; Jose, S.; Souto, E.B. Lopinavir loaded solid lipid nanoparticles (SLN) for intestinal lymphatic targeting. *Eur. J. Pharm. Sci.* **2011**, *42*, 11–18. [CrossRef] [PubMed]
7. Rao, S.; Tan, A.; Thomas, N.; Prestidge, C.A. Perspective and potential of oral lipid-based delivery to optimize pharmacological therapies against cardiovascular diseases. *J. Control. Release* **2014**, *193*, 174–187. [CrossRef] [PubMed]
8. Pantel, K.; Brakenhoff, R.H. Dissecting the metastatic cascade. *Nat. Rev. Cancer* **2004**, *4*, 448–456. [CrossRef] [PubMed]

9. Khan, A.A.; Mudassir, J.; Mohtar, N.; Darwis, Y. Advanced drug delivery to the lymphatic system: Lipid-based nanoformulations. *Int. J. Nanomed.* **2013**, *8*, 2733–2744.

10. Trevaskis, N.L.; Charman, W.N.; Porter, C.J.H. Lipid-based delivery systems and intestinal lymphatic drug transport: A mechanistic update. *Adv. Drug Deliv. Rev.* **2008**, *60*, 702–716. [CrossRef] [PubMed]

11. Porter, C.J.H.; Trevaskis, N.L.; Charman, W.N. Lipids and lipid-based formulations: Optimizing the oral delivery of lipophilic drugs. *Nat. Rev. Drug Discov.* **2007**, *6*, 231–248. [CrossRef] [PubMed]

12. Charman, W.N.A.; Stella, V.J. Estimating the maximal potential for intestinal lymphatic transport of lipophilic drug molecules. *Int. J. Pharm.* **1986**, *34*, 175–178. [CrossRef]

13. Shah, M.K.; Madan, P.; Lin, S. Preparation, in vitro evaluation and statistical optimization of carvedilol-loaded solid lipid nanoparticles for lymphatic absorption via oral administration. *Pharm. Dev. Technol.* **2014**, *19*, 475–485. [CrossRef] [PubMed]

14. Clogston, J.D.; Patri, A.K. Zeta Potential Measurement. *Methods Mol. Biol.* **2011**, *697*, 63–70. [PubMed]

15. Arami, H.; Khandhar, A.; Liggitt, D.; Krishnan, K.M. In vivo delivery, pharmacokinetics, biodistribution and toxicity of iron oxide nanoparticles. *Chem. Soc. Rev.* **2015**, *44*, 8576–8607. [CrossRef] [PubMed]

16. Shubayev, V.I.; Pisanic, T.R.; Jin, S. Magnetic nanoparticles for theragnostics. *Adv. Drug Deliv. Rev.* **2009**, *61*, 467–477. [CrossRef] [PubMed]

17. Gupta, A.K.; Gupta, M. Synthesis and surface engineering of iron oxide nanoparticles for biomedical applications. *Biomaterials* **2005**, *26*, 3995–4021. [CrossRef] [PubMed]

18. Neuberger, T.; Schöpf, B.; Hofmann, H.; Hofmann, M.; von Rechenberg, B. Superparamagnetic nanoparticles for biomedical applications: Possibilities and limitations of a new drug delivery system. *J. Magn. Magn. Mater.* **2005**, *293*, 483–496. [CrossRef]

19. Mornet, S.; Vasseur, S.; Grasset, F.; Duguet, E. Magnetic nanoparticle design for medical diagnosis and therapy. *J. Mater. Chem.* **2004**, *14*, 2161. [CrossRef]

20. Vismara, E.; Valerio, A.; Coletti, A.; Torri, G.; Bertini, S.; Eisele, G.; Gornati, R.; Bernardini, G. Non-covalent synthesis of metal oxide nanoparticle-heparin hybrid systems: A new approach to bioactive nanoparticles. *Int. J. Mol. Sci.* **2013**, *14*, 13463–13481. [CrossRef] [PubMed]

21. Bendas, G.; Borsig, L. Cancer cell adhesion and metastasis: Selectins, integrins, and the inhibitory potential of heparins. *Int. J. Cell Biol.* **2012**, *2012*, 676731. [CrossRef] [PubMed]

22. Smorenburg, S.M.; Hettiarachchi, R.J.; Vink, R.; Büller, H.R. The effects of unfractionated heparin on survival in patients with malignancy—A systematic review. *Thromb. Haemost.* **1999**, *82*, 1600–1604. [PubMed]

23. Casu, B.; Naggi, A.; Torri, G. Re-visiting the structure of heparin. *Carbohydr. Res.* **2015**, *403*, 60–68. [CrossRef] [PubMed]

24. Min, K.A.; Yu, F.; Yang, V.C.; Zhang, X.; Rosania, G.R. Transcellular Transport of Heparin-coated Magnetic Iron Oxide Nanoparticles (Hep-MION) Under the Influence of an Applied Magnetic Field. *Pharmaceutics* **2010**, *2*, 119–135. [CrossRef] [PubMed]

25. Caliph, S.M.; Charman, W.N.; Porter, C.J. Effect of short-, medium-, and long-chain fatty acid-based vehicles on the absolute oral bioavailability and intestinal lymphatic transport of halofantrine and assessment of mass balance in lymph-cannulated and non-cannulated rats. *J. Pharm. Sci.* **2000**, *89*, 1073–1084. [CrossRef]

26. Turcheniuk, K.; Tarasevych, A.V.; Kukhar, V.P.; Boukherroub, R.; Szunerits, S. Recent advances in surface chemistry strategies for the fabrication of functional iron oxide based magnetic nanoparticles. *Nanoscale* **2013**, *5*, 10729. [CrossRef] [PubMed]

27. Gershkovich, P.; Hoffman, A. Uptake of lipophilic drugs by plasma derived isolated chylomicrons: Linear correlation with intestinal lymphatic bioavailability. *Eur. J. Pharm. Sci.* **2005**, *26*, 394–404. [CrossRef] [PubMed]

28. Olbrich, C.; Müller, R.H. Enzymatic degradation of SLN-effect of surfactant and surfactant mixtures. *Int. J. Pharm.* **1999**, *180*, 31–39. [CrossRef]

29. Shimpi, S.L.; Mahadik, K.R.; Paradkar, A.R. Study on mechanism for amorphous drug stabilization using gelucire 50/13. *Chem. Pharm. Bull. (Tokyo)* **2009**, *57*, 937–942. [CrossRef] [PubMed]

30. Date, A.A.; Vador, N.; Jagtap, A.; Nagarsenker, M.S. Lipid nanocarriers (GeluPearl) containing amphiphilic lipid Gelucire 50/13 as a novel stabilizer: Fabrication, characterization and evaluation for oral drug delivery. *Nanotechnology* **2011**, *22*, 275102. [CrossRef] [PubMed]

31. Dubray, O.; Jannin, V.; Demarne, F.; Pellequer, Y.; Lamprecht, A.; Béduneau, A. In-vitro investigation regarding the effects of Gelucire 44/14 and Labrasol ALF on the secretory intestinal transport of P-gp substrates. *Int. J. Pharm.* **2016**, *515*, 293–299. [CrossRef] [PubMed]

32. Sachs-Barrable, K.; Thamboo, A.; Lee, S.D.; Wasan, K.M. Lipid excipients Peceol and Gelucire 44/14 decrease P-glycoprotein mediated efflux of rhodamine 123 partially due to modifying P-glycoprotein protein expression within Caco-2 cells. *J. Pharm. Pharm. Sci.* **2007**, *10*, 319–331. [PubMed]

33. Trevaskis, N.L.; Kaminskas, L.M.; Porter, C.J.H. From sewer to saviour—Targeting the lymphatic system to promote drug exposure and activity. *Nat. Rev. Drug Discov.* **2015**, *14*, 781–803. [CrossRef] [PubMed]

34. Chatterjee, B.; Hamed Almurisi, S.; Ahmed Mahdi Dukhan, A.; Mandal, U.K.; Sengupta, P. Controversies with self-emulsifying drug delivery system from pharmacokinetic point of view. *Drug Deliv.* **2016**, *23*, 3639–3652. [CrossRef] [PubMed]

35. Valdiglesias, V.; Fernández-Bertólez, N.; Kiliç, G.; Costa, C.; Costa, S.; Fraga, S.; Bessa, M.J.; Pásaro, E.; Teixeira, J.P.; Laffon, B. Are iron oxide nanoparticles safe? Current knowledge and future perspectives. *J. Trace Elem. Med. Biol.* **2016**, *38*, 53–63. [CrossRef] [PubMed]

36. Soenen, S.J.H.; de Cuyper, M. Assessing cytotoxicity of (iron oxide-based) nanoparticles: An overview of different methods exemplified with cationic magnetoliposomes. *Contrast Media Mol. Imaging* **2009**, *4*, 207–219. [CrossRef] [PubMed]

37. Pisanic, T.R.; Blackwell, J.D.; Shubayev, V.I.; Fiñones, R.R.; Jin, S. Nanotoxicity of iron oxide nanoparticle internalization in growing neurons. *Biomaterials* **2007**, *28*, 2572–2581. [CrossRef] [PubMed]

38. Licciardi, M.; Scialabba, C.; Fiorica, C.; Cavallaro, G.; Cassata, G.; Giammona, G. Polymeric Nanocarriers for Magnetic Targeted Drug Delivery: Preparation, Characterization, and in vitro and in vivo evaluation. *Mol. Pharm.* **2013**, *10*, 4397–4407. [CrossRef] [PubMed]

39. Jiao, Y.; Ubrich, N.; Hoffart, V.; Marchand-Arvier, M.; Vigneron, C.; Hoffman, M.; Maincent, P. Anticoagulant activity of heparin following oral administration of heparin-loaded microparticles in rabbits. *J. Pharm. Sci.* **2002**, *91*, 760–768. [CrossRef] [PubMed]

40. Mahajan, S.; Koul, V.; Choudhary, V.; Shishodia, G.; Bharti, A.C. Preparation and in vitro evaluation of folate-receptor-targeted SPION-polymer micelle hybrids for MRI contrast enhancement in cancer imaging. *Nanotechnology* **2013**, *24*, 015603. [CrossRef] [PubMed]

Sample Availability: Samples of the compounds are available from the authors.

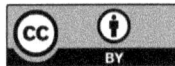

molecules

MDPI

Article

Albumin and Hyaluronic Acid-Coated Superparamagnetic Iron Oxide Nanoparticles Loaded with Paclitaxel for Biomedical Applications

Elena Vismara [1,*], Chiara Bongio [1], Alessia Coletti [1], Ravit Edelman [2], Andrea Serafini [1], Michele Mauri [3], Roberto Simonutti [3], Sabrina Bertini [4], Elena Urso [4], Yehuda G. Assaraf [5] and Yoav D. Livney [2,*]

[1] Department of Chemistry, Materials and Chemical Engineering "G. Natta", Politecnico di Milano, 20131 Milano, Italy; chiara.bongio@polimi.it (C.B.); alessia.coletti08@gmail.com (A.C.); andrea.serafini@polimi.it (A.S.)
[2] Biotechnology and Food Engineering Department, Technion-Israel Institute of Technology, Haifa 3200000, Israel; sravitm@gmail.com (R.E.); roberto.simonutti@unimib.it (R.S.)
[3] Department of Materials Science, University of Milan Bicocca, 20125 Milano, Italy; michele.mauri@mater.unimib.it
[4] Istituto scientifico di chimica e biochimica "G. Ronzoni", 20133 Milano, Italy; bertini@ronzoni.it (S.B.); urso@ronzoni.it (E.U.)
[5] Biology Department, Technion-Israel Institute of Technology, Haifa 3200000, Israel; assaraf@technion.ac.il
* Correspondence: elena.vismara@polimi.it (E.V.); livney@technion.ac.il (Y.D.L.); Tel.: +39-022-399-3088 (E.V.); +9-724-829-4225 (Y.D.L.); Fax: +39-022-399-3180 (E.V.); +9-724-829-3399 (Y.D.L.)

Academic Editors: Jawed Fareed, Giangiacomo Torri and Diego Muñoz-Torrero
Received: 22 May 2017; Accepted: 16 June 2017; Published: 22 June 2017

Abstract: Super paramagnetic iron oxide nanoparticles (SPION) were augmented by both hyaluronic acid (HA) and bovine serum albumin (BSA), each covalently conjugated to dopamine (DA) enabling their anchoring to the SPION. HA and BSA were found to simultaneously serve as stabilizing polymers of $Fe_3O_4 \cdot DA\text{-}BSA/HA$ in water. $Fe_3O_4 \cdot DA\text{-}BSA/HA$ efficiently entrapped and released the hydrophobic cytotoxic drug paclitaxel (PTX). The relative amount of HA and BSA modulates not only the total solubility but also the paramagnetic relaxation properties of the preparation. The entrapping of PTX did not influence the paramagnetic relaxation properties of $Fe_3O_4 \cdot DA\text{-}BSA$. Thus, by tuning the surface structure and loading, we can tune the theranostic properties of the system.

Keywords: super paramagnetic iron oxide nanoparticles (SPION); hyaluronic acid (HA); bovine serum albumin (BSA); $Fe_3O_4 \cdot DA\text{-}BSA/HA$; paclitaxel (PTX); magnetic resonance imaging (MRI)

1. Introduction

Nanotechnology has opened the way to an incredibly high number of new composite materials. As part of the growing field of nanomedicine [1], composite nanoscale biomaterials are based on assembling nanoparticles with biomolecules. The palette of available nanoparticles is large and matched by an equally large number of biomolecules [2]. Iron oxide nanoparticles are among the most extensively studied types of nanoparticles (NPs) [3]. Superparamagnetic iron oxides nanoparticles (SPIONs), composed by magnetite (Fe_3O_4) or maghemite ($\gamma\text{-}Fe_2O_3$), have been explored in view of their potentiality in biomedical applications [4]. In fact, a key advantage of iron oxide nanoparticles in comparison to other heavy metal-based NPs is their natural integration into tissue physiology. They can be part of superparamagnetic materials, whose suspensions are generally referred to as ferrofluids, clinically investigated as MRI contrast agents [5,6]. An overview has been published both on the many possibilities to prepare SPIONs suitable for enhancing with biomolecules and for potentially engineering for biomedical applications [7]. The authors of reference [8] have already described the logic of SPION-developed biomedical applications in recent years. SPION-appropriate surface coatings can be studied for various biomedical applications, such as magnetic resonance imaging, hyperthermia, drug delivery, tissue repair, cell and tissue targeting, and transfection. Development of coated and loaded SPIONs is a promising theranostic approach. In fact, following a quite similar approach, we pursued multitasking nanostructures—using cyclodextrin as a vector of antitumor drugs and low molecular weight heparins, covalently linked to cyclodextrin—that were thought to target the nanostructures to the tumor mass, according to heparanase and growth factors inhibition mechanisms [9]. We then progressed to iron oxide and heparin-based materials to introduce the diagnostic functionality [10,11]. Since 2005, magnetic NPs have been considered of great interest for biomedical applications, and, among them, iron oxide NPs have been considered the more promising [12]. Additionally, depending on particle size, positive or negative contrast agents can be prepared [13,14]. Even though SPIONs have been clinically approved metal oxide NPs, the potential toxicity of SPION has been thoroughly investigated [14]. Although there is no intrinsic risk associated with SPION per se, adverse biological effects and safety issues could be associated with specific SPIONs. Ref. [15] argues about issues that need be addressed by the scientific community prior to approving their clinical use. We already cited that SPION-appropriate surface coatings divert SPION towards different biomedical applications. In advance, SPION coating has been used to modulate their biocompatibility and to reduce their toxicity. This is the case of Bovine Serum Albumin (BSA) protein [16]. The same authors from Reference [16] are working today on human serum albumin, for better biocompatibility, thus supporting the crucial role that protein corona can play [17].

The common challenge of engineered SPION for biomedical applications is that the material used for surface coating of the magnetic particles must not only be nontoxic and biocompatible but also enable selective targeted delivery of the particles to the location of the disease. Passive targeting of long circulating nanoparticles via the enhanced permeability and retention (EPR) effect is one of the mechanisms by which such coated nanoparticles can reach solid tumors. Decoration of engineered magnetic nanoparticles with targeting molecules that selectively bind to target proteins overexpressed on the target cells could significantly enhance the selectivity of their targeting to these cells [18,19]. Magnetic nanoparticles can deliver drugs and an external magnetic field can be applied to guide them to the target site. Different polymers/molecules have been used for nanoparticle coating to stabilize the suspensions of magnetic nanoparticles under in vitro and in vivo situation and selected proteins/targeting ligands have been used for derivatizing magnetic nanoparticles. It is noteworthy that magnetic drug targeting employing nanoparticles as carriers is a promising cancer theranostic treatment, avoiding the side effects of conventional chemotherapy [3]. Molecular imaging is one of the most promising applications of targeted iron oxide nanoparticles, and various applications using targeted iron oxide nanoparticles have been evaluated in vitro and in animal experiments [20]. Looking forward, the fact that targeted superparamagnetic iron oxide nanoparticles can be used for early detection of cancer has to be considered a plus [21]. On the other hand, the challenges associated with penetration of nanoparticles across cell and tissue barriers have been recently reviewed [22]. Therefore, current understanding led us to the conclusion that the combination of a diagnostic imaging aid along with a targeted therapeutic compound loaded onto the same NP systems is a promising route of drug delivery.

The challenge of our study was to design and build new theranostic SPION systems starting from a magnetic iron oxide core decorated with bovine serum albumin (BSA) and hyaluronic acid (HA), where each component was selected to play its peculiar role and where the SPION systems could include paclitaxel (PTX) as a drug. Hyaluronic acid (HA) is a natural linear anionic glycosaminoglycan (molecular weight (MW) 5–10^4 kDa), composed of repeating disaccharide units of D-glucuronic acid and N-acetyl-D-glucosamine linked via alternating β-1,4 and β-1,3 glycosidic bonds. Owing to its biocompatibility and biodegradability, HA has been extensively investigated for medical applications. In particular, HA can specifically bind to various cancer cells that overexpress CD44 receptors.

Molecules **2017**, 22, 1030

In this regard, different considerations concerning the utile length of HA oligomers must be reported. Selecting HA oligosaccharides long enough to bind to more than one CD44 receptor but too short to bind to the hyaluronic acid receptor for endocytosis (HARE) receptors in the liver (preferably <10 kDa) may enable the formation of an HA-based CD44-targeted carrier that avoids hepatic elimination while achieving tumor targeting [23]. Recently, this enhanced tumor-targeting ability as well as higher therapeutic efficacy compared to free anti-cancer agents has been reported [24]. Therefore, several HA-conjugates containing anticancer agents (such as paclitaxel or doxorubicin) have already been designed [25]. Over the years, ever new functions of the CD44 protein have been found, but the main one for our purposes is the recognition of hyaluronic acid as a component of the extracellular matrix in particular areas, such as embryonic connective tissues and the outline of invasive cancerous lesions. Most HA-drug conjugates have been developed for cancer chemotherapy as macromolecular prodrugs. HA has also been conjugated onto various drug-loaded nanoparticles for use as a targeting moiety. Hyaluronic acid was bound to the initially dextran-coated SPIONs by esterification [26].

Bovine serum albumin (BSA) protein was used to improve the colloidal stability of the nanoparticles. BSA has been one of the most extensively studied proteins because of its sequence and structural homology with human serum albumin (HSA). HSA could be considered the most suitable protein for biocompatible coating of nanoparticles for biomedical applications. Herein we used BSA as a model for HSA, with the aim of ultimately using HSA for future clinical stages. BSA is an abundant serum protein with a MW of ~66 kDa. The primary physiological function of serum albumin (SA) is to transport lipids and metabolites present in blood plasma; hence, it is a suitable carrier for hydrophobic drugs. Due to the high protein binding of various drugs, it could be used for effective incorporation of these compounds. It has an extraordinary ligand binding capacity, providing a depot for a wide variety of compounds with favorable monovalent reversible binding characteristics for transport in the body and release at the cell surface. Folate–bovine serum albumin-functionalized polymeric micelles loaded with superparamagnetic iron oxide nanoparticles have been proposed for tumor targeting and magnetic resonance imaging [27,28]. Ultrasound-triggered BSA/SPION hybrid nanoclusters investigated for liver-specific magnetic resonance imaging support the interest in the use of SA in the field of nanomedicine [29].

Paclitaxel (PTX) is a medication used to treat a number of types of cancer, including ovarian cancer, breast cancer, lung cancer, and pancreatic cancer, among others. Its clinical application is hampered by poor solubility in water and other pharmaceutically acceptable solvents (<2 µg/mL). To increase its bioavaibility, various alternative formulation approaches have been explored, including emulsions, nanoparticles, polymeric micelles, cyclodextrins, liposomes, etc. [30]. Of note, hyaluronic acid-anchored PTX nanocrystals have been found to improve chemotherapeutic efficacy and inhibit lung metastasis in tumor-bearing rat models [31].

The aim of this study was to design and develop a new theranostic nanosystem, named $Fe_3O_4 \cdot DA$-BSA/HA, suitable for loading PTX (see Scheme 1). The iron core and HA were selected according to the specific roles they can play in therapy, diagnosis and targeting, while BSA could make stable, biocompatible and non-toxic the hybrid $Fe_3O_4 \cdot DA$-BSA/HA system. The iron core was decorated irreversibly by BSA and HA [32]. This is the reason why dopamine (DA) is a fundamental part of the system. Covalent linkage of both BSA and HA with DA was built up, DA being identified as the specific anchoring molecule to the inorganic core. BSA-DA and HA-DA were both linked to the surface of the iron core, in order to obtain a strong interaction between the bioorganic layer and the inorganic core. Scheme 1 summarizes the schematic protocol to $Fe_3O_4 \cdot DA$-BSA/HA that was thought to be as simple as possible, reproducible, and suitable for scaling up. The choice of HA and BSA was also in agreement with the final challenge of the work, that is the loading of $Fe_3O_4 \cdot DA$-BSA/HA with the real anticancer PTX drug. The rational of the PTX $Fe_3O_4 \cdot DA$-BSA/HA inclusion can also be supported by the fact that, on 6 September 2013, the Food and Drug Administration (FDA) approved PTX albumin-stabilized nanoparticle formulation and also partially by Ref. [31].

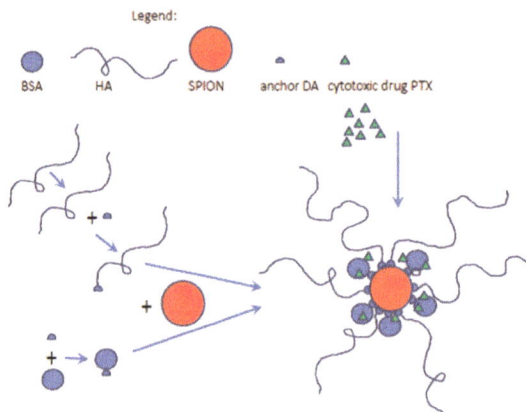

Scheme 1. A schematic protocol of the envisioned $Fe_3O_4 \cdot DA\text{-}BSA/HA$ nanoparticle, where DA means dopamine, loaded with paclitaxel (PTX), BSA—bovine serum albumin; HA—hyaluronic acid.

2. Results

2.1. Preparation and Characterization

2.1.1. Synthesis of BSA-DA Adduct

Since DA and BSA respectively possess amine and carboxylic moieties, the common carbodimmide cross-linker chemistry was explored. The condensation between DA and BSA was performed by employing 1-ethyl-3-(3'-dimethyl-aminopropyl)-carbodiimide (EDC).

The DA:BSA degree of substitution was evaluated by means of MALDI–TOF analysis (Figure 1). The spectrum shows a large peak at mass-to-charge (m/z) values of about 70,000 Da, corresponding to the medium average derivatization of 20:1 (20 molecules of DA for each molecule of BSA).

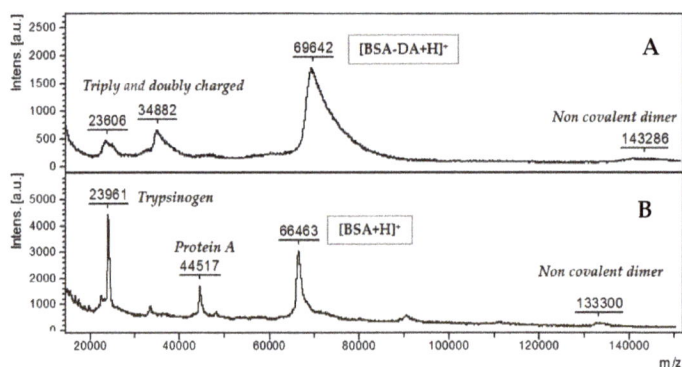

Figure 1. Matrix-assisted laser desorption/ionization (MALDI)-time of flight (TOF) spectra of (**A**) bovine serum albumin-dopamine (BSA-DA) and (**B**) BSA protein, protein A and trypsinogen.

2.1.2. Synthesis of HA-DA Adduct

Commercial low molecular weight hyaluronic acid (HA, 5400 Da) and dopamine hydrochloride were reacted to form HA-DA conjugates using EDC as the activating agent of carboxyl groups of the HA chain. The crude HA-DA was dialyzed before characterization.

Structural characterization of the starting material (HA) and the obtained HA-DA adduct was performed by LC–MS chromatography and NMR. Concerning HA, the LC–MS based method allowed the elution and identification of oligomer dispersion from 4 mer (with a molecular weight of about 700 Da) to 40 mer (with a molecular weight of about 7600 Da). Almost all the species eluting in the labelled chromatographic peaks (Figure S1) were identified; assignment is reported in Table S1. At any rate, the elution of several isomers was observed, confirming the presence of species with the same molecular weight but different sequences. As expected, the regular chains distribution on (G-ANAc)$_n$, that means hyaluronic acid disaccharide repeating unit, 4-β-D-glucuronic acid (1–3) N-acetyl β-D-glucosamine, seems to be the most abundant, but relevant contribution arises from the other species.

While the LC–MS analysis of intact HA provided good chromatographic separation of numerous species and their identification with very high mass accuracy, the analysis of its DA conjugate (HA-DA) showed several issues, due to the presence of unreacted starting hyaluronic acid, eventual reagents carried by the interaction with the polymer and the elution of less strongly retained derivatized oligomers under the unreacted HA chains, which cannot be quantified with this technique. Expanded portions of the chromatograms (Figure 2) allow for detecting the appearance of several mass signals corresponding to derivatized HA chains observed in the extracted ion chromatograms (Figure 3).

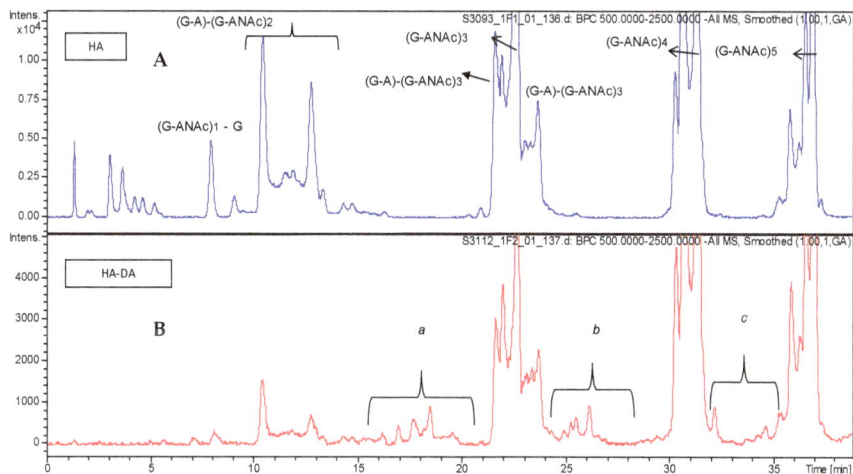

Figure 2. Partial HPLC–MS profiles: (**A**) intact hyaluronic acid (HA) and (**B**) HA-DA.

The elution of these derivatized components at lower retention times than the non-derivatized ones agrees with the behaviour of reversed-phase ion pair chromatography using alkylammonium as the ion pair when masking the negative charge of glucuronic acid is accomplished by reaction with DA.

Due to the extremely high complexity of the HA-DA material, we attempted to assign the structures of these signals (Table S2); data show that about the same modification, corresponding to a mass addition of about 534 Daltons, was observed in all HA components from 5 mer to 20 mer, suggesting the formation of modified HA chains containing at least three DA molecules. This first level of investigation appeared to be enough to confirm the HA derivatization with DA in the HA-DA material, as supported by parallel NMR analysis. No information can be provided via LC–MS analysis about the formation of the non-covalent HA/DA complex.

Structural characterization of HA-DA material was also performed using ^{1}H- and ^{13}C-NMR with mono- and bidimensional techniques such as COSY, TOCSY, DOSY, HSQC, and HMBC. Table 1 shows the chemical shifts and assignments of the signals.

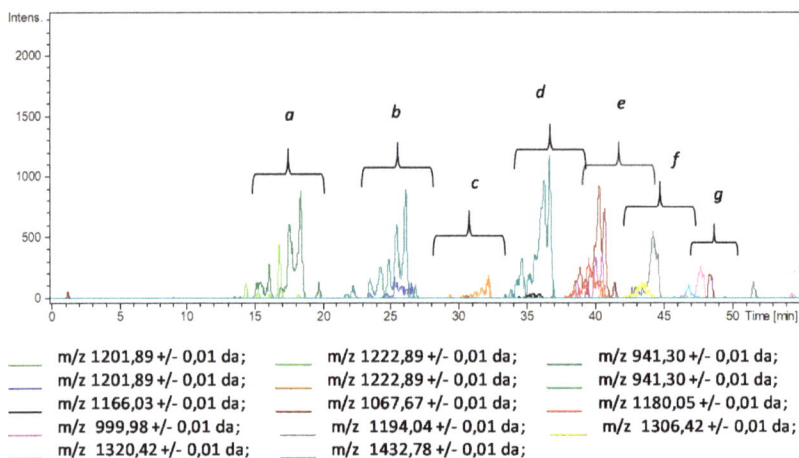

Figure 3. Extracted ion chromatograms (EIC) of mass signals identified as derivatized HA chains (HA-DA) ranging from 5-mer oligomers (Mw ~1500) to 20-mer oligomers (Mw ~4300) (see Table S2).

The legend of Figure 3:

m/z 1201,89 +/- 0,01 da;   m/z 1222,89 +/- 0,01 da;   m/z 941,30 +/- 0,01 da;
m/z 1201,89 +/- 0,01 da;   m/z 1222,89 +/- 0,01 da;   m/z 941,30 +/- 0,01 da;
m/z 1166,03 +/- 0,01 da;   m/z 1067,67 +/- 0,01 da;   m/z 1180,05 +/- 0,01 da;
m/z 999,98 +/- 0,01 da;   m/z 1194,04 +/- 0,01 da;   m/z 1306,42 +/- 0,01 da;
m/z 1320,42 +/- 0,01 da;   m/z 1432,78 +/- 0,01 da;

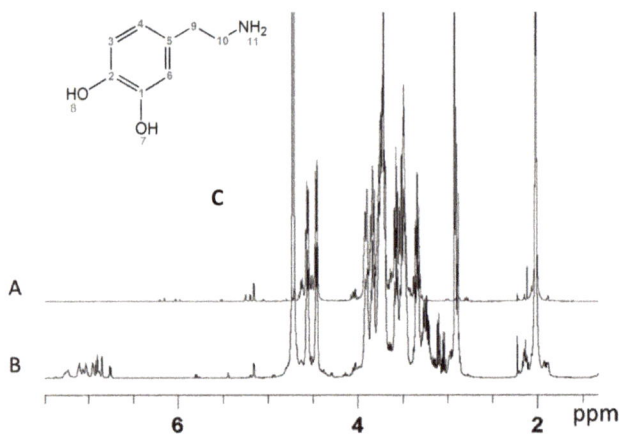

Figure 4. Proton spectra of HA (**A**) and HA-DA (**B**), (**C**) the DA chemical structure.

The HA ^{1}H-NMR (Figure 4A) spectrum signals a low molecular weight structure. The main signals are sharper than the usual polymeric HA ones, while minor signals are due to the reducing and non-reducing terminal chain residues. Both the glucosamine and the glucuronic acid show their terminal reducing residues, suggesting a non-enzymatic chemical degradation. Integration values of easily detectable reduced end signals correspond to an average of chains centred between nine and ten disaccharide units. Free NH$_2$ glucosamine is also detected, in the range of 1.5%. The spectrum of the product shows traces of minor components.

The HA-DA derivative presents a simplified ^{1}H-NMR spectrum (Figure 4B) with respect to the corresponding HA spectrum induced by the derivatization procedure. The reducing anomeric pattern and other minor signals have disappeared or are significantly lowered, corresponding to a loss of the shortest HA oligomers. The quantification of reducing end anomeric signals is no longer possible due to the occurred derivatization. The main spectrum signals are unmodified, while the new signals in the expected region of the DA signals appear to be minor, in agreement with the planned derivatization degree. The ratio between the aromatic and the anomeric signals allows for estimating an average ratio of 2 DA for each 10 disaccharide building blocks. A high complexity in these spectral regions is observed.

Table 1. Proton ^{1}H and carbon ^{13}C structure-chemical shift assignment of hyaluronic acid (HA) and HA-dopamine (DA). Italics: free DA. The numbers used for the attribution of DA signals refer to the DA structure reported in Figure 4.

HA (ppm)		Glucosamine	HA-DA (ppm)	
^{1}H	^{13}C		^{1}H	^{13}C
5.16	93.8	A1α	5.16	93.9
4.71	97.6	A1β	4.71	97.6
5.22	95.1	A1NH$_2$α	-	-
4.56	103.3	A1	4.56	103.4
3.84	57.1	A2	3.83	57.2
3.72	85.5	A3	3.71	85.5
3.52	71.3	A4	3.51	71.3
3.48	78.3	A5	3.46	78.3
3.76	63.4	A6	3.75	63.4
3.92		A6′	3.90	
2.02	25.4	ME	2.02	25.4
-	177.8	N-CO	-	177.7
		Glucuronic Acid		
5.26	94.9	G1$_{red\,α}$	5.20	94.9
3.01	57.1	G2$_{red\,α}$	nd	nd
4.61	98.9	G1$_{red\,β}$	4.62	99.0
2.77	59.7	G2$_{red\,β}$	nd	nd
4.46	106.0	G1	4.45	105.8
3.45	75.4	G2	3.33	75.3
3.58	76.5	G3	3.56	76.5
3.74	82.8	G4	3.71	85.5
3.71	79.2	G5	3.71	79.2
-	176.9	G6	-	176.9
		Dopamine		
2.87	32.0	CH$_2$ (9)	2.98–2.93	34.8
			2.96–2.87	
3.22	40.0	CH$_2$-Nr (10)	3.27	43.3
			3.23	39.5
6.75	123.0	4	6.88	124.7
			6.93	124.2
			6.76	124.1
-	130.1	5		138.9
				141.3
				131.9
6.90	117.4	3	7.10	130.7
			7.26	125.8
			7.23	125.7
			6.91	119.4
6.85	117.4	6	7.02	121.2
			7.09	126.7
			6.85	119.5
-	145.0	1 and 2		132.1
	143.8			140.2
				149.9
				150.7
				151.1
				147.1
				145.9

At least three different structures are detectable at the level of the aromatic signals (Figure S2). One appears with sharp signals, and the chemical shift of the signals corresponds to the free dopamine's surviving the dialysis step, probably because of salt effect with HA. These signals were not considered for quantitative evaluations. The two other observable structures present similar signal patterns, but both show deshielded signals, in different degrees, with respect to the free DA. Furthermore, the signals appear as broad ones, due to their incorporation in a polymeric structure. This interpretation was supported by a DOSY NMR experiment that allows identification of homogeneous molecules through their diffusion coefficients, which depend on the size and shape of the molecule. The experiment shows the polymeric chain signals containing the linked aromatic ones all aligned and having similar low diffusion coefficients, while the small components show different distributions. The discriminating spectrum of the DOSY experiment shows that the free DA component is lost while the DA-HA linked components survive (see Figure 5).

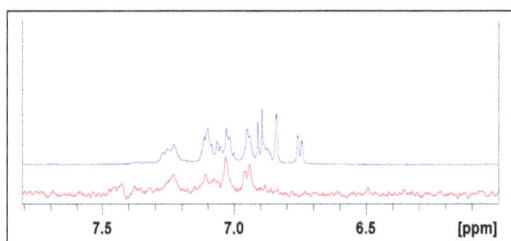

Figure 5. Comparison of aromatic proton sector of normal NMR spectrum (blue) with a DOSY section (red) taken in the correspondence of the polymeric chain signals.

The ^{13}C spectrum and the multiple bond correlation experiment (HMBC) associated with the heteronuclear correlation (HSQC) was determinant for the identification of the quaternary carbons and their correlations with the protons of the structure. It was possible to identify the correlations, in addition to the HA structural components, of quaternary aromatic carbons of DA substituent (Figure 6) with the aliphatic CH_2 of the linkage sequence $-CH_2-NHR$. They showed chemical shifts between 3.2 and 3.3, while CH_2 linked to the aromatic residue showed values between 2.8 and 3.0 ppm.

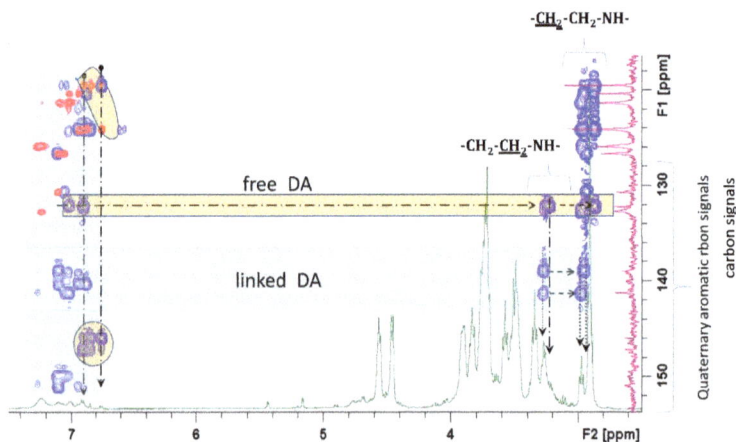

Figure 6. HMBC partial spectrum of HA-DA aromatic quaternary carbon correlation signals (blue) superimposed on the HSQC (red) and ^{1}H spectrum (green). Correlations of the DA polymeric components are underlined in the light blue areas while the free form is evidenced in the yellow area.

2.1.3. Synthesis of $Fe_3O_4 \cdot OA$ Nanoparticles

The synthesis of magnetite-oleate nanoparticles ($Fe_3O_4 \cdot OA$, SPION1) was performed according to the following description. The magnetite was prepared by coprecipitation of a Fe^{2+} and Fe^{3+} salt solution ($FeCl_2 \cdot 4H_2O$ and $FeCl_3 \cdot 6H_2O$, respectively) with the introduction of ammonia as an alkaline agent. No post-treatment procedure was required, since the oleic acid was introduced as a reactant during the crystallization. The FTIR spectrum (Figure S3) confirmed the formation of the product due to the presence of the bands typical for the symmetric and antisymmetric stretching vibration of oleate (1407 cm^{-1} and 1520 cm^{-1}, respectively) and the signal at 600 cm^{-1}, which is representative of Fe–O bond in the crystalline lattice of magnetite. Concerning the morphological characterization, dynamic light scattering (DLS) measurements showed that the averaged hydrodynamic diameter (Z_{av}) of obtained oleate-nanocrystals is 31.12 ± 0.41, with a good polydispersity index (PDI) of 0.219 (Table 2). TEM images allow estimation of the size of the iron cores throughout the steps leading to the nanoassemblies. As depicted in Figure 7, their diameter is around 5 nm, and it is conserved in subsequent steps. DLS is more informative on the structure of the assemblies: the solvodynamic diameter of 30 nm of the $Fe_3O_4 \cdot OA$ in hexane indicates that the loose assemblies appearing in the dry samples (Figure 7 and Table S3) are representative of the aggregation state seen in dispersion. Furthermore, different samples obtained with the same synthetic procedure over time highlighted good reproducibility of the size values.

Table 2. Zeta average (Z_{av}) and polydispersity index (PDI) of nanosystems, superparamagnetic iron oxide nanoparticle (SPION) 1–5.

Sample	Z_{av} (d. nm)	PDI
SPION1	31.1 ± 0.4	0.22
SPION2	77.5 ± 1.3	0.28
SPION3	83.9 ± 0.9	0.28
SPION5	75.0 ± 1.3	0.29
SPION6	79.4 ± 0.7	0.28

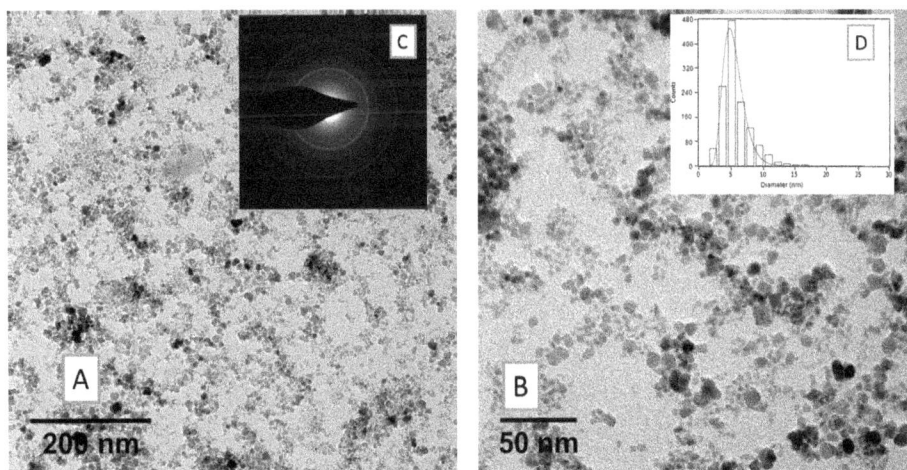

Figure 7. TEM measurements on nanocrystals of magnetite-oleate nanoparticles ($Fe_3O_4 \cdot OA$, SPION1) (**A**) low and (**B**) high magnification bright field micrographs; (**C**) relevant selected-area electron diffraction (SAED) pattern and (**D**) size distribution histogram of the nanoparticles ensemble.

2.1.4. Synthesis of $Fe_3O_4 \cdot DA$-BSA/HA Nanoparticles

Once the BSA-DA and HA-DA adducts were prepared, they were employed in a one-pot reaction procedure by using cetyl trimethylammonium bromide (CTAB), which acts as a phase transfer agent, allowing the dispersion of magnetite-oleate nanoparticles ($Fe_3O_4 \cdot OA$, SPION1) in water and the contemporary ligand exchange reaction with BSA-DA and HA-DA adducts, giving sample SPION2. Figure 8 shows the FTIR spectrum of SPION2, which is representative of all $Fe_3O_4 \cdot DA$-BSA/HA.

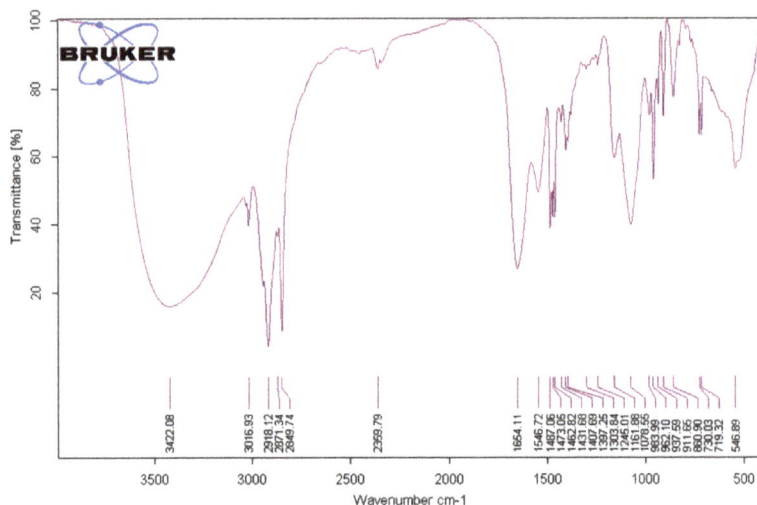

Figure 8. Fourier transform infrared spectroscopy (FTIR) spectrum of SPION2.

It is possible to identify the presence of DA, HA, BSA, and cetyl trimethylammonium cation (CTA) structures and the core Fe–O by diagnostic wavenumbers per every component: ν_{max} cm^{-1}: 3422.08 (O–H sym stretching, N–H stretching amide); 3016.93 (aromatic sym C–H stretching); 2918.1, 2871, 2849 (CH$_3$ asymmetric stretching and $-N^+(CH_3)_3$ symmetric stretching vibrations, CTA), 1654.11 CONH (C=O stretching); 1546.72 (aromatic sym C–C stretching); 1487.06 (benzene ring vibrations); 1473.05; 1462.82 (CH$_2$ bending); 1431.68; 1397.25 (aromatic C=C bonds); 1303.84 (aromatic C–O asym bending); 1245.01 (aromatic C–O sym bending); 1161.88 (C–O alcohol); 1078.55 (C–O alcohol) 962.10 (aromatic C–C–H sym bending); 937 (–CH=CH–ring); 730.03 (C–C–C asym bending); 719.32 (C–C–C asym bending); 546.89 (Fe–O).

The bands at 1481, 1333, and 1258 cm^{-1} have been assigned as diagnostic signals in the infrared spectrum of the bidentate ligand catechol bound to TiO$_2$ [33]. Accordingly, we tentatively assigned the bands at 1487.06, 1397.25, and 1245.01 to the bidentate ligand DA bound to Fe. Bands at 2918.1, 2871, 2849, and 1462.82 were assigned to CTA, in keeping with a very recent article, "Electrochemistry and surface-enhanced Raman spectroscopy of CTAB modulated interactions of magnetic nanoparticles with biomolecules", strictly related to our work [34]. Both TEM (Figure 9) and DLS (Z_{av} = 77.51 ± 1.32, PDI = 0.28, Table 2) depicted a significant change in the morphology of the system. The overall dimensions grew and took the shape of multiple small cores coated by shells of organic material.

Since organic layer size could interfere with MRI detection by shielding the iron core, the amount of HA was decreased, giving SPION3 and SPION4 with different relative amounts of HA and BSA (20% and 10% HA, respectively, in comparison with SPION2): see the TEM images in Figures 10 and 11. The choice to modulate HA content depends on the fact that HA is the real targeting component of $Fe_3O_4 \cdot DA$-BSA/HA. Hence, the availability of SPIONs 2–4 could endow $Fe_3O_4 \cdot DA$-BSA/HA with different targeting properties. Table 3 summarizes the different amounts of BSA and HA.

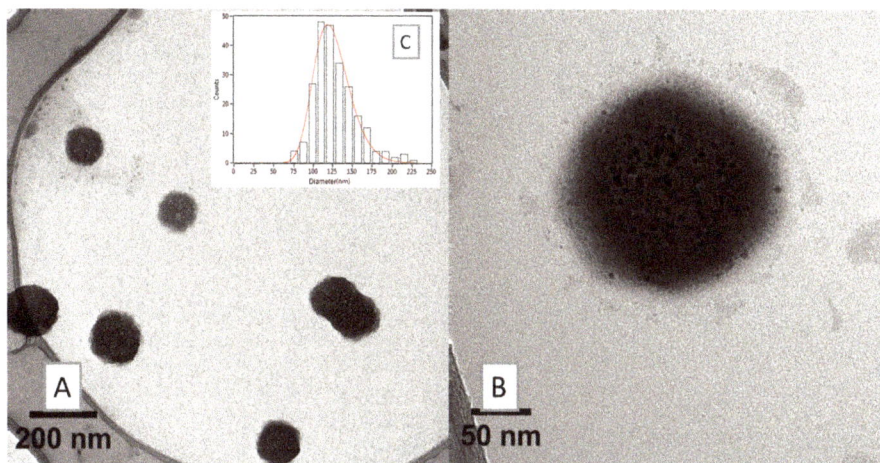

Figure 9. TEM analysis on SPION2: (**A**) low- and (**B**) high-magnification bright field micrographs and (**C**) size distribution histogram of the nanosystems.

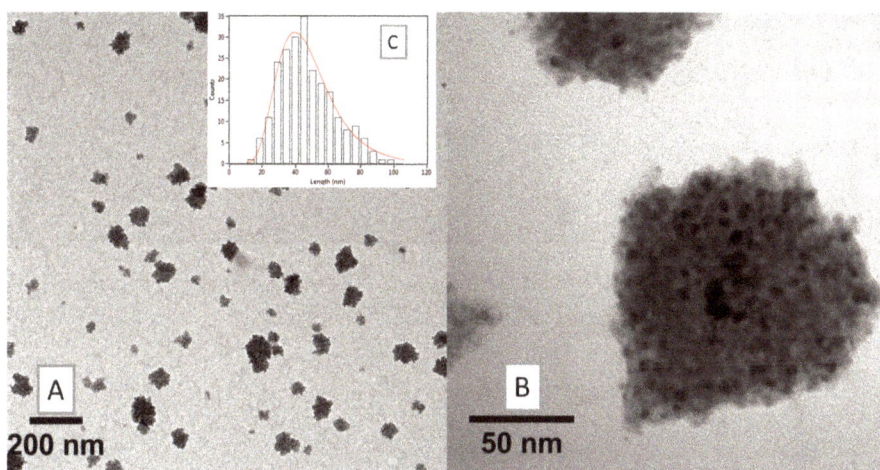

Figure 10. TEM analysis on SPION3: (**A**) low and (**B**) high-magnification bright field micrographs, and (**C**) size distribution histogram of the nanosystems.

Table 3. Different HA amounts (mg) used for the preparation of $Fe_3O_4 \cdot DA\text{-}BSA/HA$ nanoparticles.

$Fe_3O_4 \cdot OA$ (SPION1)	BSA	HA	Samples
		250	SPION2
100	250	50	SPION3
		25	SPION4

The huge decrease of HA organic components appeared to provoke a loss in the homogeneous morphology of SPION4 (as is clearly detectable from the TEM image, Figure 11). For these reasons, SPION4 was discarded for subsequent evaluations. Concerning SPION2 and SPION3, minor differences in nanoparticle size were noticed in DLS measurements (Table 2 and Figure 12).

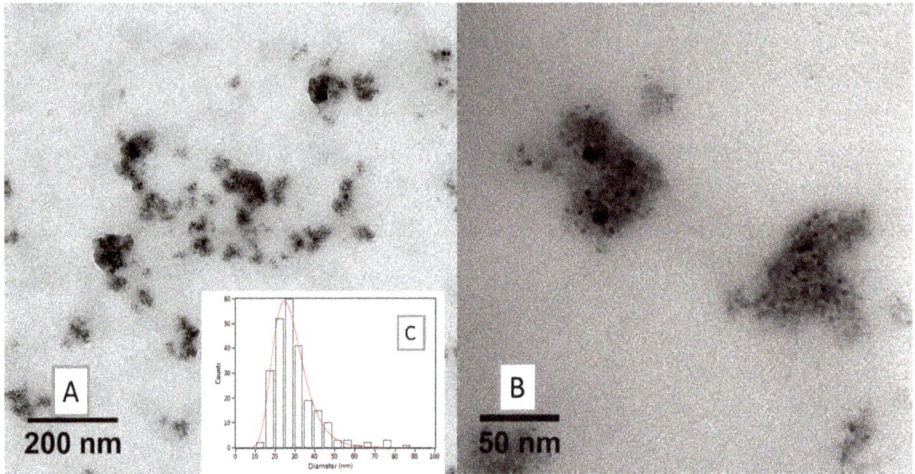

Figure 11. TEM analysis on SPION4: (**A**) low and (**B**) high magnification bright field micrographs, and (**C**) size distribution histogram of the nanosystems.

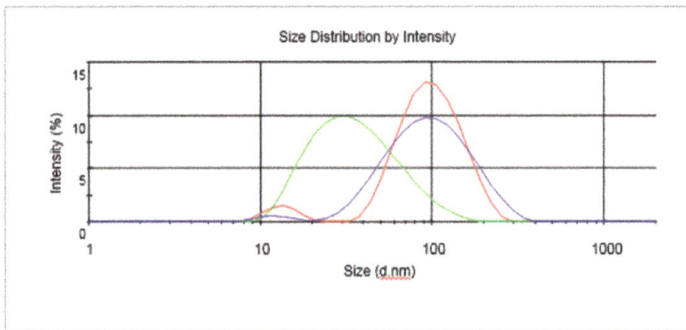

Figure 12. Dynamic light scattering (DLS) profiles of SPION1 (green), SPION2 (red), and SPION3 (blue).

Concerning the evaluation of the surface charges of the nanosystem, Table 4 reports Z potential (ξ) values of different samples. Both of the functional organic molecules (HA and BSA) own an overall negative surface charge, which is slightly decreased as a result of the covalent linkage with dopamine moiety. The positive ξ values of SPIONs depend on the surface charge due to the CTA [34].

Table 4. Zeta potential (ξ) values for HA, BSA, BSA-DA, HA-DA, and SPION2, 3, and 6.

	ξ (mV)
Hyaluronic Acid (HA)	−30.8 ± 1.74
Bovine Serum Albumin (BSA)	−26.4 ± 1.51
BSA-DA	−6.14 ± 1.30
HA-DA	−2.17 ± 0.83
SPION2	+15.3 ± 1.01
SPION3	+19.2 ± 1.16
SPION6	+17.5 ± 2.21

2.2. Inclusion of Paclitaxel and Drug Release

2.2.1. Fe$_3$O$_4$·DA-BSA/HA Nanoparticles with Paclitaxel (PTX)

The antimitotic drug Paclitaxel (PTX) was included in both Fe$_3$O$_4$·DA-BSA/HA nanoparticles, resulting in samples SPION5 and SPION6, obtained from SPION2 and SPION3, respectively.

A dispersion of PTX was slowly added to progressive volumes of Fe$_3$O$_4$·DA-BSA/HA nanoparticles in PBS (until 1:3 *v/v*). The efficiency of the entrapment was firstly verified due to the visual disappearance of water-insoluble PTX crystals. No significant changes in the structure of the assemblies (Z$_{av}$ in Table 2 and Figure S7), in their morphology (TEM, Figure S8) and in their superficial electric potential (ξ, Table 4) were observed.

2.2.2. PTX Release Kinetics

SPION6 was used as the pilot nanosystem in order to test a preliminary kinetic profile of the PTX release over time. In particular, an aliquot of SPION6 colloidal solution containing PTX was submitted to a dialysis-based assay. The amount of released PTX into the dialysis solution was monitored by means of quantitative UV-Vis spectrophotometry. A gradual almost total release of the drug was observed, as detectable by plotting the percentage of released PTX versus times (Figure 13). More details are reported in the experimental part (see Section 4.4).

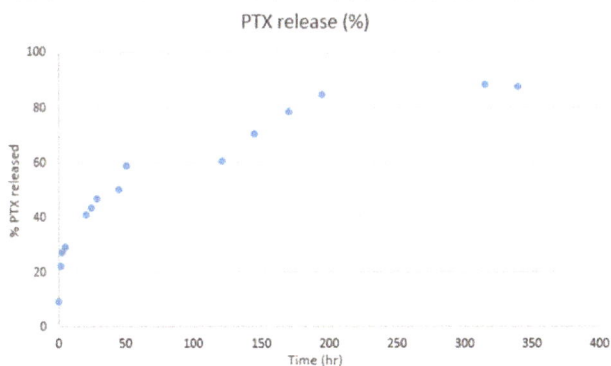

Figure 13. Percentage of released PTX plotted against time (hours). Data were obtained with UV-Vis experiments performed on SPION6 (see Figure S4).

2.3. Time-domain (TD)-NMR Experiments

The solution behavior of contrast agents is often used to screen their potential before animal testing [35]. Thus, relaxation times T$_1$ and T$_2$ were calculated for all preparations at several different dilutions, starting from saturated dispersions of samples SPION2 and SPION3. Additionally, we tested corresponding preparations where PTX was added. For the base dispersions, we measured the amount of nanoparticles, expressed in weight, by drying. In addition, we determined the Fe atomic content of SPION2 and SPION3 by inductively coupled plasma (ICP) spectrometry. The results, expressed in % wt, are 1.38% and 5.45% for SPION2 and SPION3, respectively. Addition of the PTX was performed by adding 1 mL of PTX solution to 3 mL nanoparticle solution.

All NMR experimental data were well fitted by monomodal decay functions (Figure S5). An absence of multimodal decay indicates the system is in rapid exchange regime, with relaxation averaged by fast molecular motion between bulk solvent and nanoparticle surface. Iron nanoparticles are covered by a HA/BSA layer that makes them compatible with water as well as with each other.

The coexistence of these interactions makes the grafted particles stick together into hierarchical superstructures, as is clearly detectable from TEM images (Figures 10 and 11). Microscopically, they are loose assemblies where water molecules can move easily throughout the soft and hydrophilic particle organic cover, coming in proximity of the paramagnetic iron oxide cores dispersed within with high rate. This is very promising for future study on renal clearance, a desirable goal for nanoparticle design since it avoids iron buildup within the body. This kind of clearance is usually limited to nanoparticles with less than a 5.5 nm hydrodynamic radius [36], a much smaller value than that measured by DLS for the present samples. Still, it is well known that soft and flexible particles can squeeze through the renal nodules [37]. Furthermore, while the present samples are stable in PBS solution, their hierarchical nature provides the opportunity to further tune the surface for stimuli-responsive decomposition [13], ultimately separating component particles which are in the range of 3–5 nm.

Relaxation rates R_1 and R_2, defined as the inverse of relaxation times T_1 and T_2, respectively, were plotted against the molar concentration of Fe, as exemplified by Figure 14A, which shows a comparison between the R_2 values for samples SPION2 and SPION3. The resulting plots were highly linear ($R^2 > 0.99$); thus, molar relaxivities r_1 and r_2 could be calculated as slopes of the linear fitting and are indicated in Table 5. Firstly, the high linearity indicates that the aggregates are stable, since any phenomenon of aggregation or splitting of the nanoassemblies would qualitatively change the interaction with water. The values in Fe molar concentration for the two samples span different ranges because the nanoparticle concentration in the dispersions is the same, but the nanoassemblies prepared with lower amounts of HA have a higher content in Fe cores. This is apparent in Figure 14B, where we instead plot the same relaxivity values against the amount of nanoparticles (not of Fe). Due to the higher Fe loading potential of SPION3, this compound could be the most suitable for medical applications.

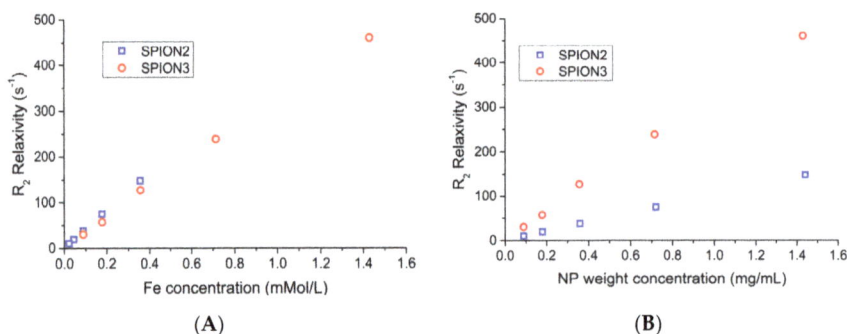

Figure 14. Dependence of R_2 relaxation rates for unloaded NP over (**A**) Fe concentration and (**B**) amount of nanoparticles.

Table 5. Longitudinal relaxation R_1 of SPION2, SPION5, SPION3 and SPION6.

Sample	Composition	$r_1 \pm SD$ (s^{-1} Mm^{-1})	$r_2 \pm SD$ (s^{-1} Mm^{-1})	$r_2/r_1 \pm SD$
SPION2	$Fe_3O_4 \cdot DA\text{-}BSA/HA$	76.8 ± 1.4	414 ± 4	5.41 ± 0.03
SPION5	SPION2 + PTX	81.2 ± 1.4	396 ± 5	4.88 ± 0.04
SPION3	$Fe_3O_4 \cdot DA\text{-}BSA/HA_{20\%}$	61.1 ± 0.7	321 ± 6	5.26 ± 0.04
SPION6	SPION3 + PTX	62.9 ± 1.2	333 ± 6	5.29 ± 0.005

On the other hand, the similarity of the values plotted against Fe concentration indicates that the particles have fundamentally the same interactions with water regardless of the BSA/HA ratio.

Later, we also verified the effect of the presence of PTX. From the data presented in Table 5 (see also figures), it is apparent that there is no effect. Similar plots were prepared for longitudinal relaxation R_1; those values are also reported in Table 5.

The high molar relaxivity values show high promise for application as an MRI agent, since both the r_1 and r_2 values are comparable to top end commercial contrast agents [38]. In addition, the inclusion of PTX did not significantly influence the relaxometric parameters, suggesting theranostic applications. Since current MRI techniques are based on achieving contrast in different T_1 and T_2 experiments, the R_2/R_1 ratio is often used to evaluate the applicability of a system for use as a black or white contrast agent [39]. The present samples have values of around 5, indicating a preferential usage as a dark contrast agent, but also some possible applications for white contrast, a field currently dominated by Gd contrast agents, which have high effectivity but some well-known side effects including deposition in brain tissue and a risk of nephrogenic fibrosis.

Figure 15 shows that SPIONs have a darkening effect on T2w scans, as expected, dilution of the sample with PBS decreased the signal of the SPIONs as the iron concentration decreased. The concentration of Fe_3O_4 in the samples was insufficient for significant signal because HA unexpectedly caused a lightening effect in the MRI, which counteracted the SPION signal reducing the signal darkening effect. A significant signal darkening was observed for the original samples of SPION3 and SPION4, but, after 50-fold dilution, the signal of SPION3 was dramatically less dark compared to SPION4, which corresponds to the fact that HA concentration of SPION4 was half the concentration of SPION3. We can conclude from this experiment that decreasing HA concentration significantly improved the ability of the SPIONs to serve as good contrast agents in MRI.

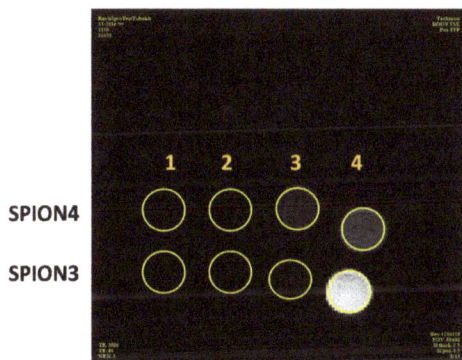

Figure 15. In vitro MRI T2w scans of samples SPION3 and SPION4. (**1**) Original sample; (**2**) 2-fold dilution; (**3**) 10-fold dilution; and (**4**) 50-fold dilution.

3. Discussion

The challenge of this work was to prepare $Fe_3O_4\cdot DA\text{-}BSA/HA$ nanoparticles (SPION samples) with the capability of loading PTX. We pursued this investigation to provide biologists and possibly clinics with new theranostic tools. We depicted SPION features and potentialities, starting with the design, passing from the synthesis to the structural and physicochemical characterization of both the final adducts and the intermediates, going on with TD-NMR investigation, and ending with the loading and release of PTX.

As anyone can recognize in current research, the nanomedicine field is becoming immeasurable. It could be compared to a dark forest where it is very difficult to find one's bearings. As an example, a scholar intending to update the enhanced permeability and retention (EPR) of nanoparticles in tumors could not avoid considering the paper of Nichols and Bae, published in 2014, where they presented a solid overview of EPR limits and perspectives [40]. We offer these remarks to clarify the thinking we followed to project $Fe_3O_4\cdot DA\text{-}BSA/HA$. First, we judge that the theranostic approach is still valid to fight cancer, and that its rationale is the best to pursue, as far as we know. Additionally, we decided that, in this war, our chemical approach must be not too sophisticated, while structural and physicochemical characterization needed to be as in-depth as possible. The synthetic strategy for creating SPIONs was based on well-known reactions. Dopamine (DA) has been shown to easily bind to Fe_3O_4 as a bidentate enediol ligand [41] and to be a robust and stable anchor group to functionalize iron oxide nanoparticles with functional molecules [42]. In $Fe_3O_4 \cdot DA$-BSA/HA, dopamine (DA) is the spacer between BSA and HA and the iron core. Furthermore, DA is very convenient as a bifunctional molecule suitable to functionalize the terminal amino group, for example by condensation with the carboxylic group of glycosaminoglycans [43] and of proteins [44]. BSA and HA were separately cross-linked to DA by an amide bond, affording BSA-DA and HA-DA, as detailed in the result and experimental sections. Of note, a dialysis procedure was used to remove nonpolymeric materials and undesired byproducts from the BSA-DA and HA-DA crude reactions. The reagents ratio employed for HA/BSA and DA crosslinking was decided with the aim of not functionalizing all the carboxylic groups of DA and HA, because in our minds HA and BSA have to maintain their biological and physical properties to act by targeting glycosaminoglycan (HA) and biocompatible protein (SA). It is well known that charges are crucial for the electrostatic interaction so important in biological environments.

A significant effort was made to characterize both the dialyzed crude reactions, putting in evidence the amido linkage formation and estimating the substitution degree of the HA and BSA carboxylic groups with DA: see Sections 2.1.1 and 2.1.2 The medium average derivatization of BSA was estimated 20 molecules of DA for each molecule of BSA. The medium average derivatization of HA was estimated at two molecules of DA for each 10 disaccharide building blocks.

BSA-DA and HA-DA solutions were used in a one-pot reaction to perform ligand exchange on iron oleate (OA) nanoparticles, $Fe_3O_4 \cdot OA$, prepared in organic solvent [45,46]: see Sections 2.1.3 and 2.1.4. Oleic acid coating was used to stabilize and enhance the exchange with DA adducts. $Fe_3O_4 \cdot OA$ ligand exchange with DA-BSA and DA-HA provided $Fe_3O_4 \cdot DA$-BSA/HA as a bioactive adduct suitable for suspensions in buffer solution [47]. As far as we know, $Fe_3O_4 \cdot DA$-BSA/HA is a new nanostructure, in terms of its covalent DA linkages and DA chelation of Fe. HA and BSA undergo strong interactions that could be associated with significative bioactivities and synergic effects in stabilizing SPION and targeting citotoxic drugs to tumor mass. Different $Fe_3O_4 \cdot DA$-BSA/HA (SPIONs) were prepared by changing the DA-HA:DA-BSA ratios: see Table 3 and Section 4.2.4. We assume that modified DA reactivity towards Fe does not depend on the cross-linked polymers. This assumption is justified by the high affinity between DA and Fe and by the fact that steric effects are, in our opinion, not very important because of the distance between the diol and the amino group. Therefore, the initial DA-HA:DA-BSA ratio affords $Fe_3O_4 \cdot DA$-BSA/HA composition. SPIONs were all characterized by IR spectroscopy that supports the $Fe_3O_4 \cdot DA$-BSA/HA structure and gives evidence of CTA as positive counter ions of the carboxylic groups not involved in the amidation. The relevant rule that CTAB plays in modulating the interactions of magnetic nanoparticles with biomolecules [34] is noteworthy.

For convenience, the SPION2 spectrum is shown and detailed: see Figure 8. TEM images were reported in Figures 9–11 and partly discussed in the results. Before further discussing SPION2-6 TEM and DLS results, let us have a look to SPION1, which is the precursor of $Fe_3O_4 \cdot DA$-BSA/HA. SPION1 could be described as a nanostructured organic salt or complex. Its morphology is shown in Figure 7. It shows iron cores surrounded by the organic layer of oleic acid. After the ligand exchange, the situation dramatically changes. The $Fe_3O_4 \cdot DA$-BSA/HA morphology resembles a pomegranate, with several iron cores covered by a single organic envelopment. The size of the iron cores does not seem to vary significantly in the different SPIONs. On the other hand, SPION size distribution depends on the different ratios between the inorganic and organic parts, as reported in Table 3. SPION2 was prepared starting from same amount of HA-DA and BSA-DA. In SPION3 preparation, the amount of HA-DA was strongly reduced, and this was even less for SPION4. SPION2 presents a much higher size distribution than SPION3; SPION4 shows the same trend. From TEM, it appears that SPION2 and SPION3 have quite the same morphology (see Figures 9 and 10). We can argue that SPION2 and SPION3 are representatives of the $Fe_3O_4 \cdot DA$-BSA/HA nanosystem, where both HA-DA and HA-BSA contributes to the morphology. This is not true for SPION4 (see Figure 11). In other words, SPION4 cannot be described as a $Fe_3O_4 \cdot DA\text{-}BSA/HA$ nanosystem.

SPION DLS analysis was also provided and summarized in Table 2 and Figure 12. They confirm the difference between SPION1 and the other SPIONS. The DLS data correspond well to most of the engineered SPIONs proposed in the literature. After ligand exchange, the hydrodynamic radius of the newly formed HA/BSA SPIONs increases to 70 nm. Table 2 shows that all the different $Fe_3O_4 \cdot DA\text{-}BSA/HA$ fall in the range of standard SPION (50–150 nm). Noteworthy SPION that are 10–100 nm in size are considered to be optimal for intravenous administration [15]. This observation makes $Fe_3O_4 \cdot DA\text{-}BSA/HA$ promising for future biomedical applications. Since the iron cores are not modified, this confirms that the assembly of large particles, as seen in Figure 9, is modulated by the interaction between biomolecular coronas and water, resulting in complex hierarchical (pomegranate) structures. Looking to the SPIONs' morphology and size distribution, we argue that some $Fe_3O_4 \cdot DA\text{-}BSA/HA$ properties could be modulated by changing the ratios between HA and DA and between them and Fe. Note especially the zeta potential (ξ) values reported in Table 4 for HA, BSA, BSA-DA, HA-DA, and SPION2, 3 and 6. The ξ values change from negative, for HA-DA and BSA-DA, to positive for SPION2 and SPION3, perfectly agreeing with surface charges due to the CTA cation [34]. The presence of CTA as counter ion can be correlated with a very good colloidal stability as observed in Ref. [34]. Furthermore, the magnetic properties of our SPIONs discussed on the base of their TD-NMR results support the biomedical diagnostic potentiality of the system $Fe_3O_4 \cdot DA\text{-}BSA/HA$ plus CTA.

SPION2 and SPION3 were loaded with PTX to obtain SPION5 and SPION6, as explained in Section 2.2.1. PTX was easily dispersed by the SPION2 and SPION3 suspensions. Both of the SPION5 and SPION6 DLS and TEM measurements of the obtained drug vehicle did not highlight any significant morphological variation (see Table 2 and Figures S7 and S8). Zeta potential values were also not affected ($\xi = 17.5 \pm 2.21$ mV, Table 4). The maintenance of size, morphology and ξ support the PTX loading within SPION2 and SPION3 affording SPION5 and SPION6. In advance, the $Fe_3O_4 \cdot DA\text{-}BSA/HA$ capability to load PTX can be correlated with the PTX hydrophobic interaction with BSA. Since the nanoparticle albumin-bound paclitaxel has been discovered, many approaches have been attempted to put it in more complex systems to avoid the undesired effects of PTX anticancer drug. As a matter of fact, unfortunately the nanoparticle albumin-bound paclitaxel alone cannot solve the PTX limits and drawback. Layer-by-layer assembly of hierarchical nanoarchitectures has been investigated to enhance the systemic performance of nanoparticle albumin-bound paclitaxel [48]. The biodegradability has been pursued in one-step fabrication of agent-loaded biodegradable microspheroids for drug delivery and imaging applications [49]. A quite similar approach has been the thermoreversible gelation of poly(ethylene glycol)/poly(ester anhydride) triblock copolymer nanoparticles for injectable drug delivery systems [50]. Nanoparticle albumin-bound paclitaxel has been loaded into a nanoporous solid multistage nanovector to enhance therapeutic efficacy [51]. Finally, drug-induced self-assembly of modified albumins has been proposed for tumor-targeted combination therapy [52]. The rational of our approach to load PTX within $Fe_3O_4 \cdot DA\text{-}BSA/HA$ perfectly agrees with References [48–52] and enhances the BSA role in $Fe_3O_4 \cdot DA\text{-}BSA/HA$ structures.

As shown in Figure 13, PTX was released by SPION6 at 90% in nine days: see Section 2.2.2. In about one day, 60% of PTX was released. Both the PTX loading and the preliminary release data associated with the physicochemical characterization of SPION5 and SPION6 are strongly encouraging for the development of $Fe_3O_4 \cdot DA\text{-}BSA/HA$ as PTX delivery nanosystems, where loaded PTX was made bioavailable in buffer solution and matched with the $Fe_3O_4 \cdot DA\text{-}BSA/HA$ targeting potentiality according to the hope of reducing the PTX administered dose.

Section 2.3 reports the results obtained by TD-NMR experiments and highlights useful comments. In particular, the SPIONs' magnetic properties appear crucial to recognition that $Fe_3O_4 \cdot DA\text{-}BSA/HA$ can also be tested as an innovative contrast agent: see Table 5 and Figure 14. Figure 14b shows the very important result about the R_2 relaxation of SPION2 compared with SPION3: the same NP weight concentration, but different Fe contents (SPION3 > SPION2), corresponds to a higher R_2 relaxation for SPION3 than for SPION2.

SPIONs were reported to be excellent MRI T2 contrast agents. As excepted, in vitro T2w MRI scanning of SPION3 and SPION4 demonstrated significant dark signal having a great potential for targeted imaging. The approximate blood volume of a mouse is 77–80 µL/g weight. After IV injection (200 µL) to mice, the sample is diluted in the blood stream (1.9–2 mL) and concentrated in the tumor so the dilution of the sample is up to 10 fold. From the MRI in vitro result (Figure 15), even after 10-fold dilution the darkening effect of SPION3 and SPION4 is significant, thus we can deduct from this experiment that a sufficient signal will be presumably observed in mice. Moreover, at higher dilution, SPION4 has a better darkening signal due to its lower concentration of HA.

We can argue not only that SPION3 could be more suitable as contrast agent, but also that the synthetic strategy approached in this paper can modulate $Fe_3O_4 \cdot DA\text{-}BSA/HA$ properties. The TD-NMR experiments also confirm $Fe_3O_4 \cdot DA\text{-}BSA/HA$ stability, a feature that is essential for further developments. Finally, the fact that the inclusion of PTX did not at all modify the magnetic properties of $Fe_3O_4 \cdot DA\text{-}BSA/HA$ strongly supports the achievement of using $Fe_3O_4 \cdot DA\text{-}BSA/HA$ as theranostic agent.

4. Materials and Methods

4.1. General

Chemicals: Ferric chloride hexahydrate ($FeCl_3 \cdot 6H_2O$), ferrous chloride tetrahydrate ($FeCl_2 \cdot 4H_2O$), sodium chloride (NaCl), potassium chloride (KCl), sodium hydrogenphosphate (Na_2HPO_4), potassium dihydrogen phosphate (KH_2PO_4), dopamine hydrochloride (DA·HCl), bovine serum albumine (BSA), cetyl trimethylammonium bromide (CTAB), *N*-(3 dimethylaminopropyl)-*N'*-ethylcarbodiimide hydrochloride (EDC·HCl), hydrochloric acid (HCl, 37%), sodium hydroxide (NaOH), and paclitaxel (PTX) were purchased from Sigma Aldrich (St. Louis, MO, USA). Oleic acid ≥85% and sodium oleate were purchased from Tokyo Chemical Industry (TCI), Tokyo, Japan. Sodium hyaluronate (5400 Da) was purchased from Lifecore Biomedical, Inc., Chaska, MN, USA.

Materials: Dialysis sacks were purchased from Sigma Aldrich (MWCO: 12,000 Da) (St. Louis, MO, USA) and from SpectrumLabs (Spectra/Por 3 Dialysis Tubing, MWCO: 3500 Da). Syringe filters (25 mm, 0.22 µm) were purchased from VWR International, Milan, Italy.

4.2. Synthetic Procedures

4.2.1. Synthesis of BSA-DA Adduct

The reaction flask was obscured to prevent denaturation of the BSA protein. First, 250 mg of BSA were dissolved in 20 mL of PBS buffer solution (NaCl 137 mM, KCl 3 mM, Na_2HPO_4 10 mM and KH_2PO_4 2 mM. pH = 7.4). Then 527.5 mg of 1-ethyl-3-(3'-dimethyl-aminopropyl)-carbodiimide (EDC) were added, under magnetic stirring. After a few minutes, 500 mg of dopamine hydrochloride were added to the solution, which rapidly became darker. The reaction lasted 20 h. The final mixture was dialyzed against several changes (6 × 1 L) of PBS buffer solution (MWCO: 12,000 Da). The recovered mixture was analyzed by MALDI–TOF.

4.2.2. Synthesis of HA-DA Adduct

The first 250 mg of Sodium Hyaluronate (5400 Da) were dissolved with 20 mL of PBS solution (pH = 7.4). A few drops of aqueous solution of HCl (1M) were added to adjust the pH to the value of 5–5.5. Then, 120 mg of Dopamine hydrochloride and 100 mg of EDC were added. The pH of the solution rapidly increased up to 8.0, and several drops of HCl 1M were added to the solution over time in order to keep the pH values between 5.0 and 6.0 during the reaction time (3 h). After 3 h, the pH no longer increased and the reaction was considered finished. The final mixture was dialyzed against several changes (3 × 1 L) of PBS buffer solution (MWCO: 3500 Da).

4.2.3. Synthesis of $Fe_3O_4 \cdot OA$ Nanoparticles (SPION1)

The magnetite gel was formulated by coprecipitation. First, 3.44 g of $FeCl_2 \cdot 4H_2O$ and 9.40 g of $FeCl_3 \cdot 6H_2O$ were dissolved in 160 mL of distilled water under nitrogen gas with vigorous stirring, at 80 °C for 30 min. Next a mixture composed of 24 mL of NH_4OH solution (25% NH_3 in H_2O), 4 mL of oleic acid, and 4 mL of acetone was slowly added to the solution. The color of the reaction mixture immediately turned to black. Stirring lasted 30 min and then the solution was heated again, to 80 °C, for 30 min. $Fe_3O_4 \cdot OA$ nanoparticle precipitation was promoted by adding 200 mL of EtOH 99% and putting a magnet under the reaction flask. The transparent liquid phase was removed and the recovered black solid material was dissolved in hexane (150 mL) and reprecipitated with ethanol (200 mL), with the simultaneous promoted magnetic sedimentation. After the removal of liquid supernatant, a last washing of the nanoparticles was performed by using acetone in an ultrasonic bath for 10 min. The SPIONs were collected and dissolved in hexane, a solvent that allows their storage for a long time avoiding any aggregation phenomena. The chemical structure of dried $Fe_3O_4 \cdot OA$ nanoparticles (SPION1) was investigated by FTIR analysis; TEM and DLS characterization was also performed.

4.2.4. Synthesis of $Fe_3O_4 \cdot DA$-BSA/HA Nanoparticles (SPION2, SPION3, SPION4)

Once DA-BSA and DA-HA adducts were prepared, the exchange reaction between them and the oleic acid coating of nanoparticles was performed in a one-step procedure. In addition, 100 mg $Fe_3O_4 \cdot OA$ (SPION1) were dispersed in 7 mL of chloroform. These dispersed nanoparticles were added to a solution of 1.33 g of cetyl trimethylammonium bromide (CTAB) in 66.5 mL of PBS buffer. Chloroform was carefully removed under reduced pressure. Suspended $Fe_3O_4 \cdot OA$ nanoparticles were added, drop by drop and under vigorous stirring, to different mixtures of dissolved DA-BSA and DA-HA adducts in PBS (50:50, 80:20 and 90:10, respectively) in order to perform the ligand exchange reaction, resulting in the samples SPION2, SPION3, and SPION4, respectively. The products were soluble in PBS and the solid CTAB and the oil had to be discarded through centrifugation (9000 rpm, 30 min, r.t.). The final mixtures were dialyzed against several changes (3 × 1 L) of PBS buffer solution (MWCO: 12,000 Da). The samples were characterized with FTIR, DLS, and TEM and then submitted to further evaluations by means of TD-NMR experiments.

4.2.5. Inclusion of PTX in $Fe_3O_4 \cdot DA$-BSA/HA Nanoparticles (SPION5, SPION6)

An aliquot of milky aqueous dispersion of paclitaxel (0.5 mg/mL) was added to $Fe_3O_4 \cdot DA$-BSA/HA NPs (SPION2 or SPION3) within a starting volumetric ratio of 1:1 (*v/v*). The preparation was sonicated for 10 min. Then, a further aliquot of NPs was added, with a final 1:3 (*v/v*) ratio (PTX:NPs). After a further sonication of 10 min, the system was maintained for approximately 48 h under constant stirring.

4.3. Characterization Methods

4.3.1. Fourier Transform Infrared Spectroscopy (FTIR)

The solid phase FTIR spectra of the powdered sample with infrared grade KBr were generated using an ALPHA spectrometer (Bruker, Bremen, Germany). Data were analyzed using OPUS software, version 7.0 (Bruker, Bremen, Germany).

4.3.2. Transmission Electron Microscopy (TEM)

TEM micrographs and selected area electron diffraction (SAED) patterns were acquired using a Philips CM200 Field emission gun transmission electron microscope (Koninklijke Philips N.V., Eindhoven NETHERLANDS) operating at 200 kV. The suspensions of iron oxide nanoparticles and supraparticles were deposited onto a 200 mesh holey carbon-coated copper grid and let dry a few hours before the analysis. Image analyses of TEM micrographs were performed using ImageJ software, Research Services Branch (RSB) of the National Institute of Mental Health (NIMH) [53], which is quite useful for estimating the dimension and shape of nanoparticles and supraparticles. In particular, the mean values and widths of the statistical asymmetric distribution ($\sigma-$, $\sigma+$) of particles were evaluated by fitting the experimental values with a log-normal function (Table S4).

4.3.3. Dynamic Light Scattering (DLS)

Hydrodynamic diameter (Z_{av}) and zeta potential (ξ) values of nanosystems were measured using the Zetasizer Nano ZS (Malvern, Worcestershire, UK) with a fixed 173° scattering angle and a 633-nm-helium-neon-laser. Data were analyzed using Zetasizer software, version 7.11 (Malvern, Worcestershire, UK). The temperature was set at 298 K. SPION1 was collected from the bulk mixture after the first dispersion with hexane and directly submitted to DLS measurement. SPION2 and SPION3 were passed through a 0.22 μm syringe filter, sonicated for 10 min, and then submitted to DLS measurements. SPION5 and SPION6 were directly collected and analyzed after 10 min of sonication.

4.3.4. MALDI–TOF Measurements

Measurements of BSA samples and their corresponding dopamine derivatives were performed using an UV-MALDI–TOF Autoflex mass spectrometer (Bruker, Bremen, Germany) equipped with an ultraviolet laser (λ = 232 nm) operating in linear and positive ion mode in the mass range from 10 to 150 kDa. Each spectrum was recorded by averaging about 300 shots after appropriate mass range calibration performed with commercial standard proteins mixture (trypsinogen, protein A, albumin-bovine). The matrix solution, used either for analytes or standard proteins solution, was freshly prepared as a saturated solution of sinapinic acid (SA) in water 0.1% TFA:acetonitrile 2:1 (*v/v*). The analyte solutions were prepared at a concentration of 5–7 mg/mL in water (corresponding to about 100 pmol/μL of BSA protein) and mixed with the matrix solution in a 1:1 (*v/v*) ratio; then, 1 μL of this matrix/analyte mixture was loaded on the stainless steel probe and left to dry at room temperature.

4.3.5. HPLC/Mass Spectrometry Measurements

Analyses of hyaluronic acid and its dopamine derivative were performed on an HPLC system (Platin Blue, Knauer, Berlin, Germany) coupled to ESI-Q-TOF mass spectrometer (impact II, Bruker). Because of the polyanionic nature of hyaluronic acid, chromatographic separation of the numerous components contained in extremely complex mixture of the hyaluronic acid sample was performed by ion pairing reversed-phase liquid chromatography (IP RP LC method) using alkylamine for ion pairing.

The sample solution was prepared at a concentration of 1 mg/mL. 2 μL were injected on a 2.1 × 100 mm Kinetex reversed-phase C18 column with 2.6 μm particles (Phenomenex, Aschaffenburg, Germany) hold at 35 °C and run at a flow rate of 0.15 mL/min, by the mobile phases A (dibutylamine 10 mM, acetic acid 10 mM in water) and B (dibutylamine 10 mM, acetic acid 10 mM in methanol) according to the following gradient: isocratic step at 10% B for 5 min, followed by a first linear gradient from 10% to 31% B in 30 min and a second slower gradient from 31% to 45% B in 30 min; then, column washing at 90% B for 5 min and reconditioning in the initial conditions were performed.

The mass spectrometry detector was set to negative polarity (capillary voltage: +3500 V) in the mass range from m/z 140 to m/z 2500; nitrogen gas used as nebulizer and heater gases was set at 1.8 bar and 7.0 L/min, respectively.

Mass calibration was performed by using sodium formate solution (water–isopropanol 1:1 *v/v* solution containing HCOOH 0.2% and NaOH 5×10^{-3} N).

4.3.6. NMR Experiments

NMR spectra were recorded at 30 °C using a Bruker Avance HD spectrometer (500 MHz) equipped with a high sensitivity 5 mm TCI cryoprobe. Samples were dissolved in ^2H_2O (99.996%) and in 0.5 M NaCl, pH 7.4 and placed in 5-mm NMR tubes. Proton spectra were recorded with presaturation of the residual water signal with a recycle delay of 12 s and 8–16 scans. Bidimensional double quantum filter-COSY and two-dimensional Total Correlation Spectroscopy (TOCSY) spectra were acquired using 16 scans per series of 2048_320 data points with zero filling in F1 and F2 (4096_2048), and a shifted ($\pi/2$) squared cosine function was applied prior to Fourier transformation.

Heteronuclear single quantum coherence (HSQC) spectra were obtained in phase sensitivity-enhanced pure absorption mode with decoupling in the acquisition period and 24 scans while heteronuclear multiple bond correlation spectra (HMBC) were obtained with 64 scans. The matrix size of both experiments was 1024_320 data points and was zero-filled to 4096_2048 by application of a shifted ($\pi/2$) squared cosine function prior to Fourier transformation. Diffusion-ordered spectroscopy (DOSY) spectra were acquired using 32 scans and a series of 16 spin echo spectra registered with a time domain of 16 K zero-filled to 64 K.

4.3.7. ICP Experiments

For the experiments, 14.4 mg of both SPION2 and SPION3 (obtained by lyofilization) were mineralized with nitric acid (HNO_3) and subsequently analyzed using inductively coupled plasma (ICP) spectrometry. The employed instrument was a Perkin Elmer Optica 2300 (Perkin Elmer, Milan, Italy).

4.3.8. Time-Domain (TD) NMR Experiments

A 0.5 T Bruker Minispec was used for relaxometry. This instrument is a low-resolution NMR spectrometer with proton larmor frequency of 19.65 MHz, equipped with static probe and a BVT3000 temperature control unit working with nitrogen gas. The temperature was calibrated using an external thermometer with an accuracy of ±1 K. The precision was 0.1 K; in these conditions, the temperature is stable within that range during the measurement.

All of the experiments were performed at a temperature of 303 K (29.85 °C), obtained using a Eurotherm nitrogen gas thermal apparatus (Como, Italy). Samples were prepared outside the NMR tube, and then 150 µL of each solution was inserted in a 10 mm o.d. tube, positioned in the magnet with the sample in the volume of maximum homogeneity of the B_0 and B_1 fields. All of the samples were thermalized for 10 minutes before performing the experiments.

For the $\pi/2$ and π, the pulse lengths were set to 2.07 µs and 4.15 µs, respectively. A good signal-to-noise ratio was obtained within a few scans, but due to the analytical nature of this work, each sample was measured with 128 scans during Carr–Purcell–Meiboom–Gill (CPMG) experiments and 64 scans per point during saturation recovery experiments.

For T_2 measurements, we made use of CPMG pulse sequence with parameters optimized for analytical use at low field [54]. This sequence consisted of a first 90° pulse followed by a train of equally spaced 180° pulses. The signal is measured in the midpoint between each pair of 180° pulses and the obtained decaying curve is fitted against $A \exp(-t/T_2)$.

For T_1, we implemented a saturation recovery sequence [55], a sequence composed by a pulse train that is optimized for defocusing the magnetization of the sample. Longitudinal magnetization was then measured using a single $\pi/2$ pulse after a set waiting time. Signal recovery as a function of time was then interpreted using the following equation:

$$M_z = M_0 \left[1 - exp\left(-\frac{t}{T_1}\right) \right]. \tag{1}$$

4.4. PTX-Release Experiments

SPION6 (4 mL) was placed in a dialysis sack (MWCO: 3500 Da) and dialyzed against 30 mL of mixture containing 70% PBS buffer and 30% methanol. The experiment was conducted in a shaking water bath (SW22, Julabo) at room temperature and with a shaking frequency of 100 rpm. The amount of released PTX over time was monitored through quantitative UV-Vis (UV-spectrophotometer JASCO v-650; Cremella LC, Italy), SpectraManager software (Cremella LC, Italy). Several aliquots of dialysate mixture were collected at different times and immediately submitted to UV acquisitions, and then replaced in the mixture of the dialysis experiment. The calibration curve employed for the quantitative conversion of data over time was taken from existing literature ($y = 0.04x - 0.0626$; $R^2 = 0.9931$) [56,57].

4.5. In Vitro MRI

SPION3, SPION 4 and dilutions of those samples were scanned using a 9.4 T preclinical MRI scanner (Bruker, Bremen, Germany). Echo Time (TE) and Repetition Time (TR): TR/TE = 3000/60.

5. Conclusions

Our work was successful in identifying the synthetic strategy to obtain $Fe_3O_4 \cdot DA\text{-}BSA/HA$ of 70–90 nm size containing different iron cores of 5 nm, quite homogenous and capable to afford well-dispersed and stable colloidal system. The synthetic strategy is quite easy, reproducible and up-scalable. Huge efforts were successfully done to modulate $Fe_3O_4 \cdot DA\text{-}BSA/HA$ both in terms of the ratio between the inorganic core and the bioorganic layer, and the ratio between bovine serum albumin (BSA) and hyaluronic acid (HA) content in the bioorganic layer. Great attention was dedicated to structural and morphological characterization aspects. $Fe_3O_4 \cdot DA\text{-}BSA/HA$ was capable of entrapping paclitaxel (PTX). Its physical-chemical characterization and preliminary release tests open the way to use $Fe_3O_4 \cdot DA\text{-}BSA/HA$ as PTX delivery system. Noteworthy, $Fe_3O_4 \cdot DA\text{-}BSA/HA$ increased the PTX bioavailability. $Fe_3O_4 \cdot DA\text{-}BSA/HA$ gave good results in TD-NMR experiments to demonstrating their suitability to be developed as contrast agents in MRI.

Supplementary Materials: Supplementary materials are available online.

Acknowledgments: Blerina Gjocka (Politecnico) and Gabriele Colombo (Ronzoni) for experimental works; Cesare Cosentino for NMR experiments. Bioiberica S.A., Barcelona Spain, for the contribution to the publication costs. Edith Suss-Toby, Ortal Schwartz and or Perlman for the professional assistance with the MRI experiments. La presente pubblicazione è stata realizzata con il contributo del Ministero degli Affari Esteri (MAE), Italy. (MAE, partial funding QUADRUGNOSTIC Project, MAE02674642013-11-27, bilateral project with Technion Department of Biotechnology and Food Engineering, Technion-Israel Institute of Technology, Haifa, 32000, Israel).

Author Contributions: E.V. was the main researcher, scientifically responsible and the supervisor of the MAE project. C.B., A.C. were devoted to synthesis, characterisation aspects, results and discussion. A.S. conducted the TEM experiments and wrote the discussion. M.M.R.S. was an expert researcher for the TD-NMR experiments and the discussion. S.B. was an expert researcher for DLS, Zeta Potential analysis, NMR experiments and the discussion. E.U. was an expert researcher for NMR and MALDI-TOF experiments and the discussion. R.E. conducted the in vitro MRI experiments. Y.G.A. was the Israeli partner involved in project conception and biological aspect supervision. Y.D.L. was the Israeli principal investigator and a partner from project conception, who was also responsible for the scientific co-supervision of the project.

Conflicts of Interest: The authors declare no conflicts of interest.

References

1. Pelaz, B.; Alexiou, C.; Alvarez-Puebla, R.A.; Alves, F.; Andrews, A.M.; Ashraf, S.; Balogh, L.P.; Ballerini, L.; Bestetti, A.; Brendel, C.; et al. Diverse applications of nanomedicine. *ACS Nano* **2017**, *11*, 2313–2381. [CrossRef] [PubMed]

2. Sapsford, K.E.; Algar, W.R.; Berti, L.; Gemmill, K.B.; Casey, B.J.; Oh, E.; Stewart, M.H.; Medintz, I.L. Functionalizing nanoparticles with biological molecules: Developing chemistries that facilitate nanotechnology. *Chem. Rev.* **2013**, *113*, 1904–2074. [CrossRef] [PubMed]

3. Laurent, S.; Forge, D.; Port, M.; Roch, A.; Robic, C.; Vander Elst, L.; Muller, R.N. Magnetic iron oxide nanoparticles: Synthesis, stabilization, vectorization, physicochemical characterizations, and biological applications. *Chem. Rev.* **2008**, *108*, 2064–2110. [CrossRef] [PubMed]

4. Tartaj, P.; Morales, M.P.; Veintemillas-Verdaguer, S.; Gonzalez-Carreno, T.; Serna, C.G. Synthesis, properties and biomedical applications of magnetic nanoparticles. *Handb. Magn. Mater.* **2006**, *16*, 403–482.

5. Ramimoghadam, D.; Bagheri, S.; Hamid, S.B.A. Stable monodisperse nanomagnetic colloidal suspensions: An overview. *Colloids Surf. B Biointerfaces* **2015**, *133*, 388–411. [CrossRef] [PubMed]

6. Iyer, S.R.; Xu, S.; Stains, J.P.; Bennett, C.H.; Lovering, R.M. Superparamagnetic iron oxide nanoparticles in musculoskeletal biology. *Tissue Eng. Part B Rev.* **2017**. [CrossRef] [PubMed]
7. Gupta, A.K.; Gupta, M. Synthesis and surface engineering of iron oxide nanoparticles for biomedical applications. *Biomaterials* **2005**, *26*, 3995–4021. [CrossRef] [PubMed]
8. Gupta, A.K.; Naregalkar, R.R.; Vaidya, V.D.; Gupta, M. Recent advances on surface engineering of magnetic iron oxide nanoparticles and their biomedical applications. *Nanomedcine* **2007**, *2*, 23–39. [CrossRef] [PubMed]
9. Bertini, S.; Ferro, M.; Pizzolato, D.; Torri, G.; Valerio, A.; Vismara, E. Low molecular weight heparin-vectorized beta-cyclodextrin nanostructures. In Proceedings of the NSTI Nanotech Nanotechnology Conference and Trade Show, Technical Proceedings, Boston, MA, USA, 1–5 June 2008; Laudon, M., Romanowicz, B., Eds.; CRC Press: Boca Raton, FL, USA, 2008; Volume 2, pp. 487–490.
10. Bava, A.; Cappellini, F.; Pedretti, E.; Rossi, F.; Caruso, E.; Vismara, E.; Chiriva-Internati, M.; Bernardini, G.; Gornati, R. Heparin and carboxymethylchitosan metal nanoparticles: An evaluation of their cytotoxicity. *Biomed. Res. Int.* **2013**, *2013*, 1–10. [CrossRef] [PubMed]
11. Vismara, E.; Valerio, A.; Coletti, A.; Torri, G.; Bertini, S.; Eisele, G.; Gornati, R.; Bernardini, G. Non-covalent synthesis of metal oxide nanoparticle–heparin hybrid systems: A new approach to bioactive nanoparticles. *Int. J. Mol. Sci.* **2013**, *14*, 13463–13481. [CrossRef] [PubMed]
12. Huber, D.L. Synthesis, properties, and applications of iron nanoparticles. *Small* **2005**, *1*, 482–501. [CrossRef] [PubMed]
13. Gossuin, Y.; Gillis, P.; Hocq, A.; Vuong, Q.L.; Roch, A. Magnetic resonance relaxation properties of superparamagnetic particles. *Wiley Interdiscip. Rev. Nanomed. Nanobiotechnol.* **2009**, *1*, 299–310. [CrossRef]
14. Wei, H.; Bruns, O.T.; Kaul, M.G.; Hansen, E.C.; Barch, M.; Wiśniowska, A.; Chen, O.; Chen, Y.; Li, N.; Okada, S.; et al. Exceedingly small iron oxide nanoparticles as positive MRI contrast agents. *Proc. Natl. Acad. Sci. USA* **2017**, *114*, 2325–2330. [CrossRef] [PubMed]
15. Singha, N.; Jenkins, G.J.S.; Asadib, R.; Doaka, S.H. Potential toxicity of superparamagnetic iron oxide nanoparticles (SPION). *Nano Rev.* **2010**, *1*, 5358. [CrossRef] [PubMed]
16. Zaloga, J.; Janko, C.; Nowak, J.; Matuszak, J.; Knaup, S.; Eberbeck, D.; Tietze, R.; Unterweger, H.; Friedrich, R.P.; Duerr, S. Development of a lauric acid/albumin hybrid iron oxide nanoparticle system with improved biocompatibility. *Int. J. Nanomed.* **2014**, *9*, 4847–4866. [CrossRef] [PubMed]
17. Poller, J.M.; Zaloga, J.; Schreiber, E.; Unterweger, H.; Janko, C.; Radon, P.; Eberbeck, D.; Trahms, L.; Alexiou, C.; Friedrich, R.P. Selection of potential iron oxide nanoparticles for breast cancer treatment based on in vitro cytotoxicity and cellular uptake. *Int. J. Nanomed.* **2017**, *12*, 3207–3220. [CrossRef] [PubMed]
18. Shapira, A.; Livney, Y.D.; Broxterman, H.J.; Assaraf, Y.G. Nanomedicine for targeted cancer therapy: Towards the overcoming of drug resistance. *Drug Resist. Updat.* **2011**, *14*, 150–163. [CrossRef] [PubMed]
19. Livney, Y.D.; Assaraf, Y.G. Rationally designed nanovehicles to overcome cancer chemoresistance. *Adv. Drug Deliv. Rev.* **2013**, *65*, 1716–1730. [CrossRef]
20. Wang, Y.X.J. Superparamagnetic iron oxide based MRI contrast agents: Current status of clinical application. *Quant. Imaging Med. Surg.* **2011**, *1*, 35–40. [PubMed]
21. Bakhtiary, Z.; Saei, A.A.; Hajipour, M.J.; Raoufi, M.; Vermesh, O.; Mahmoudi, M. Targeted superparamagnetic iron oxide nanoparticles for early detection of cancer: Possibilities and challenges. *Nanomedicine* **2016**, *12*, 287–307. [CrossRef] [PubMed]
22. Barua, S.; Mitragotri, S. Challenges associated with penetration of nanoparticles across cell and tissue barriers: A review of current status and future prospects. *Nano Today* **2014**, *9*, 223–243. [CrossRef] [PubMed]
23. Journo-Gershfeld, G.; Kapp, D.; Shamay, Y.; Kopecek, J.; David, A. Hyaluronan oligomers-HPMA copolymer conjugates for targeting paclitaxel to CD44-overexpressing ovarian carcinoma. *Pharm. Res.* **2012**, *29*, 1121–1133. [CrossRef] [PubMed]
24. Choi, K.Y.; Chung, H.; Min, K.H.; Yoon, H.Y.; Kim, K.; Park, J.H.; Kwon, I.C.; Jeong, S.Y. Self-assembled hyaluronic acid nanoparticles for active tumor targeting. *Biomaterials* **2010**, *1*, 106–114. [CrossRef] [PubMed]
25. Misra, S.; Heldin, P.; Hascall, V.C.; Karamanos, N.K.; Skandalis, S.S.; Markwald, R.R.; Ghatak, S. HA/CD44 interactions as potential targets for cancer therapy. *FEBS J.* **2011**, *278*, 1429–1443. [CrossRef] [PubMed]
26. Unterweger, H.; Tietze, R.; Janko, C.; Zaloga, J.; Lyer, S.; Dürr, S.; Taccardi, N.; Goudouri, O.M.; Hoppe, A.; Eberbeck, D.; et al. Development and characterization of magnetic iron oxide nanoparticles with a cisplatin-bearing polymer coating for targeted drug delivery. *Int. J. Nanomed.* **2014**, *9*, 3659–3676. [CrossRef] [PubMed]

27. Li, H.; Yan, K.; Shang, Y.; Shrestha, L.; Liao, R.; Liu, F.; Li, P.; Xu, H.; Xu, Z.; Chu, P.K. Folate-bovine serum albumin functionalized polymeric micelles loaded with superparamagnetic iron oxide nanoparticles for tumor targeting and magnetic resonance imaging. *Acta Biomater.* **2015**, *15*, 117–126. [CrossRef] [PubMed]

28. Zhang, B.; Li, Q.; Yin, P.; Rui, Y.; Qiu, Y.; Wang, Y.; Shi, D. Ultrasound-triggered BSA/SPION hybrid nanoclusters for liver-specific magnetic resonance imaging. *ACS Appl. Mater. Interfaces* **2012**, *4*, 6479–6486. [CrossRef] [PubMed]

29. Lv, W.; Cheng, L.; Li, B. Development and evaluation of a novel TPGS-mediated paclitaxel-loaded PLGA-mPEG nanoparticle for the treatment of ovarian cancer. *Chem. Pharm. Bull.* **2015**, *63*, 68–74. [CrossRef] [PubMed]

30. Wang, W.; Wang, M.; Zhang, J.; Liu, H.; Pan, H. Cloud point thermodynamics of paclitaxel-loaded microemulsion in the presence of glucose and NaCl. *Colloids Surf. A Physicochem. Eng. Asp.* **2016**, *507*, 76–82. [CrossRef]

31. Sharma, S.; Singh, J.; Verma, A.; Teja, B.V.; Shukla, R.P.; Singh, S.K.; Sharma, V.; Konwarb, R.; Mishra, P.R. Hyaluronic acid anchored paclitaxel nanocrystals improves chemotherapeutic efficacy and inhibits lung metastasis in tumor-bearing rat model. *RSC Adv.* **2016**, *6*, 73083–73095. [CrossRef]

32. Zaloga, J.; Pöttler, M.; Leitinger, G.; Friedrich, R.P.; Almer, G.; Lyer, S.; Baum, E.; Tietze, R.; Heimke-Brinck, R.; Mangge, H.; et al. Pharmaceutical formulation of HSA hybrid coated iron oxide nanoparticles for magnetic drug targeting. *Eur. J. Pharm. Biopharm.* **2016**, *101*, 152–162. [CrossRef] [PubMed]

33. McWhirter, M.J.; Bremer, P.J.; Lamont, I.L.; McQuillan, A.J. Siderophore-mediated covalent bonding to metal (oxide) surfaces during biofilm initiation by pseudomonas aeruginosa bacteria. *Langmuir* **2003**, *19*, 3575–3577. [CrossRef]

34. Delina, J.; Rodriguez, R.D.; Verma, A.; Pousaneh, E.; Zahn, D.R.T.; Lang, H.; Chandra, S. Electrochemistry and surface-enhanced Raman spectroscopy of CTAB modulated interactions of magnetic nanoparticles with biomolecules. *RSC Adv.* **2017**, *7*, 3628–3634.

35. Caillé, J.M.; Lemanceau, B.; Bonnemain, B. Gadolinium as a contrast agent for NMR. *AJNR Am. J. Neuroradiol.* **1983**, *4*, 1041–1042. [PubMed]

36. Choi, H.S.; Liu, W.; Misra, P.; Tanaka, E.; Zimmer, J.P.; Itty Ipe, B.; Bawendi, M.G.; Frangioni, J.V. Renal clearance of quantum dots. *Nat. Biotechnol.* **2007**, *25*, 1165–1170. [CrossRef] [PubMed]

37. Blanco, E.; Shen, H.; Ferrari, M. Principles of nanoparticle design for overcoming biological barriers to drug delivery. *Nat. Biotechnol.* **2015**, *33*, 941–951. [CrossRef] [PubMed]

38. Bianchi, A.; Mauri, M.; Bonetti, S.; Koynov, K.; Kappl, M.; Lieberwirth, I.; Butt, H.J.; Simonutti, R. Hierarchical self-assembly of PDMA-b-PS chains into granular nanoparticles: Genesis and fate. *Macromol. Rapid Commun.* **2014**, *35*, 1994–1999. [CrossRef] [PubMed]

39. Skouras, A.; Mourtas, S.; Markoutsa, E.; de Goltstein, M.C.; Wallon, C.; Catoen, S.; Antimisiaris, S.G. Magnetoliposomes with high USPIO entrapping efficiency, stability and magnetic properties. *Nanomedicine* **2011**, *7*, 572–579. [CrossRef] [PubMed]

40. Nichols, J.W.; Bae, Y.H. EPR: Evidence and fallacy. *J. Control. Release* **2014**, *190*, 451–464. [CrossRef] [PubMed]

41. Xie, J.; Chen, K.; Huang, J.; Lee, S.; Wang, J.; Gao, J.; Li, X.; Chen, X. PET/NIRF/MRI triple functional iron oxide nanoparticles. *Biomaterials* **2010**, *31*, 3016–3022. [CrossRef] [PubMed]

42. Xu, C.; Xu, K.; Gu, H.; Zheng, R.; Liu, H.; Zhang, X.; Gu, Z.; Xu, B. Dopamine as a robust anchor to immobilize functional molecules on the iron oxide shell of magnetic nanoparticles. *J. Am. Chem. Soc.* **2004**, *126*, 9938–9939. [CrossRef] [PubMed]

43. Lee, Y.; Lee, H.; Kim, Y.B.; Kim, J.; Hyeon, T.; Park, H.; Messersmith, P.B.; Park, T.G. Bioinspired surface immobilization of hyaluronic acid on monodisperse magnetite nanocrystals for targeted cancer imaging. *Adv. Mater.* **2008**, *20*, 4154–4157. [CrossRef] [PubMed]

44. Montalbetti, C.A.G.N.; Falque, V. Amide bond formation and peptide coupling. *Tetrahedron* **2005**, *61*, 10827–10852. [CrossRef]

45. Zhang, L.; He, R.; Gu, H.C. Oleic acid coating on the monodisperse magnetite nanoparticles. *Appl. Surf. Sci.* **2006**, *253*, 2611–2617. [CrossRef]

46. Liu, X.; Kaminski, M.D.; Guan, Y.; Chen, H.; Liu, H.; Rosengart, A.J. Preparation and characterization of hydrophobic superparamagnetic magnetite gel. *J. Magn. Magn. Mater.* **2006**, *306*, 248–253. [CrossRef]

47. Wang, X.; Tilley, R.D.; Watkins, J.J. Simple ligand exchange reactions enabling excellent dispersibility and stability of magnetic nanoparticles in polar organic, aromatic, and protic solvents. *Langmuir* **2014**, *30*, 1514–1521. [CrossRef] [PubMed]

48. Ruttala, H.B.; Ramasamy, T.; Shin, B.S.; Cho, H.-C.; Yong, C.S.; Kim, J.O. Layer-by-layer assembly of hierarchical nanoarchitectures to enhance the systemic performance of nanoparticle albumin-bound paclitaxel. *Int. J. Pharm.* **2017**, *519*, 11–21. [CrossRef] [PubMed]

49. Heslinga, M.J.; Willis, G.M.; Sobczynski, D.J.; Thompson, A.J.; Eniola-Adefeso, O. One-step fabrication of agent-loaded biodegradable microspheroids for drug delivery and imaging applications. *Colloids Surf. B Biointerfaces* **2014**, *116*, 55–62. [CrossRef] [PubMed]

50. Liang, Y.; Qiao, Y.; Guo, S.; Wang, L.; Xie, C.; Zhai, Y.; Deng, L.; Donga, A. Thermoreversible gelation of poly(ethylene glycol)/poly(ester anhydride) triblock copolymer nanoparticles for injectable drug delivery systems. *Soft Matter* **2010**, *6*, 1915–1922. [CrossRef]

51. Tanei, T.; Leonard, F.; Liu, X.; Alexander, J.F.; Saito, Y. Redirecting Transport of Nanoparticle Albumin-Bound Paclitaxel to Macrophages Enhances Therapeutic Efficacy against Liver Metastases. *Cancer Res.* **2016**, *76*, 429–439. [CrossRef] [PubMed]

52. Chen, Q.; Wang, X.; Wang, C.; Feng, L.; Li, Y.; Liu, Z. Drug-Induced Self-Assembly of Modified Albumins as Nano-Theranostics for Tumor-Targeted Combination Therapy. *ACS Nano* **2015**, *9*, 5223–5233. [CrossRef] [PubMed]

53. Schneider, C.A.; Rasband, W.S.; Eliceiri, K.W. NIH Image to ImageJ: 25 years of image analysis. *Nat. Methods* **2012**, *9*, 671–675. [CrossRef] [PubMed]

54. Mauri, M.; Mauri, L.; Causin, V.; Simonutti, R. A method based on time domain nuclear magnetic resonance for the forensic differentiation of latex gloves. *Anal. Methods* **2011**, *3*, 1802–1809. [CrossRef]

55. Braun, S.; Kalinowski, H.O.; Berger, S. *150 and More Basic NMR Experiments: A Practical Course*, 2nd ed.; Wiley-VCH: Weinheim, Germany, 1998; p. 295.

56. Zhang, M.; Yilmaz, T.; Boztas, A.O.; Karakuzu, O.; Bang, W.Y.; Yegin, Y.; Luo, Z.; Lenox, M.; Cisneros-Zevallos, L.; Akbulut, M. A multifunctional nanoparticulate theranostic system with simultaneous chemotherapeutic, photothermal therapeutic, and MRI contrast capabilities. *RSC Adv.* **2016**, *6*, 27798–27806. [CrossRef]

57. Kesharwani, P.; Jain, K.; Tekade, R.K.; Gajbhiye, V.; Jain, N.K. Spectrophotometric estimation of paclitaxel. *Int. J. Adv. Pharm. Sci.* **2011**, *2*, 29–32.

Sample Availability: Samples of the compounds are not available from the authors.

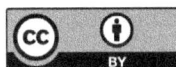

molecules

MDPI

Article

Structural Characterization of the Low-Molecular-Weight Heparin Dalteparin by Combining Different Analytical Strategies

Antonella Bisio [1,*], Elena Urso [1], Marco Guerrini [1], Pauline de Wit [1,2,†], Giangiacomo Torri [1] and Annamaria Naggi [1]

[1]   Istituto di Ricerche Chimiche e Biochimiche G. Ronzoni, 20133 Milan, Italy; urso@ronzoni.it (E.U.); guerrini@ronzoni.it (M.G.); pdewit@nl.aspenpharma.com (P.d.W.); torri@ronzoni.it (G.T.); naggi@ronzoni.it (A.N.)
[2]   Department of Cell and Applied Biology, Faculty of Science, Radboud University Nijmegen, 6525 HP Nijmegen, The Netherlands
*   Correspondence: bisio@ronzoni.it; Tel.: +39-02-7064-1630
†   Current address: Aspen Oss B.V., Kloosterstraat 6, 5349 AB Oss, The Netherlands.

Received: 31 May 2017; Accepted: 22 June 2017; Published: 24 June 2017

Abstract: A number of low molecular weight heparin (LMWH) products are available for clinical use and although all share a similar mechanism of action, they are classified as distinct drugs because of the different depolymerisation processes of the native heparin resulting in substantial pharmacokinetic and pharmacodynamics differences. While enoxaparin has been extensively investigated, little information is available regarding the LMWH dalteparin. The present study is focused on the detailed structural characterization of Fragmin® by LC-MS and NMR applied both to the whole drug and to its enzymatic products. For a more in-depth approach, size homogeneous octasaccharide and decasaccharide components together with their fractions endowed with high or no affinity toward antithrombin were also isolated and their structural profiles characterized. The combination of different analytical strategies here described represents a useful tool for the assessment of batch-to-batch structural variability and for comparative evaluation of structural features of biosimilar products.

Keywords: low-molecular-weight heparin; dalteparin; NMR; LC-MS; affinity chromatography

1. Introduction

Low molecular weight heparins (LMWHs) are heterogeneous mixtures of sulfated glycosaminoglycans with notable pharmacological activity. They were developed as alternative therapies to heparin in the prophylaxis and treatment of venous and arterial thrombotic disorders, to overcome its uncommon but potentially serious side effects, such as bleeding and thrombocytopenia, and relative unpredictability [1]. LMWHs are derived from unfractionated heparin (UFH) through controlled chemical or enzymatic depolymerization processes to yield fragments which are approximately one third the size of the original chains with Mws ranging from 1000 to 10,000 Da [2,3]. Owing to their lower molecular size they typically possess more predictable pharmacological action, better bioavailability and longer half-life [4,5]. Depending on manufacturing process, marketed LMWHs mainly differ in degree of depolymerisation, and in the chemical structure of their terminal units, as well as their therapeutic and pharmacological properties.

Apart from characteristic terminal residues [6], their linear internal sequences are primarily composed by 1,4-linked repeating trisulfated disaccharides units containing 2-*O*-sulfated iduronic acid (I_{2S}) and *N*-sulfated glucosamine 6-*O*-sulfated ($A_{NS,6S}$). These trisulfated regions alternate with undersulfated sequences containing non-sulfated uronic acids—iduronic (I) and in lower proportion glucuronic (G)—which are usually preceded by *N*-acetylated glucosamine units (A_{NAc}). The specific pentasaccharide sequence -$A_{NAc,6S}$-G-$A_{NS,3S,6S}$-I_{2S}-$A_{NS,6S}$-(AGA*IA), present only in some of the chains, constitutes the antithrombin binding site (AT-bs), essential for a high anticoagulant and antithrombotic activity of LMWHs, such as that of UFH. LMWH structures can also include traces of the linkage region (LR), the non-sulfated sequence G-Gal-Gal-Xyl which links the original heparin chain to the core protein of its natural proteoglycan precursor through a serine (Ser) residue [7].

Due to the structural diversity and heterogeneity arising from the different methods of preparation, the LMWHs available for clinical use are regarded as chemically and pharmacologically distinct entities, each one with its own unique efficacy and safety profile, and their therapeutic interchange is considered inappropriate. Correlating the biological properties with particular structural motifs has been the most important challenge in the design of new LMWHs as well as in the development of generic versions of these drugs [6].

For the LMWH dalteparin, approved indications include the prevention of venous thromboembolism (VTE) in patients undergoing hip replacement or abdominal surgery and in acutely ill medical patients with severely restricted mobility, in long term secondary prevention of VTE, in patients with VTE and cancer, and in acute coronary syndromes as unstable angina and non-Q wave myocardial infarction [8].

Dalteparin is produced from porcine intestinal mucosa through a relatively simple and low cost method based on a controlled deaminative cleavage with nitrous acid followed by reduction, resulting in the formation of an anhydromannitol (aM.ol) ring at the reducing end. The complete structural characterization of dalteparin, such as of all LMWHs, should supply information on the size of the chains, the monosaccharide composition in terms of iduronic/glucuronic acid, *N*-sulfated/*N*-acetylated glucosamine content and sulfation pattern and the sequence of these residues along the chains. No single technique is able to fulfil all these requirements and only a combination of orthogonal analytical approaches can provide a thorough characterization. Among the analytical approaches used for structure investigation of LMWHs, NMR spectroscopy and mass spectrometry (MS) represent the most effective techniques [3]. In particular, a growing interest has been registered in the last two decades in the application of MS, by increasingly sophisticated instruments with higher mass resolution and accuracy. A relevant contribution to the analysis of very complex mixtures such as LMWHs was provided by the direct connection of mass spectrometry to liquid chromatography systems (LC-MS) [9–11]. Among the most recent academic studies, fingerprint analysis by reversed-phase ion-pairing ultra-performance liquid chromatography coupled to high resolution mass spectrometry (RPIP-UHPLC–MS), has been proved to be a very important analytical method to ensure, in a very fast way, drug quality and collection of extremely interesting information about oligosaccharide structure, chain length and chemical modification [12,13]. Nevertheless, due to the extremely high complexity of samples exhibiting large polydispersity over a large molecular weight distribution together with several isomers, further approaches are necessary to obtain a detailed understanding of the samples and make ensure the comparability between different samples and lot-to-lot variability. Heparin/heparan sulfate fragment mapping by enzymatic digestion either with either heparinase I, II and III or using a mixture of them is a very common strategy reported in several studies and different analytical methods to run the depolymerized solutions and record interesting information in function to the technique used are often described [14–18]. Moreover, it was recently described that the quantitative NMR-HSQC analysis, applied to determine the mono- and disaccharide composition of heparin and LMWHs, can be used for detailed structural comparison studies between generic or biosimilar drugs with the reference product [19].

The present work describes the in-depth structural characterization of dalteparin by 2D-NMR and LC-MS techniques, applied both to intact chains and to their enzymatic products. The sample depolymerization by two strategies involving the exhaustive digestion with a cocktail of heparinases I, II and III and heparinase III bottom up fragment mapping, allows one to obtain samples of reduced complexity and at the same time point out eventual structural motifs. As a further level of detailed analysis, investigation of appropriate size-exclusion chromatography fractions, such as octa- and decasaccharides, and of their sub-fractions endowed of high affinity (HA) or no affinity (NA) for antithrombin was performed. The overall analytical approach here described represents an effective strategy for comparative purposes of structural features of different lots of dalteparin samples either concerning the appraisal of batch-to-batch variability or the evaluation of biosimilar products.

2. Results and Discussion

2.1. NMR Characterization

The mono/disaccharide percentage content of eleven different batches of Fragmin® was determined by applying a recently validated method [19]. The HSQC spectrum reported in Figure 1 shows all major and minor signals used for integration. Results are presented in Table 1.

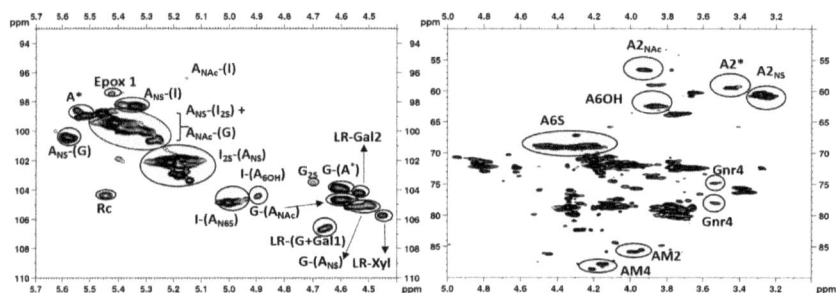

Figure 1. Anomeric (left) and ring (right) regions of ^{1}H/^{13}C HSQC NMR spectrum of Frag-5. AM corresponds to aM.ol.

Table 1. Percent content of variously substituted glucosamine and uronic acid residues in different disaccharide sequences of Fragmin® samples, together with typical linkage region residues.

	Frag-1	Frag-2	Frag-3	Frag-4	Frag-5	Frag-6	Frag-7	Frag-8	Frag-9	Frag-10	Frag-11
Amines											
A_{NS}-(I_{2S})	55.7	56.6	55.2	55.8	57.2	58.1	56.3	57.2	59.0	55.2	55.7
A_{NS}-I	7.6	5.9	7.0	7.6	6.6	6.8	6.9	7.1	6.5	7.5	8.1
A_{NS}-(G)	5.9	6.0	5.8	5.9	5.9	5.6	6.0	5.9	5.7	5.6	5.6
A*	5.9	5.5	6.1	5.3	5.6	4.9	5.5	5.2	4.7	5.5	5.1
A_{NAc}-(G)	9.4	9.5	9.0	9.5	9.3	9.2	9.2	9.3	8.9	9.7	9.7
A_{NAc}-(I)	nd	nd	nd	nd	nd	nd	nd	nd	nd	nd	nd
A_{NH2}	nd	nd	nd	nd	nd	nd	nd	nd	nd	nd	nd
A-epox	nd	nd	0.8 *	0.6 *	0.6 *	0.7 *	0.8 *	0.6 *	nd	1.1 *	nd
A-(GalA)	1.6	1.9	1.4 *	1.0 *	1.1 *	1.1 *	0.5 *	1.0 *	0.9 *	2.0	1.4
A_{6S}	90.7	90.5	90.6	90.4	89.9	90.3	90.6	89.8	90.2	91.0	90.8
aM.ol	12.9	13.3	13.5	13.3	12.9	12.6	13.9	12.7	13.2	12.7	13.3
Rc	1.0 *	1.2 *	1.0 *	0.9 *	0.8 *	1.0 *	1.0 *	0.9 *	1.1 *	0.7 *	1.2 *
Uronic acids											
I_{2S}	75.3	77.3	76.4	76.9	76.2	76.5	75.8	76.6	76.7	73.2	74.1
I-(A_{6S})	8.3	7.2	7.4	7.2	7.0	7.4	7.1	7.0	7.0	8.3	8.6
I-(A_{6OH})	0.6	0.7 *	0.8 *	1.0 *	0.7 *	0.7 *	0.9 *	0.9 *	0.7 *	0.8 *	0.9 *
G-(A*)	4.9	4.4	4.4	4.4	4.4	4.5	4.7	4.4	4.5	5.0	4.7
G-(A_{NS})	6.0	5.2	5.8	5.8	5.9	5.4	5.8	5.3	5.7	5.7	6.8
G-(A_{NAc})	3.9	4.6	3.9	4.1	4.5	4.7	4.9	4.5	5.3	4.1	3.8
Gnr	nd	nd	nd	nd	nd	nd	nd	nd	nd	nd	nd
epox	nd	nd	0.8 *	0.6 *	0.6 *	0.6 *	0.7 *	0.6 *	nd	1.0 *	nd
GalA	1.1	0.7 *	0.5 *	nd	0.5 *	nd	nd	0.7 *	nd	1.7	1.1 *
Linkage region											
Gal1+G	1.6 *	1.2 *	1.6	2.1	2.0	1.8	2.1	2.0	1.9	1.3 *	1.4
Gal2	1.3 *	1.0 *	1.3 *	1.6	1.5	1.4 *	1.6	1.4	1.6	1.2 *	1.0 *
Xyl-Ser-ox	0.8 *	0.6 *	0.8 *	0.9 *	0.9 *	1.0 *	1.0 *	0.9 *	1.1	0.6 *	0.7 *
Xyl-Ser	nd	nd	nd	nd	nd	nd	nd	nd	nd	nd	nd

nd indicates values under the limit of detection (LOD); * indicates values under the limit of quantification (LOQ); Gnr indicates glucuronic acid located at the non-reducing end.

The main structural features of dalteparin revealed by HSQC NMR analysis were the presence of an anhydromannitol ring as the only detectable residue at the reducing end, the relatively high content of sulfated monosaccharides and a substantial percentage of G-(A*) marker of the binding site for antithrombin, in agreement with previous results [20], the absence of N-acetylated glucosamine linked to non-sulfated iduronic acid [A_{NAc}-(I)] and a modest presence of linkage region. Moreover, traces of anomalous structures were also detected, such as epoxide and 2-deoxy-2-C-hydroxymethylpentafuranosidic residues. The former is the result of alkaline treatments possibly suffered by the parent heparin and are identified by typical H2/C2 and H3/C3 signals at 3.74/54.2 and 3.82/53.3 ppm, respectively. Such epoxides can convert to L-galacturonic acid (GalA) during the processes for preparation of both unfractionated heparin and LMWH and this structure was identified too. The latter structure is a side effect of nitrous acid treatment of heparin used to obtain dalteparin. Actually, some internal glucosamine residues can undergo a deamination to give, by ring contraction (Rc), a 2-deoxy-2-C-hydroxymethylpentafuranosidic residue, which hexocyclic CH_2 groups are identified by the typical chemical shift at 5.45/104.5 ppm [21].

2.2. Chain Mapping

The eleven Fragmin® samples were subjected to LC-MS analysis of the whole intact mixture. The UHPLC method, using pentylamine as ion reagent in the ion pair reversed phase (IPRP) liquid chromatography, provided a good chromatographic separation of numerous components in a relatively short time range (less than 30 min). Mass spectral information allowed us to calculate oligosaccharide composition, in terms of chain length, number of sulfate and/or acetyl groups, and chemical modifications induced by the production process. The structure hypothesis was expressed using a code consisting of a letter indicating the non-reducing residue, such as U (uronic acid) or A (glucosamine) followed by three numbers indicating monosaccharide residues, sulfate groups and N-acetyl groups, respectively, followed by the aM.ol symbol for the fragment residues terminating with 2,5-anhydro-D-mannitol. All samples displayed highly similar UHPLC/MS profiles in terms of number and shape of peaks; in Figure 2 a representative base peak chromatogram (BPC) is reported. Mass spectra details of the main signals detected in all dalteparin samples are reported in Table S1.

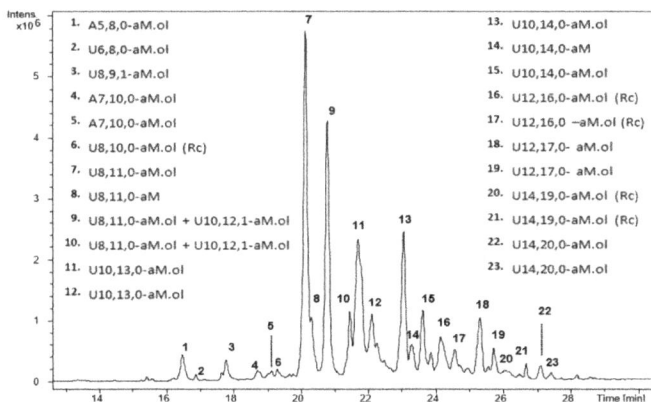

Figure 2. LC-MS profile (BPC) of a representative Fragmin® sample (Frag-5). Mass signals assignment of the main components is reported. LC conditions: isocratic step at 15% B for 1 min, followed by a linear gradient from 15% to 40% B in 31 min; then, column washing and reconditioning in the initial conditions were performed.

Twentythree main species ranging from pentamer to tetradecamer were detected. It is important to underline that the intensity of peaks observable in Figure 2 is not related to the content of oligomeric species. Actually, the ion desorption efficiency in mass spectrometry ionization source is strongly affected by structure and molecular weight of components. In general, the higher the molecular weight of a species the lower the MS response is. This explains the apparent discrepancy between the LC-MS profile displayed in Figure 2 and the oligomeric composition profiles obtained by size exclusion chromatography (Section 2.5, Figures S3–S5).

The main species detected are associated to anhydromannitol derivative structures, most of them having a high degree of sulfation and no acetyl group. Almost all the oligosaccharides have a high degree of sulfation, but a few monoacetylated species were also observed. Odd species (penta- and heptasaccharides) were detected as minor components. Since they have a glucosamine residue at the non-reducing end, they represent original terminal chains of the parent heparin which dalteparin was derived from.

Interestingly, a number of fully sulfated oligosaccharides were detected, such as U8,11,0-aM.ol, U10,14,0-aM.ol, U12,17,0-aM.ol and U14,20,0-aM.ol. They are expected to correspond to regular sequences made up of trisulfated disaccharides (I_{2S}-Glc$_{NS,6S}$) and terminating with the typical anhydromannitol moiety, i.e., (I_{2S}-Glc$_{NS,6S}$)$_n$-I_{2S}-aM.ol$_{6S}$, where n range from 3 to 6. Nevertheless, for each of the above oligomers at least two isomers were found: for U8,11,0-aM.ol in particular, two isomers were recorded as main components under the peaks 7 and 9, and a third one as minor species in the peak 10. Different isomers could contain a G-A* sequence in different positions (positional isomers).

The molecular mass of dalteparin oligosaccharides terminating with 2,5-anhydro-D-mannitol shows a loss of 15 Da with respect to the MW of unmodified heparin oligosaccharides, corresponding to the loss of an amino group produced by the depolymerization process.

Mass signals corresponding to a further loss of 15 Da can be often observed, suggesting an additional deamination, most probably occurred on glucosamine residues within the chain, with no subsequent depolymerization. In agreement with NMR data, such signals were associated to a ring contracted (Rc) unit, derived from a glucosamine residue [21]. Structures with the Rc unit were observed in nearly all peaks of the chromatogram. As reported in Figure 2, the presence of all these structures has been verified in peaks 6, 16, 17, 20 and 21. Minor mass signals corresponding to the expected molecular mass with 2 Daltons less were detected and identified as an aldehyde form (aM) produced by an incomplete reduction to the 2,5-anhydro-D-mannitol terminal residue.

2.3. Building Blocks Analysis by Heparinases I, II, III Digestion

Under exhaustive digestion conditions, 23 major entities were typically observed (Figure 3). Mass spectra details of the main signals detected in all dalteparin samples are reported in Table S2. Regular unsaturated disaccharides with different sulfation degree, but also monoacetylated and saturated disaccharides were observed. In particular, two isomers of the saturated disaccharide U2,3,0 were detected under the peak of the main trisulfated disaccharide ΔU2,3,0, suggesting the presence of the following isomers I_{2S}-A$_{NS,6S}$ and G-A* (Figure 3). Accordingly, a number of dalteparin chains starting with G-A* sequence at the non-reducing end are expected.

Several anhydromannitol residues were identified in different chains ranging from disaccharides to hexasaccharides. Minor signals were assigned to disaccharide ΔU2,1,0-aM.ol, ΔU2,2,0-aM.ol and to hexasaccharide ΔU6,6,1-aM.ol. The highest component in the tetrasaccharides region was attributed to ΔU4,5,0-aM.ol with five sulfate groups and the anhydro derivative at the reducing end glucosamine, followed by ΔU4,4,1 with four sulfates and an acetyl group. The former could be interpreted as ΔU$_{2S}$-A$_{NS,6S}$-I_{2S}-aM.ol$_{6S}$ and its survival can be explained by the presence of anhydromannitol derivative; the latter can be explained as ΔU-A$_{NAc,6S}$-G-A*. In fact, the presence of 3-O-sulfate glucosamine renders the glycosidic bond between N-acetylated, 6-O-sulfated glucosamine and the unsulfated glucuronic acid impervious to the action of heparinases [22]. This effect can be used to obtain interesting structural information, mainly in the tetra-hexasaccharides region. Actually, among the minor tetrasaccharide species, two interesting structures were detected such as ΔU4,5,0 and ΔU4,5,1, both deriving from the possible fragmentation of two structural variants of the binding site. Their most probable sequence interpretations are as follows: ΔU-A$_{NS,6S}$-G-A* and ΔU$_{2S}$-A$_{NAc,6S}$-G-A*, respectively.

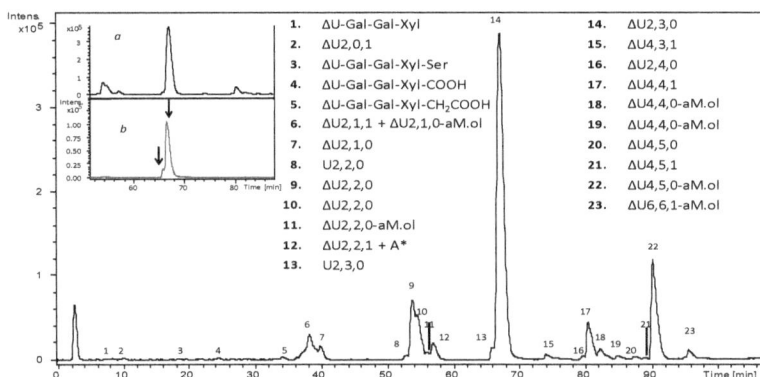

Figure 3. LC-MS profile (BPC) of a representative Fragmin® sample (Frag-5) depolymerized by a cocktail of Heparinase I, II, III. Mass signals assignment of the main components is reported. *Inset*: expansion of chromatogram portion with the main unsaturated trisulfated disaccharide (ΔU$_{2S}$-A$_{NS,6S}$) eluted (panel a); extracted ion chromatograms (EIC) of *m/z* 594.0 attributed to saturated trisulfated disaccharide (panel b): as indicated by arrows, two positional isomers were detected. LC elution conditions: isocratic step at 2% B for 10 min, followed by a linear gradient to 60% B in 90 min and final steps of column washing and reconditioning.

2.4. Bottom up Analysis by Heparinases III Digestion

Heparinase III cleaves the linkage between N-acetylated glucosamine A$_{NAc}$, with or without 6-O-sulfate, and glucuronic or iduronic acid, with preference for the former. As expected, all the fully sulfated oligosaccharides and their isomers, identified by the previous chain mapping analysis, were not recognized by this enzyme. The LC-MS profile and mass spectra assignment (Figure 4) show several oligosaccharides arising from the intact parent Fragmin® (with *m/z* values accounting for oligomers ranging from hexa- to hexadecasaccharides). Mass spectra details of the main signals detected in all dalteparin samples are reported in Table S3.

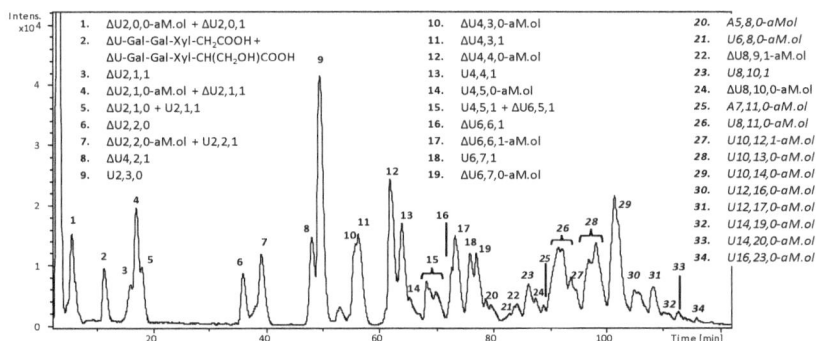

Figure 4. LC-MS profile (BPC) of a representative Fragmin® sample (Frag-5) following digestion with heparinase III. Mass signals assignment of the main components is reported. Components identified in the parent sample, before the enzymatic digestion, are indicated in italic font. LC elution conditions: isocratic at 10% B for 5 min, linear gradient from 10% to 50% B in 55 min, linear gradient from 50% to 90% B in 80 min, followed by column washing and reconditioning.

Highly sulphated odd intact structures were also observed and identified as pentasaccharide A5,8,0-aM.ol and heptasaccharide A7,11,0-aM.ol. Confirmation of the sum formula of both oligosaccharides was provided by Ion Cyclotron Resonance-FT-MS (ICR-FT-MS) analysis (Figures S2 and S3, Supplementary Material). These unusual oligosaccharide composition can be explained by the presence of I_{2S}-A* sequence inside their chain, $(A_{NS,6S}-I_{2S})_{1or2}$-A*-$I_{2S}$-aM.ol$_{6OS}$. Such interpretation would be in agreement with the previous building blocks results where the disaccharide $\Delta U2,4,0$, compatible with the structure ΔU_{2S}-A*, was detected.

2.5. Isolation of Octasaccharide and Decasaccharide Fractions

Fractionation of dalteparin by size exclusion chromatography into size homogeneous oligomeric fractions can be achieved both by Biogel P6 and Biogel P10 [20]. For the present work, all the analysed dalteparin samples underwent chromatographic fractionation on Biogel P6, to obtain a fingerprint of their overall oligomeric composition: their highly similar chromatographic profiles are compared in Figures S3–S5 (Supplementary Material). A series of peaks were resolved with each peak corresponding to a size-homogeneous oligomeric family. In particular, octa- and decasaccharide fractions were isolated from Frag-11 by implementing three chromatographic runs which yielded, after desalting, 27.6 mg of octasaccharides and 60.5 mg of decasaccharides, corresponding to 3.1% and 7.8%, respectively, of the whole sample.

2.6. Affinity Chromatography Separation of NA and HA Components

The isolated size-homogeneous oligosaccharide fractions were fractionated with regards to their ability to interact with AT-Sepharose column. Affinity chromatography of octa- and decasaccharides resulted in the separation of two components: the first one, considered devoid of affinity for AT as eluting at lower ionic strength (NA); the second one endowed of high affinity for AT as eluting at higher ionic strength (HA). The relative content of HA components for octa and decasaccharides with respect to the total fraction, were 5% and 6% respectively.

2.7. NMR Characterization of Octasaccharide and Decasaccharide Fractions and of their NA and HA Components

The isolated octa and decasaccharide fractions and their corresponding NA and HA components were studied through the quantitative compositional analysis method based on HSQC ^{1}H-^{13}C correlation measurement already applied for parent LMWH. The average monosaccharide content of all samples is presented in Table 2.

Table 2. Percent content of variously substituted glucosamine and uronic acid residues in octa and decasaccharide fractions, and in their corresponding HA and NA components. n.d. = not detected.

	Octa	HA-Octa	NA-Octa	Deca	HA-Deca	NA-Deca
Amines						
A_{NS}-(I_{2S})	56.6	34.5	58.6	58.1	27.0	59.8
A_{NS}-I	2.8	4.1	2.3	4.6	13.8	4.1
A_{NS}-(G)	4.4	10.3	2.8	5.3	9.0	5.1
A*	10.5	21.9	8.1	6.4	20.3	5.0
A_{NAc}-(G)	2.2	7.2	2.0	4.4	11.6	3.3
A_{NAc}-(I)	n.d.	n.d.	n.d.	n.d.	n.d.	n.d.
A_{NH2}	n.d.	n.d.	0.8	n.d.	n.d.	n.d.
A-epox	n.d.	n.d.	n.d.	n.d.	n.d.	n.d.
A-(GalA)	0.9	n.d.	0.8	0.9	n.d.	n.d.
A_{6S}	98.5	99.5	98.8	97.0	99.5	97.4
aM.ol	20.8	21.6	22.6	19.0	18.2	18.7
Rc	1.0	n.d.	1.0	1.3	n.d.	1.5

Table 2. *Cont.*

	Octa	HA-Octa	NA-Octa	Deca	HA-Deca	NA-Deca
Uronic acids						
I_{2S}	84.7	69.7	88.2	81.6	66.0	81.8
$I-(A_{6S})$	2.7	3.2	2.5	4.7	14.2	3.9
$I-(A_{6OH})$	n.d.	n.d.	n.d.	0.7	n.d.	0.6
$G-(A^*)$	8.2	22.6	6.1	5.8	17.5	5.0
$G-(A_{NS})$	2.9	4.4	2.4	4.8	2.3	5.1
$G-(A_{NAc})$	0.6	n.d.	n.d.	1.5	n.d.	2.1
Gnr	4.6	traces	4.2	1.5	traces	2.9
G_{2S}	n.d.	traces	n.d.	n.d.	n.d.	n.d.
epox	n.d.	n.d.	n.d.	n.d.	n.d.	n.d.
GalA	0.9	n.d.	0.7	0.9	n.d.	1.4

Given the length of oligosaccharide sequences, additional structural information with respect to whole Fragmin® samples was determined (Table 1) such as the percent content of glucuronic acid located at the non-reducing end (Gnr). Whereas no significant differences were detected between octa- and decasaccharide composition, the most important diversities were displayed by each NA and HA components with respect to the parent oligosaccharides. Signals of residues associated with the AT-binding pentasaccharide sequence, e.g., A*, G-(A*) and A_{NAc}-(G), increased in HA components and their percentage content turned out to be about two-three times higher with respect to parent oligosaccharide fractions. Monodimensional ^{1}H-NMR spectra of HA and NA components of the two oligosaccharide fractions clearly revealed the main structural differences above mentioned (Figure 5). In both HA sub-fractions a substantial increase of the typical signals of AT-bs ($A_{NS,3S}$, GlcA and acetyl group) appeared accompanied by the expected decrease of N-sulfated glucosamine, A_{NS}. Additionally, in HA-deca, a significant increase of non-sulfated iduronic acid, which is expected to precede the AGA*IA sequence, was also observed and quantified. No trace of linkage region was detected in parent oligosaccharides or their derived components. Interestingly, despite a small amount of ring contracted unit (Rc) and galacturonic acid were detected in total octasaccharide and decasaccharide fractions, no traces of these structures appeared in both octa-HA and deca-HA components. The presence of anomalous monosaccharide units in so short sequences would impair definitely their interaction with AT.

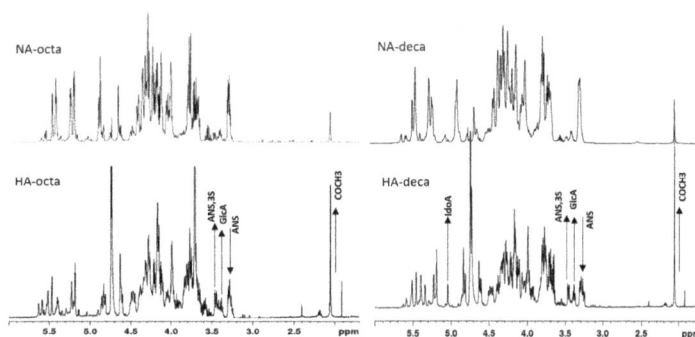

Figure 5. ^{1}H-NMR spectra of HA and NA components of octa and decasaccharide fractions. The direction of arrows, up or down, indicates the increase or decrease respectively of some characteristic signals in spectra of HA components.

2.8. LC-MS Analysis of Octasaccharide and Decasaccharide fractions

The compositional profiles of the isolated octa- and decasaccharide fractions are presented in Figure 6, together with the list of the main oligomeric species detected in BPCs. In the octasaccharide fraction, different octameric sequences were detected with a number of sulfate groups ranging from 9 to 11. In particular, nona- and decasulfated species, U8,9,1-aM.ol and U8,10,1-aM.ol respectively, contained also an acetyl group, whereas undecasulfated sequences, i.e., U8,11,0-aM.ol, accounted for a regular fully sulfated sequence. Two out of ten species are the most represented sequences, all accounting for the fully sulfated octasaccharide U8,11,0-aM.ol. A few species present in minor peaks, whose *m/z* ratio accounted for nona- and decasaccharides, coeluted with octasaccharides, including two isomers of a highly sulfated nonasaccharide sequence bearing 13 and 14 sulfate groups, respectively (A9,13,0-aM.ol and A9,14,0-aM.ol). As previously discussed, oligosaccharides with a glucosamine residue located at the non-reducing end represent the original terminal chains of the parent heparin.

The decasaccharide fraction turned out to be composed by eight main species bearing from 12 to 14 sulfate groups and including three monoacetylated dodecasulfated isomers. A sequence containing a ring contracted unit (Rc) was also detected. As for octasaccharide fraction, also in this case two isomers of the fully sulfated sequence U10,14,0-aM.ol were detected.

As already discussed in "Chain mapping" paragraph, together with octa and decasaccharides with regular structure $(I_{2S}-A_{NS,6S})_n-I_{2S}-aM.ol_{6S}$ (n = 3 or 4 respectively), isomers containing a G-A* in different positions are expected. Such oligosaccharides could either contain a fully sulfated AT-bs or a fragment if it. Actually, the presence of a G-A* located at the non-reducing terminal chain would be in agreement with the presence of Gnr detected by NMR in both oligosaccharide fractions.

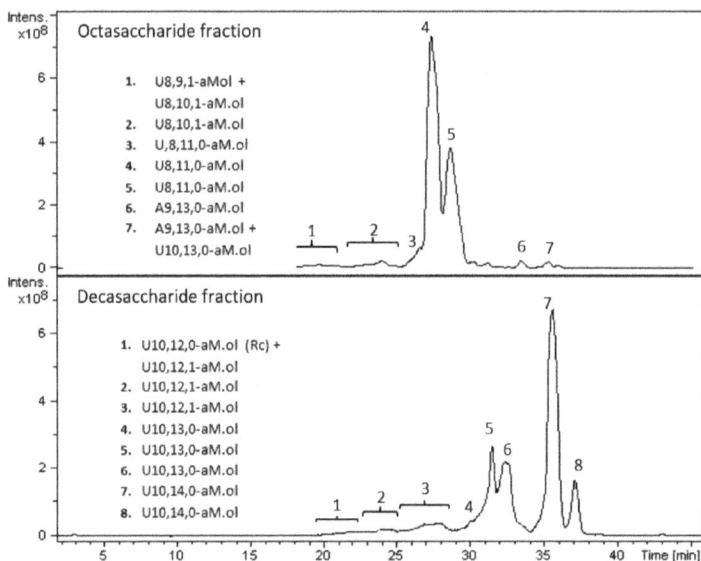

Figure 6. LC-MS profiles (BPC) of exemplary octasaccharide and decasaccharide fractions isolated from of Frag-5. Mass signals assignment of the main components is reported. LC elution conditions: linear gradients from 50% B to 57% B in 5 min and from 57% B to 80% B in 52 min, followed by column washing at 90% B and reconditioning in the initial conditions.

In principle, fully sulfated octa and decasaccharides could contain also $G_{2S}-A_{NS,6S}$ sequences in alternative to the prevailing trisulfated disaccharide. Nevertheless, the presence of G_{2S} residue was not detected by NMR spectra, possibly because under the sensitivity of the technique (Table 2). Further experiments are required to prove our hypothesis. Anyway, although such structural details were of great concern, their understanding did not meet the scope of the present paper.

2.9. LC-MS Analysis of NA and HA components of Octasaccharide and Decasaccharide fractions

It is important to underline that the sub-fractionation of oligosaccharide fractions based on their interaction with AT-Sepharose column, and then the composition of the resulting NA and HA components, greatly depend on the elution conditions applied (e.g., type of salt, salt concentration, type of gradient, etc.).

The compositional profiles of the obtained NA and HA components of both octa and decasaccharides greatly differed each other for the number and intensity of peaks (Figure 7). The reduced complexity of both sub-fractions allowed to detect also some species that were not observed in the whole corresponding oligosaccharide fractions, such as A7,9,1-aM.ol and A7,10,0-aM.ol in HA-octa, U8,8,1-aM.ol in NA-octa, and A11,15,0-aM.ol in HA-deca. In HA-octa sub-fraction five main octameric species were revealed including (i) two monoacetylated sequences (U8,9,1-aM.ol; U8,10,1-aM.ol), which are expected to contain the AGA*IA sequence; (ii) three fully sulfated octasaccharides, possibly containing an AT-bs with all N-sulfated glucosamines (U8,11,0-aM.ol) [23]; (iii) two coeluted heptasaccharides, a fully sulfated one, A7,10,0-aM.ol and the monoacetylated A7,9,1-aM.ol.

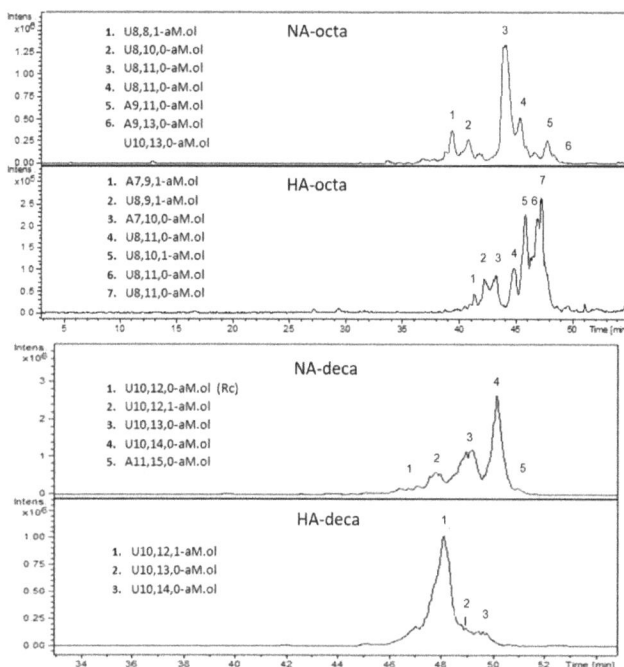

Figure 7. LC-MS profiles (BPC) of HA and NA components of octa- and decasaccharide fractions. Mass signals assignment of the main components is reported. LC elution conditions: isocratic at 20% Solvent B for 20 min, gradient elution from 20% B to 40% B for 10 min followed by a 20 min gradient from 40% B to 90% B; subsequently, 90% B was kept for 10 min.

In agreement with NMR data (Table 2) and building block analysis results (Figure 3), the structure of the main species detected in HA-octa fraction can be interpreted as shown in Table 3.

Heptasaccharides 1 and 3 are both compatible with the presence of AT-binding region, bearing an acetyl group or a sulfate group on the reducing glucosamine, respectively. Two possible interpretations have been reported for octasaccharide 2 (U8,9,1-aM.ol), both containing the AGA*IA pentasaccharide located in two different positions.

Table 3. Structure assignment of species detected in octa-HA sub-fraction.

Peak	Composition	Saccharide Sequence
1	A7,9,1-aM.ol	$A_{NAc,6S}$-G-A*-I_{2S}-$A_{NS,6S}$-I_{2S}-aM.ol$_{6S}$
2	U8,9,1-aM.ol	I-$A_{NAc,6S}$-G-A*-I_{2S}-$A_{NS,6S}$-I_{2S}-aM.ol$_{6S}$ and/or I_{2S}-$A_{NS,6S}$-I-$A_{NAc,6S}$-G-A*-I_{2S}-aM.ol$_{6S}$
3	A7,10,0-aM.ol	$A_{NS,6S}$-G-A*-I_{2S}-$A_{NS,6S}$-I_{2S}-aM.ol$_{6S}$
5	U8,10,1-aM.ol	I_{2S}-$A_{NS,6S}$-I-$A_{NAc,6S}$-I_{2S}-A*-I_{2S}-aM.ol$_{6S}$
4, 6, 7	U8,11,0-aM.ol	I_{2S}-$A_{NS,6S}$-G-A*-I_{2S}-$A_{NS,6S}$-I_{2S}-aM.ol$_{6S}$ I_{2S}-$A_{NS,6S}$-I_{2S}-$A_{NS,6S}$-G-A*-I_{2S}-aM.ol$_{6S}$ G-A*-I_{2S}-$A_{NS,6S}$-I_{2S}-$A_{NS,6S}$-I_{2S}-aM.ol$_{6S}$

The octasaccharides U8,10,1-aM.ol, one of the most important peaks, could be explained by hypothesizing the presence of a I_{2S}-A* sequence instead of G-A*, in agreement with the previous detection of ΔU2,4,0 building block. Interestingly, a synthetic octasaccharide containing the sequence I_{2S}-A*-I_{2S} was found to be endowed of high binding affinity to AT [24]. As concerns the highly sulfated octasaccharide isomers U8,11,0-aM.ol two of the proposed structures contain the fully *N*-sulfated AT-binding region preceded by a 2-*O*-sulfated iduronic acid, and located in two different positions. Following cleavage with heparinase cocktail, these oligosaccharides are expected to generate the corresponding resistant tetrasaccharides U4,6,0 and ΔU4,6,0 respectively, which turned out to be almost undetectable in the whole dalteparin sample. Nevertheless, it is likely that the significant decreasing of structure polydispersity, such as in HA-Octa sub-fraction with respect to parent LMWH, allows the detection also of very minor sequences. The third undecasulfated isomer was interpreted as G-A*-I_{2S}-$A_{NS,6S}$-I_{2S}-$A_{NS,6S}$-I_{2S}-aM.ol$_{6S}$, which is in agreement with the finding of traces of non-reducing glucuronic acid in HA-Octa (Table 2). Despite such octasaccharide was expected to have a moderate AT-affinity, its presence in HA fraction is compatible with the elution conditions of AT-Sepharose column here applied, as the NA component was recovered at relatively very low salt concentration (50 mM NaCl). A possible additional or alternative interpretation of the third isomer U8,11,0-aM.ol, could be the presence of a G_{2S} instead of I_{2S}, taking into account that traces of 2-*O*-sulfated glucuronic acid were detected by NMR, but further investigation is required to confirm the exact structure. In the deca-HA subfraction three main decameric species were detected: U10,12,1-aM.ol, which is supposed to contain the I-$A_{NAc,6S}$-G-A*-I_{2S}-$A_{NS,6S}$ sequence; U10,13,0-aM.ol and U10,14,0-aM.ol, where both containing the fully N-sulfated AT-bs. As anticipated by the NMR results, the decasaccharide species containing a ring contracted unit (Rc) was recovered in the deca-NA fraction.

3. Materials and Methods

3.1. Materials

Dalteparin samples used in the present study were from different lots of injectable Fragmin® (Pfizer), named as follows: Frag-1 (lot 96223A51), Frag-2 (lot 96218B51), Frag-3 (lot 96231A51), Frag-4 (lot 96238A51), Frag-5 (lot 96240B51), Frag-6 (lot 96242A51), Frag-7 (lot 96228A51), Frag-8 (lot 96235A51), Frag-9 (lot 96225A51), Frag-10 (lot 96246A51) and Frag-11 (lot Z06358). Heparinases I (EC 4.2.2.7), II and III (EC 4.2.2.8) were purchased from Grampian Enzymes (Aberdeen, Scotland, UK). Dibutylamine (>99.5%), methanol (LC-MS grade), acetonitrile (LC-MS grade), acetic acid (glacial 99.9%), formic acid (98-100%), ammonium chloride (>99.5%), potassium phosphate monobasic were purchased from Sigma-Aldrich (Milan, Italy); sodium acetate was from Merck (Milan, Italy), and calcium acetate (>97%) from BDH (VWR Milan, Italy).

3.2. Fractionation by Size-Exclusion Chromatography

Fractionation by SEC to isolate octasaccharide and decasaccharide fractions was performed either on Biogel P10, as previously described [20] or Biogel P6. Briefly, on Biogel P6 column (5 × 190 cm) 300-350 mg sample dissolved in 5 mL purified water were loaded and eluted with 0.25 M NH$_4$Cl at a flow rate of 1.8 mL/min. The flow-through was collected in about 8 ml fractions and their UV absorbance was detected at 210 nm. Elution profile obtained by Biogel P6 is presented in additional material. Fractions of interest were collected and pooled. The pool volume was reduced to approximately 5 mL by evaporation under reduced pressure.

3.3. Desalting of Oligosaccharide Fractions

Desalting was performed using TSK-gel HW40S Toyopearl (Tosoh Bioscience, Yamaguchi, Japan) column 2.6 cm × 60 cm, particle size 20–40 μm. Samples were loaded onto the column and elution was performed in 10% EtOH in water at a flow rate of 1.4 mL/min. Two-point-one ml fractions were collected using a fraction collector. Absorbance at 210 nm was evaluated for each fraction. Fractions of interest were collected, pooled and lyophilized.

3.4. Affinity Chromatography on AT-Sepharose

Fifteen mg of octa and decasaccharide samples were dissolved in 5 mL equilibrium buffer (Tris-HCl 50 mM, pH 7.4, NaCl 50 mM), loaded onto a 30 mL of AT-Sepharose column (2 × 9.5 cm) and eluted first with 90 ml of equilibrium buffer to recover a fraction devoid of affinity for AT (NA), then with 90 mL of Tris-HCl 0.05M pH 7.4, 2.5 M NaCl, to recover a high affinity fraction (HA), at a flow rate of 0.5 mL/min. The flow-through was collected into 26 sub-fractions, 13 for NA and 13 for HA. Each sub-fraction was analysed for the uronic acid content [25]. HA and NA fractions were desalted as previously described [20].

3.5. NMR

Samples (8–20 mg) were dissolved in deuterium oxide containing 0.12 mM TSP (0.6 mL). NMR spectra were measured on a Bruker AVANCE III 600 MHz spectrometer or on a Bruker AVANCE IIIHD 500 MHz spectrometer (Bruker, Karlsruhe, Germany), both equipped with a 5 mm TCI cryo-genic probe. Proton spectra were measured with water suppression (decoupling power corresponding to 5 Hz linewidth). HSQC experiments (hsqcetgpsisp2.2 Bruker pulse sequence) were performed at 303 K, by using 32 dummy scans; from 60 to 48 scans; 2 s (500 MHz) or 2.5 s (600 MHz) relaxation delay; 8 ppm (F2) and 80 ppm (F1) spectral width; transmitter offset was set at 4.7 ppm(F2) and 80 ppm (F1); 1024 points were collected in F2 and 320 increments in F1. Zero filling was applied to 4k in F2 and, in F1, linear prediction to 640 points and zero filling to 1k; a 90 shifted squared sine bell-function was applied in both dimensions. Spectra were integrated by using the standard Topspin routine using rectangular integration domains with manual adjustment of regions according data published [19].

3.6. Exhaustive enzymatic Depolymerization with Heparin Lyases

Heparinase I, II, III. Each sample (20 μL of a 20 mg/mL solution in water) was incubated at 25 °C for 48 h in a total volume of 160 μL, containing 20 μL hep.ase I, II and III (0.4 IU/mL of each heparinase in 10 mM K$_2$HPO$_4$ buffer, pH 7.0) and 120 μL of 100 mM sodium acetate buffer pH 7.0, containing 2 mM of calcium acetate and 0.1 mg/mL bovine serum albumin (BSA).

Heparinase III. Each sample (20 μL of a 20 mg/mL solution in water) was incubated at 25 °C for 48h in a total volume of 160 μL, containing 20 μL hep.ase III (0.4 IU/mL 10 mM K$_2$HPO$_4$ buffer, pH 7.0) and 120 μL of 100 mM sodium acetate buffer pH 7.0, containing 2 mM of calcium acetate and 0.1 mg/mL BSA.

Enzyme inactivation. At the end of each incubation, enzymes were inactivated by a 2-min heating at 100 °C, and sample solutions were filtered onto 0.22 μm membrane.

3.7. LC-MS Analysis

Chain mapping analyses of intact samples were run on UHPLC system (Platin Blue, Knauer, Berlin, Germany) coupled to ESI-Ion Trap mass spectrometer (amaZon SL, Bruker Daltonics, Bremen, Germany). 5 µL of sample solution, prepared at the concentration of about 5 mg/mL, was injected on C_{18} Blue Orchid (150 mm × 2.0 mm i.d., 1.8 µm particle size, Knauer) column (maintained at 40 °C) and run at the flow rate of 0.3 mL/min, by the mobile phases A (10 mM pentylamine, 10 mM acetic acid in water/acetonitrile 95:5 *v/v*) and B (10 mM pentylamine, 10 mM acetic acid in acetonitrile) according to the following gradient: isocratic step at 15%B for 1 min, followed by a linear gradient from 15% to 40% B in 31 min; then, column washing by a gradient until 100% B kept for 5 min and reconditioning in the initial conditions were performed. The electrospray interface was set in negative ionization mode (Spray Voltage +4200 V), to record total ion current profiles in the *m/z* 300–2000 mass range. Nitrogen was used as a drying (9 L/min) and nebulizing gas (30 p.s.i.) and the ion transfer capillary was kept at 200 °C.

Building blocks composition and fragment mapping analyses were run on HPLC system (Ultimate 3000, Dionex, Sunnyvale, CA, USA) connected to ESI-Q-TOF mass spectrometer (micrOTOF$_Q$, Bruker Daltonics). Sample solutions at the concentration of 2 mg/mL in water were injected on C_{18} KINETEX column (100 mm × 2.1 mm i.d., with 2.6 µm particles, Phenomenex, Aschaffenburg, Germany) hold at room temperature and run by mobile phases A (10 mM dibutylamine and 10 mM acetic acid in water) and B (10 mM dibutylamine and 10 mM acetic acid in methanol) at 0.1 mL/min. Analyses of heparinases I, II, III digestion products were performed by injecting 5 µL of sample solution and eluting according to the following gradient: isocratic step at 2% B for 10 min, followed by a linear gradient to 60% B in 90 min and final steps of column washing and reconditioning. The separation method of heparinase III digestion products (injection volume of 10 µL) comprised an isocratic step of 5 min at 10% B, a linear gradient from 10% to 50% B in 55 min and a second linear gradient from 50% B to 90% B in 80 min, followed by column washing and reconditioning.

Mass spectrometry detector was set in negative polarity (Capillary voltage: +3200 V) in the mass range from *m/z* 200 to *m/z* 2000; nitrogen gas, used as nebulizer and heater gases, was set at 0.9 bar and 7.0 L/min, respectively; the ion transfer capillary was held at 180 °C.

Oligosaccharide fractions were run on Agilent 1100 HPLC system (Agilent Technologies, Santa Clara, CA, USA) coupled to ESI FT-ICR mass spectrometer (Solarix, Bruker Daltonics). Sample solutions at concentration of 10 mg/mL were injected (2 µL) on C_{18} KINETEX column (100 mm × 2.1 mm i.d., 2.6 µm partcles size, Phenomenex) held at room temperature and run by mobile phases containing 10 mM dibutylamine and 10 mM acetic acid (A: in water 100%, B: in methanol 100%) at 0.1 mL/min according to the following steps of linear gradient: from 50% B to 57% B in 5 min, from 57% B to 80% B in 52 min , from 80% B to 90% B in 16 min; then, 90% B was kept for 10 min and followed by column conditioning in the initial conditions. MS conditions were: capillary voltage at + 3200 V, nebulizer gas 1.0 bar, drying gas 3.7 liters/min, ion transfer capillary temperature 180 °C, mass range 200–3000 *m/z*.

Calibration of ESI-Q-TOF mass spectrometer was performed by using water -isopropanol 1:1 *v/v* solution containing HCOOH 0.2% and 5 mM NaOH; the ESI FT-ICR MS system was calibrated using sodium trifluoroacetate solution (0.05 mg/mL in water: acetonitrile 50:50 *v/v*), while low concentration tuning mix (Agilent Technologies) was employed for the mass range calibration of the ion trap detector. The LC-MS profiles and mass spectra were elaborated using the DataAnalysis software (Bruker Daltonics).

Octa-HA, octa-NA, deca-HA and deca-NA were run on an Agilent 1100 HPLC system (Agilent Technologies) coupled to an Esquire 3000 Plus (Bruker) as mass detector. Reversed-phase separation of LMWH fractions was carried out on a C_{18} KINETEX column (100 mm × 2.1 mm i.d., 2.6 µm partcles size, Phenomenex). Typically, 10 µg of each LMWH fraction was injected onto the column. The column was first eluted in isocratic conditions with 80% Solvent A (20 mM dibutylamine, 20 mM acetic acid in water) and 20% Solvent B (20 mM dibutylamine, 20 mM acetic acid in methanol) for 20 min. Then gradient elution gradient from 20% B to 40% B was applied followed for 10 min. The column was eluted at 40% B for 10 min. Subsequently, a 20 min gradient from 40% B to 90% B was applied and once 90% B was reached, this was kept for 10 min. Column conditioning for subsequent injections was established by a 5 min gradient from 90 % B to 20 % B and a 30 min equilibration at this solvent mixture. The flow rate and column temperature were maintained at 0.15 mL/min and 25 °C, respectively, throughout the run. The Chemstation software (Agilent Technologies) was used for instrument control.

Mass spectrometric analysis were performed on an Esquire 3000 Plus electrospray ion trap (Bruker Daltonics). Acquisition parameters for ESI-ion trap mass spectrometer were (set) negative polarity, mass range 300–1000 *m*/*z*, capillary +3166 V, nebulizer gas 60.0 psi, dry gas 12.0 L/min, dry temperature 350 °C.

4. Conclusions

In the present work, a combination of different methods for detailed structural investigation of dalteparin was proposed. The strategy involves a first analysis of the whole samples through a bi-dimensional NMR study, to determine the molar percentage of all differently substituted glucosamine and uronic acids. In parallel, high resolution LC-MS study was performed both on the whole samples and on their fragments obtained by digestion with a cocktail of heparinases I, II, III and heparinase III alone. For a more in-depth investigation, the same combined NMR and LC-MS approach was applied also to two size homogeneous oligosaccharide fractions, precisely octa and decasaccharides, and further on their sub-fractions endowed with and devoid of affinity toward AT. High resolution LC-MS approach applied provided information that was complementary to that produced by HSQC NMR, allowing to obtain an accurate and detailed picture of the oligomeric composition of dalteparin. The application of orthogonal analytical methods to the study of size homogeneous oligomeric families and of their HA and NA components permitted to identify a number of sequences, especially among the octasaccharide components endowed of affinity to AT.

The overall analytical approach here reported represents an effective strategy for comparative studies of dalteparin samples, either concerning the assessment of batch-to-batch variability or the appraisal of biosimilar drugs.

Supplementary Materials: The following are available online. Figure S1: LC-MS analysis of dalteparin Frag-5 following heparinase III digestion: confirmation of A5,8,0-aM.ol composition by ICR-FT-MS. Figure S2: LC-MS analysis of dalteparin Frag-5 following heparinase III digestion: confirmation of A7,11,0-aM.ol composition by ICR-FT-MS. Figure S3: Elution profiles on Biogel P6 of dalteparin samples Frag-1–Frag-4. Figure S4: Elution profiles on Biogel P6 of dalteparin samples Frag-5–Frag-8. Figure S5: Elution profiles on Biogel P6 of dalteparin samples Frag-9–Frag-11. Table S1: Oligosaccharide family identified by LC-MS chain mapping in all the analysed dalteparin samples Frag-1–Frag-11: mass signal assignment. Table S2: Oligosaccharide fragments produced by heparinases I, II, III digestion observed in all the analysed dalteparin samples Frag-1–Frag-11: mass signal assignment. Table S3: Oligosaccharide fragments produced by heparinase III digestion observed in all the analysed dalteparin samples Frag-1–Frag-11: mass signal assignment. (*) In blue, species observed in the untreated sample too.

Acknowledgments: The authors thank Opocrin SpA for funding part of the work and Bioiberica for supporting the costs of publication.

Author Contributions: A.B. drew up the research plan and together with E.U., M.G., G.T. and A.N. discussed the experimental data; P.d.W. isolated oligosaccharide fractions, H.A. and N.A. sub-fractions; E.U. and M.G. performed LC-MS and NMR studies, respectively. A.B. and E.U. wrote the paper and together with M.G. edited and revised the manuscript. All the authors read and approved the final manuscript.

Conflicts of Interest: The authors declare no conflict of interest.

References

1. Fareed, J.; Jeske, W.; Hoppensteadt, D.; Clarizio, R.; Walenga, J.M. Low-molecular-weight heparins: Pharmacologic profile and product differentiation. *Am. J. Cardiol.* **1998**, *82*, 3L–10L. [CrossRef]
2. Bisio, A.; Mantegazza, A.; Vecchietti, D.; Bensi, D.; Coppa, A.; Torri, G.; Bertini, S. Determination of the molecular weight of low-molecular-weight heparins by using high-pressure size exclusion chromatography on line with a triple detector array and conventional methods. *Molecules* **2015**, *20*, 5085–5098. [CrossRef] [PubMed]

3. Guerrini, M.; Bisio, A. Low-molecular-weight heparins: Differential characterization/physical characterization. In *Heparin-A Century of Progress*; Lever, R., Mulloy, B., Page, C.P., Eds.; Springer: London, UK, 2012; pp. 127–157.

4. Hirsh, J.; Bauer, K.A.; Donati, M.B.; Samama, M.M.; Weitz, J.L. Parenteral anticoagulants: American college of chest physicians evidence-based clinical practice guidelines (8th edition). *Chest* **2008**, *133* (Suppl. 6), 141S–159S. [CrossRef] [PubMed]

5. Fareed, J.; Hoppensteadt, D.; Schultz, C.; Ma, Q.; Kujawski, M.F.; Neville, B.; Messmore, H. Biochemical and pharmacologic heterogeneity in low molecular weight heparins. Impact on the therapeutic profile. *Curr. Pharm. Des.* **2004**, *10*, 983–999. [CrossRef] [PubMed]

6. Guerrini, M.; Guglieri, S.; Naggi, A.; Sasisekharan, R.; Torri, G. Low molecular weight heparins: Structural differentiation by bidimensional nuclear magnetic resonance spectroscopy. *Semin. Thromb. Hemost.* **2007**, *33*, 478–487. [CrossRef] [PubMed]

7. Iacomini, M.; Casu, B.; Guerrini, M.; Naggi, A.; Pirola, A.; Torri, G. "Linkage region" sequence of heparin and heparan sulfate: Detection and quantification by nuclear magnetic resonance spectroscopy. *Anal. Biochem.* **1999**, *274*, 50–58. [CrossRef] [PubMed]

8. Fragmin (dalteparin sodium injection) Product Monograph, Pfizer Canada Inc, issued April 2016. Available online: www.pfizer.ca/sites/g/files/g10028126/f/201605/FRAGMIN_PM_193875_27April2016_E.pdf (accessed on 23 June 2017).

9. Henricksen, J.; Ringborg, L.H.; Roepstorff, P. On-line size-exclusion chromatography/mass spectrometry of low molecular mass heparin. *J. Mass Spectrom.* **2004**, *39*, 1305–1312. [CrossRef] [PubMed]

10. Korir, A.; Larive, C.K. Advances in the separation, sensitive detection, and characterization of heparin and heparan sulfate. *Anal. Bioanal. Chem.* **2009**, *393*, 155–169. [CrossRef] [PubMed]

11. Zaia, J. On-line separations combined with MS for analysis of glycosaminoglycans. *Mass Spectrom. Rev.* **2008**, *28*, 254–272. [CrossRef] [PubMed]

12. Langeslay, D.J.; Urso, E.; Gardini, C.; Naggi, A.; Torri, G.; Larive, C.K. Reversed-phase ion-pair ultra-high-performance-liquid chromatography-mass spectrometry for fingerprinting low-molecular-weight heparins. *J. Chromatogr. A* **2013**, *1292*, 201–210. [CrossRef] [PubMed]

13. Alekseeva, A.; Casu, B.; Torri, G.; Pierro, S.; Naggi, A. Profiling glycol-split heparins by high-performance liquid chromatography/mass spectrometry analysis of their heparinase-generated oligosaccharides. *Anal. Biochem.* **2013**, *434*, 112–122. [CrossRef] [PubMed]

14. Zhang, Q.; Chen, X.; Zhu, Z.; Zhan, X.; Wu, Y.; Song, L.; Kang, J. Structural analysis of low molecular weight heparin by ultraperformance size exclusion chromatography/time of flight mass spectrometry and capillary zone electrophoresis. *Anal. Chem.* **2012**, *85*, 1819–1827. [CrossRef] [PubMed]

15. Wang, B.; Buhse, L.F.; Al-Hakim, A.; Boyne li, M.T.; Keire, D.A. Characterization of currently marketed heparin products: Analysis of heparin digests by RPIP-UHPLC-QTOF-MS. *J. Pharm. Biomed. Anal.* **2012**, *67–68*, 42–50. [CrossRef] [PubMed]

16. Galeotti, F.; Volpi, N. Novel reverse-phase ion pair-high performance liquid chromatography separation of heparin, heparan sulfate and low molecular weight-heparins disaccharides and oligosaccharides. *J. Chromatogr. A* **2013**, *1284*, 141–147. [CrossRef] [PubMed]

17. Ouyang, Y.; Wu, C.; Sun, X.; Liu, J.; Linhardt, R.J.; Zhang, Z. Development of hydrophilic interaction chromatography with quadruple time-of-flight mass spectrometry for heparin and low molecular weight heparin disaccharide analysis. *Rapid Commun. Mass Spectrom.* **2016**, *30*, 277–284. [CrossRef] [PubMed]

18. Sun, X.; Guo, Z.; Yu, M.; Lin, C.; Sheng, A.; Wang, Z.; Linhardt, R.J.; Chi, L. Hydrophilic interaction chromatography-multiple reaction monitoring mass spectrometry method for basic building block analysis of low-molecular-weight heparins prepared through nitrous acid depolymerization. *J. Chromatogr. A* **2017**, *1479*, 121–128. [CrossRef] [PubMed]

19. Mauri, L.; Boccardi, G.; Torri, G.; Karfunkle, M.; Macchi, E.; Muzi, L.; Keire, D.; Guerrini, M. Qualification of HSQC methods for quantitative composition of heparin and low molecular weight heparins. *J. Pharm. Biomed. Anal.* **2017**, *136*, 92–105. [CrossRef] [PubMed]

20. Bisio, A.; Vecchietti, D.; Citterio, L.; Guerrini, M.; Raman, R.; Bertini, S.; Eisele, G.; Naggi, A.; Sasisekharan, R.; Torri, G. Structural features of low-molecular-weight heparins affecting their affinity to antithrombin. *Thromb. Haemost.* **2009**, *102*, 865–873. [CrossRef] [PubMed]

21. Alekseeva, A.; Casu, B.; Cassinelli, G.; Guerrini, M.; Torri, G.; Naggi, A. Structural features of glycol-split low-molecular-weight heparins and their heparin lyase generated fragments. *Anal. Bioanal. Chem.* **2014**, *406*, 249–265. [CrossRef] [PubMed]

22. Yamada, S.; Yoshida, K.; Sugiura, M.; Sugahara, K.; Khoo, K-H.; Morris, H.R.; Dell, A. Structural studies on the bacterial lyase-resistant tetrasaccharides derived from antithrombin III-binding site of porcine intestinal heparin. *J. Biol. Chem.* **1993**, *268*, 7, 4780–4787.

23. Loganathan, D.; Wang, H.M.; Mallis, L.M.; Linhardt, R.J. Structural variation in the antithrombin III binding region and its occurrence in heparin from different sources. *Biochemistry* **1990**, *29*, 4362–4368. [CrossRef] [PubMed]

24. Wang, Z.; Hsieh, P.-H.; Xu, Y.; Thieker, D.; En Chai, E.J.; Xie, S.; Cooley, B.; Woods, R.; Chi, L.; Liu, J. Synthesis of 3-*O*-sulfated oligosaccharides to understand the relationship between structures and functions of heparan sulfate. *J. Am. Chem. Soc.* **2017**, *139*, 5249–5256. [CrossRef] [PubMed]

25. Bitter, T.; Muir, H.M. A modified uronic acid carbazole reaction. *Anal. Biochem.* **1962**, *4*, 330–334. [CrossRef]

Sample Availability: Samples of the compounds are not available from the authors.

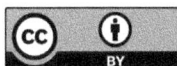

Article

Characterization of Danaparoid Complex Extractive Drug by an Orthogonal Analytical Approach

Cristina Gardini [1], Elena Urso [2], Marco Guerrini [2], René van Herpen [3], Pauline de Wit [3] and Annamaria Naggi [2,*] (ORCID)

[1] Centro Alta Tecnologia Istituto di Ricerche Chimiche e Biochimiche G. Ronzoni S.r.l., via G. Colombo 81, 20133 Milan, Italy; gardini@cat-ronzoni.it

[2] Istituto di Ricerche Chimiche e Biochimiche G. Ronzoni S.r.l., via G. Colombo 81, 20133 Milan, Italy; urso@ronzoni.it (E.U.); guerrini@ronzoni.it (M.G.)

[3] Aspen Oss B.V., Kloosterstraat 6, 5349 AB Oss, The Netherlands; rvanherpen@nl.aspenpharma.com (R.v.H.); pdewit@nl.aspenpharma.com (P.d.W.)

* Correspondence: naggi@ronzoni.it; Tel.: +39-02-70641626

Received: 31 May 2017; Accepted: 2 July 2017; Published: 5 July 2017

Abstract: Danaparoid sodium salt, is the active component of ORGARAN, an anticoagulant and antithrombotic drug constituted of three glycosaminoglycans (GAGs) obtained from porcine intestinal mucosa extracts. Heparan sulfate is the major component, dermatan sulfate and chondroitin sulfate being the minor ones. Currently dermatan sulfate and chondroitin sulfate are quantified by UV detection of their unsaturated disaccharides obtained by enzymatic depolymerization. Due to the complexity of danaparoid biopolymers and the presence of shared components, an orthogonal approach has been applied using more advanced tools and methods. To integrate the analytical profile, 2D heteronuclear single quantum coherence (HSQC) NMR spectroscopy was applied and found effective to identify and quantify GAG component signals as well as those of some process signatures of danaparoid active pharmaceutical ingredient (API) batches. Analyses of components of both API samples and size separated fractions proceeded through the determination and distribution of the molecular weight (Mw) by high performance size exclusion chromatographic triple detector array (HP-SEC-TDA), chain mapping by LC/MS, and mono- (^{1}H and ^{13}C) and bi-dimensional (HSQC) NMR spectroscopy. Finally, large scale chromatographic isolation and depolymerization of each GAG followed by LC/MS and 2D-NMR analysis, allowed the sequences to be defined and components to be evaluated of each GAG including oxidized residues of hexosamines and uronic acids at the reducing ends.

Keywords: danaparoid sodium; low molecular weight glycosaminoglycans; orthogonal multi-analytical methods; sequence and compositional investigations; component quantitative analysis

1. Introduction

Danaparoid sodium, constituted by a mixture of Low Molecular Weight (LMW) heparan sulfate (HS), dermatan sulfate (DS), and chondroitin sulfate (CS), extracted from porcine intestinal mucosa, is the active component of ORGARAN an anticoagulant and antithrombotic drug approved for prophylaxis of post-operative deep-vein thrombosis. Its beneficial effect upon factor IIa (thrombin) is shown by the anti-factor Xa/IIa ratio more than that of heparin [1–3].

A weight/weight (w/w) percentage maximum of 8.5% of CS and in the range of 8.0% up to 16.0% for DS, have been specified and quantified by an enzymatic method reported in the danaparoid monograph of the EC-Pharmacopoeia [4]. The chondroitinase selective depolymerization of galactosaminoglycans to UV detectable unsaturated disaccharides was originally developed to quantify

CS and DS present in API heparin batches. Alternative more feasible NMR quantifications have been developed for the components of danaparoid API batches [5] and for heparin composition [6].

The linear polymers HS, CS, and DS are the most abundant mucopolysaccharides in the body and ubiquitous components of connective tissue and cartilages. As other extracted and purified glycosaminoglycans (GAGs), they show high size, mean molecular weight (Mw) 50 kDa and heterogeneous chains [7] too great to be fully characterized as they are. Therefore, they must be partially/fully depolymerized by enzymatic or chemical methods. Lyase enzymes generally cleave hexosamine–uronic acid bonds and the final products of their exhaustive digestion are disaccharides bearing at the non-reducing end (NRE) a 4,5-unsaturated (Δ) uronic acid. Nitrous acid is also used to cleave hexosamine N-sulfated bonds at pH 1.5 and free hexosamine at pH 4.0 [8] leading to an anhydromannose at the reducing end (RE) of the depolymerized fragments. CS-A and CS-C, bearing a common repeating unit of D-glucuronic acid β-3-D-N-acetylgalactosamine β-4 (GlcA β-3-GalNAc β4) differ in sulfation degree of the 4-O and 6-O positions of GalNAc. DS, also known as CS-B, is a variant bearing a number of GlcA units epimerized to L-iduronic acid (L-IdoA), some of them 2-O sulfated (IdoA2S). HS, expressed on cell surface and basement membranes is a linear, highly heterogeneous, acidic GAG, in nature mainly bound to core proteins in proteoglycans. Depending on the core protein, cell types and cellular environment, the HS polysaccharides show an average chain size ranging from 5 up to 50 KDa and a polydispersity of 1.05–1.6 [7]. In the Golgi apparatus of most mammalian cells the HS precursor, constituted by the alternating (1–4) linked β-D-glucuronic acid α-N-Acetyl D-glucosamine (GlcA-GlcNAc) is synthesized. In the following complex biosynthetic steps some GlcA units are epimerized to IdoA and partially 2-O-sulfated (IdoA2S) while some GlcNAc are N-deacetylated, N-sulfated as well as 3-O and/or 6-O-sulfated leading to a plethora of diverse HS chains. Porcine intestinal mucosa is a source of HS usually in a mixture with CS and DS, remaining after the extraction of heparin [9].

To define compositional and structural characteristic of API samples an orthogonal analytical approach, already adopted for detecting potential contaminants in API heparin batches, was applied for this study [10,11].

At first, danaparoid API was characterized using NMR spectroscopy, mass spectrometry, and molecular weight determination. This allowed a general picture to be obtained of the API in which HS was observed to be the most abundant component in danaparoid. With the aim of also investigating the galactosaminoglycan component, a study was carried out. The structural information here obtained was fundamental for the subsequent part, where two paths were followed to go deeper into the characterization work: (1) fractionation of danaparoid by size and (2) isolation of the two GAG families, which are HS and CS/DS. Both groups of fractions were fully characterized as the parent sample, benefitting from the complementary information coming from the applied analytical methods.

2. Results

2.1. Danaparoid API Samples

Seven danaparoid API batches and their related size separated fractions were submitted for a full characterization by nuclear magnetic resonance experiments, mass spectrometry, and molecular weight determination.

A study in depth of digested products obtained by chondroitinase ABC (ChABC) digestion treatment (Section 2.2) and the pilot study on size exclusion chromatography (SEC) fractions, described in the first part of Section 2.3.3, were conducted only on one sample.

2.1.1. Determination of Molecular Weight Parameters

Analysis of molecular weight distribution was performed on seven API samples of danaparoid using high performance size-exclusion chromatography (HP-SEC) on polymeric columns, combined with a triple detector array (TDA) and UV detector. Using a 0.1 M $NaNO_3$ aqueous mobile phase, comparable Gaussian profiles exemplified in Figure 1a, were obtained by refractive index, viscometer, and right-angle laser light scattering [12,13].

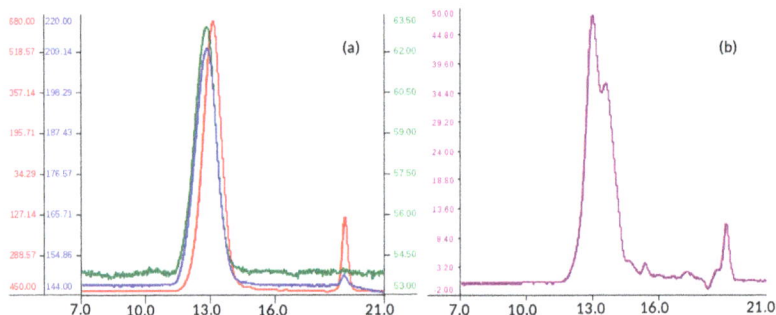

Figure 1. Size-exclusion chromatography profile of a danaparoid sample (CAT272): (**a**) red—refractive index (mV), blue—viscometer (mV) and green—right-angle laser light scattering (mV) detectors; (**b**) UV (mV) detector.

The software processed data of number average molecular weight (Mn), weight average Mw, and polydispersity (Pd) of analyzed samples were calculated as the mean of two runs. The values of Mn, Mw, and Pd ranging between 3300–3400 Da, 4200–4600 Da, and 1.27–1.36 respectively, indicate for the danaparoid analyzed samples small variation, near to the experimental error (5%).

The non-Gaussian profiles, obtained by UV detection at 260 nm (the eluent suppressed the lower λ signals) (Figure 1b) suggest an inhomogeneous distribution of different components of the complex GAG mixture. This could be ascribed to galactosaminoglycans that are present in high concentration in the higher Mw chains eluted which contain higher molar concentration of UV absorbing N-acetyl groups in comparison to the HS chains of lower Mw and N-acetyl content.

2.1.2. Determination of Sulfate to Carboxylate Ratio

The sulfate-carboxylate ratio, expressing the average disaccharide charge density, was determined in duplicate for all samples by a conductimetric titration method previously reported [14].

The resulting mean ratio of each sample, comprised in the narrow interval 1.19–1.32, indicated a substantial sample equivalence for the sulfation degree, considering the intrinsic variability of the extracted natural GAG components of API danaparoid.

Over the last forty years, the mean ratio values of several analyzed GAG samples, determined in our laboratories with the same method, were found in the range of 1.0–1.2 for CS and DS, 1.0–1.8 for HS and 2.1–2.8 for API porcine mucosal heparin.

2.1.3. Compositional Analysis by 1D and 2D NMR Spectroscopy

Both ^{1}H and ^{13}C one-dimensional NMR spectra of the samples have similar profiles, in Figures 2 and 3 a proton and a carbon spectra are displayed as examples.

In the proton spectra, the most evident difference is detected in the region of N-acetyl signals at 2.0–2.1 ppm which is correlated to the variable content of galactosaminoglycan components among samples [10,11,15]. Signals of N-acetyl galactosamine of CS are observed at 2.02 ppm, while that of DS is at 2.08 ppm. On the other hand, GlcNAc signals of HS are detected at 2.04 and 2.06 ppm, while those of oxidized N-acetyl hexosamine (ANAc-ox) are at 2.1 ppm (Figure 2b) [16–18]. A comparison between acetyl regions of different samples is reported in Figure S1.

^{13}C-NMR spectral analysis allowed signals to be attributed to each danaparoid component (Figure 3) confirmed by HSQC NMR spectra (Figure 4) and comparison with the corresponding literature data [15].

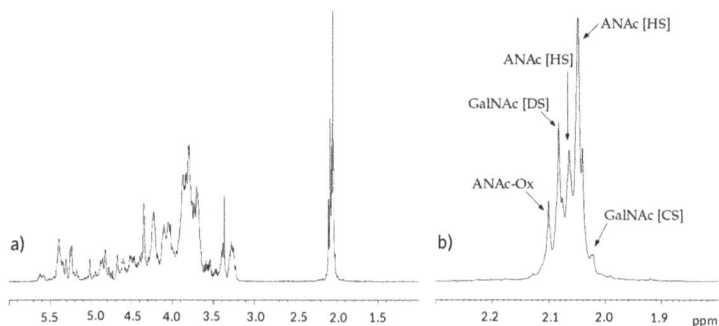

Figure 2. Example of ^{1}H-NMR spectrum of a danaparoid sample (CAT272): (**a**) whole spectrum; (**b**) expansion of the acetyl region.

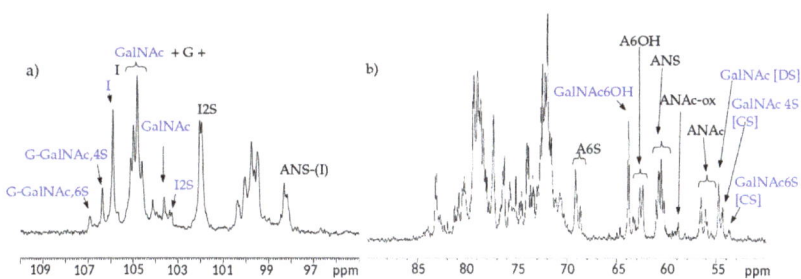

Figure 3. Example of ^{13}C-NMR spectrum of a danaparoid sample (CAT272): (**a**) anomeric region; (**b**) ring carbon region. Black: signals attributed to heparan sulfate (HS); Blue signals attributed to chondroitin sulfate (CS) and dermatan sulfate (DS).

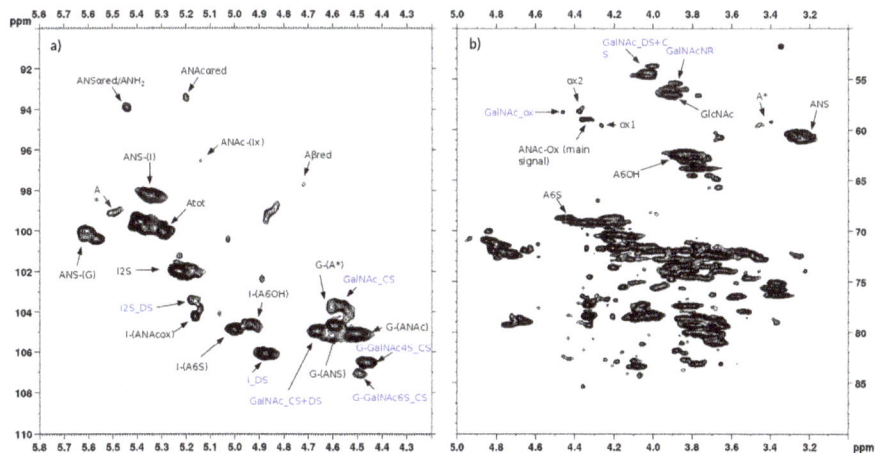

Figure 4. Example of 2D Heteronuclear Single Quantum Coherence (HSQC) NMR of a danaparoid sample (CAT272): (**a**) anomeric region; (**b**) ring region. Black: signals attributed to HS; Blue: signals attributed to DS and CS. Abbreviations in Table S1.

Heteronuclear single quantum coherence spectroscopy (HSQC) 2D NMR experiments on danaparoid samples were recorded by adapting the method recently validated for heparin samples [6].

The qualitative observation of 2D NMR spectra (Figure 4) allows the observation that the majority of peaks can be attributed to the HS component. In the ring region different signals correspond to glucosamines with various sulfation and acetylation substitution (such as ANS, A2*, ANAc, A6OH, and A6S, abbreviations in Table S1); moreover, the signals corresponding to N-acetylated galactosamines and their NRE are present and shown as GalNAc and GalNAc_NR.

In the area 4.6–4.2/57–61 ppm peaks associated to H2/C2 of N-acetyl hexosamine oxidized at the RE due to a bleaching process are observed. The assignments of this group of signals are done based on both literature [17–19] and experimental data: the cross-peak at 4.47/58.3 ppm is attributed to the oxidized N-acetylgalactosamines of CS/DS component (GalNAc-ox), whereas the signal at 4.37/58.9 ppm, shown as ANAc-ox, is assigned to oxidized reducing end (N-acetylglucosaminic acid) as described in [16,17]. The other peaks in the same area, displayed as ox1 and ox2, are associated with HS component because they are absent in the enriched CS/DS fractions described in Section 2.4. The hypothesis is that they can be associated to similar oxidized reducing ends on different oligosaccharidic sequences.

In the anomeric region, together with the HS signals, peaks related to DS and CS are displayed (I_DS, I2S_DS, G-GalNAc,4S and G-GalNAc,6S): the uronic acids of both components are useful for the characterization of the API samples.

The assignment of the peak at 5.18/104.2 ppm, previously reported [18], is confirmed as H1/C1 α-L-iduronic acid linked to oxidized N-acetylglucosamine (abbreviation I-(ANAcox)) by 2D NMR experiments.

The integration of characteristic signals of each component allows every contribution to be calculated and produces a detailed characterization of HS in a sample as shown in Tables 1 and 2.

For the analyzed samples, HS, DS, and CS the percentage ranged from 77.6–88.4%, from 9.0–16.8% and from 2.3–8.0%, respectively. The present NMR quantification was useful for the comparability of API batches. The comparability of the NMR method with the EU Pharmacopeia enzymatic method is ongoing. The NMR method should be not compared equally to the EU Pharmacopeia enzymatic method.

The composition of HS in different danaparoid batches was found very similar, supporting the validity of the process used to extract and purify the product. Moreover, the low percentage of 6-O-sulfation, agrees with the typical composition of an HS structure [20]. The sulfation degree, calculated from the NMR data, confirm the similarity of the HS composition. Values are in the range between 1.62 and 1.70 with an average value of 1.65. The IdoA/IdoA2S ratio of DS and CS-A/CS-C ratio is also similar to that of galactosaminoglycans extracted from porcine mucosa (Table 3) [21].

Table 1. Percentage of glucosamine residues of heparan sulfate (HS) of one danaparoid sample (CAT272). A* corresponds to 3-O,N-sulfated glucosamine according with the abbreviations shown in Table S1.

A*	ANAc αred	ANAc-(I)	ANAc-(G)	ANAc-ox	ANS αred	ANS βred	ANS-(G)	ANS-(I)	ANS-(I2S)	A6S
2.2	0.9	0.3	23.4	4.4	1.7	0.4	11.4	19.3	33.5	48.4

"A *" means 3-O,N-sulfated glucosamine according with the abbreviations in Table S1.

Table 2. Percentage of uronic acid residues and sulfation degree of HS of one danaparoid (CAT272). (Abbreviations are in Table S1.)

I2S	I-(A6S)	I-(A6OH)	I-(ANAcox)	G-(ANS)	G-(ANAc)	Sulfation Degree
43.5	11.2	6.7	3.2	13.3	22.1	1.63

Table 3. Sulfate distribution (percentage) of dermatan sulfate (DS) and chondroitin sulfate (CS) of one danaparoid sample (CAT272). (Abbreviations in Table S1.)

DS		CS	
I2S	I	G-(GalNAc,4S)	G-(GalNAc,6S)
8.7	91.3	80.0	20.0

2.1.4. Chain Mapping by HPLC/ESI MS

An optimized LC/MS method allowed fingerprints of all the samples to be recorded and compared. The ion pair reversed phase high performance liquid chromatography (IPRP-HPLC) coupled to electrospray ionization mass spectroscopic (ESI-TOF MS) detection achieved partial separation of chain components and first level structural assignment. The presence in danaparoid GAGs of epimeric hexosamines required an optimization of the method successfully applied for chain mapping of LMWHs [22,23].

Dibutylamine, the ion pair in the mobile phase, interacting with sulfate groups allowed a better peak resolution when an initial isocratic mode was followed by a linear gradient elution (Figure S2). Good repeatability in three consecutive days and inter-day precision of LC/MS chromatograms was obtained and shown in Figure S3.

Comparable profiles were obtained for all the samples showing common oligosaccharidic peaks ranging from 1200 up to 7000 Da. Complete base peak chromatogram of sample CAT272 was shown in Figure 5a: minor fluctuations were observed for some samples in the chromatogram portions at 30–40 min and at 75–85 min.

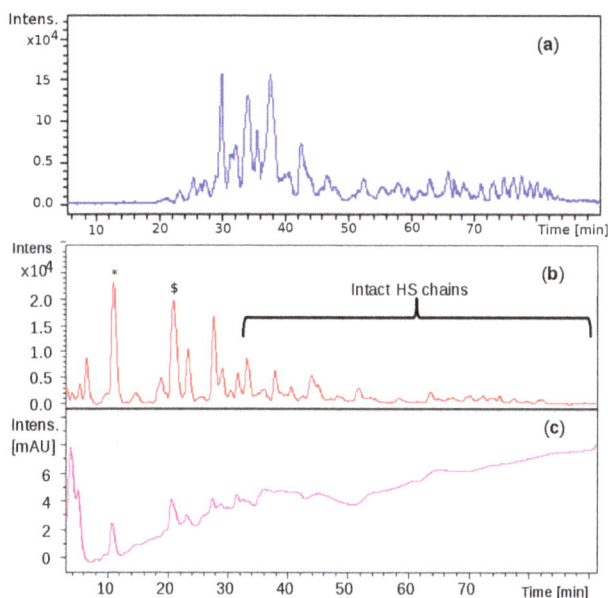

Figure 5. Liquid Chromatography-Mass Spectrometry (LC-MS) profiles: (**a**) one danaparoid sample CAT272; (**b**) ChABC danaparoid digestion product CAT469; (**c**) UV chromatogram at 232 nm of CAT469.

Only the most representative mass signals were attributed to the HS structures: several even and odd chains having 16 additional mass units than the regular oligosaccharidic sequences were identified and, supported by the previous NMR data that highlighted the presence of oxidized residues at the reducing ends, identified as 1-carboxy N-acetyl hexosamine [17,18].

2.2. Structural Study of One Danaparoid Sample

Compared to the natural porcine HS, the major component of danaparoid showed some structural modifications that could occur on galactosaminoglycan minor components of danaparoid and need to be further investigated.

One API sample was submitted to digestion with ChABC, the digest was analyzed by ^{1}H-NMR and its main signals were assigned to HS sequences. Comparing the N-acetyl region signals with those of the starting material a reduction of DS contribution (Figure S4) became evident; while at 5.9–6.0 ppm the signals of 4,5- unsaturated (Δ) uronic acids at the NRE produced by lyase were observed.

The same mixture was analyzed by LC-MS: the profile showed that the first eluted species (0 to 30 min) generated by the depolymerization of CS/DS could be detected at 232 nm for the presence of 4,5- unsaturated uronic acid due to the lyase action, followed by intact HS species detectable only by MS (Figure 5b,c).

This phase was focused on CS/DS oligosaccharides and among them two species with mass value of 934 (m/z 466 (z-2) RT 10′) and 1050 (m/z 524.0 (z-2) RT 20′) were detected (Figure 5b) and submitted to MS/MS fragmentation. Two species were identified: one as an unsaturated disulfated, di-N-acetyl tetrasaccharide bearing at the RE an oxidized N-acetyl galactosamine residue (ΔU4,2,2(T1)) and an unsaturated disulfated, di-N-acetyl pentasaccharide with a remnant (Ra) at the RE (ΔU5,2,2(Ra)) (Figure 6).

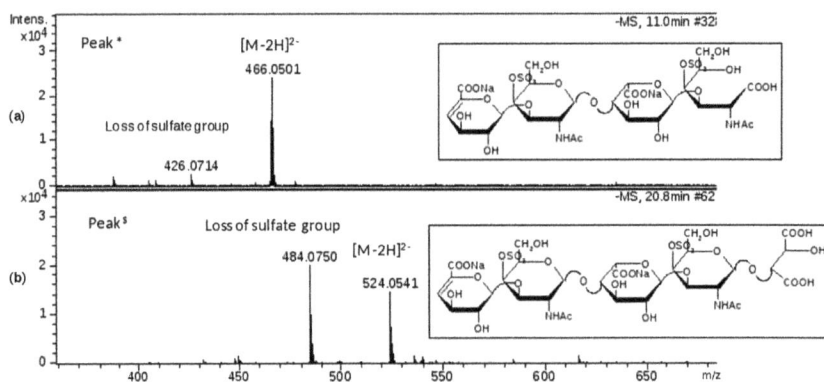

Figure 6. Mass spectra of chromatographic peaks * and $, respectively (as labelled in Figure 5b) and corresponding to structures identified by MS/MS fragmentation experiment (data shown in supplementary material Figures S5 and S6): (a) fragment at m/z 466.0501 (z-2; M 934) attributed to ΔU4,2,2(T1); (b) fragment at m/z 524.0541 (z-2; M 1050) attributed to ΔU5,2,2(Ra). The substitution pattern of DS was used.

The MS/MS spectra show the fragmentation pattern obtained by collision induced dissociation (CID) and structure annotation of numerous product ions allowed to elucidate the structure of the unknown parent ion (Figures S5 and S6). In particular, the characteristic ion product at m/z 316.0 (z-1) in the MS/MS spectrum of the first tetrasaccharide (M 934), revealed the oxidized galactosamine residue (ANAc,S +O labelled T1) which differs by 16 mass units from its regular form, as similarly observed for HS in Section 2.1.4. While the CID product ion at m/z 352.1 (z-1) generated from the second oligosaccharide (M 1050) resulted in being particularly informative for the confirmation of Ra terminal (ANAc + $C_4H_4O_5$).

Considering the whole profile, the main peaks were integrated and their assignments underlined such that the expected final product of the enzymatic cleavage ΔU2,1,1 was accompanied by the variant bearing a remnant Ra at the reducing end ΔU3,2,1(Ra). Other peaks were assigned to sequences having modified terminals T1 or Ra such as the oligosaccharides ΔU6,2,3(T1) and ΔU7,2,3(Ra), but also odd regular species such as the hexosamine A1,1,1, and trisaccharides A3,2,2 and A3,3,2 as well as the pentasaccharide ΔU5,2,2 bearing a uronic acid at the RE.

Since the digestion products detected in the mixture highlighted the presence of oligomers longer than the expected disaccharides, the conditions for an exhaustive depolymerization with ChABC were verified using a higher quantity of enzyme and repeating the reaction on the same sample, without improvement as checked by NMR. Therefore, the enzymatic efficiency was likely decreased by the presence of oxidized and remnant residues at the RE.

This study allowed the presence of unusual reducing ends on CS/DS component to be highlighted: the experimental data agreed in that T1 modification was observed on the galactosamine at the reducing end, while the terminal Ra occurred on uronic acid at the RE.

2.3. Preparative Size Exclusion Chromatography of API Danaparoid Samples

Seven batches of danaparoid (CAT271-277) were submitted to preparative gel filtration (SEC) on a Biogel P6 column. Comparable UV curves were detected for all the samples, an example with the indication of the collected fractions is displayed in Figure 7: the molecular weight decreases from A to N.

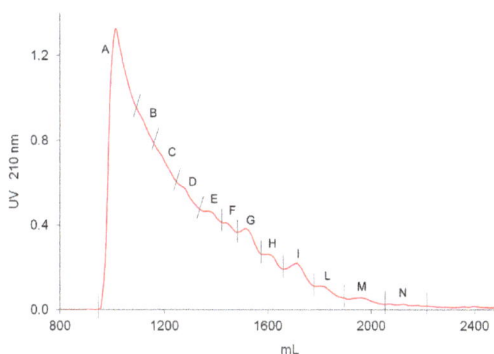

Figure 7. Preparative size exclusion chromatography (SEC) fractionation chromatographic UV 210 nm profile of a danaparoid (CAT277).

2.3.1. Determination of the Mw Distribution of SEC Fractions

The Mw distribution of fractions A, B, and C of all the seven API samples was determined and the results, reported in Table 4, showed comparable ranges of weight average Mw and polydispersity. The fraction A, constituted by the highest Mw components, was at the limit of the Biogel P6 chromatographic separation efficiency.

Table 4. Ranges of weight average molecular weight (Mw) and polydispersity (Pd) of SEC fractions of seven danaparoid Active Pharmaceutical Ingredient (API) samples.

Fractions	Mw (Da)	Pd
A	8200–8800	1.14–1.17
B	5300–5700	1.06–1.11
C	4400–4700	1.05–1.11

All SEC fractions (A–N) obtained from one danaparoid sample (CAT277) were analyzed for the determination of molecular weight parameters (Table 5): components of the subsequent fractions showed decreasing Mw and very low Pd values; the partial overlapping between adjacent fractions was displayed by their Refractive Index (RI) profiles in Figure 8.

Table 5. Weight average Mw and polydispersity (Pd) of SEC fractions of danaparoid Active Pharmaceutical Ingredient (API) sample CAT277.

Fractions	A	B	C	D	E	F	G	H	I	L	M	N
Mw (kDa)	8.2	5.4	4.4	3.9	3.3	3.0	2.8	2.5	2.3	2.1	2.1	1.9
Pd	1.17	1.06	1.06	1.04	1.05	1.06	1.05	1.05	1.05	1.04	1.04	1.01

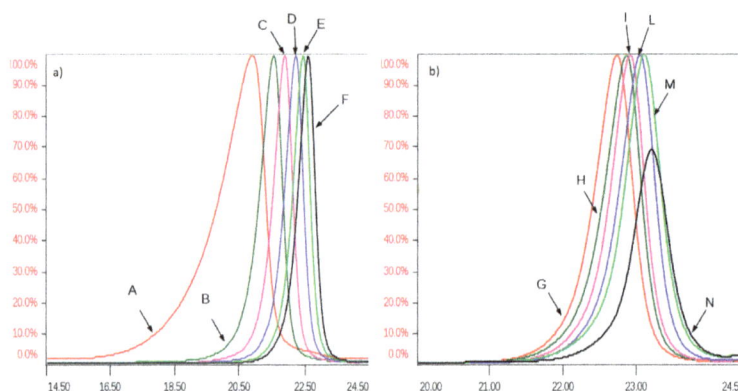

Figure 8. Overlapping of normalized Refractive Index (RI) profiles of SEC fractions of a danaparoid sample (CAT277): (**a**) fractions A–F, range volume 14–24.5 mL; (**b**) fractions G–N, range volume 20–24.5 mL.

2.3.2. 2D-NMR Spectroscopic Analysis of SEC Fractions of Danaparoid Samples

The 2D-NMR spectra of the danaparoid SEC fractions, considering some signals characteristic for each component, allowed it to be underlined how the proportion of GAG species varies over fractions.

Inspection of the H2/C2 region displays that the galactosamine (CS/DS) signals had more or equal intensity than those of glucosamine (HS) in the high Mw oligomers corresponding to fractions A and B followed by a progressive decrease in the subsequent fractions up to being absent in fractions L, M, and N.

The signal of C2/H2 of NS,3S,6S glucosamine (A2*) is present with variable intensity in almost all fractions, up to being undetected or in traces in fractions A and B.

The peaks related to oxidized RE residues at 4.6–4.2/57–61 ppm were variably present in almost all fractions.

The comparison between fractions obtained from different APIs was performed by analyzing the anomeric regions of the HSQC spectra (Figure S7), considering the peculiar disaccharides, IdoA2S-GlcN for HS, IdoA-GalNAc for DS and GlcA-GalNAc 4 and/or 6 sulfated for CS.

By visual inspection the highest content of CS and DS components was found in fraction A, the intensity of their cross-peaks being superior to those of IdoA2S of HS, then decreasing gradually in all the danaparoid samples, while the HS oligosaccharides increased upwards to become the sole components in fractions L to N. The DS components seemed to be more abundant than those of CS which disappeared early, as the signals of GlcA linked to GalN6S in comparison with those of GlcA linked to GalN4S. Variation of the CS/DS component content and distribution was qualitatively evaluated in HSQC spectra and summarized as scores in Table 6, resulting in being slightly different among the seven API danaparoid samples. This is considered normal for a natural extraction product.

Table 6. Variation of dermatan sulfate and chondroitin sulfate among SEC fractions of seven API batches by qualitative observation of peculiar HSQC anomeric signals.

		A	B	C	D	E	F	G	H	I	L	M	N
CAT271	DS	+++	+++	+++	+++	++	++	++	++	+	−	−	−
	CS	+++	+++	+++	+++	++	++	++	+	−	−	−	−
CAT272	DS	+++	+++	+++	+++	++	++	++	++	++	−	−	−
	CS	+++	+++	+++	+++	++	++	++	+	+	−	−	−
CAT273	DS	+++	+++	++	++	++	++	++	+	−	−	−	−
	CS	+++	+++	++	++	++	++	−	−	−	−	−	−
CAT274	DS	+++	+++	++	++	++	++	+	−	−	−	−	−
	CS	+++	+++	++	++	+	−	−	−	−	−	−	−
CAT275	DS	+++	+++	++	++	++	++	+	−	−	−	−	−
	CS	+++	+++	++	++	+	−	−	−	−	−	−	−
CAT276	DS	+++	+++	++	++	++	+	+	−	−	−	−	−
	CS	+++	+++	++	+	−	−	−	−	−	−	−	−
CAT277	DS	+++	+++	+++	+++	++	++	++	++	+	−	−	−
	CS	+++	+++	+++	+++	++	++	++	+	−	−	−	−

Where '−' = absent; '+' = traces; '++' = present; '+++' = more present.

2.3.3. Sequencing of Danaparoid SEC Fractions by LC/MS Analysis

A pilot study by the IPRP-HPLC/MS method was addressed to sequence the SEC fractions of a danaparoid sample (CAT277) (Figure 7) to achieve a first level structural assignment of components and identify probable modified structures on shorter chains. This explorative study was conducted by analyzing a restricted portion of each SEC fraction of the danaparoid sample, with the aim of simplifying the expected complexity of sequences and eventually identifying structure modifications. These selective analyses provided only a partial picture of the whole fractions but also the detection of minor modified sequences useful for the study.

This approach led to the identification in the fractions E to N of few HS regular sequences and a majority of HS chains bearing oxidized residues at the reducing end, likely 1-carboxylated glucosamines, shown as T1 in Figure 9 [17–19] applying the code already used for the similar modification on CS/DS (Section 2.2). Less abundant modifications were observed and displayed as T2, T3, T4 and T5 (Figure 9).

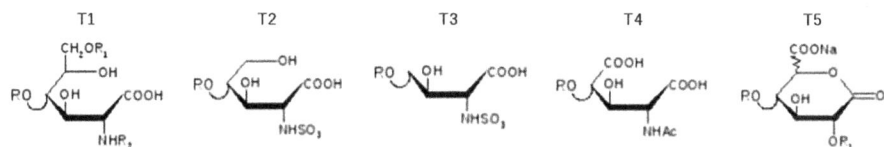

where R= GAG chain; R_1=H or SO_3; R_2=H, SO_3 or Ac

Figure 9. Structures of oxidized Reducing End (RE) residues compatible with the observed *m/z* values (the substitution pattern was in accordance with the observed species listed in Table 7).

In particular, the species exhibiting T2 and T3 end residues, detected in a minor peak of fraction N, can be explained by further oxidation of the secondary alcohol and decarboxylation steps of terminal T1 (Figure 10). Confirmation of the molecular formula is supported by a very low error (<10 ppm) between experimental and theoretical mass values.

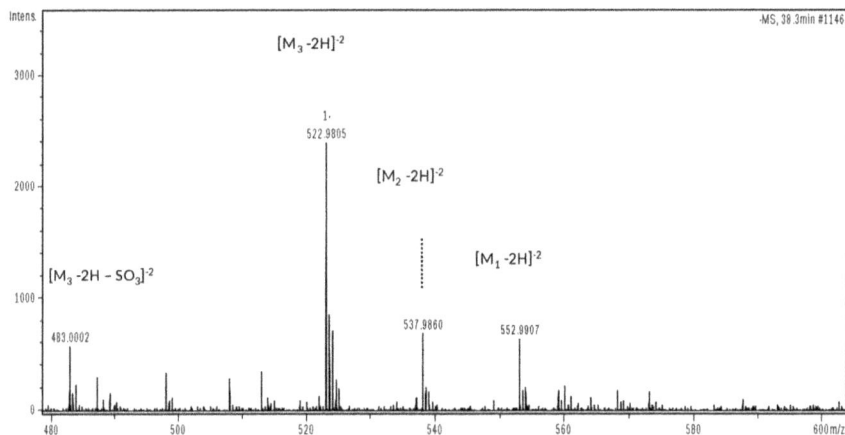

Figure 10. Mass spectrum displaying the different oxidation forms of oligosaccharide U4,5,0 from M_1 to M_3 derivative: m/z 552.9907 (z-2, M_1 1108) identified as U4,5,0 (T1); m/z 537.9860 (z-2, M_2 1078) identified as U4,5,0 (T2); m/z 522.9805 (z-2, M_3 1048) identified as U4,5,0 (T3).

Concerning the T4 modification, observed in fraction H, only a high resolution MS measurement allowed this oxidized residue to be discriminated from a regular structure.

The experimental mass signal at m/z 881.086 (z-2), shown in Figure 11, at first sight seemed to correspond to the regular hexasaccharide U6,6,3 (sum formula $C_{42}N_3O_{52}H_{65}S_6$). A more detailed mass investigation, revealing a high mass error between experimental and theoretical values (22 ppm), suggested another possible structure modification as U6,6,3(T4) corresponding to a sum formula of $C_{41}N_3O_{53}H_{61}S_6$, showing a good overlap of mass signals with a decrease of the error to 2 ppm.

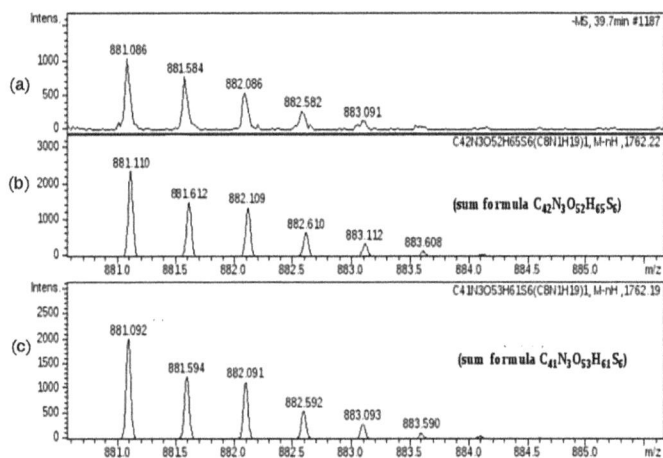

Figure 11. Mass signal at m/z 881.086 (z-2): (**a**) experimental m/z and isotopic distribution; (**b**) theoretical m/z and isotopic distribution corresponding to the regular structure of U6,6,3 (sum formula $C_{42}N_3O_{52}H_{65}S_6$); (**c**) theoretical m/z and isotopic distribution corresponding to the oxidized structure U6,6,3(T4) (sum formula $C_{41}N_3O_{53}H_{61}S_6$).

In fractions F, H, and L, some mass values differing by two Daltons (-2H) with respect to the HS regular sequences were observed. The hypothesis was that after the oxidation of carbon 1 a water loss occurred to give the lactone (T5 in Figure 9) and lacking 2 Da. The mass accuracy of both T1 and T5 modifications found in fraction F was verified also by ESI-FT MS: the error on theoretical mass was minor or equal to 1.5 ppm.

After the pilot study the same analytical method was applied to the SEC fractions isolated from seven API samples. A qualitative observation of the LC profiles of the corresponding fractions showed a good similarity mainly among fractions D to N, containing LMW chains. A higher variability was observed among the first eluted fractions (A to C), containing mainly CS/DS high Mw chains endowed with an intrinsic heterogeneity of natural extractive GAGs such as danaparoid and whose content varied among API samples. A compositional analysis was performed integrating the main peaks where the principal detected species were investigated: the structures were the same inside each fraction group, while different oligomers were observed in different fractions.

The list of main species found in SEC fractions is shown in Table 7, together with the GAG assignment and eventual additional species previously identified in the pilot study. Components are indicated by: A for hexosamines or U for uronic acids as NRE residues, followed by three numbers referring respectively to oligosaccharidic units, sulfate, and N-acetyl groups. The number of oligosaccharidic units includes both RE and/or NRE variants (T1–T5 and Ra), examples of sequences are shown in Figure 12. The assignment of the m/z value to a single GAG component was based on the knowledge of their N-acetylated, N-, O-sulfated degrees.

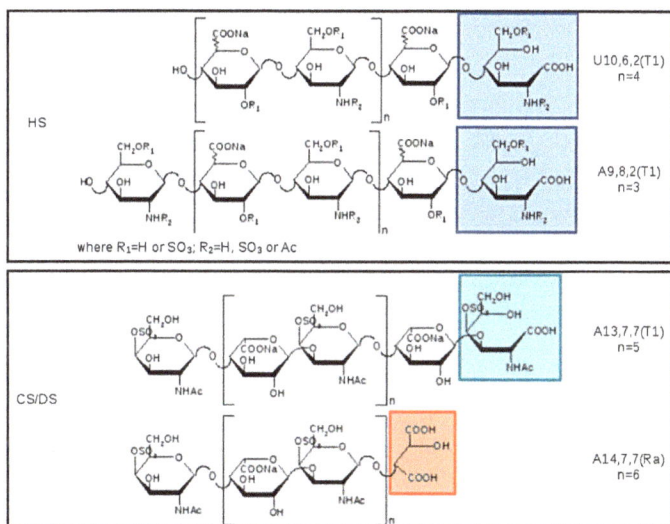

Figure 12. Example of structures detected in SEC fractions, the modified RE are highlighted in the boxes: HS sequences are displayed in the upper panel with the terminal T1 at the RE and with the uronic acid or the glucosamine at the non reducing end (NRE) in even or odd oligomers, respectively. CS/DS structures are shown in the lower panel (the substitution pattern of DS is used as example because it is more abundant than CS): two possibly reducing ends are T1 and Ra, the galactosamine is placed at the NRE.

The main components of fractions A–C were assigned to CS/DS, and those of fractions D to N to HS components. Some unassigned mass values were present, but detected in all samples.

Almost all the detected species showed a structural modification of the reducing end residue. Oxidized hexosamine T1 was present in both CS/DS and HS sequences, while the remnant Ra, of oxidized uronic acid, seems to be present only on CS/DS chains.

In principle, oxidation of reducing end residues can occur both on hexosamine and uronic acid [24]. Actually, whereas for odd sequences experimental mass data permitted the certain identification of ending residues thus confirming the presence of T1 on RE hexosamine, for even sequences terminal RE and NRE residues cannot be distinguished, and oxidized residues were not precisely assigned accordingly. Considering the literature data [17,18], in Table 7 and Figure 12 the variant T1 was attributed to the RE hexosamine of even sequences bearing a uronic acid at the NRE.

The terminal T5 (lactonized form of T2) was observed on both even and odd sequences as shown in Figure 9 and Table 7.

Table 7. Main species detected in fractions A–N of 7 API samples.

Fraction	Main Species in the Woul Fraction	GAG	Species Detect at the Top of the Fraction (Pilot Study)
A	A19,10,10(T1) to A27,14,14(T1); A20,10,10(Ra) to A26,13,13(Ra)	CS/DS	-
B	A17,9,9(T1) to A21,11,11(T1); A16,8,8(Ra) to A22,11,11(Ra)	CS/DS	-
C	A13,7,7(T1) to A15,11,8(T1); A14,7,7(Ra) to A18,9,9(Ra)	CS/DS	-
D	U10,9,3 to U10,10,3; A7,10,0(T1); A11,10,6(T1) to A11,11,6(T1); U10,10,3(T1) to U10,13,3(T1)	HS	-
E	U8,8,3(T1) to U8,10,3(T1); A11,8,2(T1) to A11,14,2(T1)	HS	U8,10,2(T1); A11,14,1(T1)
F	U10,6,2(T1) to U10,8,2(T1); U10,8,1(T1) to U10,13,1(T1)	HS	U7,8,1(T5) to U7,10,1(T5); U10,8,0(T5)
G	A9,4,2(T1) [#] to A9,8,2(T1); A9,8,1(T1) to A9,13,1(T1)	HS	-
H	U8,6,1(T1) to U8,10,1(T1); U6,6,3(T4) to U6,8,3(T4)	HS	A9,6,2; A9,9,1 and A9,10,1; U8,6,0(T5)
I	A7,6,1 and A7,7,1; A7,5,1(T1) to A7,10,1(T1); U6,4,1 to U6,5,1; U6,6,1(T1)	HS	A7,5,2(T1); U7,4,0(T5)
L	A7,6,1; A5,5,1; A7,5,2 [#] to A7,6,2; U6,5,1(T1) to U6,7,1(T1); U6,6,1(T5) [#]	HS	U6,3,0(T5) and U6,4,0(T5); A7,7,1; A7,8,0 to A7,9,0; A7,9,1
M	A5,4,1; U6,5,1 to U6,6,1; U6,6,0 to U6,9,0; A5,4,1(T1) to A5,7,1(T1); A5,7,0(T1)	HS	A5,8,1(T1)
N	A5,5,0 to A5,9,0; A5,5,1 and A5,6,1; A5,5,1(T1); U4,5,0(T3)	HS	U4,5,0(T1); U4,5,0(T2)

[#] species not detected in one sample.

2.4. Isolation of GAG Components of Danaparoid and Compositional Analysis

Three danaparoid samples were chosen to perform the isolation of HS and CS/DS components, based on their different content of HS-DS-CS that range from 78.0–87.2%, from 9.8–14.0% and from 3.0–8.0%, respectively (NMR data).

The parent samples were submitted to complementary procedures to depolymerize selectively the two GAG families of danaparoid: for the isolation of HS the chondroitinase ABC was applied, while the isolation of CS/DS was performed using heparin lyase III followed by a chemical reaction using nitrous acid.

The depolymerization methods, described in Section 5, led to the isolation of three enriched fractions of HS and CS/DS. The weight recovery for the enriched HS fractions was about 78–81%, while those of CS/DS range from 15–26%.

Both components were fully characterized by NMR, molecular weight distribution, LC-MS chain mapping and only for HS fractions by LC-MS disaccharidic analysis as subsequently reported herein.

2.4.1. Molecular Weight Data

Molecular weight distribution was determined by triple detector array (TDA) for both families of samples: the enriched CS/DS fractions range from 6200 to 7100 Da, while for those enriched HS components the Mw varies from 3300 to 3500 Da and is consistent with the data of the SEC fractions. The polydispersity is lower for the HS species (1.13) than for the CS/DS ones (1.19), both are lower than the API samples.

In Figure 13 The Refractive Index (RI) profile overlay of a parent API sample and its enriched HS and CS/DS fractions displays the presence of CS/DS components in the higher Mw with respect to the API, as already observed in the NMR and MS data regarding the SEC study. On the other hand, the enriched HS fraction is observed in the mid–lower Mw range.

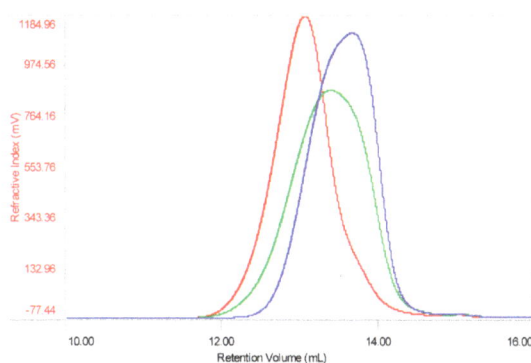

Figure 13. Refractive Index profile overlay of a danaparoid sample (CAT272 in green), its enriched CS/DS (red) and HS (blue) fractions.

2.4.2. NMR Observations

The 2D-NMR-HSQC assignments of the CS/DS component were done according to literature data [19,25,26] as shown in the spectra of one CS/DS enriched fraction (Figure 14a): the chemical shifts of 4.36/85.4 ppm and 4.19/76.8 ppm, in red, were in agreement with the positions C4′ and C5′ of remnant Ra. While the CS/DS fraction does not contain signals of HS, the spectrum of the HS fraction also shows signals typical of CS/DS oligomers, highlighted in red in Figure 14b.

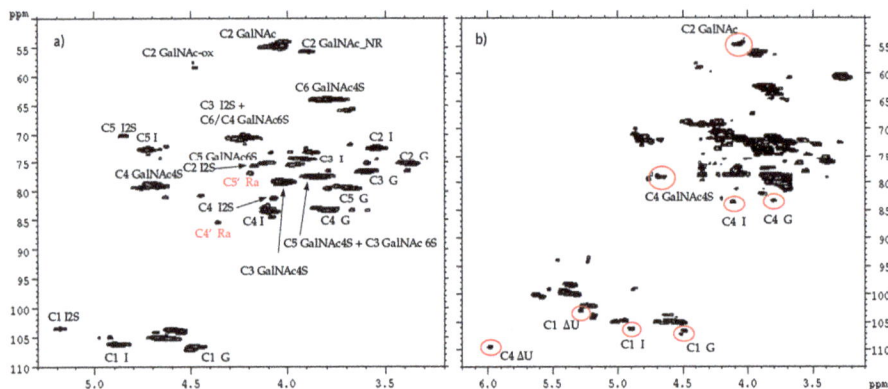

Figure 14. HSQC NMR spectra of CS/DS (**a**) and HS (**b**) fraction of danaparoid CAT272. Signals belonging to CS/DS are circled in red.

The superimposition of the HSQC spectra of HS and CS/DS fractions with that of the danaparoid starting material allows some peaks to be assigned correctly: signal at 3.90/55.5 ppm belongs to the C2 of the NRE GalNAc residue of CS/DS [25]. The signals in the oxidized region at 4.39/58.1 ppm and 4.27/59.5 ppm (shown as ox1 and ox2 in Section 2.1) belong to HS, being absent in the spectrum of the CS/DS fraction (Figure 15).

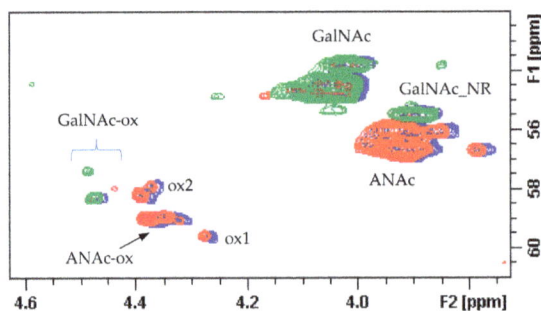

Figure 15. Superimposition of HSQC spectra (C2 region) of a danaparoid sample (CAT272 in blue), its enriched HS (red) and CS/DS fractions (green).

The composition of HS and CS/DS in the corresponding enriched fractions is very similar to that found in the parent danaparoid samples, demonstrating the robustness of the methods of separation.

The enriched CS/DS fractions, free from HS, display DS as the most abundant species ranging from 63–76%. On the contrary, the enriched HS fractions include a part of CS/DS that varies between 5% and 14%.

2.4.3. LC-MS Chain Mapping Analysis of CS/DS Fractions

The LC-MS analysis of enriched CS/DS fractions show the simplification of the region of short chains (RT 20–40 min) due to the removal of the HS component by the analytical depolymerization/purification procedure, and contemporarily the enrichment of CS/DS species in the region of long chains (RT 50–90 min).

The investigation in depth of mass spectra at the apex of each peak allows the main mass signals (Figure 16) to be assigned: CS/DS chains from A6,2,3 to A30,15,15 oligomers were identified (Table S2), almost all of them having both the oxidized variants T1 and Ra remnant due to the production process. These results are in agreement with the data obtained by SEC fractions in which the CS/DS sequences from A13,7,7 to A27,14,14 were identified. The isolation of the CS/DS component allowed their shorter oligomers previously masked by the HS component in the API danaparoid sample to be detected.

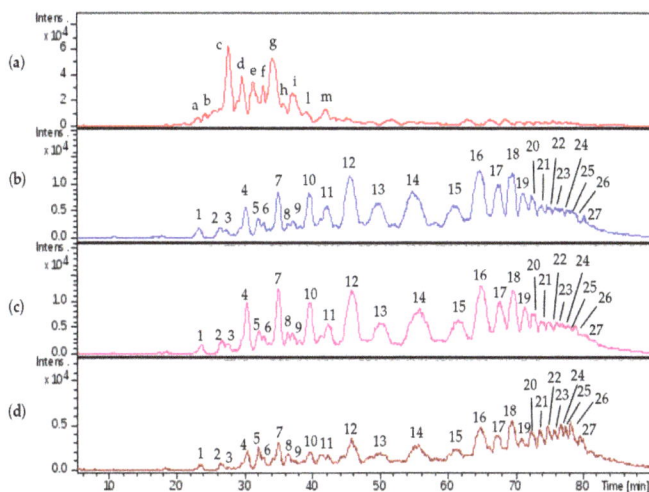

Figure 16. LC-MS profiles comparison: (**a**) danaparoid sample CAT272; (**b**) CS/DS isolated from CAT271; (**c**) CS/DS isolated from CAT272; (**d**) CS/DS isolated from CAT275.

The qualitative comparison of LC-MS profiles of the three isolated CS/DS samples underlines a good similarity between the CS/DS fractions isolated from CAT272 and CAT271, while for those isolated from CAT275 the lower molecular weight species (from 20 to 60 min) are less represented with respect to the higher Mw ones eluting from 60 to 85 min in comparison with the other two samples. This observation is in agreement with SEC data in which the variation of CS/DS content is displayed as scores in Table 6 and for CAT275 their reduction is observed in longer fractions than for CAT271 and CAT272.

2.4.4. LC-MS Chain Mapping Analysis of HS Enriched Fractions

The enriched HS fractions were also analyzed by LC-MS and compared with danaparoid (Figure 17).

The assignments were reported in accordance with the retention time, the majority of the peaks (n.7–15) were attributed to HS oligomers with the modification T1. Regular sequences of HS were observed with less intensity assigned to A5,6,0; A7,6,1; A7,5,0.

The comparison of the region from 30 to 45 min for the three isolated samples displayed slight differences in the intensity of the peaks.

The comparison of isolated HS and danaparoid (Table S3) allowed the correspondence of HS sequences in the isolated HS (peaks n.7–15) and in danaparoid (peaks from 'c' to 'm') to be observed; in the range of shorter species (peaks n.1–6 and at 29.1 min) there were pentasaccharides with 3 acetyl and hexa- and hepta-saccharides with a double bond on uronic acid, not present in the parent danaparoid that should be related to the residual presence of CS/DS fragments from the enzymatic process and not removed by purification steps (as already observed in NMR spectra).

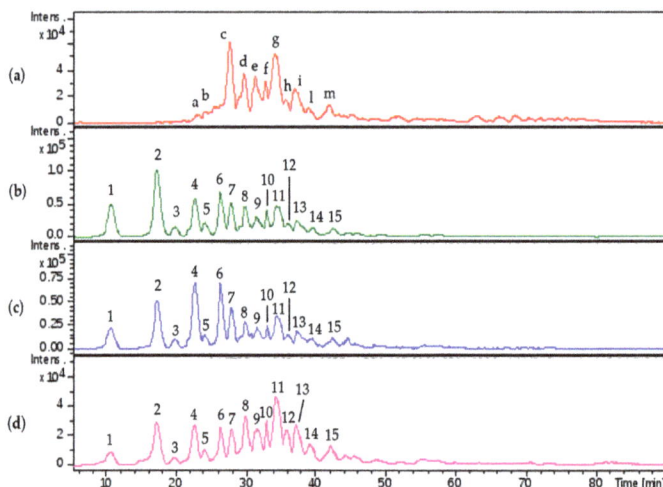

Figure 17. LC-MS profiles comparison: (**a**) danaparoid sample CAT272; (**b**) HS isolated from CAT271; (**c**) HS isolated from CAT272; (**d**) HS isolated from CAT275.

To complete the compositional analysis, the HS enriched fractions, along with a nadroparin and a heparin samples were submitted to enzymatic digestion using a mixture of heparinase I, II, III.

A qualitative inspection of the profiles highlighted a comparable oligosaccharidic composition among the digestion products of all the enriched HS fractions, some differences were observed in the nadroparin and heparin digest components (Figure 18).

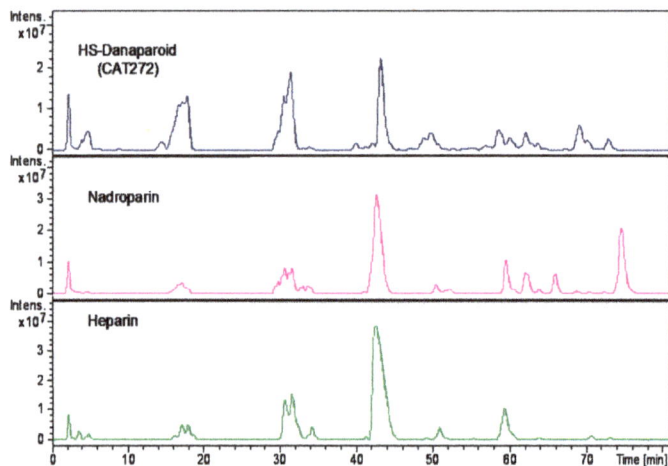

Figure 18. LC-MS profiles of HS danaparoid (CAT272), nadroparin and heparin digested by heparinases I, II, III.

The peaks identified by comparison with commercial standard disaccharides, were detected in all digested samples. As regards the species obtained from the enriched HS fractions regular unsaturated oligomers were observed together with some saturated odd and even sequences. Confirming the previously described data, some tetrasaccharides with the variant T1 at RE were present, only a very low peak corresponding to an unsaturated monosulfated, *N*-acetyl disaccharide bearing the T1 at the RE was detected supporting the hypothesis that the variants at RE inhibit the lyases.

An unsaturated tetrasaccharide with one acetyl and four sulfates was observed together with some species, Δ4,3,1, A3,4,0, and A3,5,0 that should be related to the sequence AGA*IA not cleaved by lyases [27,28].

Based on the ratio between N-acetylated and N-sulfated disaccharides, calculated by the commercial standard disaccharides peaks, the enriched HS fractions were compared with nadroparin and heparin. The data shown as percent in Table 8 allow the substantial different nature of heparin to be underlined in respect of the glucosaminoglycan component of danaparoid that has an HS structure [29,30]. This semi-quantitative analysis of N-acetylated/N-sulfated disaccharides ratio was performed on extracted ion chromatograms (EIC) of mass signals corresponding to mass values of disaccharides (the sum of ΔU-ANAc, ΔU-ANAc6S, ΔU2S-ANAc, ΔU2S-ANAc6S with respect to the sum of ΔU-ANS, ΔU-ANS6S, ΔU2S-ANS, ΔU2S-ANS6S percent).

Table 8. Ratio percentage between disaccharides N-acetylated and N-sulfated.

Sample	Ratio % N-acetylated/N-sulfated Disaccharides
HS-CAT271	41.4
HS-CAT272	39.0
HS-CAT275	39.2
nadroparin	16.8
heparin	13.2

3. Discussion

The danaparoid characterization was focused on a compositional study of intact API samples in obtaining their general picture, followed by the study of fractions differing in size and of their GAG components. Both APIs and their fractions were analyzed with complementary techniques following an orthogonal analytical approach.

The analyzed API samples resulted in similar data for every applied technique such as NMR spectra, LC-MS profiles, and HP-SEC-TDA curves; their variability was included in the natural variation typical of extractive products.

Danaparoid was a low-molecular-weight mixture of HS, CS, and DS, confirmed by experimental weight average molecular weight (Mw) ranging from 4200 to 4600 Da. The charge density determined as sulfate-to-carboxylate ratio was between 1.19 and 1.32.

By analyzing the NMR spectra, it was confirmed that the main species is an HS glucosaminoglycan, based on the sulfation/acetylation pattern. Dermatan sulfate and chondroitin sulfate were present quantitatively as secondary and tertiary components, respectively. Among the peaks relative to regular mono- or disaccharides of GAGs, some signals connected to the bleaching process were detected and attributed to oxidized gluco-/galactosamine at the reducing end (shown as T1). This modification, corresponding to the addition of one oxygen to the mass values of regular sequences, was confirmed by mass spectrometry both on HS and CS/DS. During the in-depth study on the galactosaminoglycan component, the remnant 3-O tartaric acid (Ra) at the RE was also detected.

The size fractionation was performed for all danaparoid batches and their fractions were submitted for further studies. NMR spectra were evaluated by means of the main characteristic signals of each component of danaparoid, through the variation of their anomeric peaks in every fraction and then among the starting batches: for all APIs the highest quantity of CS/DS component was found in the higher molecular weight fraction A, then decreasing down to fractions L, M, and N containing only HS. The different CS/DS content as well as their different distribution could be explained by variation in the starting natural sources. The presence of HS component in all fractions was ascertained by NMR.

The MS data of SEC fractions were evaluated qualitatively from the chromatographic profiles. These showed slight variations among batches in the range of longer chains where the major variability was expected. From the compositional point of view, the chain size decreased and sequences varied from fraction A to N, the main species found in the fraction of the same size of different API batches had an analogue composition.

In particular, investigating the main mass values, the fractions A to C showed CS/DS sequences having both T1 and Ra variants at RE; while in the subsequent fractions, structures attributed to HS were identified and characterized not only by the most abundant reducing end variant T1 but also by regular sequences and, less representative but structural interesting, variants T2, T3, T4, and T5. The majority of the HS components of all fractions were found to be odd oligosaccharides with a glucosamine (A) at the NRE; in fractions F and H only even sequences were identified; in the fractions containing shorter chains odd and even sequences were in similar abundance. Odd oligosaccharidic chains were not usually found in extractive GAG sequences even if present in low amounts in the LMWHs, enoxaparin and dalteparin [23] and highly represented in parnaparin [31] and γ-heparin [32] obtained by radical depolymerization.

The Mw range of fraction components, determined by MS is comparable with that obtained by the HP-SEC-TDA method which underlined also the closeness of contiguous fraction components, in particular for F to N included from 3000 to 1900 Da.

The isolation of components starting from three intact API samples was performed applying depolymerization procedures, using the proper enzyme and/or chemical reaction, followed by multiple purification steps. All of them were submitted for full characterization: Mw distribution, NMR, chain mapping, and only for HS fractions disaccharidic analysis by LC-MS.

The isolated CS/DS fractions were pure and the molecular weight analysis confirmed that the galactosaminoglycans were mainly present in the high molecular weight range of danaparoid, having a weight average molecular weight (Mw) from 6200 to 7100 Da. On the other hand, the HS fractions should be considered enriched HS fractions with CS/DS still being present (5–14%), their weight average Mw was found in the range from 3300 to 3500 Da, consistent with SEC fractions data.

Analyzing their NMR spectra, the fractions isolated from the three API samples showed a composition similar to that of the corresponding species present in the parent API samples, supporting the robustness of the separation procedures. Taking advantage of the purity of CS/DS fractions, some NMR signals were correctly assigned to the right component such as the C2/H2 of the NRE GalNAc residue at 3.90/55.5 ppm. In the region of oxidized residues two signals ox1 and ox2, hypothetically belonging to sequences similar to that bearing T1 variant, were attributed to HS because they were not observed in the isolated CS/DS fractions. The content of DS was evaluated by NMR in the isolated CS/DS fractions compared with that of CS and resulted ranging from 63% to 76%.

Moreover, also the LC-MS profiles of isolated CS/DS fractions were simplified by the removal of HS component, in the region of both short and long oligomers. The observed oligomeric size distribution was in good agreement with the SEC data and allowed the detection of higher oligomers (range 1271 (dp6) to 8282 Da (dp30)) bearing the variants T1 or Ra at the RE.

The study of enriched HS fractions allowed the confirmation of components already observed in danaparoid (dp5 to dp8) and the disaccharidic analysis, performed in comparison with nadroparin and heparin samples, provided compositional data in accordance with SEC data. Moreover, the evaluation of N-acetyl and N-sulfate ratio underlined that the glucosaminonoglycan component of danaparoid is heparan sulfate differing from those obtained from nadroparin and heparin samples.

4. Materials and Methods

4.1. Reagents and Starting Materials

Seven danaparoid API batches (CAT271-277), one heparin sodium USP and one Nadroparin calcium samples were provided by Aspen Oss B.V., Oss, Netherlands. Heparin lyases I (EC 4.2.2.7), II and III (EC 4.2.2.8) were purchased from Grampian Enzymes, Aberdeen, UK. Chondroitin ABC lyase from *Proteus vulgaris* (EC 4.2.2.4), ammonium acetate (≥98%), sodium azide (≥99.0%), sodium nitrate (≥99.0%), sodium dihydrogen phosphate monohydrate (>98%), sodium hydrogen phosphate dihydrate (≥99.0%), trimethylsilyl-3-propionic acid (TSP 98% D), dibutylamine (≥99.5%), acetic acid (glacial, 99.9%), acetonitrile (LC-MS grade), methanol (LC-MS grade), ammonium chloride (≥99.5%), sodium nitrite (>95%), sodium tetraborate (≥98%), hydrochloric acid (≥37%) were purchased from Sigma Aldrich (Milan, Italy); calcium acetate (≥97%) from BDH; sodium acetate (≥99%) and NaOH (≥99%) from Merck (Kenilworth, NJ, USA); Amberlite IR 120 H⁺ and 0.1 M NaOH from Fluka Analytical (Milan, Italy).

Ethanol (96%) was purchased from Girelli Alcool (Milan, Italy); ethylenediaminetetraacetic acid (EDTA D16, 98%) from Cambridge Isotope Laboratories (Tewksbury, MA, USA) and deuterium oxide (≥99.9%) from Euriso-top (Saint-Aubin, France). Deionized water (conductivity less than 0.15 μS) was prepared with an osmosis inverse system (Culligan, Milan, Italy).

4.2. Molecular Weight Determination

Molecular weight determinations were performed using an HPLC system combined with a Viscotek mod. 305 Triple Detector Array [12,13]. The HPLC Viscotek equipment was made up by a Knauer Smartline 5100 pump, a Biotech Degasser model 2003, and an HTA autosampler model HT310L. The detector system was composed of right angle laser light scattering (90° angle geometry), refractive index and viscometer; all detectors and the separation columns were contained in an oven compartment.

Two chromatographic conditions were applied: (I) for SEC fractions (Section 2.3.1) two silica columns G3000SWXL+G4000SWXL TSK GEL (7.8 mm ID × 30 cm, Tosoh Bioscience S.r.l., Rivoli, Torino, Italy) preceded by precolumn TSK GEL SWXL GUARD (7 μm, 6.0 × 40 mm, Tosoh Bioscience) were used eluting with ammonium acetate 0.1 M, sodium azide 0.02% at 0.6 mL/min ± 10% setting up the temperature at 30 °C; (II) for API samples (Section 2.1.1) and isolated fractions CS/DS and HS (Section 2.4.1) the chromatographic elution was performed at 0.6 mL/min ± 10% with sodium nitrate 0.1 M, sodium azide 0.05% on two polymeric columns G3000PWXL+G2500PWXL TSK GEL (7.8 mm ID × 30 cm, Tosoh Bioscience) at 40 °C.

The samples were dissolved with a concentration between 8 and 12 mg/mL in the mobile phase used for the elution; 100 μL of each solution was injected. All chromatographic systems were calibrated using for (I) a pullulan (PSS, Mainz, Germany) and for (II) a polyethylene oxide (Agilent Technologies, Santa Clara, CS, USA), both are certified standards of known Mw, polydispersity and intrinsic viscosity. The data elaboration was performed with OmniSEC software, version 4.6.2 (Malvern, UK).

4.3. Sulfation Degree Determination

The sulfation degree of all samples, expressed as sulfate to carboxylate molar ratio, was determined in duplicate by conductimetric titration following the method proposed by Casu et al. [14]. A sample of ~75 mg of the acidic form of danaparoid, previously exchanged on Amberlite IR 120 H+, in 100 mL of distilled water was titrated with 0.1 M NaOH using an automatic titrator (Titrando 888, Metrohm Italiana S.r.l., Origgio, Varese, Italy) equipped with a conductivity cell (constant = 0.76 cm⁻¹).

4.4. NMR

About 250 mg of API batches were dissolved in 2.5 mL of D_2O, and analyzed by using a Bruker AV 500 MHz (125 MHz for ¹³C) NMR spectrometer (Karlsruhe, Germany). The carbon spectra were recorded with a pulse delay of 1 s and 20 k scans.

About 35 mg of danaparoid samples were dissolved in 0.6 mL of buffer solution pH 7.1 (buffer phosphate 0.15 M, EDTA-D16 0.3 mM) in D_2O with 0.12 mM TSP; while the fractions isolated (20 or 35 mg) during the experimental activity were dissolved in 0.6 mL of D_2O. Both groups of samples were analyzed by using a Bruker Avance III HD NMR spectrometer operating at 500 MHz (¹H) equipped with TCI cryoprobe (Karlsruhe, Germany). The proton spectra were acquired with presaturation of residual HDO signal, 16 scans and 12 s of pulse delay. The Heteronuclear Single Quantum Coherence

(HSQC) spectra were recorded with the library Bruker pulse sequence hsqcetgpsisp2.2, a pulse delay of 2–5 s and 8–24 scans. The spectra elaboration was done using Bruker TopSpin software, version 3.2 (Karlsruhe, Germany).

4.5. LC-MS Analysis

LC-MS analysis of all of samples was performed using ion-pair reversed-phase separation on a Kinetex-C18 column (2.1 mm × 100 mm, ODS 2.6 μm, 100 Å, Phenomenex, Aschaffenburg, Germany) with pre-column filter (Phenomenex, Aschaffenburg, Germany) at room temperature coupled with mass spectrometer. The injected volume was 5 μL at a concentration of about 5 mg/mL.

A binary solvent system was used for a multi-step gradient elution using solvent A (dibutylamine 10 mM, acetic acid 10 mM in water) and solvent B (dibutylamine 10 mM, acetic acid 10 mM in acetonitrile) with the following schedule: (I) for SEC fractions of pilot study (first part of Section 2.3.3) at flow rate of 0.1 mL/min, 15% B for 5 min, linear gradient from 15% to 26% B in 25 min, 26% B for 20 min, linear gradient from 26% to 40% B in 35 min, fast linear gradient from 40% to 60% in 13 min, hold 60% B for 10 min, then return to 15% B in 2 min and hold for 30 min 15% B; (II) for API batches, isolated fractions of CS/DS and HS and all SEC fractions at flow rate of 0.15 mL/min, 15% B for 5 min, linear gradient from 15% to 24% B in 22 min, 24% B for 23 min, linear gradient from 24% to 40% B in 50 min, fast linear gradient from 40% to 60% B for 3 min, then 60% B for 10 min, then return to 15% B in 2 min and hold for 20 min at 15% B.

The samples were analyzed on an Ultimate 3000 HPLC-UV system (Dionex, Sunnyvale, CA, USA) coupled to an ESI-Q-TOFMS MicrOTOF-Q (Bruker Daltonics, Bremen, Germany). The mass spectrometer setting was as follows: ESI in negative ion mode (capillary voltage +3.2 kV); nitrogen, used as nebulizer and heater gas, flowed at 7 L/min, +180 °C and pressure 0.9 bar; mass range of 200–2000 *m/z*. Only the SEC fractions F, I–N were analyzed on an HPLC-UV system (Agilent Technologies, Santa Clara, CA, USA) coupled to an ESI FT-ICR MS Solarix (Bruker Daltonics, Bremen, Germany) using the elution schedule (II) and MS conditions were set up in negative polarity with a capillary voltage of +3.2 kV, nitrogen at the flow rate of 3.7 L/min, temperature of +180 °C and pressure of 1 bar, mass range 200–3000 *m/z*.

The MS^2 fragmentation experiments were performed on selected ions isolated in the quadrupole collision cell by a width of 5 Da and activated by collision-induced dissociation (CID) at the collision energy of 25 eV.

LC-MS analyses of enzymatic digested mixture (Section 2.4.4) were performed on an ESI-IT amaZon SL (Bruker Daltonics, Bremen, Germany) using solvent A (dibutylamine 10 mM, acetic acid 10 mM in water) with solvent C (dibutylamine 10 mM, acetic acid 10 mM in methanol) at flow rate of 0.1 mL/min, 10% C for 5 min, linear gradient from 10% to 35% C in 35 min, linear gradient from 35% to 50% C in 45 min, from 50% to 90% in 13 min, then hold at 90% C for 5 min, then return to 10% C in 2 min and hold for 25 min 10% C. The mass spectrometer parameters were as follows: ESI in negative ion mode with a capillary voltage of +3.8 kV, nitrogen at +200 °C, 9 L/min with a nebulizer pressure of 30 psi, mass range 200–1500 *m/z*.

4.6. Size-Exclusion Chromatography

The fractionation method was applied to seven API samples: about 250 mg dissolved in 2.5 mL of H_2O were loaded onto two columns in series (5.0 × 90 cm each) of Bio-Gel P6 (BIO-RAD Laboratories S.r.l., Milan, Italy), the elution was performed with 0.25 M ammonium chloride solution at a flow rate of 1.8 mL/min. Tubes of 18 mL were collected, and their absorbance at 210 nm was monitored using a variable-wavelength UV detector (Varian Cary 50scan, Agilent Technologies, Santa Clara, CA, USA). Based on the profile, twelve fractions with decreasing molecular weight were recovered (labelled from A to N).

Two desalting/purification methods were applied and described as follows: (I) one column (5.0 cm × 90 cm) filled with TSK HW40S resin (Tosoh Bioscience S.r.l., Rivoli, Torino, Italy) was eluted with 10% aqueous ethanol at the flow rate of 5 mL/min, samples elution was monitored by absorbance at 210 nm, positive fractions were pooled concentrated and lyophilized; (II) about 90–120 mg of sample were injected in a volume of 2.5 mL onto HPLC system made up by two glass columns in series (3.0 × 48 cm + 2.0 × 83 cm) filled with the resin Superdex 30 preparative grade (GE Healthcare Life Science, Milan, Italy) and a pump, a manager unit and a UV detector (KNAUER, Smartline, models 1050, 5050; and 2500, respectively) set up at 210 nm, the elution was performed with 0.25 M ammonium chloride solution at 5 mL/min, the system is managed by Clarity Chrom Preparative software, version 2.6 (Knauer, Berlin, Germany).

4.7. Depolymerization of CS/DS for the Isolation of HS Component

About 100 mg of danaparoid API sample was dissolved in phosphate sodium acetate buffer 50 mM pH 8, the enzyme Chondroitin ABC lyase was added to have a ratio enzyme/substrate equal to 7 mU/mg. The reaction was driven at 37 °C under magnetic stirring for 72 h.

At the end, to eliminate the enzyme by denaturation, the solution was heated at 95–100 °C for 5–10 min, after cooling the solution was filtered on 0.22 μm (Merck Millipore, Billerica, MA, USA), concentrated by reduced pressure and then purified by size-exclusion chromatography systems, applying TSK HW40S column, Superdex 30 and finally TSK HW40S column (Section 4.6).

4.8. Depolymerization of HS for the Isolation of CS/DS Component

About 500 mg of danaparoid API sample was dissolved in buffer 100 mM sodium acetate +10 mM calcium acetate pH 7 and incubated with the enzyme Heparinase III with a ratio of enzyme/substrate equal to 20 mU/mg, at 37 °C for 48 h under magnetic stirring. Then the solution was heated at 90–100 °C for 5–10 min for enzyme denaturation, subsequently it was cooled and filtered on 0.22 μm (Merck Millipore, Billerica, MA, USA). The solution was submitted to chemical reaction with nitrous acid twice following the procedure here described: the sample (500 mg) was dissolved in 20 mL of water, cooled to 4 °C and added to 140 mg of $NaNO_2$ dissolved in 1 mL of water. The pH was adjusted to 1.7 with HCl 4% (*w/v*) and the solution was stirred for 20 min. Then portions of $NaNO_2$ were added (140, 100 and 100 mg, respectively), after each addition the solution was stirred for 20 min. Subsequently, the pH was adjusted to 7 with NaOH 1 M and the solution was conditioned to room temperature. $NaBH_4$ was added as solid (400 mg) in several portions with stirring. After 2 h, the pH solution was adjusted to 4 with HCl 4% and then neutralized with NaOH 1M. The obtained product was purified by SEC systems such as TSK HW40S column, Superdex 30 and finally TSK HW40S column (Section 4.6).

4.9. Depolymerization of HS for the Isolation of CS/DS Component Exhaustive Enzymatic Digestion with Lyases I, II and III

Each isolated HS fraction was depolymerized using heparinases I, II, and III according to the USP method [33]. Each sample was solubilized in water to obtain a concentration of 20 mg/mL and 20 μL (400 μg) that were then digested in sodium/calcium acetate buffer pH 7.0 by using a mixture 1:1:1 of Heparinases I, II, and III prepared by mixing a solution 0.4 IU per mL of each one. The reaction mixture was stirred (Thermo shaker TS-100, Biosan, Riga, Latvia) at 25 °C for 48 h, then each digestion solution was boiled for two minutes at 100 °C and passed through a filter having a porosity of 0.20 μm and analyzed by LC-MS.

5. Conclusions

For the present work an orthogonal analytical approach based on complementary techniques, allowed a compositional comparison and first structural assignment of the components of different batches of danaparoid.

The in depth studies conducted on SEC fractions and on isolated CS/DS and HS components produced much structural information that completed the characterization of the starting API samples and allowed the similarity of analyzed batches to be established, ascribing slight differences to the intrinsic heterogeneity of extractive products such as danaparoid.

From the compositional point of view, both NMR and MS data confirmed the presence of different GAGs variably distributed over fractions/molecular weights, the CS/DS component represents the higher Mw species of danaparoid. LMW heparan sulfate was confirmed to be the major component of the API samples.

NMR and LC-MS analysis underlined the fact that a majority of the analyzed species showed oxidized hexosamines as T1 variant at the RE of both CS/DS and HS chains and a remnant (Ra) of an oxidized uronic acid at the reducing end of CS/DS species. Minor further oxidation products (T2, T3, T4, and T5) were present on the HS chains. Some NMR signals were correctly assigned to GAG species by studying the isolated components.

The exemplification of species through size fractionation and isolation of components allowed a good correspondence in terms of composition with the parent danaparoid samples to be observed, supporting the robustness of the separations methods and analytical tools.

Supplementary Materials: Supplementary Materials are available online.

Acknowledgments: The authors thank Edwin Kellenbach (Aspen Oss B.V.) and Giuseppe Cassinelli (G. Ronzoni Institute) for the critical reading of the manuscript.

Author Contributions: A.N., R.v.H. and P.d.W. conceived and designed the experiments; C.G. performed the experiments; E.U. performed and analyzed mass experiments; M.G. analyzed NMR experiments; C.G., A.N., R.v.H,. and P.d.W. analyzed the data; C.G. and A.N. wrote the paper.

Conflicts of Interest: R.v.H and P.d.W. declare that they are employed by Aspen Oss B.V. and that the study was paid for by Aspen Oss B.V.

References

1. Acostamadiedo, J.M.; Iyer, U.G.; Owen, J. Danaparoid sodium. *Expert Opin. Pharmacother.* **2000**, *1*, 803–814. [CrossRef] [PubMed]
2. Nurmohamed, M.T.; ten Cate, H.; ten Cate, J.W. Low molecular weight heparin(oid)s. Clinical investigations and practical recommendations. *Drugs* **1997**, *53*, 736–751. [CrossRef] [PubMed]
3. Skoutakis, V.A. Danaparoid in the prevention of thromboembolic complications. *Ann. Pharmacother.* **1997**, *31*, 876–887. [CrossRef] [PubMed]
4. Council of Europe; European Pharmacopoeia Commission. *European Pharmacopoeia*, 6th ed.; Strasbourg Council of Europe: Strasbourg, France, 2007; pp. 1644–1646.
5. Üstün, B.; Sanders, K.B.; Dani, P.; Kellenbach, E.R. Quantification of chondroitin sulfate and dermatan sulfate in danaparoid sodium by ^{1}H-NMR spectroscopy and PLS regression. *Anal. Bioanal. Chem.* **2011**, *399*, 629–634. [CrossRef] [PubMed]
6. Mauri, L.; Boccardi, G.; Torri, G.; Karfunkle, M.; Macchi, E.; Muzi, L.; Keire, D.; Guerrini, M. Qualification of HSQC methods for quantitative composition of heparin and low molecular weight heparins. *J. Pharm. Biomed. Anal.* **2016**, *136*, 92–105. [CrossRef] [PubMed]
7. Casu, B. Structure and biological activity of heparin. *Adv. Carbohydr. Chem. Biochem.* **1985**, *43*, 51–134. [PubMed]
8. Conrad, H.E. *Heparin-Binding Proteins*; Academic Press: New York, NY, USA, 1997.
9. Casu, B.; Moretti, M.; Oreste, P.; Riva, A.; Torri, G.; Vercellotti, J.R. Glycosaminoglycans from pig duodenum. *Arzneimittelforschung* **1980**, *30*, 1889–1892. [PubMed]
10. Guerrini, M.; Zhang, Z.; Shriver, Z.; Naggi, A.; Masuko, S.; Langer, R.; Casu, B.; Linhardt, R.J.; Torri, G.; Sasisekharan, R. Orthogonal analytical approaches to detect potential contaminants in heparin. *Proc. Natl. Acad. Sci. USA* **2009**, *106*, 16956–16961. [CrossRef] [PubMed]
11. Guerrini, M.; Shriver, Z.; Bisio, A.; Naggi, A.; Casu, B.; Sasisekharan, R. The tainted heparin story: An update. *Thromb. Haemost.* **2009**, *102*, 907–911. [CrossRef] [PubMed]
12. Bertini, S.; Bisio, A.; Torri, G.; Bensi, D.; Terbojevich, M. Molecular weight determination of heparin and dermatan sulfate by size exclusion chromatography with a triple detector array. *Biomacromolecules* **2005**, *6*, 168–173. [CrossRef] [PubMed]

13. Bisio, A.; Mantegazza, A.; Vecchietti, D.; Bensi, D.; Coppa, A.; Torri, G.; Bertini, S. Determination of the molecular weight of low-molecular-weight heparins by using high-pressure size exclusion chromatography on line with a triple detector array and conventional methods. *Molecules* **2015**, *20*, 5085–5098. [CrossRef] [PubMed]

14. Casu, B.; Gennaro, U. A conductimetric method for the determination of sulphate and carboxyl groups in heparin and other mucopolysaccharides. *Carbohydr. Res.* **1975**, *39*, 168–176. [CrossRef]

15. Holme, K.R.; Perlin, A.S. Nuclear magnetic resonance spectra of heparin in admixture with dermatan sulfate and other glycosaminoglycans. 2-D spectra of the chondroitin sulfates. *Carbohydr. Res.* **1989**, *186*, 301–312. [CrossRef]

16. Kellenbach, E.; Sanders, K.; Michiels, P.J.; Girard, F.C. ^{1}H-NMR signal at 2.10 ppm in the spectrum of KMnO$_4$-bleached heparin sodium: Identification of the chemical origin using an NMR-only approach. *Anal. Bioanal. Chem.* **2011**, *399*, 621–628. [CrossRef] [PubMed]

17. Becatti, D.; Roy, S.; Yu, F.; Gunay, N.S.; Capila, I.; Lech, M.; Linhardt, R.J.; Venkataraman, G. Identification of a novel structure in heparin generated by potassium permanganate oxidation. *Carbohydr. Polym.* **2010**, *82*, 699–705. [CrossRef] [PubMed]

18. Mourier, P.A.; Guichard, O.Y.; Herman, F.; Viskov, C. Heparin sodium compliance to the new proposed USP monograph: Elucidation of a minor structural modification responsible for a process dependent 2.10 ppm NMR signal. *J. Pharm. Biomed. Anal.* **2011**, *54*, 337–344. [CrossRef] [PubMed]

19. Panagos, C.; Thomson, D.; Bavington, C.D.; Uhrín, D. Structural characterisation of oligosaccharides obtained by Fenton-type radical depolymerisation of dermatan sulfate. *Carbohydr. Polym.* **2012**, *87*, 2086–2092. [CrossRef]

20. Griffin, C.C.; Linhardt, R.J.; Van Gorp, C.L.; Toida, T.; Hileman, R.E.; Schubert, R.L., II; Brown, S.E. Isolation and characterization of heparan sulfate from crude porcine intestinal mucosal peptidoglycan heparin. *Carbohydr. Res.* **1995**, *276*, 183–197. [CrossRef]

21. Huckerby, T.N.; Nieduszynski, I.A.; Giannopoulos, M.; Weeks, S.D.; Sadler, I.H.; Lauder, R.M. Characterization of oligosaccharides from the chondroitin/dermatan sulfates. ^{1}H-NMR and ^{13}C-NMR studies of reduced trisaccharides and hexasaccharides. *FEBS J.* **2005**, *272*, 6276–6286. [CrossRef] [PubMed]

22. Langeslay, D.J.; Urso, E.; Gardini, C.; Naggi, A.; Torri, G.; Larive, C.K. Reversed-phase ion-pair ultra-high-performance-liquid chromatography-mass spectrometry for fingerprinting low-molecular-weight heparins. *J. Chromatogr. A* **2013**, *1292*, 201–210. [CrossRef] [PubMed]

23. Alekseeva, A.; Casu, B.; Cassinelli, G.; Guerrini, M.; Torri, G.; Naggi, A. Structural features of glycol-split low-molecular-weight heparins and their heparin lyase generated fragments. *Anal. Bioanal. Chem.* **2014**, *406*, 249–265. [CrossRef] [PubMed]

24. Vismara, E.; Pierini, M.; Guglieri, S.; Liverani, L.; Mascellani, G.; Torri, G. Structural modification induced in heparin by a Fenton-type depolymerization process. *Semin. Thromb. Hemost.* **2007**, *33*, 466–477. [CrossRef] [PubMed]

25. Mascellani, G.; Liverani, L.; Prete, A.; Bergonzini, G.L.; Bianchini, P.; Silvestro, L.; Torri, G.; Bisio, A.; Guerrini, M.; Casu, B. Active Sites of Dermatan Sulfate for Heparin Cofactor II. Isolation of a Nonasaccharide Fragment Containing Four Disaccharide Sequences [α-L-Iduronic Acid 2-O-Sulfate (1, 3)-β-D-N-Acetylgalactosamine 4-Sulfate]. *J. Carbohydr. Chem.* **1995**, *14*, 1165–1177. [CrossRef]

26. Mucci, A.; Schenetti, L.; Volpi, N. [1]H and ^{13}C nuclear magnetic resonance identification and characterization of components of chondroitin sulfates of various origin. *Carbohydr. Polym.* **2000**, *41*, 37–45. [CrossRef]

27. Naggi, A.; Gardini, C.; Pedrinola, G.; Mauri, L.; Urso, E.; Alekseeva, A.; Casu, B.; Cassinelli, G.; Guerrini, M.; Iacomini, M.; et al. Structural peculiarity and antithrombin binding region profile of mucosal bovine and porcine heparins. *J. Pharm. Biomed. Anal.* **2016**, *118*, 52–63. [CrossRef] [PubMed]

28. Zhao, W.; Garron, M.L.; Yang, B.; Xiao, Z.; Esko, J.D.; Cygler, M.; Linhardt, R.J. Asparagine 405 of heparin lyase II prevents the cleavage of glycosidic linkages proximate to a 3-O-sulfoglucosamine residue. *FEBS Lett.* **2011**, *585*, 2461–2466. [CrossRef] [PubMed]

29. Gallagher, J.T.; Walker, A. Molecular distinctions between heparan sulphate and heparin. Analysis of sulphation patterns indicates that heparan sulphate and heparin are separate families of N-sulphated polysaccharides. *Biochem. J.* **1985**, *230*, 665–674. [CrossRef] [PubMed]

30. Toida, T.; Yoshida, H.; Toyoda, H.; Koshiishi, I.; Imanari, T.; Hileman, R.E.; Fromm, J.R.; Linhardt, R.J. Structural differences and the presence of unsubstituted amino groups in heparan sulphates from different tissues and species. *Biochem. J.* **1997**, *322*, 499–506. [CrossRef] [PubMed]

31. Vismara, E.; Pierini, M.; Mascellani, G.; Liverani, L.; Lima, M.; Guerrini, M.; Torri, G. Low-molecular-weight heparin from Cu^{2+} and Fe^{2+} Fenton type depolymerisation processes. *Thromb. Haemost.* **2010**, *103*, 613–622. [CrossRef] [PubMed]

32. Bisio, A.; De Ambrosi, L.; Gonella, S.; Guerrini, M.; Guglieri, S.; Maggia, G.; Torri, G. Preserving the original heparin structure of a novel low molecular weight heparin by γ-irradiation. *Arzneimittelforschung* **2001**, *51*, 806–813. [CrossRef] [PubMed]

33. U.S. Pharmacopeia–National Formulary (USP–NF). *Test for 1,6-anhydro Derivative for Enoxaparin Sodium*; U.S. Pharmacopeial Convention: Rockville, MD, USA, 2009; pp. 1–7.

Sample Availability: Samples of the compounds are not available.

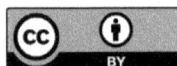

molecules

MDPI

Article

New Insights in Thrombin Inhibition Structure–Activity Relationships by Characterization of Octadecasaccharides from Low Molecular Weight Heparin[†]

Pierre A. J. Mourier, Olivier Y. Guichard, Fréderic Herman, Philippe Sizun and Christian Viskov *

Sanofi, 13 Quai Jules Guesde, 94403 Vitry sur Seine, France; pierre.mourier@sanofi.com (P.A.J.M.);
olivier.guichard@sanofi.com (O.Y.G.); frederic.herman@sanofi.com (F.H.); philippe.sizun@sanofi.com (P.S.)
* Correspondence: christian.viskov@sanofi.com; Tel.: +33-1-5893-8638
† *In Memoriam*: The authors would like to respectfully dedicate this article to Pr. B. Casu, a brilliant pioneer in glycosaminoglycan chemistry and analysis, who passed away on 11 November 2016.

Academic Editors: Giangiacomo Torri and Jawed Fareed
Received: 13 February 2017; Accepted: 3 March 2017; Published: 8 March 2017

Abstract: Low Molecular Weight Heparins (LMWH) are complex anticoagulant drugs that mainly inhibit the blood coagulation cascade through indirect interaction with antithrombin. While inhibition of the factor Xa is well described, little is known about the polysaccharide structure inhibiting thrombin. In fact, a minimal chain length of 18 saccharides units, including an antithrombin (AT) binding pentasaccharide, is mandatory to form the active ternary complex for LMWH obtained by alkaline β-elimination (e.g., enoxaparin). However, the relationship between structure of octadecasaccharides and their thrombin inhibition has not been yet assessed on natural compounds due to technical hurdles to isolate sufficiently pure material. We report the preparation of five octadecasaccharides by using orthogonal separation methods including size exclusion, AT affinity, ion pairing and strong anion exchange chromatography. Each of these octadecasaccharides possesses two AT binding pentasaccharide sequences located at various positions. After structural elucidation using enzymatic sequencing and NMR, in vitro aFXa and aFIIa were determined. The biological activities reveal the critical role of each pentasaccharide sequence position within the octadecasaccharides and structural requirements to inhibit thrombin. Significant differences in potency, such as the twenty-fold magnitude difference observed between two regioisomers, further highlights the importance of depolymerisation process conditions on LMWH biological activity.

Keywords: thrombin inhibition; LMWH; antithrombin; heparin oligosaccharides; ternary complex

1. Introduction

Low Molecular Weight Heparins (LMWH) are lifesaving anticoagulant drugs which have been used for several decades in the prevention and treatment of venous and arterial thromboembolism [1]. LMWH are industrially derived from the starting material heparin, a complex mixture of mammalian polysaccharides extracted from porcine mucosa. The centenary of the discovery of heparin has been widely celebrated around the world and many symposia, such as the 24th Glycosaminoglycans Symposium, held in September 2016 (Villa Vigoni, Loveno di Menaggio—Italy, the first symposia of these series was initiated by Pr Casu), were dedicated to this endeavor. Even with state of the art analytical methods, this "ever young life-saving drug" [2] is also one of the most complex products to analyze, as direct characterization of the polysaccharidic chains is still not feasible. Heparin is a mixture of heteropolymeric chains having a mean molecular weight around 15,000 Dalton. It consists of alternating units of 2-deoxy-2-sulfamido-α-D-glucopyranose (possibly *O*-sulfated,

N-sulfated or *N*-acetylated) and *O*-sulfated uronic acids (α-L-iduronic acid or β-D-glucuronic acid). The specific structure of each polysaccharidic chain, built up of these alternating motifs, is governed by enzymatic machinery of the host mast cells where it is stored [3]. Heparin interacts with about one hundred proteins [4] but its anticoagulant activity is mainly mediated indirectly through activation of antithrombin, a serine protease inhibitor, member of the serpin family [5]. The activation of antithrombin induces a protein conformational change and dramatically accelerates the inhibition of the Stuart factor (FXa) [6]. The discovery of the antithrombin (AT) binding pentasaccharide was the hallmark of a new era of understanding of the structure activity of this complex medicine [7,8], and the so-called AGA*IA sequence (GlcN$_{NAc/NS,6S}$-GlcA-GlcN$_{NS,3S,6S}$-IdoUA$_{2S}$GlcN$_{NS,6S}$) was identified as the specific binding sequence of heparin [7]. Then, several variants of the consensus pentasaccharide sequence were discovered and reported a posteriori [9–11]. The evolution of analytical methodologies has also permitted the identification of longer AT binding oligosaccharides from LMWH [12]. Structure-activity studies on octa to octadecasaccharides have demonstrated that interaction with antithrombin is more complex than initially envisioned and that flanking saccharide units play an important role in the modulation of the AGA*IA affinity (the synthetic version of AGA*IA, drug substance commercially known as fondaparinux was used as reference) [13]. They may affect the Kd variation by three orders of magnitude when compared to fondaparinux (Kd = 21 nM) [14], either strengthening or destabilizing this complex.

Furthermore, semuloparin an experimental drug for which development was stopped in 2012 was designed with a depolymerisation process which preserves the AT binding region from β-eliminative cleavage and increases their concentration in this particular LMWH [15]. Therefore, it allowed the isolation of unexpected multiple of two and three consecutive AGA*IA sequences in the dodecasaccharide ΔIIa-II$\underline{s}$-I$\underline{s}$-IIa-II$\underline{s}$-I$\underline{s}$ [16] and the octadecasaccharide **1** ΔIIa-II$\underline{s}$-I$\underline{s}$-IIa-II$\underline{s}$-I$\underline{s}$-IIa-II$\underline{s}$-I$\underline{s}$ [17], respectively (structural symbols are listed in Table 1; previous studies had concluded the possible presence of two AT binding sites on a single heparin chain without isolation and structural elucidation [18]). This compositional specificity is directly due to the depolymerisation selectivity with the sterically hindered phosphazene bases. Therefore, semuloparin appears as a particularly interesting tool compound to gather new insights on structure-activity relationships.

Table 1. Structural symbols.

Structural Symbols		
ΔIVa = ΔU-GlcNAc	-IVa$_{id}$- = -IdoA-GlcNAc-	-IVa$_{glu}$- = -GlcA-GlcNAc-
ΔIVs = ΔU-GlcNS		-IVs$_{glu}$- = -GlcA-GlcNS-
Δ$\underline{IVs}$ = ΔU-GlcNS,3S		-IVs$_{glu}$- = -GlcA-GlcNS,3S-
ΔIIa = ΔU-GlcNAc,6S	-IIa$_{id}$- = -IdoA-GlcNAc,6S-	
ΔIIIa = ΔU2S-GlcNAc	-IIIa$_{id}$- = -IdoA2S-GlcNAc-	
ΔIIs = ΔU-GlcNS,6S		-IIs$_{glu}$- = -GlcA-GlcNS,6S-
Δ$\underline{IIs}$ = ΔU-GlcNS,3S,6S		-IIs$_{glu}$-= -GcA-GlcNS,3S,6S-
ΔIIIs = ΔU2S-GlcNS	-IIIs$_{id}$- = -IdoA2S-GlcNS-	
ΔIa = ΔU2S-GlcNAc,6S	-Ia$_{id}$- = -IdoA2S-GlcNAc,6S-	
ΔIs = ΔU2S-GlcNS,6S	-Is$_{id}$- = -IdoA2S-GlcNS,6S-	
Δ$\underline{Is}$ = ΔU2S-GlcNS,3S,6S	-I$\underline{s}_{id}$- = -IdoA2S-GlcNS,3S,6S-	

It is noteworthy that we have previously observed that Kd affinity and molar anti FXa activity of the dodecasaccharide was twice that of fondaparinux, suggesting a dynamic equilibrium with two antithrombin proteins, which may potentiate the anticoagulant activity of such compound series.

Although thrombin is one of the key coagulation proteases for heparin and LMWHs, structure-activity data are not available due to the challenge of isolating polysaccharides that are able to form the ternary complex with antithrombin and thrombin. In fact, until the isolation of octadecasaccharide **1** (Figure 1) [17], there was no structural data on pure natural compounds that were responsible for this important mechanism of action. Interestingly, the only structure-activity relationship evidence that existed were generated on synthetic compounds [19–21] and showed that the inhibition may be potent starting from hexadecasaccharides.

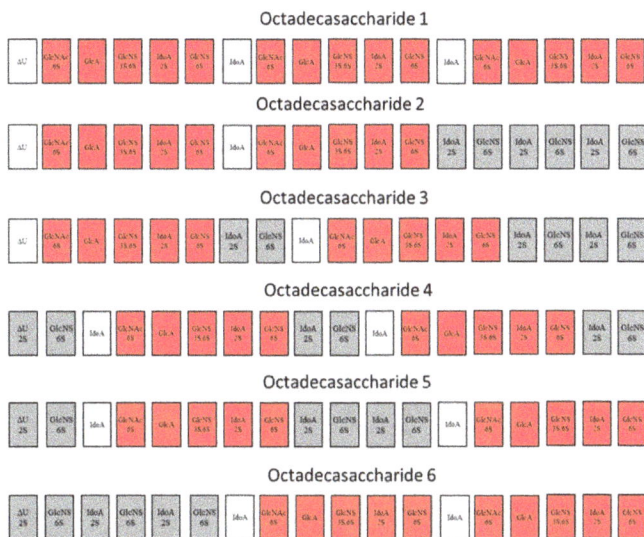

Figure 1. Studied octadecasaccharides (in red saccharide units from AGA*IA sequence). In grey, flanking saccharide units are represented. In white, additional uronic acid present in the minimal natural sequence.

With the octadecasaccharide **1**, a suitable chain length was reached so that the inhibition of the thrombin (FIIa) became possible in the case of LMWH products (no significant activity assayed on hexadecasaccharides), and activities of aFXa = 562 IU/mg and aFIIa = 8.8 IU/mg were found. Nevertheless, with respect to the whole fraction from which it was isolated (aFIIa ~20 UI/mg), the aFIIa for 1 was significantly lower than expected.

It was therefore critical to further evaluate new octadecasaccharides to increase our understanding of the electrostatic interactions with thrombin and compare them to the synthetic compounds from Petitou et al. [19–21].

For this endeavor, by using orthogonal chromatographic techniques, we have isolated five compounds from the octadecasaccharide AT affine fraction of semuloparin. Each of these compounds contain two AGA*IA sequences located at different positions within the polysaccharide chain (Figure 1). Their structure has been fully elucidated by enzymatic sequencing and NMR analysis and their anticoagulant activity was evaluated both for inhibition of factor Xa and IIa.

2. Results and Discussion

In our previous work [17], we reported the isolation from semuloparin of the first natural octadecasaccharide having AT binding affinity and able to inhibit both aFXa and aFIIa. This compound had the peculiarity to bear three consecutive AGA*IA sequences. Surprisingly, the activation of thrombin was weak (only 8.8 IU/mg; USP Heparin is about 180 IU/mg) despite the fact that it was isolated from an octadecasaccharide fraction with a specific aFIIa activity of ~20 UI/mg. All the criteria for activity were there, i.e., size of the chain, presence of AGA*IA sequences, and high anti FXa (about three times more than USP heparin) activity, but the low thrombin inhibition raised new questions. Front running hypotheses to explain low thrombin inhibition included: a lack of charge density to stabilize the ternary complex with the protein, or a dynamic equilibrium between antithrombin with all three AGA*IA sequences, which might generate in turn a steric hindrance for thrombin complexation. The later hypothesis could also explain the twofold molar aFXa activity of the compound with respect to the pentasaccharide [17]. To shed light on the origin of such biological properties, it was critical to study more compounds of these series and put in perspective the work performed on synthetic polysaccharides with dual anti FXa and thrombin inhibition potency [19,21].

2.1. Purification of Octadecasaccharide Fraction F3

The octadecasaccharide fraction was separated on an AT affinity chromatography column and five fractions F1 to F5 with increasing affinity were isolated [17]. Focus was concentrated on fraction F3, where isomers containing two AGA*IA sequences could be identified (Figure 2).

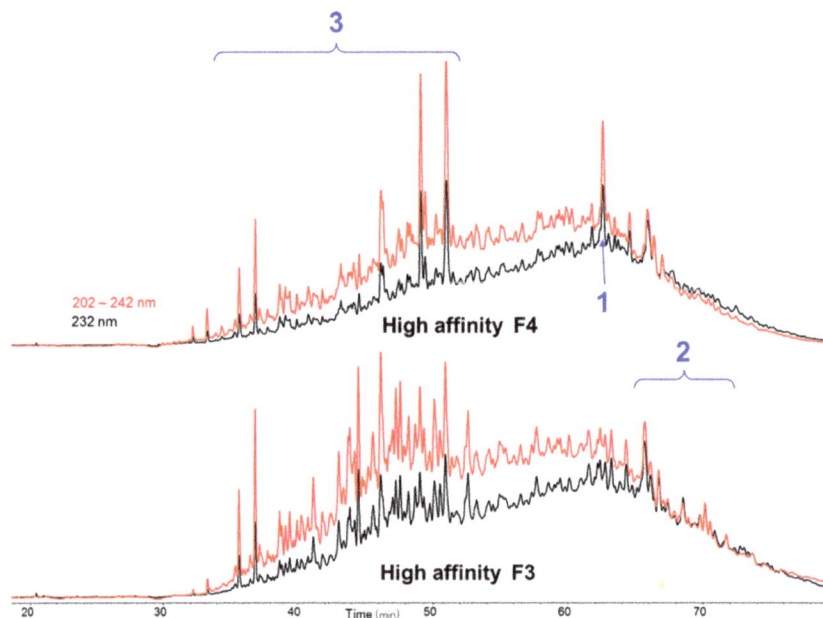

Figure 2. Cetyltrimethylammonium strong anion exchange (CTA-SAX) chromatograms of octadecasaccharide fractions F3 and F4: 1-triple site, 2-double sites, 3-glycoserine octadecasaccharides.

The overall activity was in the same order of magnitude than fraction 4 from which octadecasaccharide **1** was isolated (aFXa: F3 401 IU/mg; F4 422 IU/mg; aFIIa: F3 18.1 IU/mg; F4 19.8 IU/mg). The modest aFIIa activity may be partly related to the presence of glycoserine oligosaccharides. These oligosaccharides contain an oxidized glycoserine sequence (-GlcA-Gal-Gal-Xyl-CH$_2$-COOH) at their reducing end [22]. These compounds are eluted in the less retained part of the chromatogram (Figure 2) and represent more than 50% of the affine fractions. None of the glycoserine octadecasaccharides isolated in this study (not described here) had any measurable aFIIa activity while having aFXa. Compared to the separation of the octadecasaccharide **1**, the isolation of five regioisomers containing two AGA*IA sequences was more complex and the resolution power of ion pair chromatography was critical to enable the separation. From the key step of cetyltrimethylammonium strong anion exchange (CTA-SAX) separation (Figure 3), reconstructed ion mass LC/MS chromatograms corresponding to Mw 4957 Da (Figure 4) were used to select the fractions to be gathered. Molecular weights deduced from LC/MS analysis were sufficient to deduce the sulfate group number, *N*-acetyl number and presence or not of characteristic glycoserine moieties. These pieces of information were helpful to guide us in the last purification steps.

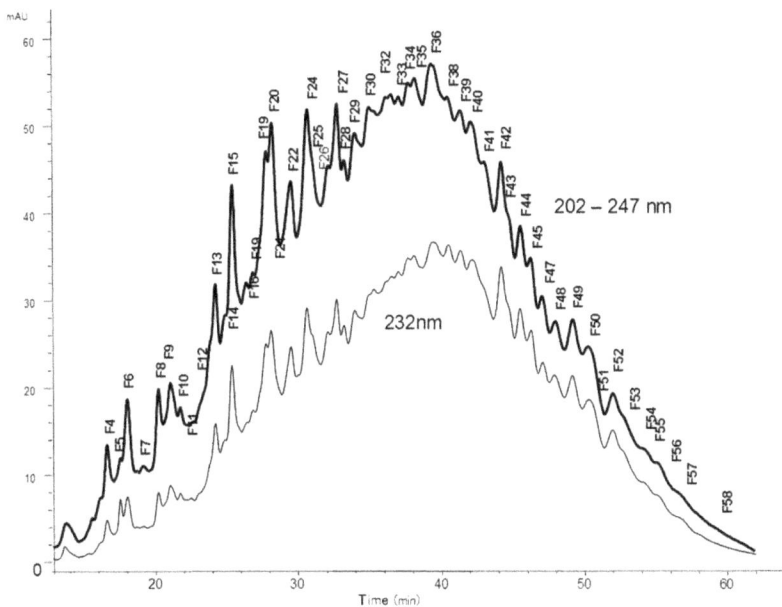

Figure 3. Preparative CTA-SAX chromatography of fraction F3.

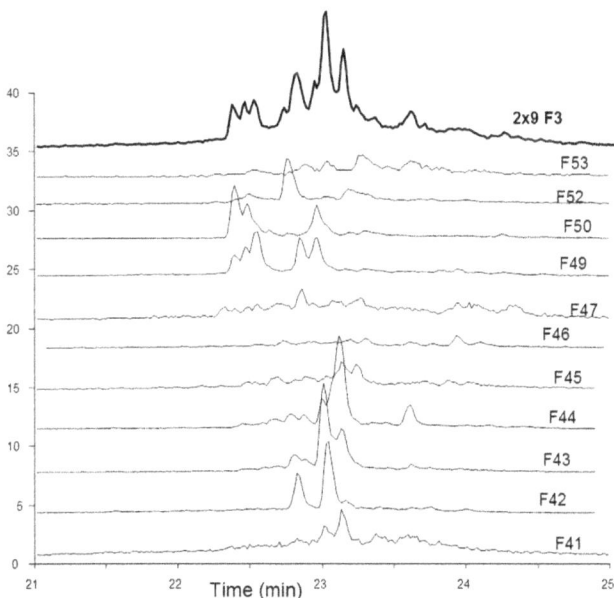

Figure 4. LC/MS reconstructed ion mass chromatograms of initial fraction F3 and sub fractions of interest corresponding to MW 4957 Da (m/z 2430.2: $(4957 + 23 \times \text{HXA} + 2\text{H})^{3+}$).

2.2. Enzymatic Sequencing

Sequencing methods based on partial or selective depolymerisation with enzymes from *Flavobacterium heparinum* and particularly heparinases have been already developed [23,24]. Monitoring of digestion and fragment analysis were done by MALDI-MS and capillary electrophoresis. Another efficient technique using a preliminary radiolabeling of the substrate, followed by partial nitrous depolymerisation and sequencing with exoenzymes has been proposed [25]. However, this method is long and most exoenzymes used in the study are not commercially available. In fact, the key element for any sequencing method is an efficient separation. This part is usually time consuming and, as already stated, requires use of many consecutive chromatographic methods with orthogonal specificities.

For long heparin-like oligosaccharides, heparinase I is the most convenient choice for sequencing experiments. Heparinase II is less selective than heparinase I and, as an exolithic enzyme, it does not generate many long fragments in detectable amounts. The full exploitation of the digestion process by heparinase I requires a good understanding of the enzyme's selectivity and behavior. Basic rules for selectivity [26] are necessary but are not sufficient to this endeavor. Know-how in that field is all the more important as current literature data may give only partially the heparinase I mechanism of digestion [27]. As a matter of fact, much evidence exists that heparinase I is not exolithic but rather endolithic [28] (also reflected in our sequencing experiments), all cleavable sites present in the chain being cleaved simultaneously. The structural determination by enzymatic sequencing of long oligosaccharides is usually a challenging experiment due to the number of saccharides bound together and to their potential arrangement. The fact that there are two AT binding sites $-\text{IIa}_{id}\text{-IIs}_{glu}\text{-Is}_{id}-$ distributed with three $-\text{Is}_{id}-$ disaccharides in an octadecasaccharide simplifies its structural elucidation. Consequently, only 10 theoretical arrangements can be found (Table 2). In addition, the UV spectrum can be used [17] to determine the beginning of the chain (either $\Delta\text{IIa-IIs}_{glu}\text{-Is}_{id}-$ or $\Delta\text{Is-}$), allowing the separation into two types of octadecasaccharides.

Table 2. Heparinase 1 cleaving sites ($\downarrow$ major sites; $\downarrow$ minor sites).

	Structure	Heparinase I Cleaving Sites
Octadeca. 2	$\Delta\text{IIa-IIs}_{glu}\text{-Is}_{id}\text{-IIa}_{id}\text{-IIs}_{glu}\text{-Is}_{id}\text{-Is}_{id}\text{-Is}_{id}\text{-Is}_{id}$	$\Delta\text{IIa-IIs}_{glu}{\downarrow}\text{Is}_{id}\text{-IIa}_{id}\text{-IIs}_{glu}{\downarrow}\text{Is}_{id}{\downarrow}\text{Is}_{id}{\downarrow}\text{Is}_{id}\text{-Is}_{id}{}^{red}$
Octadeca. 3	$\Delta\text{IIa-IIs}_{glu}\text{-Is}_{id}\text{-Is}_{id}\text{-IIa}_{id}\text{-IIs}_{glu}\text{-Is}_{id}\text{-Is}_{id}\text{-Is}_{id}$	$\Delta\text{IIa-IIs}_{glu}{\downarrow}\text{Is}_{id}{\downarrow}\text{Is}_{id}{\downarrow}\text{Is}_{id}\text{-IIa}_{id}\text{-IIs}_{glu}{\downarrow}\text{Is}_{id}\text{-Is}_{id}{}^{red}$
	$\Delta\text{IIa-IIs}_{glu}\text{-Is}_{id}\text{-Is}_{id}\text{-Is}_{id}\text{-IIa}_{id}\text{-IIs}_{glu}\text{-Is}_{id}\text{-Is}_{id}$	$\Delta\text{IIa-IIs}_{glu}{\downarrow}\text{Is}_{id}{\downarrow}\text{Is}_{id}{\downarrow}\text{Is}_{id}\text{-IIa}_{id}\text{-IIs}_{glu}{\downarrow}\text{Is}_{id}\text{-Is}_{id}{}^{red}$
	$\Delta\text{IIa-IIs}_{glu}\text{-Is}_{id}\text{-Is}_{id}\text{-Is}_{id}\text{-IIa}_{id}\text{-IIs}_{glu}\text{-Is}_{id}$	$\Delta\text{IIa-IIs}_{glu}{\downarrow}\text{Is}_{id}{\downarrow}\text{Is}_{id}{\downarrow}\text{Is}_{id}\text{-IIa}_{id}\text{-IIs}_{glu}{\downarrow}\text{Is}_{id}\text{-Is}_{id}{}^{red}$
	$\Delta\text{Is-IIa}_{id}\text{-IIs}_{glu}\text{-Is}_{id}\text{-IIa}_{id}\text{-IIs}_{glu}\text{-Is}_{id}\text{-Is}_{id}\text{-Is}_{id}$	$\Delta\text{IIs-IIa}_{id}\text{-IIs}_{glu}{\downarrow}\text{Is}_{id}\text{-IIa}_{id}\text{-IIs}_{glu}{\downarrow}\text{Is}_{id}{\downarrow}\text{Is}_{id}\text{-Is}_{id}{}^{red}$
Octadeca. 4	$\Delta\text{Is-IIa}_{id}\text{-IIs}_{glu}\text{-Is}_{id}\text{-Is}_{id}\text{-IIa}_{id}\text{-IIs}_{glu}\text{-Is}_{id}\text{-Is}_{id}$	$\Delta\text{IIs-IIa}_{id}\text{-IIs}_{glu}{\downarrow}\text{Is}_{id}{\downarrow}\text{Is}_{id}\text{-IIa}_{id}\text{-IIs}_{glu}{\downarrow}\text{Is}_{id}\text{-Is}_{id}{}^{red}$
Octadeca. 5	$\Delta\text{Is-IIa}_{id}\text{-IIs}_{glu}\text{-Is}_{id}\text{-Is}_{id}\text{-Is}_{id}\text{-IIa}_{id}\text{-IIs}_{glu}\text{-Is}_{id}$	$\Delta\text{IIs-IIa}_{id}\text{-IIs}_{glu}{\downarrow}\text{Is}_{id}{\downarrow}\text{Is}_{id}\text{-IIa}_{id}\text{-IIs}_{glu}{\downarrow}\text{Is}_{id}\text{-Is}_{id}{}^{red}$
	$\Delta\text{Is-Is}_{id}\text{-IIa}_{id}\text{-IIs}_{glu}\text{-Is}_{id}\text{-IIa}_{id}\text{-IIs}_{glu}\text{-Is}_{id}\text{-Is}_{id}$	$\Delta\text{IIs}{\downarrow}\text{Is}_{id}\text{-IIa}_{id}\text{-IIs}_{glu}{\downarrow}\text{Is}_{id}\text{-IIa}_{id}\text{-IIs}_{glu}{\downarrow}\text{Is}_{id}\text{-Is}_{id}{}^{red}$
	$\Delta\text{Is-Is}_{id}\text{-IIa}_{id}\text{-IIs}_{glu}\text{-Is}_{id}\text{-Is}_{id}\text{-IIa}_{id}\text{-IIs}_{glu}\text{-Is}_{id}$	$\Delta\text{IIs}{\downarrow}\text{Is}_{id}\text{-IIa}_{id}\text{-IIs}_{glu}{\downarrow}\text{Is}_{id}{\downarrow}\text{Is}_{id}\text{-IIa}_{id}\text{-IIs}_{glu}\text{-Is}_{id}{}^{red}$
Octadeca. 6	$\Delta\text{Is-Is}_{id}\text{-Is}_{id}\text{-IIa}_{id}\text{-IIs}_{glu}\text{-Is}_{id}\text{-IIa}_{id}\text{-IIs}_{glu}\text{-Is}_{id}$	$\Delta\text{IIs}{\downarrow}\text{Is}_{id}{\downarrow}\text{Is}_{id}\text{-IIa}_{id}\text{-IIs}_{glu}{\downarrow}\text{Is}_{id}\text{-IIa}_{id}\text{-IIs}_{glu}\text{-Is}_{id}{}^{red}$

2.2.1. Type I Octadecasaccharides

In this case of Type I octadecasaccharides, the position of the first binding site is known and the remaining question is the position of the second one. Key elements for such sequencing were described [17] for structural determination of triple site $\Delta\text{IIa-IIs}_{glu}\text{-Is}_{id}\text{-IIa}_{id}\text{-IIs}_{glu}\text{-Is}_{id}\text{-IIa}_{id}\text{-IIs}_{glu}\text{-Is}_{id}$. NaBH$_4$ preliminary reduction was used to label the reducing end.

Putative structures are listed in Table 2 as well as the heparinase I cleavage sites of the four possible isomers. Heparinase I cleaves preferentially highly sulfated moieties like $\text{-IIs}_{glu}{\downarrow}\text{Is}_{id}$ and $\text{Is}_{id}{\downarrow}\text{Is}_{id}\text{-Is}_{id}{}^{red}$ and its action on other cleavable sites like $\text{Is}_{id}{\downarrow}\text{Is}_{id}{}^{red}$ is less pronounced.

Table 3 gathers key fragments for type I octadecasaccharides. The resistance of these fragments to the action of heparinase I mainly depends on the number of cleaving sites, so that the order of increasing resistance is the following: $\Delta\text{IIa-IIs}_{glu}\text{-Is}_{id}\text{-Is}_{id}\text{-Is}_{id}\text{-IIa}_{id}\text{-IIs}_{glu}$ <

$\Delta IIa\text{-}IIs_{glu}\text{-}Is_{id}\text{-}Is_{id}\text{-}IIa_{id}\text{-}IIs_{glu} < \Delta IIa\text{-}IIs_{glu}\text{-}Is_{id}\text{-}IIa_{id}\text{-}IIs_{glu} << \Delta Is\text{-}IIa_{id}\text{-}IIs_{glu}\text{-}Is_{id}^{red}$. The sequencing details for octadecasaccharide **2** and **3** are reported in supplementary data.

Table 3. Key fragments for octadecasaccharides.

	Key Fragments for Type I Octadecasaccharides
Octadecasaccharide 2	$\Delta IIa\text{-}IIs_{glu}\text{-}Is_{id}\text{-}IIa_{id}\text{-}IIs_{glu}$; $\Delta Is\text{-}Is_{id}^{red}$
Octadecasaccharide 3	$\Delta IIa\text{-}IIs_{glu}\text{-}Is_{id}\text{-}Is_{id}\text{-}IIa_{id}\text{-}IIs_{glu}$; $\Delta Is\text{-}Is_{id}^{red}$
	Key Fragments for Type II Octadecasaccharides
Octadecasaccharide 4	$\Delta IIs\text{-}IIa_{id}\text{-}IIs_{glu}$; $\Delta IIs\text{-}IIa_{id}\text{-}IIs_{glu}\text{-}Is_{id}\text{-}Is_{id}\text{-}IIa_{id}\text{-}IIs_{glu}$; $\Delta Is\text{-}Is_{id}^{red}$
Octadecasaccharide 5	$\Delta IIs\text{-}IIa_{id}\text{-}IIs_{glu}$; $\Delta Is\text{-}IIa_{id}\text{-}IIs_{glu}\text{-}Is_{id}^{red}$
Octadecasaccharide 6	ΔIIs; $\Delta IIs\text{-}Is_{id}$; $\Delta IIs\text{-}Is_{id}\text{-}Is_{id}\text{-}IIa_{id}\text{-}IIs_{glu}$; $\Delta Is\text{-}IIa_{id}\text{-}IIs_{glu}\text{-}Is_{id}^{red}$

2.2.2. Type II Octadecasaccharides

The sequencing of type II octadecasaccharides is more challenging than that of type I. In this case, the position of the two binding sites has to be determined. Preliminary 2-O desulfatation of unsaturated acid by $\Delta^{4,5}$-glucuronate-2-sulfatase is crucial to differentiate the first AT binding site from the second one. This reaction is achieved before $NaBH_4$ reduction and heparinase I addition. It appears that the activity of the sulfatase is highly dependent on the structure and more especially on the number of disaccharide Is at the non-reducing end. Octadecasaccharides **4** and **5** are entirely transformed after one addition of sulfatase. For compound **6**, the desulfatation is very slow, and the quantity of sulfatase necessary to the transformation exceeds all other cases. The activity of O-sulfatase is found to be dependent on the substrate structure. The following order is observed: $\Delta Is\text{-}IIa_{id}\text{-}IIs_{glu}\text{-} > \Delta Is\text{-}Is_{id}\text{-}IIa_{id}\text{-}IIs_{glu}\text{-} > \Delta Is\text{-}Is_{id}\text{-}Is_{id}\text{-}IIa_{id}\text{-}IIs_{glu}\text{-}$. This enzyme has already been cloned and its selectivity studied [29,30] but the selectivity observed above was not heretofore mentioned. Table 3 gathers key fragments generated subsequently after heparinase I treatment for type II octadecasaccharides. Full details of sequencing experiments of octadecasaccharides **4**, **5** and **6** are described in the Supplementary Data.

2.3. NMR

The ^{1}H-NMR spectrum of the octasaccharide **6** is shown in Figure 5. Proton and carbon resonances of each residue were assigned using COSY (correlation spectroscopy), TOCSY (total correlation spectroscopy) and HSQC (heteronuclear single quantum coherence spectroscopy) pulse sequences (Table 4) (octadecasaccharides **2**, **3**, **4** and **5** structural assignments are reported in the Supplementary Data).

A total of 18 proton signals were observed in the anomeric region between 5.55 and 4.55 ppm, indicating that the polysaccharide is an octadecasaccharide, with only 13 different chemical shifts. As a consequence, the proton spectrum did not appear as complex as might be expected for an octadecasaccharide. This feature indicated the presence of two repeating units in the sequence of the octadecasaccharide, with many resonance superimpositions. Chemical shift analysis was compatible with a composition including nine α-D-glucosamines, six α-L-iduronic acids, two β-D-glucuronic acids (anomeric proton resonance observed between 5.53 and 5,34 ppm, 5.22 and 5.01 ppm and at 4.60 ppm, respectively), and one 4,5-unsaturated uronic acid. Two central acetyl signals are visible at 2.05 ppm. The C_i-H1 to $C_{(i+1)}$-H4 connectivity, observed in the nuclear Overhauser spectroscopy (NOESY) experiment, were used for monosaccharides sequence determination (Figure 6). The well-resolved resonance of H4-ΔU uronic acid was used as the assignment starting point. The presence of N-sulfate or N-acetyl on α-D-glucosamine residues, and the presence or absence of O-sulfate groups, was deduced from ^{1}H and ^{13}C chemical shifts.

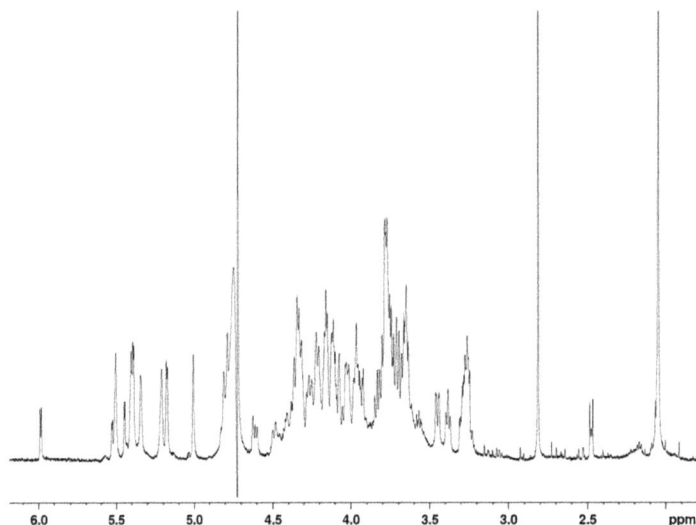

Figure 5. ^{1}H-NMR spectrum of octadecasaccharide **6** (D$_2$O, 30 °C, 600 MHz).

Table 4. Proton and carbon chemical shifts of the two pentasaccharide sequences identified inside octadecasaccharide **6**.

	ΔIs		Is$_{id}$		Is$_{id}$	
	ΔU$_{2S}$	A$_{NS,6S}$	I$_{2S}$	A$_{NS,6S}$	I$_{2S}$	A$_{NS,6S}$
1	5.51/98.4	5.40/98.1	5.21/100.4	5.41/97.8	5.22/100.4	5.34/96.6
2	4.62/75.7	3.30/58.9	4.34/76.9	3.27/59.0	4.35/76.9	3.26/59.0
3	4.31/64.0	3.65/70.8	4.22/70.2	3.66/70.8	4.20/70.4	3.65/70.8
4	5.98/107.1	3.84/79.3	4.10/77.5	3.76/77.1	4.11/77.1	3.78/77.2
5		4.03/70.0	4.81/70.5	4.02/70.3	4.81/70.5	3.96/70.4
6,6′		4.36/4.26		4.40/4.27		4.41/4.26
		67.4		67.5		67.5
CH$_3$						

	Pentasaccharide 1					
	IIa$_{id}$		IIs$_{glu}$		Is$_{id}$	
	I	A$_{Nac,6S}$	G	A$_{NS,3S,6S}$	I$_{2S}$	A$_{NS,6S}$
1	5.01/103.1	5.39/98.1	4.60/102.2	5.51/97.2	5.18/100.6	5.34/96.6
2	3.78/69.8	3.93/55.0	3.38/74.6	3.45/57.8	4.32/78.1	3.26/59.0
3	4.12/68.9	3.77/70.7	3.70/77.5	4.37/77.4	4.17/71.6	3.66/70.8
4	4.08/75.8	3.73/78.5	3.80/77.8	3.97/74.1	4.14/77.1	3.79/77.7
5	4.79/69.8	4.02/70.4	3.76/78.3	4.16/70.7	4.79/71.2	3.96/70.4
6,6′		4.34/4.21		4.49/4.26		4.46/4.23
		67.4		67.1		67.4
CH$_3$		2.05/23.2				

	Pentasaccharide 2					
	IIa$_{id}$		IIs$_{glu}$		Is$_{id}$	
	I	A$_{Nac,6S}$	G	A$_{NS,3S,6S}$	I$_{2S}$	A$_{NS,6S}$
1	5.01/103.1	5.39/98.1	4.60/102.2	5.53/97.1	5.18/100.6	4.45/92.2
2	3.78/69.8	3.93/55.0	3.39/74.6	3.45/57.8	4.31/78.1	3.27/59.0
3	4.12/68.9	3.77/70.7	3.70/77.5	4.36/77.4	4.17/71.6	3.70/70.6
4	4.08/75.8	3.73/78.5	3.80/77.8	3.97/74.1	4.16/77.2	3.78/77.6
5	4.79/69.8	4.02/70.4	3.76/78.3	4.17/70.7	4.74/71.5	4.13/69.7
6,6′		4.34/4.21		4.49/4.26		4.43/4.30
		67.4		67.1		68.0
CH$_3$		2.05/23.2				

Note: Listed as H/C in ppm.

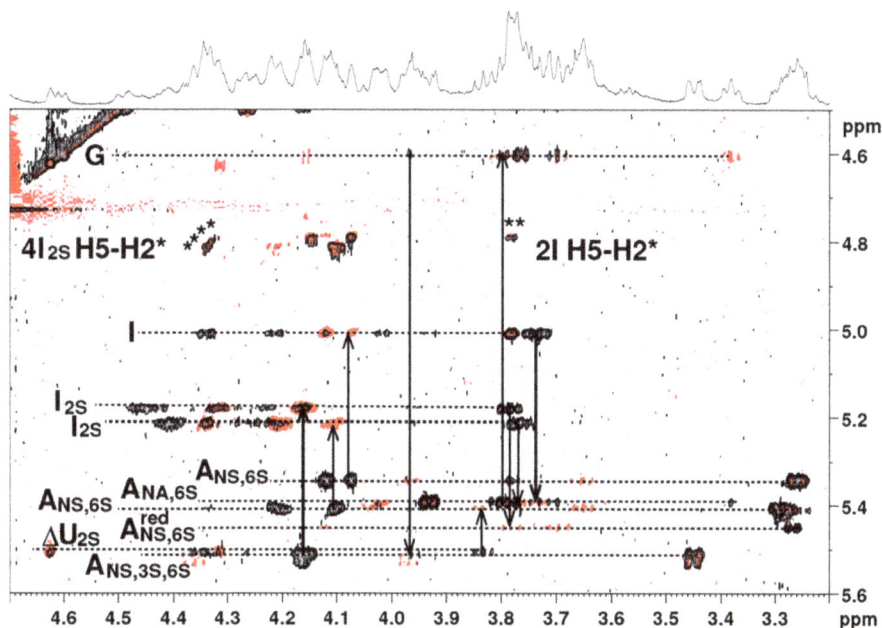

Figure 6. Superimposition of 2D nuclear Overhauser spectroscopy (NOESY) (black) and total correlation spectroscopy (TOCSY) (red) spectra for octadecasaccharide **6**: Correlations of anomeric protons. The dark lines show at start C_i-H1 to $C_{(i+1)}$-H4 connectivities on the NOESY experiment and at the arrows the C_i-H1 to C_i-H4 connectivities on the TOCSY experiment. The H5-H2 characteristic connectivity of $^2S_0$ conformation of each Iduronic acids is indicated by (*) on the NOESY experiment.

In spite of the ^{1}H signal broadness and many resonance superimpositions, it was possible to determine the main coupling constant for vicinal protons of pyranose rings in the well resolved COSY experiment. For glucosamines and glucuronic acids all $^3J_{H1-H2}$ coupling constants were superior to 8 Hz, except for the $^3J_{H1-H2}$ of glucosamines between 3and 4 Hz. Consequently, the conformational status of glucosamines and glucuronic acids was in the pure $^4C_1$ conformation. All iduronic acids signals showed small coupling constant for vicinal protons, except for the $^3J_{H2-H3}$ around 7 to 8 Hz. Besides weak-medium intensities were observed for the H5-H2 connectivities in the NOESY experiment (Figure 6). This information taken together suggested a $^1C_4 \leftrightarrow ^2S0$ equilibrium for all iduronic acids [31].

The full proton and carbon chemical shift assignments, along with all sets of inter-residue correlations observed on the 2D NOESY spectrum, fully supported the structural determination of octadecasaccharide **6** with two pentasaccharide sequences as demonstrated by the enzymatic sequencing methodology. The two AGA*IA sequences are respectively located in the middle and at the reducing end of the octadecasaccharide. The NMR assignment tables for the octadecasaccharides **2**, **3**, **4** and **5** are reported in the Supplementary Data.

2.4. aFXa and aFIIa Activities

In their previous work [19,21], Petitou et al. introduced the concepts of A domain (AT binding domain AGA*IA) and thrombin binding domain (T domain) for their synthetic heparin mimetics. At that time, pure natural structures were not available and therefore, hypotheses had to be made to figure out the AGA*IA flanking oligosaccharides, which might constitute the T domain. Their structure-activity studies showed that the T domain should be highly sulfated in order to interact with the positively charged domain of thrombin [19]. Because heparin has some highly sulfated regular regions with repetitive units of trisulfated Is disaccharides, it was therefore presumed that the T domain was an oligomer of this structural motif (Figure 7).

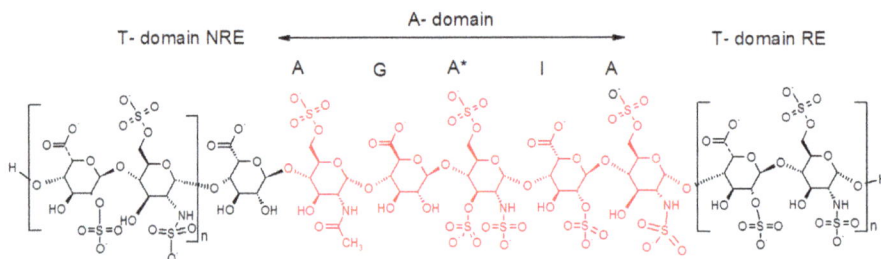

Figure 7. Model described for heparin oligosaccharides with Is disaccharide T domain extensions at reducing end (RE) and non-reducing end (NRE).

As Petitou et al. prepared modified simplified structures of both the A and T domain to generate biological data, the results are not directly comparable with those of the natural octadecasaccharide series but at least they provide us some directions. Briefly, in these synthetic oligosaccharides, *N*-sulfate groups were replaced by *O*-sulfate groups, hydroxyls were methylated in the A domain, and the T domain was built up with repeating units of 2,6-di-*O*-sulfonato β-D-glucose. The thrombin assays were performed with regioisomers of comparable chain length. When the T domain is at the reducing end, it was established that the thrombin inhibition is about 30 times less potent than when it is located at the non-reducing end (IC_{50} = 164 vs. 5 ng/mL, comparison made respectively with an octadecasaccharide and a heptadecasaccharide).

While heparin does contain sequences such as described in Figure 7, the overall picture of polysaccharide structures able to inhibit thrombin is more diverse, and the richness of activity of this collection of biosynthetic macromolecules is certainly not uniquely explained by such structures. As a matter of fact, the chromatographic complexity of the octadecasaccharide fractions speak to the diversity (Figure 2), just as well as the unexpected series of double AT binding octadecasaccharides regioisomers studied herein (Figure 1). For these, the aFXa and aFIIa were assayed by chromogenic assay and are reported in the Table 5.

Table 5. aFXa and aFIIa activities of isolated octadecasaccharides.

	Structure	aFXa Activity (IU/mg)	aFXa Activity (IU/μmol)	aFIIa Activity (IU/mg)
Octadecasaccharide 1	$\Delta IIa\text{-}IIs_{glu}\text{-}Is_{id}\text{-}IIa_{id}\text{-}IIs_{glu}\text{-}Is_{id}\text{-}IIa_{id}\text{-}IIs_{glu}\text{-}Is_{id}$	562	3090	8.8
Octadecasaccharide 2	$\Delta IIa\text{-}\overline{IIs_{glu}}\text{-}Is_{id}\text{-}IIa_{id}\text{-}\overline{IIs_{glu}}\text{-}Is_{id}\text{-}Is_{id}\text{-}\overline{Is_{id}}\text{-}Is_{id}$	371	2100	5.9
Octadecasaccharide 3	$\Delta IIa\text{-}\overline{IIs_{glu}}\text{-}Is_{id}\text{-}Is_{id}\text{-}IIa_{id}\text{-}\overline{IIs_{glu}}\text{-}Is_{id}\text{-}Is_{id}\text{-}Is_{id}$	442	2502	9
Octadecasaccharide 4	$\Delta Is\text{-}IIa_{id}\text{-}\overline{IIs_{glu}}\text{-}Is_{id}\text{-}Is_{id}\text{-}IIa_{id}\text{-}\overline{IIs_{glu}}\text{-}Is_{id}\text{-}Is_{id}$	540	3057	22.6
Octadecasaccharide 5	$\Delta Is\text{-}IIa_{id}\text{-}\overline{IIs_{glu}}\text{-}Is_{id}\text{-}Is_{id}\text{-}Is_{id}\text{-}IIa_{id}\text{-}\overline{IIs_{glu}}\text{-}Is_{id}$	517	2927	81.5
Octadecasaccharide 6	$\Delta Is\text{-}Is_{id}\text{-}\overline{Is_{id}}\text{-}IIa_{id}\text{-}\overline{IIs_{glu}}\text{-}Is_{id}\text{-}IIa_{id}\text{-}\overline{IIs_{glu}}\text{-}Is_{id}$	705	3991	119.3

Regarding aFXa inhibitory potency, these series are on molar basis 1.5 to 2.6 times more potent than the fondaparinux reference (1480 UI/μmol). This is in agreement with previous studies performed on dodecasaccharides and tetradecasaccharides where the same phenomenon was observed [32]. As a consequence, this further emphasizes that the double-site oligosaccharides are able, through a dynamic equilibrium, to engage both AGA*IA sites with antithrombin and to increase by about twofold the molar aFXa activity. At this stage however, more subtle interpretation of their ranking is difficult to assess as it is established that several parameters, either synergistic or antagonistic, might influence their potency. Among them, we could highlight the spacer length between two AGA*IA sequences, the nature of AGA*IA flanking oligosaccharides as well as their location either at RE or NRE.

Regarding thrombin activity, when the T-Domain flanking units are located at the reducing end, the potency is between 5 and 9 IU/mg. This is very low when compared to the NLT 180 IU/mg of USP Heparin. However, when T-domain flanking units are at the NRE, the thrombin activity is increasingly noteworthy. Interestingly, the octadecasaccharides **4** and **5** have the same T domain (ΔIs-IdoA) followed by an AGA*IA at the NRE but the aFIIa activities are respectively 22.6 and 81.5 IU/mg. In this case, the location of the reducing end AGA*IA plays an important role. For compound **4**, the RE pentasaccharide is not completely at the end of the chain, whereas for **5**, it is fully located at the reducing end of the octadecasaccharide. This sequence configuration provides the opportunity to maximize the chain length between at least one AGA*IA and the T-domain, which in turn strengthens the ternary complex with antithrombin and thrombin.

The octadecasaccharide **6** possesses three consecutive Is disaccharides at the NRE and one AGA*IA at the RE. This configuration maximizes both the anionic charge density for the T-domain and the spacer chain length with the reducing end AGA*IA pentasaccharide. As a consequence, the thrombin inhibition is the highest one observed in these series, with a value of 119.3 IU/mg. We conclude that between the regioisomers **2** and **6**, the thrombin inhibition potency increases by about 20 times, which is in good alignment with the results obtained on synthetic compounds. However, there are still some open questions remaining, especially when octadecasaccharide **1** is compared with octadecasaccharides **5** and **6**. For these three octadecasaccharides, there is one AGA*IA sequence fully located at the reducing end. Their differences lie in the T domain. The last two disaccharides could be considered to interact with thrombin and stabilize the complex according to Petitou et al. [19]. For octadecasaccharides **1**, **5** and **6**, there is respectively four, four and six sulfate groups. The charge density influence on thrombin inhibition could be expected for octadecasaccharides **5** and **6** but does not correlate for octadecasaccharide **1**, which is at least 10 times less potent than **5** and **6**. If we take into account that the T-domain is also an AGA*IA sequence, antithrombin could compete with thrombin and disfavor the ternary complex formation, which in turn might explain the very low potency of octadecasaccharide **1**.

3. Materials and Methods

3.1. Materials and Chemicals

Semuloparin was obtained from Sanofi (Vitry sur Seine, France). This product was prepared according to Example 2 described in a U.S. patent [33]. All other reagents and chemicals were of the highest quality available. Water was purified with a Millipore Milli-Q purification system. *Flavobacterium heparinum* heparinase I (EC 4.2.2.7) and $\Delta^{4,5}$-Glucuronate-2-sulfatase were obtained from Grampian Enzymes (Aberdeen, UK). AT used for the determination of biological activities was freeze-dried material of human origin (Instrumentation Laboratory, Le Pre Saint Gervais, France). FXa (71-nKat flask) was freeze-dried material of bovine origin (Instrument Laboratory). FIIa was freeze-dried material of human origin (Stago, Asnières sur Seine, France). FXa (S2765, Instrumentation Laboratory) and FIIa (S2238, Instrumentation Laboratory) substrates were freeze-dried materials.

3.2. Chromatographic Methods

Following the method in reference [12,17], 150 mm × 2.1 mm columns filled with Kinetex C_{18} 2.6 μm particles (Phenomenex, Le Pecq, France) were used after the CTA dynamic coating. A linear concentration gradient (0–2 M) of aqueous ammonium methane sulfonate, pH 2.5 was applied.

For the analytical control of collected fractions or chromatographic separations, a Carbopack AS11 column (250 mm × 2.1 mm) (Thermo Scientific Dionex, Courtaboeuf, France) was used with aqueous $NaClO_4$ mobile phase.

LC/MS with an ion-pairing chromatographic system (Acquity UPLC BEH C_{18} column, 2.1 mm × 150 mm, 1.7 μm, Waters, Saint-Quentin-en-Yvelines, France) was the third orthogonal method applied for deciphering the complex mixture [14,17]. The method initially described in [34] and adapted in [14] was broadened [17] to determine the number of ion-pair adducts included in the molecular ions. Briefly, each separation was duplicated, one using pentylamine (PTA) as ion pairing reagent and the second one using hexylamine (HXA). The number of adducts could be deduced from the mass shift in ion peaks obtained in parallel with both conditions. Partial degradation of 3-O sulfated glucosamines located at the reducing end was detected when working at 40 °C, and therefore, the operating column temperature was lowered to 30 °C for sequencing experiments.

3.3. Procedure for Isolation of Octadecasaccharides

The octadecasaccharide fraction was purified by gel permeation chromatography (GPC) from semuloparin as previously described [17]. 1.85 g of semuloparin were directly injected on a system equipped with two columns (100 × 5 cm (I.D.) connected in series, packed with polyacrylamide gel (Bio Gel P-30, Fine, Bio Rad, Marnes-la-Coquette, France)), and circulated at 1.7 mL/min with NaClO₄ 0.2 M. UV detection was used at 232 nm. 600 g of semuloparin were injected in fractions over about 350 runs. Selected fractions were first concentrated, desalted on Sephadex G10 columns (100 × 7 cm) and then lyophilized. Finally, 10 g of octadecasaccharides were obtained.

3.3.1. Fractionation on AT Affinity Chromatography

The octadecasaccharide fractionated by chromatography on an AT Sepharose column (30 cm × 7 cm) as previously described [17]. The column was prepared by coupling human AT (2 g) as described by Höök et al. [35]. Octadecasaccharides (80 to 150 mg) were injected in each run. The low-affinity fraction was eluted from the column with a 0.25 M NaCl solution buffered at pH 7.4 with 1 mM Tris/HCl at 12 mL/min. The five high-affinity octasaccharide fractions were eluted with a five step gradient of NaCl (0.74 M, 1.23 M, 1.71 M, 2.2 M and 3.5 M NaCl and 1 mM Tris-HCl, pH 7.4). All fractions were desalted on Sephadex–G10. After 100 injections on AT-affinity chromatography, 4.2 g were collected for the low-affinity fraction, 800 mg for F1, 1.57 g for F2, 1.02 g for F3, 616 mg for F4 and 385 mg for F5.

3.3.2. Purification of Octadecasaccharide Fraction F3

Focus was given to the separation of octadecasaccharides regioisomers with 2 AGA*IA sequences positioned differently within the chain (Figure 1). These are the components of major interest in the affine fraction F3 (Figure 2). The five octadecasaccharide series were purified by combining three chromatographic methods with orthogonal selectivities following the previously described procedure [17] namely, CTA-SAX, AS11 and ion pairing chromatography. We distinguish herein two distinct types of octadecasaccharides to guide the separation strategy. Type I octadecasaccharides (2 and 3) are devoid of 2-O sulfation at the non-reducing end's uronic acid whereas Type II compounds (4, 5 and 6) are 2-O sulfated (Figure 1). The 2-O sulfation influences the maximum of the UV spectrum and the retention behavior in CTA-SAX and AS11 chromatography. The details of the procedure are reported in the Supplementary Data.

3.4. Structural Characterization by Enzymatic Sequencing

The sequencing of octadecasaccharides (10 to 20 μg) was done by controlled depolymerisation with heparinase 1 from *Flavobacterium heparinum* following the described procedure [12,17]. The first step for Type I oligosaccharides was reduction by NaBH₄, used to selectively label the reducing end disaccharide [17]. For Type II octadecasaccharides, $\Delta^{4,5}$-glucuronate-2-sulfatase was initially applied to differentiate the non-reducing end, before the NaBH₄ reduction. The reaction was initiated by the addition of 10 μL of a 0.5 UI/mL solution of sulfatase diluted in KH₂PO₄ 10 mM pH 7 and added in combination with 2 mg/mL of bovine serum albumin (BSA). The advancement of the 2-O desulfatation was followed by analytical CTA-SAX chromatography. At the end of the reaction, the residual enzyme was destroyed by a 2 min boiling step before performing NaBH$_4$ reduction. After vacuum evaporation, reduced octadecasaccharide was diluted in a 1.7 mL HPLC vial and the pH was adjusted to 7 by addition of diluted ammonia or hydrochloric acid. Heparinase I was added (2 µL of a 0.5 UI/mL solution) and depolymerisation was performed at 16 °C. The monitoring of the fragmentation was done by injection on CTA-SAX and AS11 analytical columns. Injection in LC/MS was also performed to confirm the structure of fragments.

3.5. Mass Spectrometry Conditions

ESI mass spectra were obtained using a Waters Xevo Q-Tof mass spectrometer. The electrospray interface was set in positive ion mode with a capillary voltage of 2000 V and a sampling cone voltage of 20 V. The source and the desolvation temperatures were respectively 120 and 400 °C. Nitrogen was used as desolvation (750 L/min) and cone gas (25 L/min). The mass range used was 200–2000 Da (scan rate 0.5 s).

3.6. NMR Spectroscopy

The octadecasaccharide sample (1 mg) was dissolved in D$_2$O, freeze-dried with a final dissolution in D$_2$O (99.96% Euriso-Top, Saint-Aubin, France) and transferred into a 3-mm nuclear magnetic resonance (NMR) sample tube. One-dimensional and two-dimensional (2D) NMR (^{1}H-^{1}H and ^{1}H-^{13}C) spectra were recorded on a 600 MHz AVANCE II spectrometer (Bruker, Wissembourg, France) operating at 599.80 MHz using a 5-mm TXI cryoprobe with standard pulse sequences and a probe temperature of 30 °C. Proton spectra were recorded in 256 scans with a 2 s presaturation and a full recycle time of 6.5 s. The resolution prior zero filling was 0.2 Hz/pt. 2D-COSY and 2D-TOCSY with a mixing time value of 120 ms were acquired using 64 scans per series of 4 K × 512 W with a resolution of 1.16 Hz/pt before zero filling (4 K × 2 K) and appropriate apodization was applied prior to Fourier transformation. The 2D-nuclear Overhauser enhancement spectroscopy (NOESY) was performed in similar way with a mixing time value of 300 ms. The 2D-HSQC was performed using 64 scans per series of 1.5 K × 512 W with a resolution of 3.28 Hz/pt before zero filling (2 K × 1 K). Spectrum calibration was achieved by setting as external standard reference trimethylsilyl 2,2′3,3′-tetradeuteropropionoic acid (TSP-D$_4$) signal to 0 ppm.

3.7. Anti-Factor IIa Activity and Anti-Factor Xa Activity

AT solution of 1 IU/mL were prepared in pH 7.4 PEG 6000 buffer (0.1% PEG 6000 in pH 7.4 buffer [50 mM Tris and 150 mM NaCl adjusted by HCl to pH 7.4]). FXa was prepared to 1.8 nkat/mL in pH 7.4 PEG6000 buffer. FIIa was prepared to 5 IU/mL in pH 7.4 PEG6000 buffer. The chromogenic substrate solution for FXa and FIIa was prepared to a final concentration of 0.5 mM in pH 8.4 buffer (50 mM Tris, 175 mM NaCl, and 7.5 mM edetate disodium adjusted by HCl to pH 8.4). Semuloparin biological standard (3000ET with assigned potencies of 101.4 IU/mL for anti-FXa and 1.8 IU/mL for anti-FIIa), calibrated against the second LMWH international standard (NIBSC, code 01/608), was used for calibration.

For anti-FXa titration, the semuloparin standard solution was diluted with pH 7.4 buffer to obtain target concentrations of 0.04, 0.05, 0.06, and 0.07 IU/mL. Each concentration was assessed in duplicate (two wells filled with the same diluted solution), and two independent experiments (independent dispensing and dilutions) were conducted.

For anti-FIIa titration, the semuloparin standard solution was diluted with pH 7.4 buffer to obtain target concentrations of 0.007, 0.008, 0.010, and 0.012 IU/mL. Each concentration was assessed in duplicate (two wells filled with the same diluted solution), and three independent experiments (independent dispensing and dilutions) were conducted.

Octadecasaccharide solution was prepared to a final concentration with activities in IU/mL close to the semuloparin standard. The solution was then diluted and dispensed as for the standards.

Plates were heated at 37 °C. Solutions for analysis (20 µL) were pipetted into a 96-well plate, and 20 µL of AT solution was added. Samples were then mixed and left for 60 s before 40 µL of the FXa (or FIIa) solution were added, and the solutions were mixed and left for a further 60 s. Next, 100 µL of chromogenic substrate solution were added, mixed, and left for 240 s. Finally, 100 µL of 42% acetic acid solution were added, mixed, and left for 60 s before the optical density at 405 nm was read.

The internally developed software "Parallel", running on the Statistical Analysis System (SAS version 9.1, SAS France, Grégy-sur-Yerres, France)), was used for statistical analysis according to the European Pharmacopoeia Ph. Eur. § 5.3 for parallel-line models. Each assay result was the mean average of the independent valid tests.

4. Conclusions

The results of this study, while confirming the structure-activity relationship on synthetic compounds, also demonstrate that the overall picture for thrombin inhibition compounds may be much more complex in natural heparin sequences as well as for LMWH products. We have demonstrated that for octadecasaccharide regioisomers, built up from the same AGA*IA sequences and Is flanking disaccharides, thrombin inhibition potency may dramatically differ. Indeed, when the AGA*IA sequences are located at the reducing end vs. the non-reducing end, the octadecasaccharide becomes 20 times more potent in aFIIa activity (compound **6** vs. **2**). This is in agreement with the previous findings reported on synthetic compounds by Petitou et al. [19–21]. However, even if an AGA*IA sequence is borne at the reducing end, the presence of another one at the non-reducing end (compound **1**) obviously destabilize the complex with thrombin and decrease the potency by one log of magnitude order. The anionic charge density of T-domain is an important factor for thrombin binding but its ability to interact strongly with other proteins should be taken into consideration to improve our prediction of structure activity relationships. The findings developed in this paper pointed out that for octadecasaccharides regioisomers the sequence arrangement is critical for interaction with proteins regulating the coagulation cascade. This is emphasizing the role and the potential impact of the selectivity of the heparin depolymerization process on the overall biological properties of LMWH.

Supplementary Materials: Supplementary materials are available online.

Acknowledgments: The authors warmly thank Nathalie Karst, Andrew Van-Sickle and Marco Guerrini for their thoughtful review and recommendations to improve the manuscript as well as Min Zhang for her active contribution in the chromatographic purification of octadecasaccharides. We would like to thank also Celine Martinez for her appreciated input in the redaction of the experimental biological section, Brigitte Bordier and Monique Cherel for performing aFXa and aFIIa assay.

Author Contributions: Pierre Mourier and Christian Viskov designed the study. Pierre Mourier isolated, purified and characterized the octadecasaccharides by enzymatic sequencing. Olivier Guichard performed the mass spectrometry experiments. Philippe Sizun and Frederic Herman characterized the octadecasaccharides by NMR. Christian Viskov, Pierre Mourier, Philippe Sizun analyzed the data and reviewed the data before submission. Christian Viskov and Pierre Mourier wrote the paper.

Conflicts of Interest: The authors declare no conflict of interest.

Abbreviations

AT, antithrombin; FXa, factor Xa; FIIa, factor IIa or thrombin; SAX, strong anion exchange; CTA-SAX, cetyltrimethylammonium strong anion exchange; LMWH, low-molecular-weight heparin; GPC, gel permeation chromatography; PTA, pentylamine; HXA, hexylamine; HFIP, 1,1,1,3,3,3-hexafluoro-2-propanol; LC/MS, liquid chromatography–mass spectrometry; DQF-COSY, double-quantum-filter correlation spectroscopy; 2D-NOESY, nuclear Overhauser enhancement spectroscopy; HSQC, heteronuclear single-quantum coherence; TOCSY, total correlated spectroscopy; $GlcN_{ac}$, *N*-acetyl-α-D-glucosamine; $GlcN_{Ac,6S}$, *N*-acetylated, 6-*O*-sulfated GlcN; $GlcN_{S,6S}$, *N*,6-*O*-disulfated GlcN; $GlcN_{S,3,6S}$, *N*,3,6-*O*-trisulfated GlcN; IdoA, α-L-iduronic acid; $IdoA_{2S}$, 2-*O*-sulfated IdoA; AGA*IA, pentasaccharide sequence of $GlcN_{Ac,6S}$-GlcA-$GlcN_{S,3,6S}$-$IdoA_{2S}$-$GlcN_{S,6S}$; ΔU, 4,5-unsaturated uronic acid; $ΔU_{2S}$, 2-*O*-sulfated, 4,5-unsaturated uronic acid.

References

1. Choay, J.; Lormeau, J.-C.; Petitou, M.; Sinaÿ, P.; Casu, B.; Oreste, P.; Torri, G.; Gatti, G. Anti-Xa active heparin oligosaccharides. *Thromb. Res.* **1980**, *18*, 573–578. [CrossRef]
2. Torri, G.; Naggi, A. Heparin centenary—An ever-young live-saving drug. *Int. J. Cardiol.* **2016**, *212*, S1–S4. [CrossRef]
3. Nader, H.B.; Dietrich, C.P. Natural occurrence, and possible biological role of heparin. In *Heparin: Chemical and Biological Properties, Clinical Applications*; Lane, D.A., Lindahl, U., Eds.; CRC Press Inc.: Boca Raton, FL, USA, 1989; pp. 81–96.
4. Conrad, H.E. *Heparin Binding Proteins*; Academic Press: Millbrae, CA, USA, 1998.
5. Bock, S.C. Antithrombin and heparin cofactor II. In *Hemostasis and Thrombosis: Basic Principles and Clinical Practice*; Lippincott Williams and Wilkins: Philadelphia, PA, USA, 2006; pp. 235–248.
6. Danielsson, A.; Raub, E.; Lindahl, U.; Björk, I. Role of Ternary Complexes, in Which Heparin Binds Both Antithrombin and Proteinase, in the Acceleration of the Reactions between Antithrombin and Thrombin or Factor Xa. *J. Biol. Chem.* **1986**, *261*, 15467–15473. [PubMed]
7. Petitou, M.; Casu, B.; Lindahl, U. 1976–1983, a critical period in the history of heparin: The discovery of the antithrombin binding site. *Biochimie* **2003**, *85*, 83–89. [CrossRef]
8. Hricovini, M.; Guerrini, M.; Bisio, A.; Torri, G.; Petitou, M.; Casu, B. Conformation of heparin pentasaccharide bound to antithrombin III. *Biochem. J.* **2001**, *359*, 265–272. [CrossRef] [PubMed]
9. Loganathan, D.H.; Wang, M.; Mallis, L.M.; Linhardt, R.J. Structural variation in the antithrombin III binding site region and its occurrence in heparin from different sources. *Biochemistry* **1990**, *29*, 4362–4368. [CrossRef] [PubMed]
10. Lindahl, U.; Thunberg, L.; Bäckström, G.; Riesenfeld, J.; Nordling, K.; Bjork, I. Extension and structural variability of the antithrombin binding sequence in heparin. *J. Biol. Chem.* **1984**, *259*, 12368–12376. [PubMed]
11. Guerrini, M.; Elli, S.; Mourier, P.; Rudd, T.R.; Gaudesi, D.; Casu, B.; Boudier, C.; Torri, G.; Viskov, C. An unusual antithrombin-binding heparin octasaccharide with an additional 3-*O*-sulfated glucosamine in the active pentasaccharide sequence. *Biochem. J.* **2013**, *449*, 343–351. [CrossRef] [PubMed]
12. Mourier, P.A.J.; Viskov, C. Chromatographic analysis and sequencing approach of heparin oligosaccharides using cetyltrimethylammonium dynamically coated stationary phases. *Anal. Biochem.* **2004**, *332*, 299–313. [CrossRef] [PubMed]
13. Guerrini, M.; Mourier, P.A.J.; Torri, J.; Viskov, C. Antithrombin-binding oligosaccharides: Structural diversities in a unique function? *Glycoconj. J.* **2014**, *31*, 409–416. [CrossRef] [PubMed]
14. Guerrini, M.; Guglieri, S.; Casu, B.; Torri, G.; Mourier, P.; Boudier, C.; Viskov, C. Antithrombin-binding octasaccharides and role of extensions of the active pentasaccharide sequence in the specificity and strength of interaction: Evidence for very high affinity induced by an unusual glucuronic acid residue. *J. Biol. Chem.* **2008**, *283*, 26662–26675. [CrossRef] [PubMed]
15. Viskov, C.; Just, M.; Laux, V.; Mourier, P.; Lorenz, M. Description of the chemical and pharmacological characteristics of a new hemisynthetic ultra-low-molecular-weight heparin, AVE5026. *J. Thromb. Haemost.* **2009**, *7*, 1143–1151. [CrossRef] [PubMed]
16. Viskov, C.; Elli, S.; Urso, E.; Gaudesi, D.; Mourier, P.; Herman, F.; Boudier, C.; Casu, B.; Torri, G.; Guerrini, M. Heparin dodecasaccharide containing two antithrombin binding pentasaccharides. Structural features and biological properties. *J. Biol. Chem.* **2013**, *288*, 25895–25907. [CrossRef] [PubMed]
17. Mourier, P.A.; Guichard, O.Y.; Herman, F.; Viskov, C. Isolation of a pure octadecasaccharide with antithrombin activity from an ultra-low-molecular-weight heparin. *Anal. Biochem.* **2014**, *453*, 7–15. [CrossRef] [PubMed]
18. Jordan, R.E.; Favreau, L.V.; Braswell, E.H.; Rosenberg, R.D. Heparin with Two Binding Sites for Antithrombin or Platelet Factor 4. *J. Biol. Chem.* **1982**, *257*, 400–406. [PubMed]
19. Petitou, M.; Van Boeckel, C.A. A synthetic antithrombin III binding pentasaccharide is now a drug! What comes next? *Angew. Chem. Int. Ed. Engl.* **2004**, *43*, 3118–3133. [CrossRef] [PubMed]
20. Petitou, M.; Hérault, J.M.; Bernat, A.; Driguez, P.A.; Duchaussoy, P.; Lormeau, J.C.; Herbert, J.M. Synthesis of thrombin-inhibiting heparin mimetics without side effects. *Nature* **1999**, *398*, 417–422. [PubMed]
21. Petitou, M.; Imberty, A.; Duchaussoy, P.; Driguez, P.A.; Ceccato, M.L.; Gourvenec, F.; Sizun, P.; Hérault, J.P.; Pérez, S.; Herbert, J.M. Experimental Proof for the structure of a Thrombin-inhibiting heparin molecule. *Chem. Eur. J.* **2001**, *7*, 858–873. [CrossRef]

22. Mourier, P.; Anger, P.; Martinez, C.; Herman, F.; Viskov, C. Quantitative compositional analysis of heparin using exhaustive heparinase digestion and strong anion exchange chromatography. *Anal. Chem. Res.* **2015**, *3*, 46–53. [CrossRef]

23. Venkataraman, G.; Shriver, Z.; Raman, R.; Sasisekharan, R. Sequencing complex polysaccharides. *Science* **1999**, *286*, 537–542. [CrossRef] [PubMed]

24. Keiseri, N.; Venkataraman, G.; Shriver, Z.; Sasisekharan, R. Direct isolation and sequencing of specific protein-binding glycosaminoglycans. *Nat. Med.* **2001**, *7*, 123–128.

25. Stringer, S.E.; Kandola, B.S.; Pye, D.A.; Gallagher, J.T. Heparin sequencing. *Glycobiology* **2003**, *13*, 97–107. [CrossRef] [PubMed]

26. Desai, U.R.; Wang, H.; Linhardt, R.J. Substrate specificity of the heparin lyases from *Flavobacterium heparinum*. *Arch. Biochem. Biophys.* **1993**, *306*, 461–468. [CrossRef] [PubMed]

27. Ernst, S.; Rhomberg, A.J.; Bieman, K.; Sasisekharan, R. Direct evidence for a predominantly exolytic processive mechanism for depolymerization of heparin-like glycosaminoglycans by heparinase I. *Proc. Natl. Acad. Sci. USA* **1998**, *95*, 4182–4187. [CrossRef] [PubMed]

28. Xiao, Z.; Zhao, W.; Yang, B.; Zhang, Z.; Guan, H.; Linhardt, R.J. Heparinase I selectivity for the 3,6-di-*O*-sulfo-2-deoxy-2-sulfamido-α-D-glucopyranose (1,4) 2-*O*-sulfo-α-L-idopyranosyluronic acid (GlcNS3S6S-IdoA2S) linkages. *Glycobiology* **2011**, *21*, 13–22. [CrossRef] [PubMed]

29. Myette, J.R.; Shriver, Z.; Claycamp, C.; McLean, M.W.; Venkatarama, G.; Sasisekharan, R. The Heparin/Heparan Sulfate 2-*O*-Sulfatase from *Flavobacterium heparinum*. Molecular cloning, recombinant expression, and biochemical characterization. *J. Biol. Chem.* **2003**, *278*, 12157–12166. [CrossRef] [PubMed]

30. Raman, R.; Myette, J.R.; Shriver, Z.; Pojasek, K.; Venkataraman, G.; Sasisekharan, R. The Heparin/Heparan Sulfate 2-*O*-Sulfatase from *Flavobacterium heparinum*. A structural and biochemical study of the enzyme active site and saccharide substrate specificity. *J. Biol. Chem.* **2003**, *278*, 12167–12174. [CrossRef] [PubMed]

31. Ferro, D.R.; Provasoli, A.; Ragazzi, M.; Torri, G.; Casu, B.; Gatti, G.; Jacquinet, J.-C.; Sinaÿ, P.; Petitou, M.; Choay, J. Evidence for conformational equilibrium of the sulfated L-iduronate residue in heparin and in synthetic heparin mono- and oligo-saccharides: NMR and force-field studies. *J. Am. Chem. Soc.* **1986**, *108*, 6773–6778. [CrossRef]

32. Mourier, P.; Viskov, C. Polysaccharides Comprising Two Antithrombin III-Binding Sites, Preparation Thereof and Use Thereof as Antithrombin Medicaments. U.S. Patent 9,346,894 B2, 18 October 2016.

33. Biberovic, V.; Grondard, L.; Mourier, P.; Viskov, C. Mixture of Sulfated Oligosaccharides. U.S. Patents 8,003,623 B2 and 8,071,570 B2, 23 August 2011.

34. Doneanu, C.E.; Chen, W.; Gebler, J.C. Analysis of oligosaccharides derived from heparin by Ion-Pair Reversed-Phase Chromatography/Mass Spectrometry. *Anal. Chem.* **2009**, *81*, 3485–3499. [CrossRef] [PubMed]

35. Höök, M.; Björk, I.; Hopwood, J.; Lindahl, U. Anticoagulant activity of heparin: Separation of high-activity and low-activity heparin species by affinity chromatography on immobilized antithrombin. *FEBS Lett.* **1976**, *66*, 90–93. [CrossRef]

Sample Availability: Octadecasaccharides were prepared at 1 mg scale and are not available.

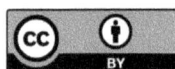

molecules

MDPI

Article

Extended Physicochemical Characterization of the Synthetic Anticoagulant Pentasaccharide Fondaparinux Sodium by Quantitative NMR and Single Crystal X-ray Analysis

William de Wildt [1], Huub Kooijman [2], Carel Funke [1], Bülent Üstün [1], Afranina Leika [1], Maarten Lunenburg [1], Frans Kaspersen [1] and Edwin Kellenbach [1,*]

[1] DTS Aspen Oss B.V., 5223BB Oss, The Netherlands; wdewildt@nl.aspenpharma.com (W.d.W.); i.funke@kpnplanet.nl (C.F.); bustun@nl.aspenpharma.com (B.Ü.); aleika@nl.aspenpharma.com (A.L.); mlunenburg@nl.aspenpharma.com (M.L.); fmkaspersen@hotmail.com (F.K.)
[2] Bijvoet Center for Biomolecular Research, Crystal and Structural Chemistry, Faculty of Science, Utrecht University, Padualaan 8, 3584 CH Utrecht, The Netherlands; Huub.Kooijman@shell.com
* Correspondence: ekellenbach@nl.aspenpharma.com; Tel.: +31-(0)6-2054-9168

Received: 31 May 2017; Accepted: 14 August 2017; Published: 17 August 2017

Abstract: Fondaparinux sodium is a synthetic pentasaccharide representing the high affinity antithrombin III binding site in heparin. It is the active pharmaceutical ingredient of the anticoagulant drug Arixtra®. The single crystal X-ray structure of Fondaparinux sodium is reported, unequivocally confirming both structure and absolute configuration. The iduronic acid adopts a somewhat distorted chair conformation. Due to the presence of many sulfur atoms in the highly sulfated pentasaccharide, anomalous dispersion could be applied to determine the absolute configuration. A comparison with the conformation of Fondaparinux in solution, as well as complexed with proteins is presented. The content of the solution reference standard was determined by quantitative NMR using an internal standard both in 1999 and in 2016. A comparison of the results allows the conclusion that this method shows remarkable precision over time, instrumentation and analysts.

Keywords: Fondaparinux sodium; extended physicochemical characterization; qNMR; single crystal X-ray structure; reference standard; iduronic acid conformation; Arixtra®

1. Introduction

Fondaparinux sodium (referred to as 'Fondaparinux' in this article; Figure 1) is a synthetic pentasaccharide [1] derived from the high affinity antithrombin III binding site in heparin, modified by a methyl group at the reducing end. It is the active pharmaceutical ingredient of GSK's anticoagulant drug Arixtra® and a selective aXa inhibitor through antithrombin III [2] and lacks aIIa activity as a result of its low molecular weight. As part of the extended physical characterization of Fondaparinux, both structure (by X-ray) and standard content (by qNMR) are described in this paper. The X-ray structures of Fondaparinux have previously been limited to co-crystals in complex with a number of proteins [3–8]. Also, related synthetic (penta) saccharides complexed with protein have been reported [9,10]. Furthermore, uncomplexed Fondaparinux (solution) structures determined by (a combination of) theoretical calculations and NMR spectroscopy have been described [11–15]. In solution, $^3J(^1H, ^1H)$ coupling constants allow to determine the conformation of the pyranose residues in heparin. The glucosamine and glucuronic acids residues adopt a stable $^4C_1$-conformation. However, the iduronate ring adopts $^1C_4$ and $^2S_0$ conformations rapidly interconverting on the NMR time scale [11,12]. Complexation by proteins locks the iduronate residue in a single $^2S_0$ conformation both in the crystal [5,6,9,10] and in solution [16]. Also in the crystal of uncomplexed Fondaparinux, the occurrence of a single iduronate conformation is foreseen. Here we report the X-ray single crystal structure of uncomplexed Fondaparinux and compare it to the conformation of Fondaparinux in solution, as well as complexed with proteins.

The content of ampoules of the Fondaparinux solution reference standard was determined in both 1999 and 2016 by quantitative NMR (qNMR) using an internal standard. The results of both determinations are discussed here. The ampoules of this standard are used to determine the Fondaparinux content of Fondaparinux batches. For consistency, the ability to assure the long-term stability of the standard content is crucial.

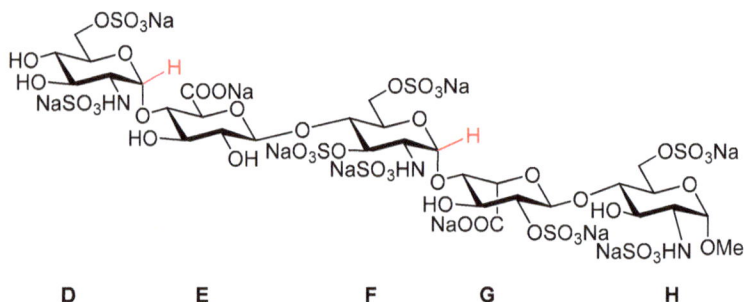

Figure 1. Structural formula of the synthetic anticoagulant pentasaccharide Fondaparinux sodium. The anomeric D1 and F1 protons used for qNMR integration have been indicated in red.

2. Results

qNMR is a well-established and accepted method for content determination [17–19] and is described in major pharmacopoeia [20–22]. The strength of qNMR lies in the fundamental property that, under the right conditions, the integrated response of a proton in ^{1}H-NMR will be identical in every molecule. This implies that a content determination can be carried out relative to a completely unrelated (but well-characterized) standard. We applied qNMR for the content determination of ampoules standard solution of the relatively complicated compound Fondaparinux using a maleic acid standard. Figure 2 shows an example of the 500 MHz ^{1}H-NMR spectrum of a mixture of the Fondaparinux standard and maleic acid in D_2O with the signals used for integration indicated. We performed these determinations on ampoules of the same standard both in 1999 and 2016 using an identical protocol which yields a unique opportunity to assess the long-term reproducibility of the qNMR method. The content determination in 1999 was performed at 400 MHz using a conventional probe whereas the content determination in 2016 was done at 500 MHz using a cryo probe. Different batches of maleic acid were used in 1996 and in 2017. For each experiment the tests were done by two different analysts and on two different days. The differences between the determinations are listed in the experimental section (Table 4).

The current analysis yields a content of 9.75 mg/mL with an SD of 0.06 mg/mL for the standard. The analysis performed in 1999 yielded a content of 9.64 mg/mL with an SD of 0.08 mg/mL. The two results are therefore not significantly different. The close correspondence between the two values obtained about 17 years apart demonstrates the intrinsic robustness of the qNMR content determination. Moreover, the differences between the two values is unlikely be due to degradation since the current content is slightly higher than the one determined 17 years ago and no signals pointing at degradation are currently detected in NMR.

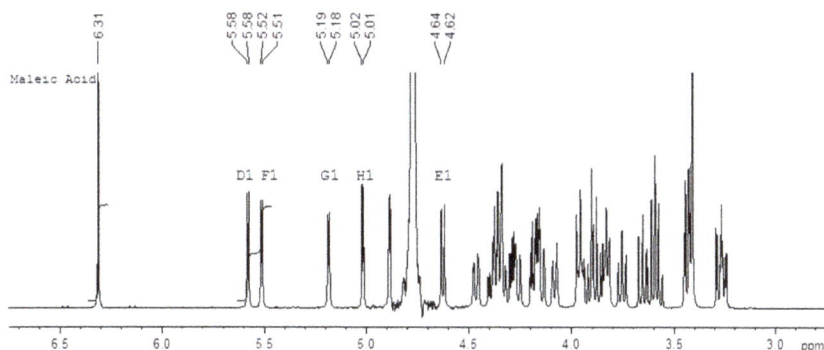

Figure 2. Example of the 500 MHz ^{1}H-NMR spectrum of a mixture of the Fondaparinux sodium standard and maleic acid in D$_2$O with the relevant integrated signals.

2.1. Fondaparinux Single Crystal X-ray Structure

Fondaparinux drug substance is industrially obtained as an amorphous powder as is evident from its X-ray powder diffractogram (XRPD; Figure 3; in green). Obtaining Fondaparinux single crystals was challenging, probably due to its inherent flexibility and linear structure. Ultimately, crystals were obtained as described in the Materials and Methods section. Several batches of crystals were produced. For a crystal from one batch, a full single-crystal structure determination was undertaken. A crystal from another batch was used for a unit-cell determination to ensure the similarity of these batches. Finally, an XRPD measurement was done for one batch of crystals see Table 7 for unit-cell comparison). In Figure 3, the blue trace shows the XRPD patterns of crystalline Fondaparinux. The XRPD pattern calculated from the crystal structure is shown as the red trace in Figure 3. A polarization microscopy image of representative crystals is displayed in Figure 4.

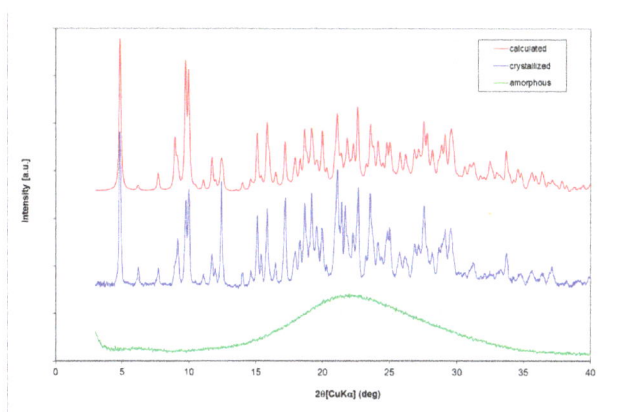

Figure 3. Comparison of the observed powder diffraction patterns of amorphous (green) and crystallized Fondaparinux (blue) with the pattern calculated from the single-crystal structure (red). The patterns are given an arbitrary displacement along the intensity axis to aid comparison. For the calculated pattern, the unit-cell parameters were refined using the Rietveld method to allow for the difference in data collection temperature. The reflection positions of observed and calculated patterns show a good correlation. The relative intensities show some differences, which are most likely due to the limited number of crystallites in the powder measurement, some preferred orientation effects and small changes in structure (especially in the water molecules) due to the temperature difference.

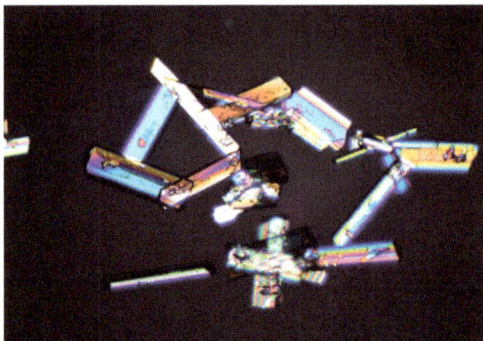

Figure 4. Polarized light microscopic picture at 40× magnification of Fondaparinux crystals formed from a water/ethanol solution.

2.2. Structural Features of the Crystal Structure

The asymmetric unit of the crystal structure of Fondaparinux contains a pentasaccharide anion, with one of the carboxylic groups protonated (vide infra), nine sodium cations, 17 water molecules coordinated to one or more sodium atoms and 15 non-coordinated water molecules. A perspective drawing of the molecular structure of the pentasaccharide Fondaparinux, along with the atomic labeling scheme of the non-hydrogen atoms and the labeling scheme of the rings is given in Figure 5.

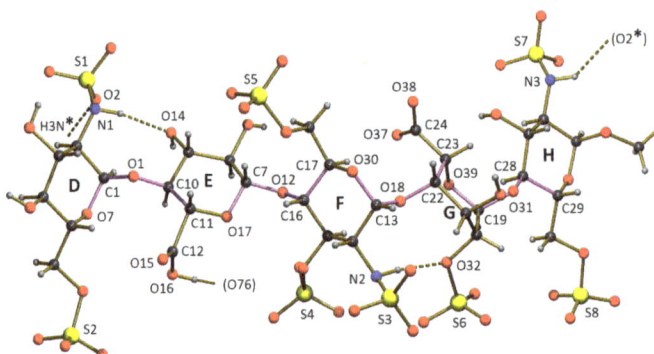

Figure 5. Perspective drawing of part of the asymmetric unit of the crystal structure of Fondaparinux. Sodium ions and water molecules (coordinated and non-coordinated) are excluded for clarity. Rings and atoms mentioned in the discussion are labelled. The bonds defining the glycosidic conformation are highlighted in pink. Hydrogen bonds are marked with dashed lines. N3-H3N donates a hydrogen bond to a translation related Fondaparinux molecule ($x - 1, y, z - 1$). The involved symmetry positions are indicated with a *. Hydroxyl O16 donates a hydrogen bond to a water molecule not shown.

The sodium ions are coordinated by numerous oxygen atoms from the pentasaccharide and extensively co-crystallized water molecules. The seven ordered sodium ions are coordinated by six oxygen atoms each. For the ordered ions, most Na...O distances fall in the range 2.3–2.7 Å. However, a small number of Na...O distances up to 2.9 Å are observed. The two disordered sodium ions are also surrounded by a total of six oxygen atoms that can be assigned to the coordination shell, but this shell is somewhat larger than that observed for the ordered sodium atoms. As a result of this, the sodium can take up several positions and some of the individual disorder components are only directly coordinated by five oxygen atoms. Full details of the observed coordination distances are given in the deposited Crystallographic Information File. Through these coordinative bonds an infinite three-dimensional structure is formed. A perspective drawing of the infinite substructure formed by sodium counter-ions, sulfate groups and coordinated water molecules is included in the Supporting Information. The final model contained no solvent accessible void. DFT calculations also indicated extensive coordination to both sodium ions and water (e.g., [13,15]).

3. Discussion

The individual glucosamine (D, F and H) rings have adopted the conventional stable $^4C_1$ chair conformation. The glucuronic acid ring (E) is in a slightly distorted $^4C_1$ chair-conformation. The iduronic acid G ring conformation has been the subject of intense debate [11–15,23–26]. Uncomplexed in solution, its structure cannot be described by a single conformer but is an equilibrium of $^1C_4$, chair and $^2S_0$. Skew-boat conformations with the equilibrium shifted to the $^2S_0$ conformation [11–15,23–26]. The conformation is $^2S_0$ in complex with antithrombin III [5,6,16].

In our crystal structure, the iduronic acid ring (G) is in a chair conformation, heavily distorted towards a half-chair conformation with the best-fitting local twofold rotation axis running through the midpoint of the bond ring O–C5 (crystal structure numbering O39–C23; see Table 1 for quantification using Cremer & Pople puckering parameters [27]). The iduronic ring conformation is therefore clearly different from the conformation reported by Johnson et al. [5], who found a skew-boat conformation (related Cremer & Pople puckering parameters are included in Table 1). A comparison of the conformations of the iduronic acid G ring in both structures is given in Figure 6. Interestingly, in the co-crystal of heparin and teichoic acid α-glycosyl transferase the iduronic acid adopts a chair conformation according to the coordinates reported by Sobhanifar et al. ([8], PDB entry 4X7R), related Cremer & Pople puckering parameters are also included in Table 1.

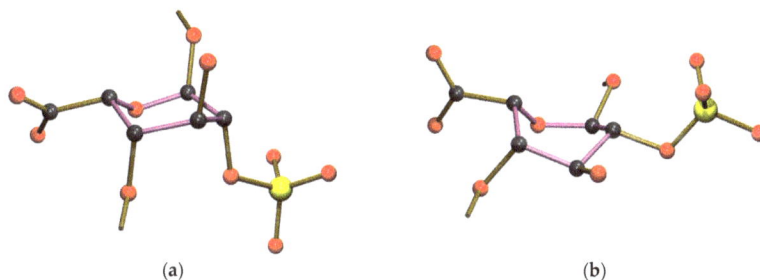

(a)   (b)

Figure 6. A comparison of the conformations of the iduronic acid G ring structures in uncomplexed Fondaparinux (**a**) and Fondaparinux co-crystallized with antithrombin (**b**); from PDB entry 2GD4 [5].

The overall conformation of the pentasaccharide can be described in terms of the torsion angles of the glycosidic links between the carbohydrate rings. An alternative description uses the dihedral angles between least-squares planes fitted through the ring atoms. Numerical data for both descriptions are given in Table 2. Table 2 contains the same set of descriptors for the pentasaccharide molecules co-crystallized with antithrombin S195A, platelet factor 4 and a glycosyl transerase as well as for the structure in solution determined by NMR. A comparison of the free and co-crystallized pentasaccharide shows only relatively small differences when the glycosidic links between adjacent sugar rings are considered. In most cases the range of torsion angles observed is approximately 30 °C. However, in combination with the conformational change of the iduronic acid, these differences add up to a substantial difference for the overall conformation of the pentasaccharide. This can be convincingly illustrated by the angle between the least-squares planes fitted through rings D and H, which shows a difference of almost 60 °C. This difference in dihedral angles (which have a defined range of 0–90 °C) corresponds to the mean planes of rings D and H being almost parallel in the crystal structure of Fondaparinux while they are almost perpendicular in complex 2GD4.

Table 1. Cremer & Pople puckering parameters for the rings in the Fondaparinux structure published here (FP). Parameters for a selection of ideal conformations are included for comparison in a separate section; *k* is an integer number [27]. For comparison, the values calculated from the published coordinates of a selection of co-crystals of proteins and heparin. These are indicated with their PDB codes: 2GD4 is antithrombin S195A with heparin [5]; 4R9W is platelet factor 4 with heparin [7], 4X7R is wall teichoic acid glycosyl transferase [8]. The last column reports the values calculated from the coordinates of a solution NMR study [28]. 2GD4 and 4X7R contain two crystallographically independent heparin molecules; values for both are included.

						Reference Values								
				θ							φ			
Chair				0 or 180							(any value)			
Half-chair				50.8 or 129.2							$k \times 60 + 30$			
Boat				90							$k \times 60$			
Skew-boat				90							$k \times 60 + 30$			

						Observed Values								
	FP		2GD4 1		2GD4 2		4R9W		4X7R 1		4X7R 2		NMR Solution	
	θ	φ	θ	φ	θ	φ	θ	φ	θ	φ	θ	φ	θ	φ
D	0	349	7	64	7	65	12	308	7	0	6	342	4	26
E	8	23	3	94	3	92	18	40	8	339	1	350	5	22
F	0	227	7	76	7	76	7	7	5	21	4	18	7	107
G	165	135	91	140	91	140	90	1	169	142	170	109	92	133
H	4	298	7	268	7	268	89	208	5	28	14	68	10	324

Table 2. Description of the overall conformation of the pentasaccharide in terms of torsion angles (deg.) of the C–O backbone in the glycosidic links (see also Figure 5 where these backbones are highlighted) and dihedral angles (deg.) between least-squares planes fitted through the ring atoms. Atom and ring labels are given in Figure 5; s.u.'s are included in parentheses. For comparison, the values for various other structures are included in the Table, see the legend of Figure 1 for details of the abbreviations used here.

Torsion Angles (deg)	FP	2GD4 1	2GD4 2	4R9W	4X7R 1	4X7R 2	NMR Solution
τ(O7–C1–O1–C10)	90.0(9)	101.4	101.4	69.5	96.4	95.5	76.9
τ(C1–O1–C10–C11)	−143.9(10)	−157.6	−158.0	−155.4	−128.2	−126.1	−151.4
τ(O17–C7–O12–C16)	−82.3(7)	−84.4	−84.3	−70.2	−94.6	−93.0	−55.2
τ(C7–O12–C16–C17)	−103.4(6)	−120.8	−121.0	−105.1	−100.5	−97.2	−111.0
τ(O30–C13–O18–C22)	88.5(7)	63.1	62.4	71.0	73.2	73.7	89.2
τ(C13–O18–C22–C23)	−145.9(6)	−157.0	−156.2	−132.0	−152.0	−146.2	−143.8
τ(O39–C19–O31–C28)	−72.0(7)	−67.8	−−67.5	−77.0	−65.2	−66.6	−73.0
τ(C19–O31–C28–C29)	−118.7(6)	−108.5	−108.7	−139.2	−106.8	−110.2	−134.0
Dihedral Angles (deg)	**FP**	**2GD4 1**	**2GD4 2**	**4R9W**	**4X7R 1**	**4X7R 2**	**NMR Solution**
χ (D,E)	57.4(5)	57.4	57.6	63.1	48.9	44.6	58.2
χ (D,H)	14.0(3)	71.3	71.4	31.7	13.6	12.7	30.3
χ (E,F)	57.3(5)	35.7	35.5	68.9	48.4	50.2	69.3
χ (F,G)	66.6(4)	78.8	78.8	89.7	69.7	72.2	84.0
χ (G,H)	39.3(4)	33.8	33.7	20.7	57.0	53.4	3.4

The intramolecular hydrogen bond between rings D and E, found in the Fondaparinux crystal structure, is also present in the co-crystal with antithrombin. In the latter, an even shorter donor-acceptor distance of 2.98 Å is found, suggesting a reasonably strong hydrogen bond. The intramolecular hydrogen bond between residues F and G (iduronic acid), found in the single-crystal structure of Fondaparinux, is not present in the pentasaccharide unit in the co-crystal. The conformational change of the iduronic acid to a twist-boat has moved the accepting sulfate out of reach of the sulfamido group. In the co-crystal, this sulfamido group rotated around the bond to which it is attached to the sugar ring so that an intramolecular hydrogen bond to the neighbouring sulfate group attached to the same sugar ring can be formed (donor-acceptor is 2.98 Å, also suggesting the presence of a reasonably strong intramolecular hydrogen bond).

The sulfamido groups play an important role in stabilizing the pentasaccharide molecule in a relatively linear conformation by forming two N-H...O intramolecular hydrogen bonds. The NH hydrogen of the sulfamido group in carbohydrate residue F is involved in an interresidue hydrogen bond to an oxygen of the 2-sulfate group residue G, as shown in Figure 5. This hydrogen bond is also found in solution [15]. Previously, in solution, an intraresidue hydrogen bond between the NH hydrogen of the sulfamido group in carbohydrate residue F and the adjacent 3-sulfo group [15,28] was found. This hydrogen bond is not observed in the crystal, possibly as a consequence of the different conformation of the iduronic acid G discussed above. Geometric details are given in Table 3.

Table 3. Geometric details of selected hydrogen bonds (Å, deg.). Standard uncertainties are given in parentheses (only available for *D*...*A* since H atoms were not freely refined). Hydrogen bond type refers to intramolecular or intermolecular hydrogen bonds. The listed hydrogen bonds are also indicated in Figure 5.

Involved Atoms	Type	*D*–H	H $\cdots$ *A*	*D* $\cdots$ *A*	*D*–H $\cdots$ *A*
N1–H1N $\cdots$ O14	intra	0.92	2.52	3.282(14)	141
N2–H2N $\cdots$ O32	intra	0.92	2.18	3.095(9)	172
N3–H3N $\cdots$ O2 ($x - 1, y, z - 1$)	inter	0.92	2.26	2.972(12)	134
O16–H16H $\cdots$ O76 (water)	inter	0.84	1.91	2.54(3)	131

Besides the items listed in Table 3, the crystal structure displays numerous hydrogen bonds, which further strengthen the infinite three-dimensional network formed by the pentasaccharide ions, sodium ions and water molecules. As can be expected in view of their acidic nature, all SO_3H groups are deprotonated, which is supported by the observed equality of the S–O bond lengths.

Interestingly, the geometry of the carboxylic acid group bonded to ring E strongly suggests a protonated, neutral acid group (d(C12–O15) = 1.09(2) Å, d(C12–O16) = 1.40(3) Å), in spite of the fact that the crystallization was carried out at neutral pH. Due to high anisotropic displacement parameters, the C–O distances appear shortened. The anisotropicity is also reflected by the accuracy of these bond lengths, which is significantly lower than that of similar bond lengths in other sections of the pentasaccharide anion. The presence of a hydrogen bond acceptor at hydrogen bonding distance from O16 (see Table 3) supports the model of a protonated acid group. However, the unfavorable value of the *D*–H $\cdots$ *A* angle (131 deg) does not suggest this is a particularly strong hydrogen bond.

The acid group bonded to ring G (iduronic acid) is deprotonated as expected, as is clearly shown by the similar lengths of the C–O bonds: d(C24–O37) = 1.242(11) Å and d(C24–O38) = 1.267(10) Å.

Based on the covalent angles between their substituents, the nitrogen atoms N1, N2 and N3 can be considered sp^3 hybridized, which is common for this type of group. The coordinates of the hydrogen atoms bonded to the nitrogen atoms were derived from the availability of hydrogen bond acceptors at reasonable distances from the nitrogen donor atoms (see "Crystal Structure Determination and Refinement").

Absolute Configuration

The Flack *x*-parameter and its standard uncertainty $u(x)$ can be used to assess absolute structure and absolute configuration [29,30]. A structure determination is considered to have strong inversion-distinguishing power if $u(x) < 0.04$. If the enantiopurity of a sample is certain, a less strict criterion is applied. When $u(x) < 0.08$, the experiment is considered to have enantiopure sufficient inversion-distinguishing power. If one of these criteria is met, a numerical value of *x* that lies within statistical fluctuation of zero, i.e., $|x| < 2\,u(x)$, assures a valid absolute structure (and absolute configuration) determination from a single crystal which is not twinned by inversion. The cited criteria are taken from Flack and Bernardinelli [31].

In this study, a value of $-0.02(11)$ was found by classical fit to all intensities, which does not satisfy the criterion for enantiopure sufficient inversion-distinguishing power. However, as argued by Parsons et al. [32] anomalous dispersion differences can be obscured by other effects, such as absorption and extinction. If these effects are filtered out as proposed by these authors, and x-value of 0.017(14) is obtained, we can classify the current structure determination as having strong inversion-distinguishing power.

As a final alternative to assess the absolute configuration, the method of Hooft et al. [33] was considered. Using Bayesian statistics, these authors offer a method that gives reliable absolute structure determinations even in cases where only weak anomalous scatterers are present. According to this method, the probability that the absolute configuration was determined correctly is calculated to be 1.00, based on the assumption of an enantiopure sample. In case the measured crystal is a racemic twin, the twin ratio, expressed as the y-parameter, comparable to Flack's x-parameter, amounts to $-0.002(14)$, further confirming the correct assignment of the absolute configuration of the enantiopure sample.

4. Materials and Methods

4.1. General Information

4.1.1. Materials

The Fondaparinux standard was prepared from a commercially manufactured Fondaparinux batch and underwent an additional ion exchange chromatography purification. Maleic acid batches were obtained from Acros (Geel, Belgium; in 1999) or Fluka (St. Louis, MO, USA; Lot BCBV2002V, in 2016) and used as such. The content of the maleic acid batches of 99.61 (1999) and 99. 99% (2016) was taken from the Certificate of Analysis from the supplier. D_2O was used as a solvent since both Fondaparinux and the standard maleic acid are charged molecules and well soluble in water. 0.01% w/v TSP-d_4 was used as a chemical shift reference at 0 ppm. The 500 MHz 1D ^1H spectrum of Fondaparinux and maleic acid is displayed in Figure 1 including the D1, F1 and maleic acid proton integrals used for content determination.

From an ampoule of Fondaparinux standard solution, 0.5 mL was transferred into an Eppendorf and 0.5 mL of a 0.67 mg/mL maleic acid standard solution was added. After stirring, the content of the Eppendorf was then frozen in a dry-ice ethanol mixture and subsequently lyophilized (>8 h, $-50\,^{\circ}C$, <300 mbar). After lyophilizing 0.7 mL D_2O was added to the freeze-dried material and subsequently stirred until complete dissolution. The solution was then transferred into a NMR tube. Five determinations were performed by two different analysts on two different days.

4.1.2. Fondaparinux Crystallization

Fondaparinux (100 mg) was dissolved in 2.5 mL of demineralized water in a flat-bottomed flask or bottle. The temperature was increased to 70 $^{\circ}C$ to dissolve the material. 5.5 mL of ethanol at room temperature was slowly added while maintaining the temperature at 70 $^{\circ}C$ to saturate the solution (the solution became slightly turbid). The solution (or even slightly turbid mixture) was then cooled to RT. No stirring was applied.

The turbidity of the mixture increased under cooling. Over time, the turbidity decreased, and in turn, an oily liquid (or drops) was formed on the bottom of the flask. After a while, the oily drops changed and crystallized (this procedure was not an optimized process and it took weeks before crystallization occurred). Various crystallization experiments of Fondaparinux (maximum concentration 16 mg/mL) were successful with an ethanol content between 70% and 90%. In addition, when available, seeding crystals were used to speed up the crystallization process.

4.2. Methods

4.2.1. qNMR

Spectrum Acquisition and Processing

^{1}H-NMR spectra were recorded on a Bruker NMR spectrometer (Bruker BioSpin, Billerica, MA, USA) according to the settings in Table 4.

Table 4. Acquisition and processing settings of the qNMR experiment.

Acquisition	1999	2016
Spectral frequency	400 MHz	500 MHz
Probe	5 mm QNP probe	TCI Cryo Probe
Temperature	25 °C/298 K	
Spinning	20 Hz	Off
Flip angle	60°	
Relaxation delay	30 s	
Dummy scans	4	2
Number of scans	128	32
Number of data points	64 k	
Processing		
Exponential line-broadening	0.5 Hz	0.3 Hz
Zero-Filling	64 k	132 k

The recorded spectra were manually phased and baseline corrected, and the signals of maleic acid and the anomeric protons D1 and F1 (indicated in red in Figure 1) were integrated as described in the protocol. The content of Fondaparinux in an ampoule was then calculated according to the formula: $C_{FP} = W_{MA}/V_{FP} \times I_{FP}/I_{MA} \times MW_{FP}/MW_{MA} \times P_{MA}/P_{FP}$ where C_{FP} = concentration of Fondaparinux in the ampoule, W_{MA} = weight of maleic acid (=concentration stock solution (mg/mL) × 0.5 mL); V_{FP} = volume of Fondaparinux taken from the ampoule (typically 0.5 mL); I_{FP} = integral of selected signals of Fondaparinux; I_{MA} = integral of maleic acid set at 2.0000 for each sample MW_{FP} = molecular weight of Fondaparinux (1728.088); MW_{MA} = molecular weight of maleic acid (116.07); P_{MA} = purity of maleic acid (99.99%); P_{FP} = purity of Fondaparinux (assumed to be 100%). The determination was performed in fivefold by two technicians on two different days and the average Fondaparinux content (mg/mL) was reported including the standard deviation and the relative standard deviation (RSD).

4.3. XRPD

X-ray powder diffractograms were obtained on a Miniflex600 diffractometer (Rikagu, Tokyo, Japan) using the settings listed in Table 5 below.

Table 5. XRPD settings.

XRPD Settings	
X-ray	40 kV, 15 mA
Goniometer	MiniFlex 600
Wavelength	Cu K$_\alpha$ (1.541 Å)
Filter	K$_\beta$ (Ni)
Scan speed/Duration time	2.0000 deg/min
Step width	0.0200 deg
Scan axis	θ/2-θ
Scan range	3.0000–40.0000 °C ambient
Temperature	Ambient

4.4. Crystal Structure Determination and Refinement

A colorless, block-shaped crystal of approximate dimensions $0.10 \times 0.20 \times 0.20$ cm was fixed to the tip of a glass capillary and transferred into the cold nitrogen stream on a kappa-CCD diffractometer (Bruker-Nonius, Billerica, MA, USA) on rotating anode. Raw data were reduced with DENZO [34]. Crystal data and details on data collection and refinement are presented in Table 6.

Table 6. Crystallographic data. Unit cell parameters are listed in Table 5.

Crystal Data	
Formula	$[C_{31}H_{44}N_3O_{49}S_8]9^- \cdot 9Na^+ \cdot 32H_2O$
Molecular weight	2282.60
Crystal system	monoclinic
Space group	$P2_1$ (No.4)
D_{calc}, g cm^{-3}	1.784
Z	2
$F(000)$	2380
μ (Mo$K\alpha$), mm^{-1}	0.401
Crystal size	$0.2 \times 0.3 \times 0.3$
Data collection	
T, K	150
θ_{min}, θ_{max}, deg	1.00, 27.49
Wavelength (Mo$K\alpha$), Å	0.71073 (graphite monochromated)
Distance crystal to detector, mm	45
X-ray exposure time, h	7.0
Refined mosaicity, deg	0.914(1)
Data set (hkl-range)	-13:13, -29:29, -24:24
Completeness at sin $\theta/\lambda = 0.6$ Å^{-1}	100.0% (no refl. missing)
Total data	81362 ($R_\sigma = 0.0498$)
Total unique data	19366 ($R_{int} = 0.0396$)
Refinement	
No. of refined parameters	1114
$wR2$	0.2211
R	0.0786 [for 16915 $F_o > 4\sigma(F_o)$]
S	1.041
w^{-1}	$\sigma^2(F^2) + (0.1328P)^2 + 11.21P$
$(\Delta/\sigma)_{av}$, $(\Delta/\sigma)_{max}$	<0.0001, 0.0002
$\Delta\rho_{min}$, $\Delta\rho_{max}$, e Å^{-3}	-0.84, 1.87 (near Na)

The unit-cell parameters were checked for the presence of higher lattice symmetry [35]. Data were not corrected for absorption. The structure was solved by automated direct methods (SHELXS86 [36]). Refinement on F^2 was carried out by full-matrix, least-squares techniques (SHELXL 2016-6 [37]); no observance criterion was applied during refinement. Two of the sodium ions and some of the water molecules coordinated with one of these sodium ions were found to be disordered. A disorder model with two positions for each of the atoms involved was introduced. The two sites for each sodium atom are close to each other. The site occupation factor of the major component refined to 0.502(11) for Na7 and 0.549(17) for Na9 and associated disordered water molecules. All hydrogen atoms were included in the refinement on calculated positions riding on their carrier atoms. The methyl hydrogen atoms and the hydroxyl hydrogen atoms were refined as rigid groups, allowing for rotation around the C–O bonds. Starting positions of the methyl hydrogen were derived from a difference Fourier map. The hydrogen atoms of the non-coordinated water solvent molecules could not be located on difference Fourier maps. Furthermore, the coordinates of these atoms could not be derived unambiguously from the distribution of potential hydrogen bond donors and acceptors. Most likely, there is extensive disorder in the hydrogen atoms of the non-coordinated water molecules. Displacement parameters of the oxygen atoms of the non-coordinated water molecules indicate that there is a slight disorder in their positions as well. Therefore, no further attempts were made to include these hydrogen atoms in the atomic model. All ordered non-hydrogen atoms were refined with anisotropic atomic displacement parameters. Atoms in the major disorder component were refined with isotropic displacement parameters, which were coupled to the isotropic displacement parameters of the related atoms in the minor component. Hydrogen atoms were refined with fixed isotropic displacement parameters related to the value of the equivalent isotropic displacement parameters of their carrier atoms by a factor of 1.5 for methyl, hydroxyl and water hydrogen atoms, and 1.2 for all other hydrogen atoms.

The Flack x-parameter [29], derived during the final structure-factor calculation, amounts to $-0.02(11)$ by classical fit to all intensities and $0.017(14)$ from 7033 selected quotients (Parsons' method, [32]). Refinement of the inverse absolute structure resulted in an x-parameter of $1.04(11)$ (value derived during final structure-factor calculation). Figures of merit for this inverted structure are $R1 = 0.0791$, $wR2 = 0.2223$ (weighting scheme not optimized) and $S = 1.0$. Refinement of a racemic twin model gave a twin ratio of reported versus inverted structure of $1.00(11):0.00$; the twin model was therefore not used.

Neutral atom scattering factors and anomalous dispersion corrections were taken from the International Tables for Crystallography [38]. Geometrical calculations and illustration were performed with PLATON [39].

Unit Cell Determination

At $T = 150$ K, a data set was collected, consisting of a scan of 20 deg of φ divided into 20 image frames, using MoKα-radiation ($\lambda = 0.71073$ Å). The unit cell was determined using DENZO [28]. Results are summarized in Table 7.

Table 7. Unit cell parameters of Fondaparinux determined for the single-crystal study, the cell check of a second batch, and the powder diffraction study. In all cases systematic absences indicate the space group is $P2_1$. s.u.'s are included in parentheses.

	Single Crystal (DW1623B)	Cell Check (DW1637A)	Powder
a, Å	10.0296(2)	10.0132(18)	10.144(3)
b, Å	23.0353(6)	23.067(5)	22.992(5)
c, Å	18.9666(7)	18.820(3)	18.626(6)
β, deg	104.1420(14)	103.731(2)	102.65(2)
V, Å^3	4249.1(2)	4222.6(2)	4238.8(4)
Refined mosaicity, deg	0.914(1)	1.626(9)	-
T, K	150	150	ambient

5. Conclusions

Both Fondaparinux structure (X-ray) and content (qNMR) have been addressed in this paper. The content of ampoules of a Fondaparinux solution standard was determined using qNMR. For consistency, the ability to assess the long-term stability of the content of the standard is crucial since the standard content is used to determine the content of Fondaparinux batches. The 2016 analysis yielded a content of 9.75 mg/mL (SD 0.06 mg/mL) whereas the analysis performed in 1999 yielded a content of 9.64 mg/mL (SD of 0.08 mg/mL). qNMR shows remarkable precision over time, instrumentation and analysts, pivotal for consistent content determination.

The determination of the single crystal X-ray structure including the absolute configuration of Fondaparinux crystals allowed an unequivocal proof of structure. The iduronic acid residue in the uncomplexed Fondaparinux adopts a chair conformation heavily distorted towards a half chair. Interestingly, this iduronic acid conformation was also found in the complex of heparin with wall teichoic acid transferase according to the coordinates published [8]. The iduronic acid conformation also provides solid evidence of the thermodynamic accessibility of this chair conformation of iduronic acid within a pentasaccharide, (and thereby helps to extend our knowledge of the available conformational space).

Supplementary Materials: Supplementary materials are available online.CCDC 1553209 contains the supplementary crystallographic data for this paper. These data can be obtained free of charge via http://www.ccdc.cam.ac.uk/conts/retrieving.html (or from the CCDC, 12 Union Road, Cambridge CB2 1EZ, UK; Fax: +44 1223 336033; E-mail: deposit@ccdc.cam.ac.uk).

Acknowledgments: The authors would like to thank Leendert van den Bos, Arno Bode and Marketta Uusi-Penttilä for carefully reading the manuscript and stimulating discussion. Judica Bootsma and Ineke Huiberts-Eeuwijk are thanked for their expert technical assistance and useful discussions. Anthony L. Spek is acknowledged for consultancy regarding the crystal structure determination. Cynthia Larive and Andrew Green made available the coordinates of their Fondaparinux solution structure [28] to us. The authors would also like to thank the referees for their critical comments and suggestions which helped us to considerably improve the original manuscript.

Author Contributions: C.F., F.K. and E.K. conceived and designed the experiments; W.d.W., M.L., A.L., H.K. and E.K. performed the experiments; H.K., B.Ü. and E.K. analyzed the data; E.K. and H.K. wrote the paper.

Conflicts of Interest: B.Ü., W.d.W., M.L., A.L. and E.K. hold positions in Aspen which commercially manufactures Fondaparinux.

References

1. Petitou, M.; van Boeckel, C.A.A. A synthetic antithrombin III binding pentasaccharide is now a drug! What comes next? *Angew. Chem. Int. Ed.* **2004**, *43*, 3118–3133. [CrossRef] [PubMed]

2. Giangrande, P.L. Fondaparinux (Arixtra): A new anticoagulant. *Int. J. Clin. Pract.* **2002**, *56*, 615–617. [PubMed]

3. Tan, K.; Duquette, M.; Liu, J.H.; Zhang, R.; Joachimiak, A.; Wang, J.H.; Lawler, J. The structures of the thrombospondin-1 N-terminal domain and its complex with a synthetic pentameric heparin. *Structure* **2006**, *14*, 33–42. [CrossRef] [PubMed]

4. Tan, K.; Duquette, M.; Liu, J.-H.; Shanmugasundaram, K.; Joachimiak, A.; Gallagher, J.T.; Rigby, A.C.; Wang, J.H.; Lawler, J. Heparin-induced *cis*- and *trans*-dimerization modes of the thrombospondin-1 N-terminal domain. *J. Biol. Chem.* **2008**, *283*, 3932–3941. [CrossRef] [PubMed]

5. Johnson, D.J.; Li, W.; Adams, T.E.; Huntington, J.A. Antithrombin–S195A factor Xa-heparin structure reveals the allosteric mechanism of antithrombin activation. *EMBO J.* **2006**, *25*, 2029–2037. [CrossRef] [PubMed]

6. Langdown, J.; Belzar, K.J.; Savory, W.J.; Baglin, T.P.; Huntington, J.A. The critical role of hinge-region expulsion in the induced-fit heparin binding mechanism of antithrombin. *J. Mol. Biol.* **2009**, *386*, 1278–1289. [CrossRef] [PubMed]

7. Cai, Z.; Yarovoi, S.V.; Zhu, Z.; Rauova, L.; Hayes, V.; Lebedeva, T.; Greene, M.I. Atomic description of the immune complex involved in heparin-induced thrombocytopenia. *Nat. Commun.* **2015**, *6*, 8277. [CrossRef] [PubMed]

8. Sobhanifar, S.; Worrall, L.J.; Gruninger, R.J.; Wasney, G.A.; Blaukopf, M.; Baumann, M.; Lameignere, E.; Solomonson, M.; Brown, E.D.; Withers, S.G.; et al. Structure and mechanism of Staphylococcus aureus TarM, the wall teichoic acid α-glycosyltransferase. *Proc. Natl. Acad. Sci. USA* **2015**, *112*, E576–E585. [CrossRef] [PubMed]

9. Li, W.; Johnson, D.J.; Esmon, C.T.; Huntington, J.A. Structure of the antithrombin–thrombin–heparin ternary complex reveals the antithrombotic mechanism of heparin. *Nat. Struct. Mol. Boil.* **2004**, *11*, 857–862. [CrossRef] [PubMed]

10. Jin, L.; Abrahams, J.P.; Skinner, R.; Petitou, M.; Pike, R.N.; Carrell, R.W. The anticoagulant activation of antithrombin by heparin. *Proc. Natl. Acad. Sci. USA* **1997**, *94*, 14683–14688. [CrossRef] [PubMed]

11. Ferro, D.R.; Provasoli, A.; Ragazzi, M.; Torri, G.; Casu, B.; Gatti, G.; Jacquinet, J.C.; Sinay, P.; Petitou, M.; Choay, J. Evidence for conformational equilibrium of the sulfated L-iduronate residue in heparin and in synthetic heparin mono-and oligo-saccharides: NMR and force-field studies. *J. Am. Chem. Soc.* **1986**, *108*, 6773–6778. [CrossRef]

12. Ragazzi, M.; Ferro, D.R.; Perly, B.; Sinaÿ, P.; Petitou, M.; Choay, J. Conformation of the pentasaccharide corresponding to the binding site of heparin for antithrombin III. *Carbohydr. Res.* **1990**, *195*, 169–185. [CrossRef]

13. Remko, M.; von der Lieth, C.W. Conformational structure of some trimeric and pentameric structural units of heparin. *J. Phys. Chem. A* **2007**, *111*, 13484–13491. [CrossRef] [PubMed]

14. Remko, M.; Van Duijnen, P.T.; Broer, R. Molecular structure of basic oligomeric building units of heparan-sulfate glycosaminoglycans. *Struct. Chem.* **2010**, *21*, 965–976. [CrossRef]
15. Hricovíni, M. Solution structure of heparin pentasaccharide: NMR and DFT analysis. *J. Phys. Chem. B* **2015**, *119*, 12397–12409. [CrossRef] [PubMed]
16. Hricovíni, M.; Guerrini, M.; Bisio, A.; Torri, G.; Petitou, M.; Casu, B. Conformation of heparin pentasaccharide bound to antithrombin III. *Biochem. J.* **2001**, *359*, 265–272. [CrossRef] [PubMed]
17. Yang, Q.; Qiu, H.; Guo, W.; Wang, D.; Zhou, X.; Xue, D.; Zhang, J.; Wu, S.; Wang, Y. Quantitative ^{1}H-NMR method for the determination of Tadalafil in bulk drugs and its tablets. *Molecules* **2015**, *20*, 12114–12124. [CrossRef] [PubMed]
18. Holzgrabe, U. Quantitative NMR Spectroscopy in Pharmaceutical R & D. In *eMagRes*; Wiley: Hoboken, NJ, USA, 2015.
19. Holzgrabe, U. *NMR Spectroscopy in Pharmaceutical Analysis*; Iwona, W., Bernd, D., Eds.; Elsevier: Amsterdam, The Netherlands, 2011; Charter 5; pp. 131–137.
20. United States Pharmacopoeia. *General Chapter <761> Nuclear Magnetic Resonance*; United States Pharmacopoeia Convention Inc.: Rockville, USA, 2017.
21. European Pharmacopoeia. *General Chapter 2.2.33. Nuclear Magnetic Resonance Spectrometry*; Council of Europe: Strasbourg, France, 2017.
22. Goda, Y. Introduction of qNMR to the Japanese Pharmacopoeia (JP) for specification of marker compounds used for standardization of herbal medicines. *Planta Medica.* **2013**, *79*, SL79. [CrossRef]
23. Torri, G.; Casu, B.; Gatti, G.; Petitou, M.; Choay, J.; Jacquinet, J.C.; Sinay, P. Mono-and bidimensional 500 MHz ^{1}H-NMR spectra of a synthetic pentasaccharide corresponding to the binding sequence of heparin to antithrombin-III: Evidence for conformational peculiarity of the sulfated iduronate residue. *Biochem. Biophys. Res. Commun.* **1985**, *128*, 134–140. [CrossRef]
24. Casu, B.; Petitou, M.; Provasoli, M.; Sinay, P. Conformational flexibility: A new concept for explaining binding and biological properties of iduronic acid-containing glycosaminoglycans. *Trends Biochem. Sci.* **1988**, *13*, 221–225. [CrossRef]
25. Casu, B.; Guerrini, M.; Torri, G. Structural and conformational aspects of the anticoagulant and antithrombotic activity of heparin and dermatan sulfate. *Curr. Pharm. Des.* **2004**, *10*, 939–949. [CrossRef] [PubMed]
26. Rudd, T.R.; Skidmore, M.A.; Guerrini, M.; Hricovini, M.; Powell, A.K.; Siligardi, G.; Yates, E.A. The conformation and structure of GAGs: Recent progress and perspectives. *Curr. Opin. Struct. Biol.* **2010**, *20*, 567–574. [CrossRef] [PubMed]
27. Boeyens, J.C. The conformation of six-membered rings. *J. Cryst. Mol. Struct.* **1978**, *8*, 317–320. [CrossRef]
28. Langeslay, D.J.; Young, R.P.; Beni, S.; Beecher, C.N.; Mueller, L.J.; Larive, C.K. Sulfamate proton solvent exchange in heparin oligosaccharides: Evidence for a persistent hydrogen bond in the antithrombin-binding pentasaccharide Arixtra. *Glycobiology* **2012**, *22*, 1173–1182. [CrossRef] [PubMed]
29. Flack, H.D. On enantiomorph-polarity estimation. *Acta. Crystallogr. Sect. A* **1983**, *39*, 876–881. [CrossRef]
30. Flack, H.D.; Gérald, B. Absolute structure and absolute configuration. *Acta. Crystallogr. Sect. A* **1999**, *55*, 908–915. [CrossRef]
31. Flack, H.D.; Bernardinelli, G. Reporting and evaluating absolute-structure and absolute-configuration determinations. *J. Appl. Crystallogr.* **2000**, *33*, 1143–1148. [CrossRef]
32. Parsons, S.; Howard, D.F.; Trixie, W. Use of intensity quotients and differences in absolute structure refinement. *Acta. Crystallogr. Sect. B* **2013**, *69*, 249–259. [CrossRef] [PubMed]
33. Hooft, R.W.; Straver, L.H.; Spek, A.L. Determination of absolute structure using Bayesian statistics on Bijvoet differences. *J. Appl. Crystallogr.* **2008**, *41*, 96–103. [CrossRef] [PubMed]
34. Otwinowski, Z.; Minor, W. Processing of X-ray diffraction data collected in oscillation mode. *Methods Enzymol.* **1997**, *276*, 307–326. [PubMed]
35. Spek, A.L. LEPAGE—An MS-DOS program for the determination of the metrical symmetry of a translation lattice. *J. Appl. Crystallogr.* **1988**, *21*, 578–579. [CrossRef]
36. Sheldrick, G.M. *SHELXS86, Program for Crystal Structure Determination*; University of Gottingen: Gottingen, Germany, 1986.
37. Sheldrick, G.M. Crystal structure refinement with SHELXL. *Acta. Crystallogr. Sect. C* **2015**, *71*, 3–8. [CrossRef] [PubMed]

38. Wilson, A.J.C. (Ed.) *International Tables for Crystallography: Mathematical, Physical, and Chemical Tables*; International Union of Crystallography: Chester, UK, 1992; Volume 3.
39. Spek, A.L. Structure validation in chemical crystallography. *Acta. Crystallogr. Sect. D* **2009**, *65*, 148–155. [CrossRef] [PubMed]

Sample Availability: Samples of Fondaparinux are available from the authors.

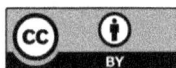

molecules

MDPI

Article

A Fluorescent Probe for Glycosaminoglycans Applied to the Detection of Dermatan Sulfate by a Mix-and-Read Assay

Melissa Rappold, Ulrich Warttinger and Roland Krämer *

Inorganic Chemistry Institute, Heidelberg University, Im Neuenheimer Feld 270, 69120 Heidelberg, Germany; melissa.rappold@aci.uni-heidelberg.de (M.R.); ulrich.warttinger@aci.uni-heidelberg.de (U.W.)
* Correspondence: kraemer@aci.uni-heidelberg.de; Tel.: +49-6221-54-8438; Fax: +49-6221-54-8599

Academic Editors: Giangiacomo Torri and Jawed Fareed
Received: 12 April 2017; Accepted: 2 May 2017; Published: 9 May 2017

Abstract: Glycosaminoglycans are complex biomolecules of great biological and medical importance. The quantification of glycosaminoglycans, in particular in complex matrices, is challenging due to their inherent structural heterogeneity. Heparin Red, a polycationic, fluorescent perylene diimide derivative, has recently emerged as a commercial probe for the convenient detection of heparins by a mix-and-read fluorescence assay. The probe also detects glycosaminoglycans with a lower negative charge density than heparin, although with lower sensitivity. We describe here the synthesis and characterization of a structurally related molecular probe with a higher positive charge of +10 (vs. +8 of Heparin Red). The superior performance of this probe is exemplified by the quantification of low dermatan sulfate concentrations in an aqueous matrix (quantification limit 1 ng/mL) and the detection of dermatan sulfate in blood plasma in a clinically relevant concentration range. The potential applications of this probe include monitoring the blood levels of dermatan sulfate after administration as an antithrombotic drug in the absence of heparin and other glycosaminoglycans.

Keywords: perylene diimide dyes; dermatan sulfate; fluorescent probe; Heparin Red; assay; dermatan sulfate; human plasma

1. Introduction

Glycosaminoglycans are complex biomolecules of great biological and medical importance. They are composed of linear, polydisperse polysaccharides with a highly variable sulfation pattern (with the exception of hyaluronate, which is not sulfated). This structural heterogeneity makes the quantification of glycosaminoglycans challenging. There is a continuous search for more convenient, precise and sensitive quantification methods, in particular for complex biological matrices. Various molecular probes for the direct optical detection of glycosaminoglycans (mainly of heparin, a widely-used antithrombotic drug) have been described [1]. Such probes enable convenient detection by photometry or fluorimetry, although their performance in complex biological matrices is often limited by interference. The fluorescent probe **Heparin Red** has recently emerged as a component of commercially available assays for the quantification of heparins in various matrices [2–4]. It is implemented in several drug development projects for the pharmacokinetic monitoring of non-anticoagulant heparins, a promising class of drug candidates [5]. **Heparin Red** is a polyamine modified, red-emissive perylene diimide fluorophore (Scheme 1, right).

It forms a supramolecular aggregate with glycosaminoglycans, resulting in contact quenching of fluorescence (Scheme 2). The strong binding of the polycationic probe to polyanionic heparin appears to be controlled by both electrostatic and aromatic π-stacking interactions [6]. While electrostatic repulsion between dye molecules prevents spontaneous aggregation in the solution, the charge neutralization by polyanionic heparin favors the formation of π-stacked complexes between the hydrophobic chromophore moieties in the ground state, leading to efficient static quenching. **Heparin Red** has also been applied to the determination of polysaccharides, such as heparan sulfate [7] and fucoidan [8], that have a lower negative charge density than heparin, but the sensitivity in a plasma matrix is significantly lower. An ultrasensitive assay with a quantification limit in the pg/mL range for the highly sulfated polysaccharide dextran sulfate in an aqueous matrix has also been described [9].

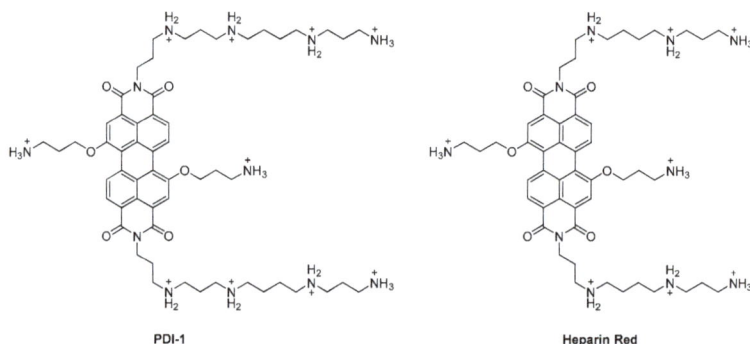

PDI-1   Heparin Red

Scheme 1. Molecular structures of the probes **PDI-1** and **Heparin Red** in their fully protonated state (charge +10 and +8, respectively).

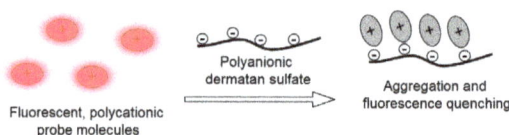

Fluorescent, polycationic probe molecules

Polyanionic dermatan sulfate

Aggregation and fluorescence quenching

Scheme 2. Schematic representation of fluorescence quenching of polycationic probe molecules in the presence of dermatan sulfate due to the formation of non-fluorescent aggregates.

Dermatan sulfate is a linear, polydisperse sulfated polysaccharide belonging to the glycosamino-glycan family. It is built of a major repeating disaccharide unit consisting of iduronic acid and galactosamine (Scheme 3). The galactosamine may be 4-*O* or 6-*O*-sulfated and the iduronic acid is 2-*O*-sulfated. Typically, the average degree of sulfation is around one per disaccharide. Dermatan sulfate is the predominant glycosaminoglycan expressed in the skin and is released at high concentrations during wound repair. It is also implicated in other biological processes [10], such as development, growth, infection, tumorigenesis and coagulation [11]. Elevated dermatan sulfate levels in plasma or urine have been suggested as a biomarker for certain types of mucopolysaccharidosis [12]. Dermatan sulfate-based drug formulations have been launched for the prevention of venous thromboembolism in Italy (marketed as Mistral) [13] and Portugal (marketed as Venorix). It is also a component of Sulodexide, a more widely-used antithrombotic agent [14]. Dermatan sulfate is produced by extraction from animal tissues, including a complex multistep purification process. The structural heterogeneity makes the direct quantification of dermatan sulfate in complex matrices such as human plasma challenging. Disaccharide analysis [15] provides both quantification and valuable information on dermatan sulfate structure, but involves tedious multistep protocols with sample pretreatment. In clinical settings, dermatan sulfate blood levels are indirectly monitored by coagulation assays [16].

We describe here the direct determination of dermatan sulfate in aqueous and plasma matrices by a new fluorescent probe, **PDI-1** (Scheme 1). The latter is structurally related to **Heparin Red** but has a higher positive molecular charge (+10 vs. +8 for Heparin Red). The enhanced performance of this probe is demonstrated by the determination of dermatan sulfate at low concentrations and in a competitive human plasma matrix.

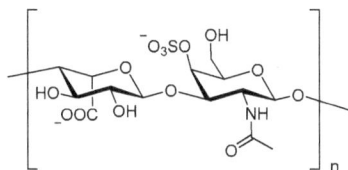

Scheme 3. Major iduronic acid-galactosamine repeating disaccharide unit of dermatan sulfate, mono-sulfated form. The sulfation pattern is variable; possible sites of sulfation are galactosamine 4-*O*, 6-*O* and iduronic acid 2-*O*. The disaccharide moiety may be unsulfated, mono- or disulfated.

2. Results and Discussion

2.1. Synthesis and Properties of the Polyamine-Functionalized Perylene Diimide Probe **PDI-1**

The synthesis of **PDI-1** is described by Scheme 4. A tetra-Boc-protected form of the pentaamine 1,5,9,14,18-pentaza-octadecane was prepared based on a procedure described in the literature [17], and combined with 1,7-dibromoperylene-3,4:9,10-tetracarboxylic acid dianhydride [18] in refluxing toluene to the perylene diimide derivative **PDI-3**. The latter was reacted further with 3-(*N*-Boc)-aminopropanol in tetrahydrofuran, using the base lithium diisopropylamide for the deprotonation of the OH-group; nucleophilic aromatic substitution of bromide led to the fully N-protected intermediate **PDI-4**. The deprotection of **PDI-4** in MeOH/HCl, purification by semi-preparative high-performance liquid chromatography (HPLC) using aqueous trifluoroacetic acid-acetonitrile as an eluent and exchange of the trifluoroacetate counterion with chloride by precipitation from acetonitrile gave the target compound [**PDI-1**]Cl$_{10}$. The probe was characterized by ^{1}H- and ^{13}C-NMR spectroscopy, electrospray mass spectrometry, UV-Vis spectroscopy, fluorimetry and analytical HPLC. The photophysical properties such as visible absorbance and fluorescence spectra ($\lambda_{max\,(Abs)}$ = 576 nm, ε (576 nm) = 35,300 M^{-1} cm^{-1}), λ_{max} = 615 nm, quantum yield ϕ_F = 0.17) in a buffered aqueous medium (pH 7) of **PDI-1** are very similar to those of **Heparin Red**.

2.2. Detection of Dermatan Sulfate in Aqueous Samples

The response of the probes to dermatan sulfate is controlled by the detection medium; while a high proportion of dimethyl sulfoxide (DMSO) suppresses any response [4], the assay becomes sensitive to dermatan sulfate at a high proportion of water. All detections were performed with spiked samples using commercially available dermatan sulfate sodium salt from porcine intestinal mucosa. A sulfation degree of 1.1 per disaccharide was calculated from the analytical data given in the certificate of the provider (S elemental analysis and water content), and refers to the repeating disaccharide unit given in Scheme 3. The resulting negative charge density per monosaccharide is −1.05, significantly lower in comparison to heparin (−1.7).

Figure 1 shows the titration of 1 μM solutions of the fluorescent probes **PDI-1** and **Heparin Red**, respectively, with dermatan sulfate in an aqueous buffer. A linear decrease of fluorescence intensity with increasing dermatan sulfate concentration was observed. To reach the endpoint of the titration, 19% more dermatan sulfate was needed in case of **PDI-1**. This is in line with the formation of charge neutral, fluorescence-quenched aggregates [6]. Since the charge of **PDI-1** in its fully protonated state is +10 but the fully protonated state of **Heparin Red** only +8, more dermatan sulfate is required for neutralization of the former. The experimental titration endpoints of 1.6 μg/mL for **Heparin Red** and 1.9 μg/mL for **PDI-1** were somewhat lower than the theoretical values of 1.7 and 2.2 μg/mL, respectively, due to the formation of charge-neutral aggregates. The probes may not be fully protonated in the aggregates under the specified conditions, since the proximity of the dye molecules (Scheme 1) could lower the pK_a value of the ammonium groups.

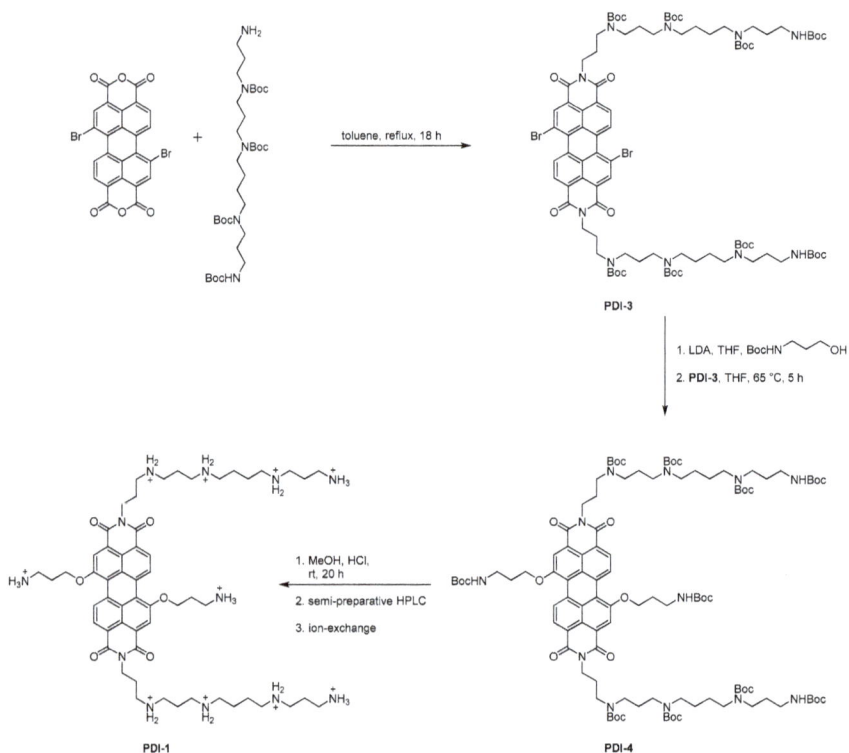

Scheme 4. Synthesis of probe **PDI-1**, chloride counterions not shown.

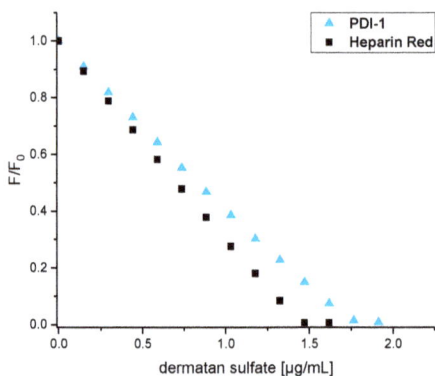

Figure 1. Normalized fluorescence response (F/F$_0$) of probes **PDI-1** and **Heparin Red** to dermatan sulfate. Excitation at 550 nm, fluorescence emission recorded at 610 nm. A solution of 1 μM probe in 10 mM MOPS pH 7 was placed into a polymethyl methacrylate (PMMA) cuvette and "titrated" with 10 μL aliquots of a 25 μg/mL dermatan sulfate solution.

We have recently described [9] a modified **Heparin Red** assay that enables the very sensitive quantification in the pg/mL range of the sulfated polysaccharide dextran sulfate in an aqueous matrix. The same protocol (see Materials and Methods for details) enables the highly sensitive detection of dermatan sulfate. Figure 2 compares the titration of a 1 nM solution of **PDI-1** and **Heparin Red**, respectively, with dermatan sulfate. Interestingly, less dermatan sulfate is required for the quenching of probe **PDI-1** under these conditions. The dermatan sulfate/**PDI-1** ratio at the titration endpoint is higher compared with the titration in Figure 1. Apparently, excess dermatan sulfate is needed to shift the equilibrium towards the aggregate at a low concentration of the components. This can only partly be interpreted with a protonation of the carboxylate groups of dermatan sulfate under the assay conditions (5 mM HCl), which may lead to a lower charge density of -0.5 per monosaccharide. Interestingly, even more dermatan sulfate is required for the quenching of **Heparin Red**. This, in contrast to the results in Figure 1, indicates a significantly higher stability of the **PDI-1**-dermatan sulfate aggregates.

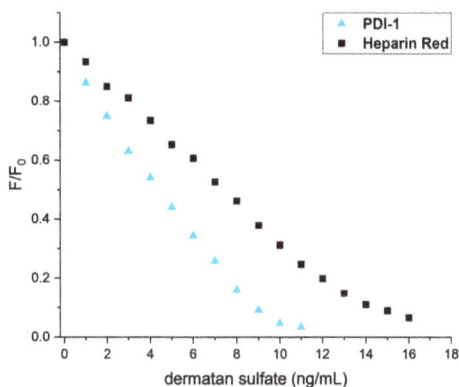

Figure 2. Normalized fluorescence response (F/F_0) of **PDI-1** and **Heparin Red** to dermatan sulfate. Excitation at 570 nm, fluorescence emission recorded at 610 nm. 2.5 mL water and 0.5 mL probe solution (6 nM in DMSO/30 mM HCl) were mixed in a polystyrene cuvette and the mixture was "titrated" with 5 µL aliquots of a 500 ng/mL dermatan sulfate solution. The indicated dermatan sulfate concentration does not correspond to the actual concentration in the reaction mixture (3 mL) but is related to the 2.5 mL aqueous portion.

Pooled normal plasma was spiked with dermatan sulfate and the standard protocol for heparin detection by the **Heparin Red** Kit was applied (Figure 3). Obviously, **PDI-1** responded more strongly than **Heparin Red** to the analyte, with about 50% fluorescence quenching at 10 µg/mL. At higher dermatan sulfate levels, the response curve flattens, possibly due to the partial, tight association of the probe with specific plasma components. Apparently, **PDI-1** forms stronger complexes with dermatan sulfate than **Heparin Red** in the human plasma matrix, and detects dermatan sulfate in the clinically relevant concentration range of 1–10 µg/mL. Like **Heparin Red**, **PDI-1** is not selective for dermatan sulfate but also responds strongly to heparin (data not shown), and interference by other glycosaminoglycans that have a similar or higher sulfation degree than dermatan sulfate is expected. A potential application of this probe is the monitoring of blood levels of dermatan sulfate after administration as an antithrombotic drug. Endogenous plasma levels of glycosaminoglycans are too low for significant interference. Only chondroitin sulfate may reach low µg/mL levels but, is present in an undersulfated form [19,20] that does not respond to **Heparin Red** in a plasma matrix.

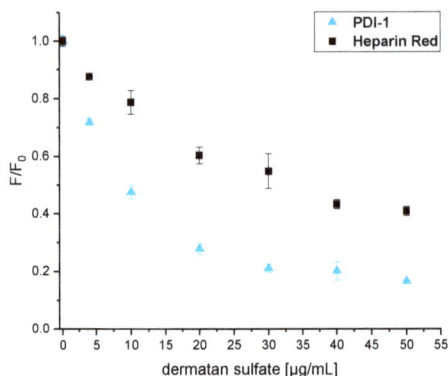

Figure 3. Normalized dose response (F/F_0) curves of **PDI-1** and **Heparin Red** to dermatan sulfate in human plasma. Spiked pooled normal plasma samples. Manually performed microplate assay was conducted, following the protocol of the supplier for the Heparin Red Kit (using 100-µM solutions of either **Heparin Red** or **PDI-1**). Excitation at 570 nm, fluorescence emission at 605 nm. Averages of duplicate determinations; error bars show standard deviation.

3. Materials and Methods

3.1. Chemicals and Reagents

Chemicals used for the synthesis were obtained from Sigma-Aldrich (Taufkirchen, Germany), Merck (Darmstadt, Germany), Acros (Nidderau, Germany), Apollo Scientific (Stockport, UK) or from the central warehouse of Heidelberg University in 95% purity or higher and were used without further purification.

Thin layer chromatography (TLC) was performed on POLYGRAM SIL G/UV$_{254}$ plates from Macherey-Nagel (Düren, Germany) and visualized by UV light. For flash chromatography, silica gel (40–63 µm, 60 Å pore size) from Macherey-Nagel (Düren, Germany) was used.

3.1.1. **Heparin Red** Kit

The **Heparin Red** Kit was a gift from Redprobes UG (Münster, Germany) [21]. Kit components included: **Heparin Red** solution (used for measurements shown in Figure 2), Product No. HR001, Lot 001-003, and Enhancer Solution, Product No. ES001, Lot 005. For the measurements shown in Figures 1 and 3, a solution of **Heparin Red**, synthesized as described in [22], was used.

3.1.2. Dermatan Sulfate

Dermatan sulfate sodium from porcine mucosa, product number C3788 (referred to as chondroitin sulfate B), batch SLBM9912V, was purchased from Sigma-Aldrich. According to the certificate of analysis of the provider, the batch contained 9% water, 6.5% S and 8.6% Na. Identity was confirmed by an ^{1}H-NMR spectrum in D$_2$O (see Supplementary Materials) and comparison with literature-reported spectra [23]. The lack of signals at >5 ppm indicates the absence of heparin and heparan sulfate. The N-Acetyl resonance and spiking experiments suggested that the sample may have contained minor impurities of chondroitin sulfate A and/or C [24].

3.1.3. Plasma

Pooled human normal plasma, applied as a matrix for the detections shown in Figure 3, was obtained from PrecisionBioLogic (Dartmouth, NS, Canada): Lot A1161, CRYOcheck. A 100 µg/mL stock solution of dermatan sulfate in plasma was prepared by mixing a 1 mg/mL aqueous dermatan sulfate solution with plasma in a volume ratio 1:9, followed by further dilution with plasma to the desired concentration. All samples were stored at $-20\,^{\circ}\text{C}$ for at least one day and up to several months, and were thawed at room temperature and vortexed before use.

3.1.4. Other

All aqueous solutions were prepared with HPLC grade water purchased from VWR (Bruchsal, Germany), product No. 23595.328. DMSO, product number 34869, Lot # STBF6384V, and hydrochloric acid (1.0 M), product number 35328, Lot # SZBF2050V, were purchased from Sigma-Aldrich.

3.2. Instrumentation

3.2.1. Analytics

Nuclear magnetic resonance spectra were recorded on a Bruker Avance III (600 MHz) spectrometer (Bruker Corporation, Billercia, MA, USA). Chemical shifts δ are given in ppm and coupling constants *J* in Hz. All spectra were recorded at 295 K and calibrated using the residual [1]H- or ^{13}C-signals of the deuterated solvents [25]. The following abbreviations were used to describe the multiplicities of the signals: s (singlet), d (doublet), m (multiplet), b (broad). Signals were assigned using COSY, HSQC and HMBC spectra. Mass spectra were recorded on a Bruker ApexQe Hybrid 9.4 FT-ICR (Bruker Corporation, Billercia, MA, USA). Semi-preparative and analytical HPLCs were performed on a Shimadzu HPLC system at 20 °C using a SPD-10Avp detector (semi-preparative) or a SPD-M20A Photodiode Array Detector (analytical), respectively. Water with 0.1% trifluoracetic acid and acetonitrile were used as eluents and C18 columns were used as the stationary phase. UV/Vis spectra were recorded on a Varian Cary 100 Bio UV/Vis and fluorescence-spectra on a Varian Cary Eclipse spectrometer (Varian Inc., Palo Alto, CA, USA) using 4.5 mL PMMA-cuvettes purchased from Sigma-Aldrich.

3.2.2. Fluorescence Measurements

Fluorescence in microplates was measured with the reader Biotek Synergy Mx (Biotek Instruments, Winooski, VT, USA), with an excitation at 570 nm, emission recorded at 605 nm, spectral band width 13.5–17 nm, gain 90–110, read height of 8 mm. Fluorescence in cuvettes was measured with either (Figure 1) Trilogy Laboratory Fluorimeter (Trilogy Modul RWT/PE, GUI Selection Green, excitation at 550 nm, emission recorded at 610 nm) or (Figure 2) the benchtop fluorimeter FluoroLog-3 (Horiba Scientific, Kyoto, Japan), with an excitation at 570 nm, emission recorded at 590–650 nm, integration time 0.4 s, average of 3 scans, and spectral band width Ex/Em 7 nm.

3.2.3. Microplates, Cuvettes, Pipettes

For fluorescence measurements, 96-well microplates, polystyrene, Item No. 655076, were purchased from Greiner Bio-One GmbH (Frickenhausen, Germany). Disposable PMMA cuvettes were used for absorbance or fluorescence measurements in aqueous medium. Disposable polystyrene fluorescence cuvettes were used for measurements in water/DMSO medium. Transferpette 0.5–10 µL, Transferpette-8 20–200 µL and Transferpette-12 20–200 µL, purchased from Brand GmbH (Wertheim, Germany). Rainin Pipettes 100–1000 µL, 20–200 µL, and 2–20 µL purchased from Mettler Toledo (Columbus, OH, USA).

3.3. Synthesis

To improve comprehensibility, simplified names were used for some synthesized compounds rather than using exact IUPAC names. 1,7-dibromoperylene-3,4:9,10-tetracarboxylic acid dianhydride [18], N^1,N^4,N^9,N^{13}-Tetra-*tert*-butyloxycarbonyl-1,16-diamino-4,9,13-triazahexadecane [17] and *N,N*'-Bis-(1-amino-4,9-diiazadodecyl)-1,7-di-(1-amino-3-hydroxypropyl)-perylene-3,4:9,10-tetracarboxydiimide

(**Heparin Red**) [2,26] were prepared according to literature-reported methods which were slightly modified [22].

3.3.1. Synthesis of *N*,*N*'-Bis-(N^1,N^4,N^9,N^{13}-tetra-*tert*-butyloxycarbonyl-1-amino-4,9,13- triazahexadecyl)-1,7-dibromperylene-3,4:9,10-tetracarboxylic acid bisimide **PDI-3**

N^1,N^4,N^9,N^{13}-Tetra-*tert*-butyloxycarbonyl-1,16-diamino-4,9,13-triazahexadecane (600 mg, 909 µmol) was dissolved in anhydrous toluene (20 mL) prior to the addition of 1,7-dibromoperylene-3,4:9,10-tetracarboxylic acid dianhydride (227 mg, 413 µmol). The reaction mixture was stirred under reflux for 18 h. Insoluble residues were removed by filtration. The filtrate was evaporated to dryness and the crude product was purified by column chromatography (SiO$_2$, CH$_2$Cl$_2$:MeOH—98:2). Compound **PDI-3** was isolated as a red powder (302 mg, 165 µmol, 40%). R_f (CH$_2$Cl$_2$:MeOH—95:5) 0.50; ^{1}H-NMR (600.13 MHz, CDCl$_3$): δ (ppm) = 9.50 (d, $^3J_{\text{H-H}}$ = 8.17 Hz, 2H, perylene-H), 8.92 (s, 2H, perylene-H), 8.71 (d, $^3J_{\text{H-H}}$ = 8.17 Hz, 2H, perylene-H), 4.17–4.27 (m, 4H, CH$_2$), 3.31–3.40 (m, 4H, CH$_2$), 3.07–3.26 (m, 24H, CH$_2$), 1.95–2.03 (m, 4H, CH$_2$), 1.73–1.83 (m, 4H, CH$_2$), 1.62–1.69 (m, 4H, CH$_2$), 1.50–1.53 (m, 8H, CH$_2$), 1.41–1.46 (m, 72H, Boc-H); ^{13}C{^{1}H}-NMR (150.91 MHz, CDCl$_3$): δ (ppm) = 138.0, 130.2, 128.6, 46.6, 44.8, 43.8, 38.6, 37.5, 28.5, 28.4, 27.6, 27.0, 25.8; MS (HR-ESI$^+$): m/z = 1853.7890 [M + Na]$^+$, calculated for C$_{90}$H$_{132}$^{79}Br$_2$N$_{10}$NaO$_{20}$$^+$: 1853.7878, m/z = 1831.8037 [M + H]$^+$, calculated for C$_{90}$H$_{133}$^{79}Br$_2$N$_{10}$O$_{20}$$^+$: 1831.8059.

3.3.2. Synthesis of *N*,*N*'-Bis-(1-amino-4,9,13-triazahexadecyl)-1,7-di-(1-amino-3-hydroxypropyl)-perylene-3,4:9,10-tetracarboxydiimide **PDI-1**

Compound **PDI-3** (20.0 mg, 19.9 µmol) was dissolved in anhydrous tetrahydrofurane (THF, 2 mL). In another flask, 3-(*N*-(*tert*-butyloxycarbonyl)-amino)1-propanol (191 mg, 1.09 mmol) was dissolved in anhydrous THF (2 mL) prior to the addition of lithium diisopropylamide (2.0 M solution in THF, 500 µL). This mixture was then added to the first flask and stirred for 5 h at 65 °C. The cooled reaction mixture was diluted with an excess of ethyl acetate. The organic layer was washed with brine and water, dried with anhydrous Na$_2$SO$_4$, and concentrated under reduced pressure. The crude product (**PDI-4**) was purified by column chromatography (SiO$_2$, CH$_2$Cl$_2$:MeOH—98:2) to afford a violet solid, which was used without further purification. R_f (CH$_2$Cl$_2$:MeOH—95:5) 0.28; MS (HR-ESI$^+$): m/z = 2045.1841 [M + Na]$^+$ calculated for C$_{106}$H$_{164}$N$_{12}$NaO$_{26}$$^+$: 2045.1850, m/z = 1034.0868 [M + 2Na]$^{2+}$ calculated for C$_{106}$H$_{164}$N$_{12}$Na$_2$O$_{26}$$^{2+}$: 1034.0849.

The crude product (**PDI-4**) was dissolved in methanol (10 mL), and concentrated HCl (1 mL) was added to remove the Boc-protecting groups. This reaction mixture was stirred for 20 h at room temperature. The solvent was removed under reduced pressure. Purification by semi-preparative HPLC (Macherey-Nagel C18 (250 mm × 10 mm), H$_2$O with 0.1% trifluoroacetic acid (TFA)/MeCN, 4 mL/min, 0–5 min—0% MeCN, 15 min—12% MeCN, 30–35 min—24% MeCN, 55 min—90% MeCN) and subsequent lyophilization yielded the TFA salt of **PDI-1** (1.53 mg, 1.50 µmol, 8%) as a violet solid.

The trifluoroacetate counterions were exchanged by dissolving the product in 0.6 M HCl followed by precipitation from acetonitrile. After washing with acetonitrile, re-dissolution in water and subsequent lyophilization, the target compound [**PDI-1**]Cl$_{10}$ was ready to use. ^{1}H-NMR (600.13 MHz, MeOD): δ (ppm) = 9.48–9.58 (m, 2H, perylene-H), 8.63 (d, $^3J_{\text{H-H}}$ = 8.28 Hz, 2H, perylene-H), 8.45 (bs, 2H, perylene-H), 4.58–4.71 (m, 4H, CH$_2$), 4.32–4.40 (m, 4H, CH$_2$), 3.32–3.35 (m, 4H, CH$_2$, superimposed by MeOD), 3.03–3.23 (m, 32H, CH$_2$, N–H), 2.47–2.53 (m, 4H, CH$_2$), 2.14–2.26 (m, 8H, CH$_2$), 2.05–2.11 (m, 4H, CH$_2$), 1.79–1.83 (m, 8H, CH$_2$); ^{13}C{^{1}H}-NMR (150.90 MHz, MeOD): δ (ppm) = 130.0, 129.5, 68.8, 48.3, 47.0, 45.7, 46.0, 38.4, 38.0, 37.9, 28.2, 25.9, 25.1, 24.0, 23.9; MS (HR-ESI$^+$): m/z = 1021.6722 [M + H]$^+$ calculated for C$_{56}$H$_{85}$N$_{12}$O$_6$$^+$: 1021.6710 m/z = 511.3395 [M + 2H]$^{2+}$, calculated for C$_{56}$H$_{86}$N$_{12}$O$_6$$^{2+}$: 511.3391; UV/Vis (H$_2$O, 10 mM MOPS, pH 7): λ$_{\text{max (Abs)}}$ (ε [M^{-1} cm^{-1}]) = 402 nm (5,900), 542 nm (24,100), 576 nm (35,300); Fluorescence (H$_2$O, 10 mM MOPS, pH 7): λ$_{\text{Ex}}$ = 530 nm, λ$_{\text{Abs(Em)}}$ = 615 nm, φ$_F$ = 0.17; Analytical HPLC: (Macherey-Nagel C18 (250 mm × 4.6 mm), H$_2$O with 0.1% TFA/MeCN, 1 mL/min, 0–5 min—0% MeCN, 15 min—12% MeCN, 30–35 min—24% MeCN, 55 min—90% MeCN) t_R = 31.6 min.

3.4. Assays

Dermatan Sulfate Assay in Aqueous and Plasma Matrix

For titrations of probe solutions with dermatan sulfate, the solutions described in the legends of Figures 1 and 2 of **PDI-1** and **Heparin Red**, respectively, were prepared using 100 µM aqueous stock solutions of the probes. Then, 6-nM probe solutions in DMSO/30 mM HCl (Figure 2) were prepared as described in detail in [9] for **Heparin Red**. Dermatan sulfate in spiked plasma samples was detected as described for heparin, following the protocol of the provider of the **Heparin Red** Kit for a 96-well microplate, using either a 100-µM aqueous solution of **Heparin Red** or of **PDI-1**. In brief, the 100-µM solution of **PDI-1** or **Heparin Red** was freshly mixed with Enhancer solution at a volume ratio of 1:90. Subsequently, 20 µL of the dermatan sulfate spiked plasma sample was pipetted into a microplate well, followed by 80 µL of the probe—Enhancer mixture. For sample numbers >10, a 12-channel pipette was used for the addition of the probe—Enhancer solution. The microplate was introduced in the fluorescence reader and mixing was performed using the plate shaking function of the microplate reader (setting "high," 3 min). Immediately after mixing, fluorescence was recorded within 1 min.

4. Conclusions

This contribution describes the synthesis and properties of the new fluorescent probe **PDI-1**, a polyamine-functionalized perylene diimide. **PDI-1** is structurally related to the commercial probe **Heparin Red**, but has in its protonated form a higher molecular charge of +10, compared to +8 for **Heparin Red**. The superior performance of **PDI-1** for sensing of a glycosaminoglycan with low negative charge density is exemplified by the detection of dermatan sulfate at a low concentration or in a competitive blood plasma matrix. A potential application of this probe is the direct monitoring of the antithrombotic drug dermatan sulfate in plasma in the absence of administered heparin and other glycosaminoglycans.

Supplementary Materials: Supplementary materials are available online.

Acknowledgments: This research was supported by Heidelberg University. We thank C. Giese for preparing the plasma spikes and Redprobes UG for a gift of the Heparin Red Kit.

Author Contributions: M.R. conceived, designed and performed the experiments, analyzed the data and wrote parts of the paper. U.W. performed the titrations in Figure 2 and analyzed the data. R.K. contributed reagents, materials and analysis tools, and wrote parts of the paper.

Conflicts of Interest: The authors declare no conflict of interest.

References

1. Bromfield, S.M.; Wilde, E.; Smith, D.K. Heparin sensing and binding—Taking supramolecular chemistry towards clinical applications. *Chem. Soc. Rev.* **2013**, *42*, 9184–9195. [CrossRef] [PubMed]
2. Szelke, H.; Schübel, S.; Harenberg, J.; Krämer, R. A fluorescent probe for the quantification of heparin in clinical samples with minimal matrix interference. *Chem. Commun.* **2010**, *46*, 1667–1669. [CrossRef] [PubMed]
3. Warttinger, U.; Giese, C.; Harenberg, J.; Holmer, E.; Krämer, R. A fluorescent probe assay (Heparin Red) for direct detection of heparins in human plasma. *Anal. Bioanal. Chem.* **2016**, *408*, 8241–8251. [CrossRef] [PubMed]
4. Warttinger, U.; Krämer, R. Quantification of heparin in complex matrices (including urine) using a mix-and-read fluorescence assay. *arXiv* **2016**, arXiv:1611.02482.
5. Galli, M.; Magen, H.; Einsele, H.; Chatterjee, M.; Grasso, M.; Specchia, G.; Barbieri, P.; Paoletti, D.; Pace, S.; Sanderson, R.D.; et al. Roneparstat (SST0001), an Innovative Heparanase (HPSE) Inhibitor for Multiple Myeloma (MM) Therapy: First in Man Study. *Blood* **2015**, *126*, 3246.
6. Szelke, H.; Schübel, S.; Harenberg, J.; Krämer, R. Interaction of heparin with cationic molecular probes: Probe charge is a major determinant of binding stoichiometry and affinity. *Bioorg. Med. Chem. Lett.* **2010**, *20*, 1445–1447. [CrossRef] [PubMed]

7. Warttinger, U.; Krämer, R. Instant determination of the potential biomarker heparan sulfate in human plasma by a mix-and-read fluorescence assay. *arXiv* **2017**, arXiv:1702.05288.

8. Warttinger, U.; Giese, C.; Harenberg, J.; Krämer, R. Direct quantification of brown algae-derived fucoidans in human plasma by a fluorescent probe assay. *arXiv* **2016**, arXiv:1608.00108.

9. Groß, N.; Arian, D.; Warttinger, U.; Krämer, R. Ultrasensitive quantification of dextran sulfate by a mix-and-read fluorescent probe assay. *arXiv* **2017**, arXiv:1703.08663.

10. Trowbridge, J.M.; Gallo, R.L. Dermatan sulfate: New functions from an old glycosaminoglycan. *Glycobiology* **2002**, *12*, 117R–125R. [CrossRef] [PubMed]

11. Benito, C.; Marco, G.; Giangiacomo, T. Structural and Conformational Aspects of the Anticoagulant and Antithrombotic Activity of Heparin and Dermatan Sulfate. *Curr. Pharm. Des.* **2004**, *10*, 939–949.

12. Mashima, R.; Sakai, E.; Tanaka, M.; Kosuga, M.; Okuyama, T. The levels of urinary glycosaminoglycans of patients with attenuated and severe type of mucopolysaccharidosis II determined by liquid chromatography-tandem mass spectrometry. *Mol. Genet. Metab. Rep.* **2016**, *7*, 87–91. [CrossRef] [PubMed]

13. Saivin, S.; Cambus, J.-P.; Thalamus, C.; Lau, G.; Boneu, B.; Houin, G.; Gianese, F. Pharmacokinetics and Pharmacodynamics of Intramuscular Dermatan Sulfate Revisited. *Clin. Drug Investig.* **2003**, *23*, 533–543. [CrossRef] [PubMed]

14. Coccheri, S.; Mannello, F. Development and use of sulodexide in vascular diseases: Implications for treatment. *Drug Des. Dev. Ther.* **2014**, *8*, 49–65. [CrossRef] [PubMed]

15. Auray-Blais, C.; Lavoie, P.; Tomatsu, S.; Valayannopoulos, V.; Mitchell, J.J.; Raiman, J.; Beaudoin, M.; Maranda, B.; Clarke, J.T.R. UPLC-MS/MS detection of disaccharides derived from glycosaminoglycans as biomarkers of mucopolysaccharidoses. *Anal. Chim. Acta* **2016**, *936*, 139–148. [CrossRef] [PubMed]

16. Vitale, C.; Berutti, S.; Bagnis, C.; Soragna, G.; Gabella, P.; Fruttero, C.; Marangella, M. Dermatan sulfate: An alternative to unfractionated heparin for anticoagulation in hemodialysis patients. *J. Nephrol.* **2013**, *26*, 158–163. [CrossRef] [PubMed]

17. Geall, A.J.; Blagbrough, I.S. Homologation of Polyamines in the Rapid Synthesis of Lipospermine Conjugates and Related Lipoplexes. *Tetrahedron* **2000**, *56*, 2449–2460. [CrossRef]

18. Boehm, A.; Arms, H.; Henning, G.; Blaschka, P. 1,7-Disubstituierte Perylen-3,4,9-10-tetracarbonsäuren, deren Dianhydride und Diimide. BASF AG Germany, Patent DE19547210A1, 19 June 1997.

19. Volpi, N.; Maccari, F. Microdetermination of chondroitin sulfate in normal human plasma by fluorophore-assisted carbohydrate electrophoresis (FACE). *Clin. Chim. Acta* **2005**, *356*, 125–133. [CrossRef] [PubMed]

20. Zinellu, E.; Lepedda, A.J.; Cigliano, A.; Pisanu, S.; Zinellu, A.; Carru, C.; Bacciu, P.P.; Piredda, F.; Guarino, A.; Spirito, R.; et al. Association between Human Plasma Chondroitin Sulfate Isomers and Carotid Atherosclerotic Plaques. *Biochem. Res. Int.* **2012**, *2012*, 281284. [CrossRef] [PubMed]

21. Mix-and-Read Assays for Heparins. Available online: www.redprobes.com (accessed on 05 May 2017).

22. Rappold, M. Perylendiimid-Basierte Fluoreszenzfarbstoffe: Synthese, Detektion von Glykosaminoglykanen und Photoinduzierte Zyklisierungsreaktionen. Ph.D. Thesis, Heidelberg University, Heidelberg, Germany, 2016.

23. Guerrini, M.; Zhang, Z.; Shriver, Z.; Naggi, A.; Masuko, S.; Langer, R.; Casu, B.; Linhardt, R.J.; Torri, G.; Sasisekharan, R. Orthogonal analytical approaches to detect potential contaminants in heparin. *Proc. Natl. Acad. Sci. USA* **2009**, *106*, 16956–16961. [CrossRef] [PubMed]

24. Carnachan, S.M.; Hinkley, S.F.R. Heparan Sulfate Identification and Characterisation: Method I. Heparan Sulfate Identification by NMR Analysis. *Bio-Protocol* **2017**, *7*, e2196. [CrossRef]

25. Fulmer, G.R.; Miller, A.J.M.; Sherden, N.H.; Gottlieb, H.E.; Nudelman, A.; Stoltz, B.M.; Bercaw, J.E.; Goldberg, K.I. NMR Chemical Shifts of Trace Impurities: Common Laboratory Solvents, Organics, and Gases in Deuterated Solvents Relevant to the Organometallic Chemist. *Organometallics* **2010**, *29*, 2176–2179. [CrossRef]

26. Poeck, A. Ionische Fluoreszenzsonden zur Heparinbestimmung: Synthese und Anwendung. Ph.D. Thesis, Heidelberg University, Heidelberg, Germany, 2013.

Sample Availability: Samples of the compounds are not available

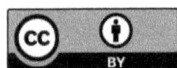

molecules

MDPI

Review

New Applications of Heparin and Other Glycosaminoglycans

Marcelo Lima [1,2,*], Timothy Rudd [2,3,*] and Edwin Yates [1,2,*]

1 Department of Biochemistry, Federal University of São Paulo (UNIFESP), Vila Clementino, São Paulo, S.P. 04044-020, Brazil
2 Department of Biochemistry, Institute of Integrative Biology, University of Liverpool, Crown Street, Liverpool L69 7ZB, UK
3 National Institute of Biological Standards and Controls (NIBSC), Blanche Lane, Potters Bar, Herts EN6 3QG, UK
* Correspondence: mlima@unifesp.br (M.L.); tim.rudd@nibsc.org (T.R.); eayates@liverpool.ac.uk (E.Y.); Tel.: +55-11-992725274 (M.L.); +44-1707-641120 (T.R.); +44-151-795-4429 (E.Y.)

Academic Editor: Giangiacomo Torri
Received: 5 April 2017; Accepted: 28 April 2017; Published: 6 May 2017

Abstract: Heparin, the widely used pharmaceutical anticoagulant, has been in clinical use for well over half a century. Its introduction reduced clotting risks substantially and subsequent developments, including the introduction of low-molecular-weight heparin, made possible many major surgical interventions that today make heparin an indispensable drug. There has been a recent burgeoning of interest in heparin and related glycosaminoglycan (GAG) polysaccharides, such as chondroitin sulfates, heparan sulfate, and hyaluronate, as potential agents in various applications. This ability arises mainly from the ability of GAGs to interact with, and alter the activity of, a wide range of proteins. Here, we review new developments (since 2010) in the application of heparin and related GAGs across diverse fields ranging from thrombosis and neurodegenerative disorders to microbiology and biotechnology.

Keywords: heparin; glycosaminoglycans; chondroitin sulfate

---

1. Introduction

Heparin, a member of the glycosaminoglycan (GAG) family of sulfated polysaccharides, is one of the most widely used pharmaceuticals, whose major role is in the inhibition of clot formation and thrombi, especially during surgery or following trauma. Beyond referring to some important historical literature, this review will attempt to survey recent (by which we mean from ca. 2010 to 2017) applications for this important and widely used drug, and will include other GAG members, which are being explored increasingly for other potential uses.

Heparin has been an established anticoagulant drug for more than 60 years for the prevention and control of thrombotic events owing to its interaction with a number of proteins of the blood clotting cascade, notably antithrombin and thrombin [1]. It consists of a linear, highly sulfated polysaccharide chain of various lengths varying from 2000 to 40,000 Da [2–4], composed of repeating disaccharide units of 1,4 linked α-L-iduronic or β-D-glucuronic acid (D-GlcA), and α-D-glucosamine (D-GlcN). The predominant substitution pattern comprises 2-O-sulfation of the iduronate residues and N- and 6-O-sulfation of the glucosamine residues [5]. Heparin is also closely related structurally to heparan sulfate (HS), which is present on cell surfaces and in the extracellular matrix. HS is generally less sulfated than heparin and is often considered to have a defined domain structure [6–8] and a lower proportion of L-iduronate residues. There are also D-GlcA and N-acetylated glucosamine (D-GlcNAc) residues, as well as variations in sulfation, including a small proportion of 3-O-sulfates on glucosamine residues. Hyaluronic acid (HA) is the only member of the GAG family that is not sulfated, being a homo-polymer consisting of beta (1→4) linked disaccharides of D-GlcA β (1→3) D-GlcNAc. Chondroitin sulfate (CS) encompasses various structures, based on repeating β (1-4) linked disaccharides of GlcA β (1→3) GalNAc containing 6-(Chondroitin sulfate-C: CS-C) and 4-sulfates (CS-A), sulfation at position-2 of the GlcA residues (GlcA2S β (1→3) GalNAc6S) (CS-D), and 4,6-di-sulfated GalNAc (GlcA β (1→3) GalNAc4, 6diS (in CS-E). The polysaccharide, dermatan sulfate (DS), which was formerly known as CS-B, contains repeating →4) L-IdoA β (1→3) D-GalNAc β (1→ units with 4-O-sulfation on the GalNAc moiety. GAG-like structures from non-mammalian sources, often marine, have become the focus of attention recently, and these, while possessing similar backbone structures, often include branches of fucose units [9], which can include non-reducing terminal fucose with sulfation at positions-2 and -3 [10].

The discovery and development of heparin as an anticoagulant agent had a tremendous impact on health because major surgical procedures became possible, especially those in which cardiopulmonary bypass (CPB), which was first demonstrated in animals in 1939 [11], were necessary. Another important medical procedure that is only possible due to the anticoagulant properties of heparin is dialysis. Indeed, unfractionated (full-length) heparin (UFH) named heparin sodium, its antidote, protamine sulfate [12], as well as a form of low-molecular-weight heparin (LMWH) [13] all appear in the World Health Organization's (WHO) List of Essential Medicines. The pharmacological activity of heparin results mainly from its ability to bind and accelerate the AT activity, thereby considerably enhancing the inhibition of coagulation factors Xa and IIa, although it interacts in concert with AT and other members of the blood clotting cascade as well, including factor IXa, XIa, and XIIa [14]. In a biological rather than a clinical context though, heparin action is more closely linked to defense against exogenous pathogens [15] and responses following tissue damage. Heparin alters cytokine levels [16], and one of its biological roles may be to dampen the effects of the sudden release of large numbers of cytokines following infection or sudden trauma.

In recent times, the majority of pharmaceutical heparin has been sourced from the intestine of pigs, and detailed studies of the sequence of heparin have involved laborious separation techniques. Recent advances in the biosynthesis of heparin-related structures employing recombinant enzymes and synthetic uridine-diphosphate-monosaccharide donors have been developed by Liu and Linhardt, allowing not only for the production of heparin sequences but also for the systematic and controlled preparation of heparin (and HS) analogues, which will be suitable for a wide-range of experimental purposes and applications [17].

2. Applications in Anticoagulation and Cancer Treatments

In current clinical use, one of the most important forms of heparin is low-molecular-weight heparin (LMWH) which consists of a complex mixture of fragments ranging from tetra to hexadecasaccharides and somewhat higher oligosaccharides [18–20] obtained by various chemical and enzymatic depolymerization processes. The main advantages of LMWHs over UFH are improved bioavailability and higher anti-factor Xa/anti-factor IIa activity ratios, with decreased hemorrhagic risk during prolonged treatments [21]. While UFH can be monitored effectively and reversed in patients undergoing surgery with extracorporeal circulation, LMWHs cannot, because neutralization with protamine sulfate is ineffective. The development of new anticoagulant agents with the beneficial properties of both UFH and LMWH is therefore still pursued and is an important area in which biosynthetic structures are being applied [22,23].

Aside from the well-known anticoagulant activities of heparin and related GAGs or GAG mixtures, such as sulodexide (a mixture of LMWH and DS in the ratio 80:20), heparin is also active in a wide range of activities in which the naturally occurring cell surface polysaccharide, heparan sulfate (HS), is a participant. Many of the proteins with which heparin interacts originate in the extracellular matrix, the best studied of which belong to the fibroblast growth factor (FGF) family. The potential use of heparin to interfere with aberrant cell–cell signaling by this route has been investigated and the relationship between sequence and activity sought [24–27].

The importance of the FGF signaling system to development and regulation, and hence when its function is impaired or altered, also to disease is one obvious area in which heparins, acting in this case as analogues for HS, can be applied. One area in which modulating FGF signaling would be desirable is cancer treatment. However, it is noteworthy that cancer-related thrombotic disorders are also well known and were first described as long ago as 1865, when the clinical association between thrombosis and an initially undiagnosed cancer was noted. Unfractionated heparin and LMWHs have been used successfully for the prophylaxis and treatment of cancer-related hemostatic disorders; however, since cancer patients have an increased risk of bleeding [28], LMWHs have gained significant ground since they produce a more predictable anticoagulant response, display improved subcutaneous bioavailability, and exhibit an extended half-life. Furthermore, heparin-induced thrombocytopenia (HIT) incidence is lower when LMWHs and the synthetic pentasaccharide, Fondaparinux, are used. Novel oral anticoagulants are under development, but their efficacy and safety in cancer-patients has yet to be proved. Despite being well recognized now, the pathogenesis is complex and results from the combination of several factors, but the expression of tumor cell-associated clotting factors is a shared characteristic. The prevention and treatment of these conditions extends beyond the ease of symptoms, it has a direct impact in cancer patient survival [29], and there are some known beneficial effects of heparin, but elucidating these is hampered by the complexity of the systems involved. The widespread use of heparin as a treatment is hindered by unwanted anticoagulant side-effects [30] (see also review by Afratis et al. [31]); however, the possibility of correcting signaling defects caused by altered HS structure (e.g., by sulf enzyme activity) in cancer [32,33] or the direct inhibition of the sulf enzymes with heparin or heparin analogues is an area of potential interest. Of direct relevance to the progression of the disease is the inhibition of a mammalian heparanase enzyme [34], while other routes are thought to influence metastasis, acting via P- and L-selections [35–37], inhibiting galectins [38], inhibiting tumorogenesis and angiogenesis through cellular receptors such as CD44 and growth factor receptors [39], or, in the case of the use of heparin as a means of ameliorating resistance to cisplatin treatment, acting through as-yet unidentified mechanisms [40], all of which are affected by heparin or heparin analogues. Among other GAGs, an example of the treatment of cancer is the use of the non-sulfated GAG, hyaluronate (HA) in pancreatic ductal adenocarcinoma [41].

3. Recovery from Nervous System Damage

Recent work shows that, while CS inhibits the regeneration of neurites in the CNS, CS-bound HB-GAM (pleiotrophin) activates them, inducing dendrite regeneration in adult cerebral cortex and axonal regeneration in adult spinal cord [42]. Chondroitin sulfate forms a barrier following nerve injury [43], but can be digested by enzymes to improve repair [44–47]. Chondroitin sulfate-E (CS-E), containing unusual 4,6 di-sulfated GalNAc residues and 4-sulfated CS in aggrecan, have been shown to be inhibitory to neurite outgrowth [48], and CS-E mediates estrogen-induced osteoanabolism [49], suggesting several potential future applications for CS and its derivatives.

4. Respiratory Diseases

GAGs and heparin in particular have been suggested as playing a protective roles in the inflammation response [50], which has been interpreted as involving (among other things) the inhibition of elastase and the interaction with several cytokines [51]. Heparin and its analogues have been proposed for the application to elastase inhibition for cystic fibrosis treatment (or other conditions, such as acute respiratory distress syndrome (ARDS). Although they do not originate from a conventional mammalian GAG, oligosaccharide fragments of the fucosylated GAG structures from the sea cucumber (*Holothuria forskali*) [9] were shown to lower neutrophil infiltration by reducing selectin interactions.

5. Neurodegenerative Diseases

There is an emerging role in Parkinson's Disease for heparin acting via cathepsin-d activity affecting α-synuclein accumulation [52], while, in Alzheimer's Disease, the inhibition of BACE-1, the key protease responsible for the generation of toxic Aβ fragments (1–42) is inhibited by heparin and its derivatives [53,54], some of which have been engineered to possess very low anticoagulant activity [55,56]. Furthermore, it is known that heparin modulates fibril formation [57], and understanding the mechanisms underlying such events may open new routes for the prevention, for instance, of toxic fibril formation and deposition.

6. Roles as Antimicrobial Agents

6.1. Viruses

GAGs might be expected, on the basis of their universal presence on cell surfaces, to serve as a broad spectrum and relatively non-specific receptors for virus binding [58]; [see also an earlier review: [59]]. Such interactions are not unexpected, since virus envelope proteins present patches of positively charged amino acids. While GAGs have been shown to attach to filoviruses [60] and CS-E, but not CS-D, and inhibit dengue virus infection [61], it is clear that GAGs are indeed of relevance to the mechanisms of viral attachment and invasion. The ability of viruses to bind cell surface HSs and, by extension, bind heparin under experimental conditions has long been known in the case of herpes simplex (HSV) and dengue (DENV) viruses. Heparin as a potential inhibitor of viral attachment follows naturally from these observations and has been demonstrated for DENV [62]. What is less clear is whether and how this knowledge can be exploited to enable GAGs to be applied as inhibitors of attachment, a process that may be able to be exploited for the well-known property of multivalency to increase the avidity of the binding of the viral particles to the GAG, perhaps immobilized in some device, or attached to multidentate ligands in a nanotechnology format (see also a review of this field: [63]). The potential importance of such applications is difficult to over-emphasize, however. Recently, viral attachment to GAGs was reported for IFNα/βBP from variola (smallpox virus), monkeypox viruses [64], and GAGs have been shown to prevent measles virus infection in cell lines via hemagglutinin protein [65]. Other viruses, including hepatitis B, have been found to bind to heparin [66] as has Japanese encephalitis virus (JEV) [67]. Thus, the interest in GAG-based intervention seems set to increase.

Heparin and derivatives have been shown to be effective in preventing the infection of cells by the influenza virus, strain H5N1 [68], and to have effects on ZIKV-induced cell death that are independent of adhesion and invasion [69]. In this case, heparin has only a modest ability to protect infection by analogy with dengue virus, which is also of the flavivirus family, and which interacts with heparin through the envelope glycoproteins [70]. Rather, heparin may be acting to protect infected cells from cytotoxic effects and cell death via the activation of cell survival signaling pathways. The ability of heparin to protect cells from programmed cell death had already been observed in human cells (non-infected) [71], and this may form an interesting new avenue for the application of GAG derivatives in itself.

6.2. Parasites

The involvement of GAGs in a parasitic disease has been studied relatively little. However, the potential for the application of GAGs remains high in cases where GAGs form a major part of the means of attachment and invasion, especially where there is the possibility of topical application. The ability of heparin and derivatives to inhibit rosetting of parasite infected erythrocytes has been noted [72] and, recently, effective inhibitors (comprising fucosylated CS (FucCS)) of cytoadherence (the process of adhesion of infected red blood cells to vascular epithelia) derived from sea cucumber have been reported [73]. Heparin is known to alter the activity of a cysteine protease in the parasite, *L. mexicana*, that causes Leishmaniasis [74] and interacts with a metalloprotease from *L.(v). braziliensis* [75]. Heparin has also been shown to accelerate protein degradation by human neutrophil elastase [76]. Several heparin-binding proteins have also been identified in *T. cruzi*, where some of them are implicated in parasite adhesion to midgut epithelial cells [77].

6.3. Bacteria

Binding of GAGs facilitates Streptococcal entry into the CNS of *Drosophila* [78] and determines disease progression [79]. In relation to the phenomenon of shock, GAGs seem to be elevated overall, perhaps originating from damaged tissue, but they also seem to neutralize antimicrobial peptides [80]. Glycosaminoglycans were studied en masse, however, without paying attention to the individual types involved. Heparin use in sepsis patients, where crosstalk between thrombosis and inflammation plays a critical role, has also been recognized. The use of heparin prevents the development of microthromboembolic disease during sepsis, impairing tissue hypoxygenation and further organ damage and dysfunction [81]. There is also literature pointing to the use of heparin-coated stents for the prevention of bacterial biofilm formation and subsequent microbe attachment [82].

7. Panceatitis

Acute pancreatitis has been reported independently by several groups to benefit from treatment with heparin [83] in rats and in patients [84–86]. Furthermore, LMW heparin has also been shown to be effective [87].

8. Roles in Rheumatoid Arthritis (RA)

Naturally occurring autoantibodies to GAGs are markers in rheumatoid arthritis [88]. The level of IgM type Ab for CS-C in serum correlates with RA, although GAG concentration alone is not a good indicator in knee injury [89] in agreement with earlier findings in horses [90].

9. Inflammation Reduction

Many of the applications of heparin mentioned in this review may stem, at least in part, from the ability of heparin to moderate inflammation. This topic has itself been reviewed in 2013 [91] and, in general, heparin is perceived as acting via several routes, which include interaction with cytokines and as an inhibitor of heparanase, to achieve reduced leukocyte recruitment.

Applications in which these properties may be important include the treatment of burns [92] and the proposed use of heparin in asthma treatment [93]. The potential, based on a projection of the ability of heparin to inhibit bacterial infection and reduce inflammation, to improve the symptoms of cystic fibrosis has also been investigated [94] but no marked improvement at low doses (50,000 IU) has been shown.

While cystic fibrosis applications acting to reduce inflammation assist sputum clearance, inhibit elastase, or act as an inhibitor of microbial attachment or growth have not been convincing, heparin derivatives were shown to be capable of acting at several points in the inflammatory process [51].

10. Alternative Sources of GAG-Like Structures with Potentially Useful Activities

This review attempts to cover not only new applications for heparin but also potential new sources of active agents among the GAGs for both old and new applications. Although not all of these structures correspond to GAGs according to the classical definitions of mammalian GAGs provided above, GAG-like structures are found in a wide range of organisms, including *Cnidaria*, *Arthropoda*, *Mollusca*, *Echinodermata*, and *Chordata* [95]. A host of polysaccharides, either GAGs in the conventional sense or polysaccharides with structural features closely resembling GAGs, usually bearing additional ramifications have been identified and linked to a variety of biological activities. These include Sea cucumber (*S. hermanni*) as an antiinflammatory [95], marine GAG analogues [96], fish cartilage as an antitumor and anti-pathognic agent [97], GAGs from starfish with antithrombotic and anti-inflammatory activities [95], and mussels (*Perna canaliculis*) as an anti-inflammatory agent [98].

11. Biotechnological and Other Applications

An emerging use of GAGs is in biotechnological applications, particularly in the field of embryonic stem cells, for the regulation of differentiation [reviewed in [99]] and neural speciation in mouse embryonic stem cells [100]. The successful fractionation of a cell population by HS epitopes has also been reported [101]. The prospect of incorporating GAGs into electrospun meshes for the purpose of supporting stem cell applications has also been undertaken [102]. A possible role is emerging in muscular dystrophy, following signs of involvement of HS sulfation in the disease process and ageing, acting via FGF-2 [103].

12. Concluding Remarks

Many a student textbook of biochemistry once dismissed the role of GAGs as merely structural; decades of intensive research led to a burgeoning of the biological roles ascribed to them and potential practical applications. The precise nature of the relationship between their structure and function remains a matter of debate, a fact that stems not only from their structural complexity, but also the difficulty of analysis, which may also indicate that new approaches are required. These approaches may need to be sensitive to as yet undefined properties, and one such property is their large-scale vibrational modes [104]. Nevertheless, even without this detailed information, it is clear that the number of roles of these versatile materials seem to set to increase in the future.

Conflicts of Interest: The authors declare no conflict of interest.

References

1. Barrowcliffe, T.W. History of heparin. *Handb. Exp. Pharmacol.* **2012**, *207*, 3–22.
2. Nader, H.B.; McDuffie, N.M.; Dietrich, C.P. Heparin fractionation by electrofocusing: presence of 21 components of different molecular weights. *Biochem. Biophys. Res. Commun.* **1974**, *57*, 488–493. [CrossRef]
3. McDuffie, N.M.; Dietrich, C.P.; Nader, H.B. Electrofocusing of heparin: Fractionation of heparin into 21 components distinguishable from other acidic mucopolysaccharides. *Biopolymers* **1975**, *14*, 1473–1486. [CrossRef] [PubMed]
4. Dietrich, C.P.; Nader, H.B.; Mcduffie, N.N. Electrofocusing of heparin: Presence of 21 monomeric and dimeric molecular species in heparin preparations. *An. Acad. Bras. Cienc.* **1975**, *47*, 301–309. [PubMed]
5. Perlin, A.S.; Mackie, D.M.; Dietrich, C.P. Evidence for a (1→4)-linked 4-*O*-(α-L-idopyranosyluronic acid 2-sulfate)-(2-deoxy-2-sulfoamino-D-glucopyranosyl 6-sulfate) sequence in heparin. *Carbohydr. Res.* **1971**, *18*, 185–194. [CrossRef]
6. Turnbull, J.E.; Gallagher, J.T. Distribution of iduronate 2-sulphate residues in heparan sulphate. Evidence for an ordered polymeric structure. *Biochem. J.* **1991**, *273*, 553–559. [CrossRef] [PubMed]
7. Maccarana, M.; Sakura, Y.; Tawada, A.; Yoshida, K.; Lindahl, U. Domain structure of heparan sulfates from bovine organs. *J. Biol. Chem.* **1996**, *271*, 17804–17810. [CrossRef] [PubMed]
8. Merry, C.L.; Lyon, M.; Deakin, J.A.; Hopwood, J.J.; Gallagher, J.T. Highly sensitive sequencing of the sulfated domains of heparan sulfate. *J. Biol. Chem.* **1999**, *274*, 18455–18462. [CrossRef] [PubMed]
9. Panagos, C.G.; Thomson, D.S.; Moss, C.; Hughes, A.D.; Kelly, M.S.; Liu, Y.; Chai, W.; Venkatasamy, R.; Spina, D.; Page, C.P.; et al. Fucosylated chondroitin sulfates from the body wall of the sea cucumber Holothuria forskali: Conformation, selectin binding, and biological activity. *J. Biol. Chem.* **2014**, *289*, 28284–28298. [CrossRef] [PubMed]
10. Pomin, V.H. Holothurian fucosylated chondroitin sulfate. *Mar. Drugs* **2014**, *12*, 232–254. [CrossRef] [PubMed]
11. Gibbon, J.G., Jr. The maintenance of life during experimental occlusion of the pulmonary artery followed by survival. *Surg Gynecol Obs.* **1939**, *69*, 602–614.
12. Warkentin, T.E.; Crowther, M.A. Reversing anticoagulants both old and new. *Can. J. Anaesth.* **2002**, *49*, S11–S25. [PubMed]

13. Johnson, E.A.; Kirkwood, T.B.; Stirling, Y.; Perez-Requejo, J.L.; Ingram, G.I.; Bangham, D.R.; Brozović, M. Four heparin preparations: Anti-Xa potentiating effect of heparin after subcutaneous injection. *Thromb. Haemost.* **1976**, *35*, 586–591. [PubMed]

14. Beeler, D.L.; Marcum, J.A.; Schiffman, S.; Rosenberg, R.D. Interaction of factor XIa and antithrombin in the presence and absence of heparin. *Blood* **1986**, *67*, 1488–1492. [PubMed]

15. Straus, A.H.; Sant'anna, O.A.; Nader, H.B.; Dietrich, C.P. An inverse relationship between heparin content and antibody response in genetically selected mice. Sex effect and evidence of a polygenic control for skin heparin concentration. *Biochem. J.* **1984**, *220*, 625–630. [CrossRef] [PubMed]

16. Call, D.R.; Remick, D.G. Low molecular weight heparin is associated with greater cytokine production in a stimulated whole blood model. *Shock* **1998**, *10*, 192–197. [CrossRef] [PubMed]

17. Liu, J.; Linhardt, R.J. Chemoenzymatic synthesis of heparan sulfate and heparin. *Nat. Prod. Rep.* **2014**, *31*, 1676–1685. [CrossRef] [PubMed]

18. Viskov, C.; Just, M.; Laux, V.; Mourier, P.; Lorenz, M. Description of the chemical and pharmacological characteristics of a new hemisynthetic ultra-low-molecular-weight heparin, AVE5026. *J. Thromb. Haemost.* **2009**, *7*, 1143–1151. [CrossRef] [PubMed]

19. Bisio, A.; Vecchietti, D.; Citterio, L.; Guerrini, M.; Raman, R.; Bertini, S.; Eisele, G.; Naggi, A.; Sasisekharan, R.; Torri, G. Structural features of low-molecular-weight heparins affecting their affinity to antithrombin. *Thromb. Haemost.* **2009**, *102*, 865–873. [CrossRef] [PubMed]

20. Zhang, Z.; Weïwer, M.; Li, B.; Kemp, M.M.; Daman, T.H.; Linhardt, R.J. Oversulfated chondroitin sulfate: Impact of a heparin impurity, associated with adverse clinical events, on low-molecular-weight heparin preparation. *J. Med. Chem.* **2008**, *51*, 5498–5501. [CrossRef] [PubMed]

21. Hoppensteadt, D.; Iqbal, O.; Fareed, J. Chapter 21—Basic and clinical differences of heparin and low molecular weight heparin treatment. *Chem. Biol. Heparin Heparan Sulfate* **2005**, *1*, 583–606.

22. Xu, Y.; Wang, Z.; Liu, R.; Bridges, A.S.; Huang, X.; Liu, J. Directing the biological activities of heparan sulfate oligosaccharides using a chemoenzymatic approach. *Glycobiology* **2012**, *22*, 96–106. [CrossRef] [PubMed]

23. Xu, Y.; Pempe, E.H.; Liu, J. Chemoenzymatic synthesis of heparin oligosaccharides with both anti-factor Xa and anti-factor IIa activities. *J. Biol. Chem.* **2012**, *287*, 29054–29061. [CrossRef] [PubMed]

24. Xu, R.; Ori, A.; Rudd, T.R.; Uniewicz, K.A.; Ahmed, Y.A.; Guimond, S.E.; Skidmore, M.A.; Siligardi, G.; Yates, E.A.; Fernig, D.G. Diversification of the structural determinants of fibroblast growth factor-heparin interactions: Implications for binding specificity. *J. Biol. Chem.* **2012**, *287*, 40061–40073. [CrossRef] [PubMed]

25. Li, Y.; Sun, C.; Yates, E.A.; Jiang, C.; Wilkinson, M.C.; Fernig, D.G. Heparin binding preference and structures in the fibroblast growth factor family parallel their evolutionary diversification. *Open Biol.* **2016**, *6*, 150275. [CrossRef] [PubMed]

26. Schultz, V.; Suflita, M.; Liu, X.; Zhang, X.; Yu, Y.; Li, L.; Green, D.E.; Xu, Y.; Zhang, F.; DeAngelis, P.L.; et al. Heparan sulfate domains required for fibroblast growth factor 1 and 2 signaling through fibroblast growth factor receptor 1c. *J. Biol. Chem.* **2017**, *292*, 2495–2509. [CrossRef] [PubMed]

27. Theodoraki, A.; Hu, Y.; Poopalasundaram, S.; Oosterhof, A.; Guimond, S.E.; Disterer, P.; Khoo, B.; Hauge-Evans, A.C.; Jones, P.M.; Turnbull, J.E.; et al. Distinct patterns of heparan sulphate in pancreatic islets suggest novel roles in paracrine islet regulation. *Mol. Cell. Endocrinol.* **2015**, *399*, 296–310. [CrossRef] [PubMed]

28. Rickles, F.R.; Falanga, A. Molecular basis for the relationship between thrombosis and cancer. *Thromb. Res.* **2001**, *102*, V215–V224. [CrossRef]

29. Nishioka, J.; Goodin, S. Low-molecular-weight heparin in cancer-associated thrombosis: Treatment, secondary prevention, and survival. *J. Oncol. Pharm. Pract.* **2007**, *13*, 85–97. [CrossRef] [PubMed]

30. Solari, V.; Jesudason, E.C.; Turnbull, J.E.; Yates, E.A. Determining the anti-coagulant-independent anti-cancer effects of heparin. *Br. J. Cancer* **2010**, *103*, 593–594. [CrossRef] [PubMed]

31. Afratis, N.; Gialeli, C.; Nikitovic, D.; Tsegenidis, T.; Karousou, E.; Theocharis, A.D.; Pavão, M.S.; Tzanakakis, G.N.; Karamanos, N.K. Glycosaminoglycans: Key players in cancer cell biology and treatment. *FEBS J.* **2012**, *279*, 1177–1197. [CrossRef] [PubMed]

32. Solari, V.; Borriello, L.; Turcatel, G.; Shimada, H.; Sposto, R.; Fernandez, G.E.; Asgharzadeh, S.; Yates, E.A.; Turnbull, J.E.; DeClerck, Y.A. MYCN-dependent expression of sulfatase-2 regulates neuroblastoma cell survival. *Cancer Res.* **2014**, *74*, 5999–6009. [CrossRef] [PubMed]

33. Vicente, C.M.; Lima, M.A.; Yates, E.A.; Nader, H.B.; Toma, L. Enhanced tumorigenic potential of colorectal cancer cells by extracellular sulfatases. *Mol. Cancer Res.* **2015**, *13*, 510–523. [CrossRef] [PubMed]

34. Vlodavsky, I.; Elkin, M.; Ilan, N. Impact of heparanase and the tumor microenvironment on cancer metastasis and angiogenesis: Basic aspects and clinical applications. *Rambam Maimonides Med. J.* **2011**, *2*, 1–17. [CrossRef] [PubMed]

35. Laubli, H.; Varki, A.; Borsig, L. Antimetastatic properties of low molecular weight heparin. *J. Clin. Oncol.* **2016**, *34*, 2560–2561. [CrossRef] [PubMed]

36. Borsig, L.; Wong, R.; Feramisco, J.; Nadeau, D.R.; Varki, N.M.; Varki, A. Heparin and cancer revisited: Mechanistic connections involving platelets, P-selectin, carcinoma mucins, and tumor metastasis. *Proc. Natl. Acad. Sci. USA* **2001**, *98*, 3352–3357. [CrossRef] [PubMed]

37. Läubli, H.; Stevenson, J.L.; Varki, A.; Varki, N.M.; Borsig, L. L-selectin facilitation of metastasis involves temporal induction of Fut7-dependent ligands at sites of tumor cell arrest. *Cancer Res.* **2006**, *66*, 1536–1542. [CrossRef] [PubMed]

38. Duckworth, C.A.; Guimond, S.E.; Sindrewicz, P.; Hughes, A.J.; French, N.S.; Lian, L.-Y.; Yates, E.A.; Pritchard, D.M.; Rhodes, J.M.; Turnbull, J.E.; et al. Chemically modified, non-anticoagulant heparin derivatives are potent galectin-3 binding inhibitors and inhibit circulating galectin-3-promoted metastasis. *Oncotarget* **2015**, *6*, 23671–23687. [CrossRef] [PubMed]

39. Karousou, E.; Misra, S.; Ghatak, S.; Dobra, K.; Götte, M.; Vigetti, D.; Passi, A.; Karamanos, N.K.; Skandalis, S.S. Roles and targeting of the HAS/hyaluronan/CD44 molecular system in cancer. *Matrix Biol.* **2016**, *59*, 1–20. [CrossRef] [PubMed]

40. Pfankuchen, D.B.; Stölting, D.P.; Schlesinger, M.; Royer, H.-D.; Bendas, G.; Bastian, D.; Philipp, D.; Schlesinger, M.; Royer, H.-D.; Bendas, G. Low molecular weight heparin tinzaparin antagonizes cisplatin resistance of ovarian cancer cells. *Biochem. Pharmacol.* **2015**, *97*, 147–157. [CrossRef] [PubMed]

41. Sato, N.; Cheng, X.-B.; Kohi, S.; Koga, A.; Hirata, K. Targeting hyaluronan for the treatment of pancreatic ductal adenocarcinoma. *Acta Pharm. Sin. B* **2016**, *6*, 101–105. [CrossRef] [PubMed]

42. Paveliev, M.; Fenrich, K.K.; Kislin, M.; Kuja-Panula, J.; Kulesskiy, E.; Varjosalo, M.; Kajander, T.; Mugantseva, E.; Ahonen-Bishopp, A.; Khiroug, L.; et al. HB-GAM (pleiotrophin) reverses inhibition of neural regeneration by the CNS extracellular matrix. *Nat. Publ. Gr.* **2016**, *6*, 33916. [CrossRef] [PubMed]

43. Siebert, J.R.; Conta Steencken, A.; Osterhout, D.J. Chondroitin Sulfate Proteoglycans in the Nervous System: Inhibitors to Repair. *Biomed Res. Int.* **2014**, *2014*, 845323. [CrossRef] [PubMed]

44. Kwok, J.C.F.; Yang, S.; Fawcett, J.W. Neural ECM in regeneration and rehabilitation. *Prog. Brain Res.* **2014**, *214*, 179–192.

45. Dick, G.; Liktan, C.; Alves, J.N.; Ehlert, E.M.E.; Miller, G.M.; Hsieh-Wilson, L.C.; Sugahara, K.; Oosterhof, A.; Van Kuppevelt, T.H.; Verhaagen, J.; et al. Semaphorin 3A binds to the perineuronal nets via chondroitin sulfate type E motifs in rodent brains. *J. Biol. Chem.* **2013**, *288*, 27384–27395. [CrossRef] [PubMed]

46. Orlando, C.; Ster, J.; Gerber, U.; Fawcett, J.W.; Raineteau, O. Perisynaptic chondroitin sulfate proteoglycans restrict structural plasticity in an integrin-dependent manner. *J. Neurosci.* **2012**, *32*, 18009–18017. [CrossRef] [PubMed]

47. Wang, D.; Ichiyama, R.M.; Zhao, R.; Andrews, M.R.; Fawcett, J.W. Chondroitinase Combined with Rehabilitation Promotes Recovery of Forelimb Function in Rats with Chronic Spinal Cord Injury. *J. Neurosci.* **2011**, *31*, 9332–9344. [CrossRef] [PubMed]

48. Gilbert, R.J.; McKeon, R.J.; Darr, A.; Calabro, A.; Hascall, V.C.; Bellamkonda, R. V CS-4,6 is differentially upregulated in glial scar and is a potent inhibitor of neurite extension. *Mol. Cell. Neurosci.* **2005**, *29*, 545–558. [CrossRef] [PubMed]

49. Koike, T.; Mikami, T.; Shida, M.; Habuchi, O.; Kitagawa, H. Chondroitin sulfate-E mediates estrogen-induced osteoanabolism. *Sci. Rep.* **2015**, *5*, 8994. [CrossRef] [PubMed]

50. Li, L.; Ling, Y.; Huang, M.; Yin, T.; Gou, S.M.; Zhan, N.Y.; Xiong, J.X.; Wu, H.S.; Yang, Z.Y.; Wang, C.Y. Heparin inhibits the inflammatory response induced by LPS and HMGB1 by blocking the binding of HMGB1 to the surface of macrophages. *Cytokine* **2015**, *72*, 36–42. [CrossRef] [PubMed]

51. Veraldi, N.; Hughes, A.J.; Rudd, T.R.; Thomas, H.B.; Edwards, S.W.; Hadfield, L.; Skidmore, M.A.; Siligardi, G.; Cosentino, C.; Shute, J.K.; et al. Heparin derivatives for the targeting of multiple activities in the inflammatory response. *Carbohydr. Polym.* **2015**, *117*, 400–407. [CrossRef] [PubMed]

52. Lehri-Boufala, S.; Ouidja, M.O.; Barbier-Chassefière, V.; Hénault, E.; Raisman-Vozari, R.; Garrigue-Antar, L.; Papy-Garcia, D.; Morin, C. New roles of glycosaminoglycans in α-synuclein aggregation in a cellular model of Parkinson disease. *PLoS ONE* **2015**, *10*, e0116641. [CrossRef] [PubMed]

53. Scholefield, Z.; Yates, E.A.; Wayne, G.; Amour, A.; McDowell, W.; Turnbull, J.E. Heparan sulfate regulates amyloid precursor protein processing by BACE1, the Alzheimer's β-secretase. *J. Cell Biol.* **2003**, *163*, 97–107. [CrossRef] [PubMed]

54. Zhang, X.; Zhao, X.; Lang, Y.; Li, Q.; Liu, X.; Cai, C.; Hao, J.; Li, G.; Yu, G. Low anticoagulant heparin oligosaccharides as inhibitors of BACE-1, the Alzheimer's β-secretase. *Carbohydr. Polym.* **2016**, *151*, 51–59. [CrossRef] [PubMed]

55. Patey, S.J.; Edwards, E.A.; Yates, E.A.; Turnbull, J.E. Heparin derivatives as inhibitors of BACE-1, the Alzheimer's β-secretase, with reduced activity against factor Xa and other proteases. *J. Med. Chem.* **2006**, *49*, 6129–6132. [CrossRef] [PubMed]

56. Ma, Q.; Cornelli, U.; Hanin, I.; Jeske, W.P.; Linhardt, R.J.; Walenga, J.M.; Fareed, J.; Lee, J.M. Heparin Oligosaccharides as Potential Therapeutic Agents in Senile Dementia. *Curr Pharm Des.* **2007**, *13*, 1607–1616. [CrossRef] [PubMed]

57. Stewart, K.L.; Hughes, E.; Yates, E.A.; Akien, G.R.; Huang, T.Y.; Lima, M.A.; Rudd, T.R.; Guerrini, M.; Hung, S.C.; Radford, S.E.; Middleton, D.A. Atomic Details of the Interactions of Glycosaminoglycans with Amyloid-β Fibrils. *J. Am. Chem. Soc.* **2016**, *138*, 8328–8331. [CrossRef] [PubMed]

58. Vigant, F.; Santos, N.C.; Lee, B. Broad-spectrum antivirals against viral fusion. *Nat. Rev. Microbiol.* **2015**, *13*, 426–437. [CrossRef] [PubMed]

59. *Nonanticoagulant Actions of Glycosaminoglycans*; Harenberg, J.; Casu, B., Eds.; Springer US: Boston, MA, USA, 2012.

60. Salvador, B.; Sexton, N.R.; Carrion, R.; Nunneley, J.; Patterson, J.L.; Steffen, I.; Lu, K.; Muench, M.O.; Lembo, D.; Simmons, G. Filoviruses utilize glycosaminoglycans for their attachment to target cells. *J. Virol.* **2013**, *87*, 3295–3304. [CrossRef] [PubMed]

61. Kato, D.; Era, S.; Watanabe, I.; Arihara, M.; Sugiura, N.; Kimata, K.; Suzuki, Y.; Morita, K.; Hidari, K.I.P.J.; Suzuki, T. Antiviral activity of chondroitin sulphate E targeting dengue virus envelope protein. *Antiviral Res.* **2010**, *88*, 236–243. [CrossRef] [PubMed]

62. Lin, Y.-L.; Lei, H.-Y.; Lin, Y.-S.; Yeh, T.-M.; Chen, S.-H.; Liu, H.-S. Heparin inhibits dengue-2 virus infection of five human liver cell lines. *Antiviral Res.* **2002**, *56*, 93–96. [CrossRef]

63. Sapsford, K.E.; Algar, W.R.; Berti, L.; Gemmill, K.B.; Casey, B.J.; Oh, E.; Stewart, M.H.; Medintz, I.L. Functionalizing nanoparticles with biological molecules: Developing chemistries that facilitate nanotechnology. *Chem. Rev.* **2013**, *113*, 1904–2074. [CrossRef] [PubMed]

64. Montanuy, I.; Alejo, A.; Alcami, A. Glycosaminoglycans mediate retention of the poxvirus type I interferon binding protein at the cell surface to locally block interferon antiviral responses. *FASEB J.* **2011**, *25*, 1960–1971. [CrossRef] [PubMed]

65. Terao-Muto, Y.; Yoneda, M.; Seki, T.; Watanabe, A.; Tsukiyama-Kohara, K.; Fujita, K.; Kai, C. Heparin-like glycosaminoglycans prevent the infection of measles virus in SLAM-negative cell lines. *Antiviral Res.* **2008**, *80*, 370–376. [CrossRef] [PubMed]

66. Schulze, A.; Gripon, P.; Urban, S. Hepatitis B virus infection initiates with a large surface protein-dependent binding to heparan sulfate proteoglycans. *Hepatology* **2007**, *46*, 1759–1768. [CrossRef] [PubMed]

67. Su, C.M.; Liao, C.L.; Lee, Y.L.; Lin, Y.L. Highly sulfated forms of heparin sulfate are involved in japanese encephalitis virus infection. *Virology* **2001**, *286*, 206–215. [CrossRef] [PubMed]

68. Skidmore, M.A.; Kajaste-Rudnitski, A.; Wells, N.M.; Guimond, S.E.; Rudd, T.R.; Yates, E.A.; Vicenzi, E. Inhibition of influenza H5N1 invasion by modified heparin derivatives. *Med. Chem. Commun.* **2015**, *6*, 640–646. [CrossRef]

69. Ghezzi, S.; Cooper, L.; Rubio, A.; Pagani, I.; Capobianchi, M.R.; Ippolito, G.; Pelletier, J.; Meneghetti, M.C.Z.; Lima, M.A.; Skidmore, M.A.; et al. Heparin prevents Zika virus induced-cytopathic effects in human neural progenitor cells. *Antiviral Res.* **2017**, *140*, 13–17. [CrossRef] [PubMed]

70. Kim, S.Y.; Zhao, J.; Liu, X.; Fraser, K.; Lin, L.; Zhang, X.; Zhang, F.; Dordick, J.S.; Linhardt, R.J. Interaction of Zika Virus Envelope Protein with Glycosaminoglycans. *Biochemistry* **2017**, *56*, 1151–1162. [CrossRef] [PubMed]

71. Hills, F.A.; Abrahams, V.M.; González-Timón, B.; Francis, J.; Cloke, B.; Hinkson, L.; Rai, R.; Mor, G.; Regan, L.; Sullivan, M.; et al. Heparin prevents programmed cell death in human trophoblast. *Mol. Hum. Reprod.* **2006**, *12*, 237–243. [CrossRef] [PubMed]

72. Skidmore, M.A.; Dumax-Vorzet, A.F.; Guimond, S.E.; Rudd, T.R.; Edwards, E.A.; Turnbull, J.E.; Craig, A.G.; Yates, E.A. Disruption of rosetting in Plasmodium falciparum malaria with chemically modified heparin and low molecular weight derivatives possessing reduced anticoagulant and other serine protease inhibition activities. *J. Med. Chem.* **2008**, *51*, 1453–1458. [CrossRef] [PubMed]

73. Bastos, M.F.; Albrecht, L.; Kozlowski, E.O.; Lopes, S.C.P.; Blanco, Y.C.; Carlos, B.C.; Castiñeiras, C.; Vicente, C.P.; Werneck, C.C.; Wunderlich, G.; et al. Fucosylated chondroitin sulfate inhibits Plasmodium falciparum cytoadhesion and merozoite invasion. *Antimicrob. Agents Chemother.* **2014**, *58*, 1862–1871. [CrossRef] [PubMed]

74. Judice, W.A.S.; Manfredi, M.A.; Souza, G.P.; Sansevero, T.M.; Almeida, P.C.; Shida, C.S.; Gesteira, T.F.; Juliano, L.; Westrop, G.D.; Sanderson, S.J.; et al. Heparin modulates the endopeptidase activity of Leishmania mexicana cysteine protease cathepsin L-like rCPB2.8. *PLoS ONE* **2013**, *8*, 602–614. [CrossRef] [PubMed]

75. De Castro Côrtes, L.; de Souza Pereira, M.; da Silva, F.; Pereira, B.A.; de Oliveira Junior, F.; de Araújo Soares, R.; Brazil, R.; Toma, L.; Vicente, C.; Nader, H.; et al. Participation of heparin binding proteins from the surface of Leishmania (Viannia) braziliensis promastigotes in the adhesion of parasites to Lutzomyia longipalpis cells (Lulo) in vitro. *Parasit. Vectors* **2012**, *5*, 142. [CrossRef] [PubMed]

76. Nunes, G.L.C.; Simões, A.; Dyszy, F.H.; Shida, C.S.; Juliano, M.A.; Juliano, L.; Gesteira, T.F.; Nader, H.B.; Murphy, G.; Chaffotte, A.F.; et al. Mechanism of heparin acceleration of tissue inhibitor of metalloproteases-1 (TIMP-1) degradation by the human neutrophil elastase. *PLoS ONE* **2011**, *6*, e21525. [CrossRef] [PubMed]

77. Oliveira, F.O.R.; Alves, C.R.; Souza-Silva, F.; Calvet, C.M.; Côrtes, L.M.C.; Gonzalez, M.S.; Toma, L.; Bouças, R.I.; Nader, H.B.; Pereira, M.C.S. Trypanosoma cruzi heparin-binding proteins mediate the adherence of epimastigotes to the midgut epithelial cells of Rhodnius prolixus. *Parasitology* **2012**, *139*, 735–743. [CrossRef] [PubMed]

78. Chang, Y.C.; Wang, Z.; Flax, L.A.; Xu, D.; Esko, J.D.; Nizet, V.; Baron, M.J. Glycosaminoglycan binding facilitates entry of a bacterial pathogen into central nervous systems. *PLoS Pathog.* **2011**, *7*, e1002082. [CrossRef] [PubMed]

79. Wang, Z.; Flax, L.A.; Kemp, M.M.; Linhardt, R.J.; Baron, M.J. Host and pathogen glycosaminoglycan-binding proteins modulate antimicrobial peptide responses in Drosophila melanogaster. *Infect. Immun.* **2011**, *79*, 606–616. [CrossRef] [PubMed]

80. Nelson, A.; Berkestedt, I.; Schmidtchen, A.; Ljunggren, L.; Bodelsson, M. Increased levels of glycosaminoglycans during septic shock: Relation to mortality and the antibacterial actions of plasma. *Shock* **2008**, *30*, 623–627. [CrossRef] [PubMed]

81. Cornet, A.D.; Smit, E.G.M.; Beishuizen, A.; Groeneveld, A.B.J. The role of heparin and allied compounds in the treatment of sepsis. *Thromb. Haemost.* **2007**, *98*, 579–586. [CrossRef] [PubMed]

82. Tenke, P.; Riedl, C.R.; Jones, G.L.; Williams, G.J.; Stickler, D.; Nagy, E. Bacterial biofilm formation on urologic devices and heparin coating as preventive strategy. *Int. J. Antimicrob. Agents* **2004**, *23*, S67–S74. [CrossRef] [PubMed]

83. Ceranowicz, P.; Dembinski, A.; Warzecha, Z.; Dembinski, M.; Cieszkowski, J.; Rembisz, K.; Konturek, S.J.; Kusnierz-Cabala, B.; Tomaszewska, R.; Pawlik, W.W. Protective and therapeutic effect of heparin in acute pancreatitis. *J. Physiol. Pharmacol.* **2008**, *59*, 103–125. [PubMed]

84. Berger, Z.; Quera, R.; Poniachik, J.; Oksenberg, D.; Guerrero, J. Heparin and insulin treatment of acute pancreatitis caused by hypertriglyceridemia. Experience of 5 cases. *Rev. Med. Chil.* **2001**, *129*, 1373–1378. [CrossRef] [PubMed]

85. Qiu, F.; Lu, X.S.; Huang, Y.K. Protective effect of low-molecular-weight heparin on pancreatic encephalopathy in severe acute pancreatic rats. *Inflamm. Res.* **2012**, *61*, 1203–1209. [CrossRef] [PubMed]

86. Trzaskoma, A.; Kruczek, M.; Rawski, B.; Poniewierka, E.; Kempiński, R. The use of heparin in the treatment of acute pancreatitis. *Pol. Przegl. Chir.* **2013**, *85*, 223–227. [CrossRef] [PubMed]

87. Lu, X.-S.; Qiu, F.; Li, J.-Q.; Fan, Q.-Q.; Zhou, R.-G.; Ai, Y.-H.; Zhang, K.-C.; Li, Y.-X. Low molecular weight heparin in the treatment of severe acute pancreatitis: A multiple centre prospective clinical study. *Asian J. Surg.* **2009**, *32*, 89–94. [PubMed]

88. Gyorgy, B.; Tothfalusi, L.; Nagy, G.; Pasztoi, M.; Geher, P.; Polgar, A.; Rojkovich, B.; Ujfalussy, I.; Misjak, P.; Koncz, A.; Pozsonyi, E.; Fust, G.; Falus, A.; Buzas, E.I. Natural autoantibodies reactive to glycosaminoglycans are disease state markers in rheumatoid arthritis and are associated with HLA. *Ann. Rheum. Dis.* **2010**, *69*, A2. [CrossRef]

89. Larsson, S.; Lohmander, L.S.; Struglics, A. Synovial fluid level of aggrecan ARGS fragments is a more sensitive marker of joint disease than glycosaminoglycan or aggrecan levels: A cross-sectional study. *Arthritis Res. Ther.* **2009**, *11*, R92. [CrossRef] [PubMed]

90. Palmer, J.L.; Bertone, A.L.; McClain, H. Assessment of glycosaminoglycan concentration in equine synovial fluid as a marker of joint disease. *Can. J. Vet. Res.* **1995**, *59*, 205–212. [PubMed]

91. Page, C. Heparin and related drugs: beyond anticoagulant activity. *ISRN Pharmacol.* **2013**, *2013*, 910743. [CrossRef] [PubMed]

92. McIntire, A.M.; Harris, S.A.; Whitten, J.A.; Fritschle-Hilliard, A.C.; Foster, D.R.; Sood, R.; Walroth, T.A. Outcomes Following the Use of Nebulized Heparin for Inhalation Injury (HIHI Study). *J. Burn Care Res.* **2017**, *38*, 45–52. [CrossRef] [PubMed]

93. Shastri, M.D.; Peterson, G.M.; Stewart, N. Non-anticoagulant derivatives of heparin for the management of asthma: Distant dream or close reality? *Expert Opin. Investig. Drugs* **2014**, *23*, 357–373. [CrossRef] [PubMed]

94. Serisier, D.J.; Shute, J.K.; Hockey, P.M.; Higgins, B.; Conway, J.; Carroll, M.P. Inhaled heparin in cystic fibrosis. *Eur. Respir. J.* **2006**, *27*, 354–358. [CrossRef] [PubMed]

95. Kozlowski, E.O.; Gomes, A.M.; Silva, C.S. Structure and Biological Activities of Glycosaminoglycan analogs from marine invertebrates: New therapeutic agents? In *Glycans in Diseases and Therapeutics, Biology of the Extracellular Matrix 158*; Pavão, M.S.G., Ed.; Springer: Berlin/Heidelberg, Germany, 2011; pp. 159–184.

96. Pavão, M.S.G. Glycosaminoglycans analogs from marine invertebrates: Structure, biological effects, and potential as new therapeutics. *Front. Cell. Infect. Microbiol.* **2014**, *4*, 123.

97. Sato, K.; Tsutsumi, M.; Nomura, Y.; Murata, N.; Kondo, N. Proteoglycan Isolated from Cartilaginous Fish and Process for Producing the Same. WO/2004/083257, 30 September 2004.

98. Brosstad, F.; Flengsrud, R.; Skjervold, P.O.; Odegaard, O.R. Glycosaminoglycan Anticoagulants Derived from Fish. US7618652 B2, 22 March 2002.

99. Holley, R.J.; Meade, K.A.; Merry, C.L.R. Using embryonic stem cells to understand how glycosaminoglycans regulate differentiation. *Biochem. Soc. Trans.* **2014**, *42*, 689–695. [CrossRef] [PubMed]

100. Pickford, C.E.; Holley, R.J.; Rushton, G.; Stavridis, M.P.; Ward, C.M.; Merry, C.L.R. Specific glycosaminoglycans modulate neural specification of mouse embryonic stem cells. *Stem Cells* **2011**, *29*, 629–640. [CrossRef] [PubMed]

101. Holley, R.J.; Smith, R.A.; van de Westerlo, E.M.A.; Pickford, C.E.; Merry, C.L.R.; van Kuppevelt, T.H. Use of flow cytometry for characterization and fractionation of cell populations based on their expression of heparan sulfate epitopes. *Methods Mol. Biol.* **2015**, *1229*, 239–251. [PubMed]

102. Meade, K.A.; White, K.J.; Pickford, C.E.; Holley, R.J.; Marson, A.; Tillotson, D.; Van Kuppevelt, T.H.; Whittle, J.D.; Day, A.J.; Merry, C.L.R. Immobilization of heparan sulfate on electrospun meshes to support embryonic stem cell culture and differentiation. *J. Biol. Chem.* **2013**, *288*, 5530–5538. [CrossRef] [PubMed]

103. Ghadiali, R.S.; Guimond, S.E.; Turnbull, J.E.; Pisconti, A. Dynamic changes in heparan sulfate during muscle differentiation and ageing regulate myoblast cell fate and FGF2 signaling. *Matrix Biol.* **2017**, *59*, 54–68. [CrossRef]

104. Holder, G.M.; Bowfield, A.; Surman, M.; Suepfle, M.; Moss, D.; Tucker, C.E.; Rudd, T.R.; Fernig, D.G.; Yates, E.A.; Weightman, P. Fundamental differences in model cell-surface polysaccharides revealed by complementary optical and spectroscopic techniques. *Soft Matter* **2012**, *8*, 6521–6527. [CrossRef]

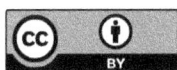

![molecules logo] *molecules*

Review

Non-Anticoagulant Heparins Are Hepcidin Antagonists for the Treatment of Anemia

Maura Poli [1], Michela Asperti [1], Paola Ruzzenenti [1], Annamaria Naggi [2] and Paolo Arosio [1,*]

[1] Department of Molecular and Translational Medicine, University of Brescia, Viale Europa 11, 25123 Brescia, Italy; maura.poli@unibs.it (M.P.); michela.asperti@unibs.it (M.A.); p.ruzzenenti001@unibs.it (P.R.)
[2] G. Ronzoni Institute for Chemical and Biochemical Research, Milan 20133, Italy; naggi@ronzoni.it
* Correspondence: paolo.arosio@unibs.it; Tel.: +39-030-371-7303; Fax: +39-030-371-7305

Academic Editor: Diego Muñoz-Torrero
Received: 21 March 2017; Accepted: 6 April 2017; Published: 8 April 2017

Abstract: The peptide hormone hepcidin is a key controller of systemic iron homeostasis, and its expression in the liver is mainly regulated by bone morphogenetic proteins (BMPs), which are heparin binding proteins. In fact, heparins are strong suppressors of hepcidin expression in hepatic cell lines that act by inhibiting the phosphorylation of SMAD1/5/8 proteins elicited by the BMPs. The inhibitory effect of heparins has been demonstrated in cells and in mice, where subcutaneous injections of non-anticoagulant heparins inhibited liver hepcidin expression and increased iron bioavailability. The chemical characteristics for high anti-hepcidin activity in vitro and in vivo include the 2O-and 6O-sulfation and a molecular weight above 7 kDa. The most potent heparins have been found to be the super-sulfated ones, active in hepcidin suppression with a molecular weight as low as 4 kDa. Moreover, the alteration of endogenous heparan sulfates has been found to cause a reduction in hepcidin expression in vitro and in vivo, indicating that heparins act by interfering with the interaction between BMPs and components of the complex involved in the activation of the BMP/SMAD1/5/8 pathway. This review summarizes recent findings on the anti-hepcidin activity of heparins and their possible use for the treatment of anemia caused by hepcidin excess, including the anemia of chronic diseases.

Keywords: heparin; hepcidin; iron homeostasis; anemia

---

1. Introduction

The biological function of heparins has not been fully established yet, but it is well known that they can bind a large number of plasma proteins with important biological roles that include growth factors, morphogens, and cytokines. This occurs because heparin shares the same binding capacity as the heparan sulfates (HSs) bound to the surfaces of all mammalian cells. The binding of growth factors and morphogens to surface HSs is important to modulate and control their functionalities, availability, and stability [1]. Most members of the TGF-beta superfamily bind heparin and HSs, and they include more than 15 types of bone morphogenetic proteins (BMPs) [2]. Among them, BMP2 and BMP4 and the homologous drosophila decapentaplegic have been extensively characterized for the binding to heparin and to the endogenous heparan sulfates, an interaction shown to be essential both for making a gradient during embryo development and for controlling local concentration [3]. The heparan sulfates have a major role for the binding and activity of FGF and VEGF and for the osteogenic activity of BMPs [2,4,5]. More recently, it was shown that the BMPs, and in particular BMP6, in the liver have the specific role of activating the expression of hepcidin, the iron-inflammation peptide hormone that regulates systemic iron homeostasis [6]. This has stimulated studies to verify if heparin can interfere with the activity of BMP6 and hepcidin expression in cells and in animals, and this led to the demonstration that non-anticoagulant heparins are efficient suppressors of hepcidin. This review summarizes the recent development on mammalian iron homeostasis, its regulation and pathological deregulations, and the possible use of heparins for treatment of anemias caused by hepcidin excess, as it occurs in inflammatory conditions.

2. Iron Homeostasis and the Role of Hepcidin

Iron is an essential micronutrient for all organisms since it acts as a cofactor for enzymes involved in vital processes including oxygen transport (hemoglobin and myoglobin), citric acid cycle and cellular respiration (Fe/S cluster proteins and cytochromes), antioxidant defense (peroxidase and catalase), DNA/RNA synthesis, and nucleotide metabolism (ribosome reductase). However, it is also potentially toxic because Fe(II) can participate in Fenton's reaction, giving rise to toxic oxygen species. As a consequence, iron homeostasis must be tightly controlled, at both the cellular and the systemic levels. The mechanism acting at the cellular level has been clarified long ago and uses the iron regulatory proteins that bind elements on the ferritin and transferrin-receptor-1 mRNA in an iron-dependent manner and that thus regulate iron storage and iron uptake in the opposite way [7]. The study of systemic iron homeostasis was more complex, and the basic mechanism has only recently been elucidated. The normal Western daily diet contains about 10–15 mg of iron, most of which is heme iron and the rest is as Fe(III) complexed to various molecules, but only a portion of this iron is absorbed to compensate the physiological losses of the body (1–2 mg/day). They are not regulated and consist in cell defoliation, sweat, and by periodic/occasional blood losses that must be balanced by an equal amount of iron intake to maintain the 4–5 g of iron needed for the synthesis of hemoglobin and the many essential iron enzymes [8]. Only under conditions of iron deprivation, most of the available iron can be taken up by the body. The mechanism used by heme iron to enter the duodenal enterocyte has not been clarified, while non-heme iron is first reduced by an epithelial ferric reductase DcytB that makes it more soluble and adapt to be taken up by the transporter named DMT1 [9]. Once in the enterocyte, the iron can enter the storage compartment of the ferritin to be lost at the end of the cell life cycle, or be transferred to circulation via the exporter named ferroportin, in a step that needs the assistance of a ferroxidase enzyme, hephestin, or ceruloplasmin to load it onto the serum transferrin. The transferrin iron is delivered via the transferrin-receptor-1 to the various organs and in particular to the bone marrow where the erythroid precursors use most of it for hemoglobin synthesis [10]. The hemoglobin iron is eventually released to the transferrin, and the red blood cells are thereafter taken up by phagocytic macrophages, mainly in the spleen, where the heme is degraded by heme-oxygenase and the iron is exported via the ferroportin. This pathway implies that the availability of systemic iron relies mostly on the cellular iron export that depends on the ferroportin, and the exported iron originates partly from the diet (1–2 mg/die) and mostly from hemoglobin recycling (20–25 mg/die). In fact, the major control of systemic iron relies on a protein hormone, named hepcidin, that binds specifically to ferroportin to induce its internalization, ubiquitination, and degradation, thus reducing systemic iron availability [11]. When hepcidin is low, iron is readily released by enterocytes and macrophages, it becomes more available and may determine iron overload in the parenchymal cells, as it occurs in hereditary hemochromatosis. If hepcidin is high, less iron is absorbed and recycled, leading to anemia and iron retention in the macrophages of the spleen. After the discovery that hepcidin is the major controller of systemic iron availability, the focus was on the mechanism of its regulation. Hepcidin is produced as a propeptide that is processed in the mature 25 amino acid form stabilized by four disulfide bonds. It is expressed mainly by the hepatocytes in an iron-dependent manner with a typical feedback manner: upregulated when body iron is high and downregulated when body iron is low. The finding that hepcidin is upregulated also by inflammation and downregulated by erythroid activity and hypoxia was important [12]. The important role of inflammation on hepcidin transcription clarified why many inflammatory conditions are accompanied by low hemoglobin, as it occurs in the anemia of chronic diseases or anemia of inflammation [13]. Dysregulations of hepcidin expression are associated with various disorders, so an understanding of the detailed mechanism of hepcidin control could lead to the development of therapies for the treatment of various iron-related disorders.

The regulation of hepcidin occurs mainly at a transcriptional level and mostly relies on the BMP6/SMAD pathway that, when activated, strongly stimulates hepcidin expression in the liver [14]. This involves the BMP receptors and requires the assistance of a specific co-receptor named hemojuvelin (HJV) that is a GPI-anchor membrane protein [15]. The BMP binding activates the Type II receptor BMPRII to phosphorylate the Type I receptor ALK2, which causes the phosphorylation of SMAD1/5/8 that then associates with SMAD4 and the complex migrates to the nucleus to bind the element at the hepcidin promoter [16]. Iron activates this pathway via a mechanism that has not been fully elucidated but is known to involve the induction of BMP6 [17]. The inflammatory stimulus acts mainly via IL6 produced by macrophages that activates the JAK/STAT3 pathway, which potentiates the BMP/SMAD pathway [18]. A further regulation is made by the presence of a liver-specific membrane serine-protease named TMPRSS6, which cleaves and inactivates HJV, thus inhibiting hepcidin expression [19]. Mutation of this gene cause a genetic iron-refractory iron-deficiency anemia (IRIDA) because of elevated hepcidin levels [20].

3. Heparins and Hepcidin Expression

In vitro studies on hepatic cells initially showed that BMP2 is a strong inducer of hepcidin, but later it was found that BMP6 is the physiological BMP dedicated to hepcidin expression based on the evidence that the major phenotype of mice deficient in BMP6 was a massive liver iron overload and that BMP6 is regulated in an iron-dependent manner [21]. After these findings, many approaches have been taken for a pharmacological control of hepcidin expression, identifying and developing both hepcidin agonists and antagonists. These studies have been described in recent reviews and include molecules that sequester hepcidin, that interfere with the BMP/SMAD or IL6/STAT3 pathways, that regulate hepcidin expression, that act on BMP co-receptors, and that mimic hepcidin and others [22–24].

Our approach started with the observation that BMPs are heparin binding proteins and thus heparin might interfere with the BMP/SMAD pathway that controls hepcidin expression. We demonstrated that commercial heparins used in clinics for their anticoagulant property are strong inhibitors of hepcidin expression in vitro in mice and in the few hospitalized patients we analyzed [25]. In vitro, we tested hepatoma HepG2 cells with unfractionated heparin (UFH), low-molecular-weight heparin (LMWH), and the pentasaccharide Fondaparinux, and we observed that UFH was the most effective in suppressing hepcidin expression at pharmacological concentrations with an effect that lasted up to 22 h. Moreover, in these cells, UFH fully suppressed hepcidin stimulation by exogenous BMP6 in a manner slightly different from that of BMP2. LMWH maintained some anti-hepcidin activity but at higher doses, while the pentasaccharide Fondaparinux was only marginally functional; thus, the potency was in the following order: UFH > LMWH >> Fondaparinux [25]. Mice treatments with pharmacological concentrations of UFH downregulated hepcidin and modified body iron status, with an increase of circulating iron and a decrease of spleen storage iron [25]. However, the use of heparin in mice was difficult because of its anticoagulant activity. To overcome this problem, the heparins were chemically modified to reduce/abolish this activity by altering the antithrombin binding site. This was done by a process of oxidation and reduction that produced Glycol-split heparins or by increasing the sulfation degree in the super-sulfated heparins [26]. The Glycol-split heparins we analyzed, named RO-82 and RO-68, were completely devoid of anti-coagulant activity and could be easily used in the mice without side effects, showing a potent hepcidin inhibitory activity [27]. The super-sulfated heparin, coded SSLMWH-19, was even more potent than the glycol-split heparins although it retained a marginal anticoagulant activity [28]. The anti-hepcidin activity of heparins, both anti-coagulant and modified ones, was always accompanied by the concomitant reduction in the pSMAD activation and the reduction in Id1 mRNA, a marker of this pathway, both in hepatoma cells and in mice. In addition, we observed that the inhibitory effect was specific for the BMP/SMAD pathway; in fact, when we stimulated hepcidin expression with an inflammatory stimulus (IL6 in cells and lipopolysaccharide in mice), heparins suppressed hepcidin induction by inhibiting only the BMP-SMAD related pathway, without any changes in the activation of the pSTAT3 inflammatory pathway [27].

Molecular weight and the degree of sulfation are the two major chemical properties of heparins that we analyzed to evaluate their effect on anti-hepcidin activity. Heparin preparations are a pool of molecules with different molecular weights. Thus, they were fractionated on gel filtration columns to obtain preparations with defined and restricted molecular weight. We found that the Glycol-split heparins with a molecular weight above 7 kDa were able to completely suppress hepcidin expression in hepatoma cells, even after BMP6 stimulation. Interestingly, the super-sulfated heparin SSLMWH-19 preserved a high anti-hepcidin activity even with molecular weight as low as 4 kDa. In vivo experiments in mice confirmed that the Glycol-split heparins above 7 kDa and the super-sulfated ones of about 4 kDa were highly effective in suppressing liver hepcidin expression [29]. We further analyzed heparins in which the sulfated groups in position 6-O and 2-O were selectively removed or were N-acetylated and we found that they had a reduced inhibitory effect on hepcidin expression both in the absence or presence of BMP6 stimulation and in mice [29]. Altogether, we showed that non-anti-coagulant Glycol-split heparins have a strong anti-hepcidin property, and to be functional they must be 2O- and 6O-sulfated and have a molecular weight > 7 kDa that corresponds to about 17 saccharide residues. Similarly, the effective super-sulfated heparins have a molecular weight >4 kDa and are made of more than 9 saccharide residues. This is in line with the finding that to exert a potent activity, these compounds should expose numerous binding sites for the interaction with different molecules or different sites of the same molecule. The heparins used in our studies and their properties are summarized in Table 1, and a scheme of the mechanism of the anti-hepcidin activity of heparin shown in Figure 1.

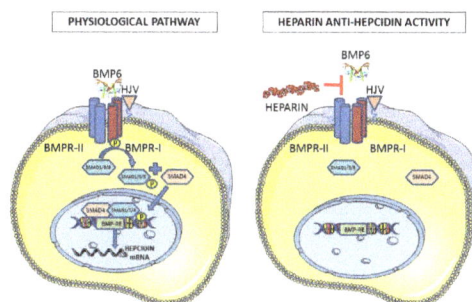

Figure 1. Scheme of the anti-hepcidin activity of heparin. In the physiological pathway, the binding of BMP6 causes the phosphorylation of Type I receptor by Type II receptor, which phosphorylates SMAD1/5/8 that associates with SMAD4, and the complex enters the nucleus to bind to the responsive element on the hepcidin promoter. The anti-hepcidin activity of heparin is thought to act by sequestering BMP6 and interfering with its binding to the receptors.

Table 1. List of the heparins tested for the anti-hepcidin property in vitro and/or in vivo. These include anti-coagulant and non-anticoagulant heparins as indicated. The main features and the anti-hepcidin potency (*** strong anti-hepcidin activity/** intermediate anti-hepcidin activity/* low anti-hepcidin activity) of the heparins are described. The fractions of fractionated heparins are coded as F plus a number.

Heparins Tested for Anti-Hepcidin Activity					
Compounds	Description	Mw (kD)	Anticoagulant	Potency	Ref.
UFH	Pig Mucosal heparin, commercial (Calciparina)	12.0–15.0	yes	***	[25,27]
PMH	Pig Mucosal heparin (API)	19.9	yes	***	[25,27]
LMWH	Commercial LMWH Enoxaparin (Clexane)	4.5	yes	**	[25,27]
FONDAPARINUX	Commercial pentasaccharide (Arixtra)	1.7	yes	*	[25,27]
RO-82	Glycol-Split,	16.0	no	***	[27,29]
RO-68	Partially 2O-desulfated,Glycol-split	16.4	no	***	[27,29]
NAc-91	N-acetylated	16.0	no	*	[27,29]
NAc-RO-00	N-Acetylated, glycol-split	15.9	no	*	[27,29]
SSLMWH-19	Super-sulfated LMW	8.8	partially	***	[27,29]
PMH-F1	PMH fraction	21.6	yes	***	[29]
PMH-F2	PMH fraction	14.4	yes	***	[29]
PMH-F3	PMH fraction	10.0	yes	***	[29]
RO-82-F1	Glycol-Split, fraction	12.0	no	***	[29]
RO-82-F2	Glycol-Split, fraction	9.2	no	***	[29]
RO-82-F3	Glycol-Split, fraction	7.8	no	**	[29]
RO-82-F4	Glycol-Split, fraction	6.8	no	**	[29]
RO-68-F1	Partially 2O-desulfated Glycol-split	7.8	no	**	[29]
RO-68-F2	Partially 2O-desulfated Glycol-split	6.2	no	**	[29]
RO-68-F3	Partially 2O-desulfated Glycol-split	3.9	no	*	[29]
SSLMWH-19-F1	Super-sulfated LMW fraction	12.9	partially	***	[29]
SSLMWH-19-F2	Super-sulfated LMW fraction	10.3	partially	***	[29]
SSLMWH-19-F3	Super-sulfated LMW fraction	6.9	partially	***	[29]
SSLMWH-19-F4	Super-sulfated LMW fraction	4.0	partially	***	[29]
2-O	PMH 2-O desulfated	-	no	*	[29]
6-O	PMH 6-O desulfated	-	no	*	[29]

4. Alternative Ways of Heparin Administration

Heparin is normally administrated subcutaneously, the absorption of which is now well characterized and known [30]. Therefore, for the treatment of mice, we use the same subcutaneous administration that produced good results in the short run [27]. However, in some cases of iron deficient anemia caused by hepcidin excess, it would take a long time to replenish the iron stores, and thus chronic treatments should probably be used. Thus, alternative ways of administration should be explored—methods that are less invasive than the daily subcutaneous injection. To this aim, we started using mice osmotic pumps, which ensure the continuous delivery of the compound for 7 or 28 days. This has already been successfully used in mice for the delivery of a non-anticoagulant heparin to study its anti-tumor activity [31,32]. This encouraged us to deliver Glycol-split heparins with an osmotic pump in mice for 7 days. The preliminary data showed that the implants and heparin delivery did not cause any evident adverse effect, but we did find a significant inhibition of liver hepcidin mRNA and of the serum hepcidin (unpublished data). These results encourage use to continue with further analysis. Oral administration of heparin is also interesting; oral heparin therapeutics for anticoagulant activity using different methods for drug delivery, such as liposomes, emulsions, or chemically modified heparin, has long been attempted, without major effects [33]. In preliminary attempts, we administrated the super-sulfated SSLMWH-19 heparin by a single oral gavage in mice and observed a significant reduction in liver hepcidin mRNA. Further studies are needed to verify if functional, low-molecular-weight heparin can diffuse across the gastrointestinal membrane and enter the circulation to exert reproducible anti-hepcidin activity.

5. Hepcidin and Endogenous Heparan Sulfates

The exogenous heparin is normally used to interfere with the physiological interactions between the ligands and endogenous heparan sulfates, thus it was of interest to verify if and how the heparan sulfates participate in the mechanism of hepcidin expression. As an approach to study this, we analyzed the effect of heparanase, the enzyme that physiologically degrades the heparan sulfates [34]. Overexpression of the enzyme in hepatic cell lines caused an inhibition of hepcidin expression and an increase of cellular iron and ferritin [35]. Mice with overexpression of heparanase were healthy, but they showed abnormal levels of hepcidin and liver iron loading [35]. In another approach, we treated HepG2 cells with sodium chlorate, a known inhibitor of heparan sulfate biosynthesis that interferes with the sulfate carrier donor PAPS (3'-phosphoadenosine 5'-phosphosulfate). This caused a strong inhibition of hepcidin expression even after stimulation with BMP6 (unpublished results). Experiments to inhibit key enzymes of heparan sulfate biosynthesis in cells and in mice are in progress. We propose a scheme of the mechanism of action of endogenous heparan sulfates involvement in hepcidin expression pathway, as shown in Figure 2.

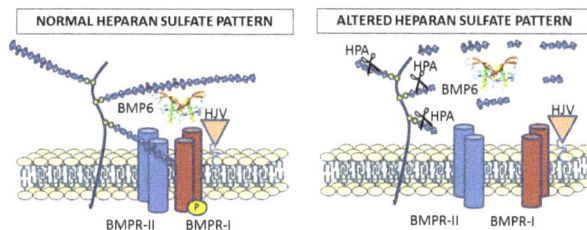

Figure 2. The heparan sulfates bound to proteoglycans cover cellular membranes and are thought to participate in the binding of BMP6 to the receptors for activation of the SMAD signaling. This is supported by the evidence that alteration of the endogenous heparan sulfate structure by heparanase overexpression strongly reduced BMP6 signaling and hepcidin expression in cells and mice. Exogenous heparins probably interfere with the roles of endogenous heparan sulfates.

6. BMP6 and Heparin Binding

Most BMPs bind heparin, and in fact they were originally purified from heparin columns [36]. A major heparin binding domain has been identified in BMP2 by site-directed mutagenesis [37–39], and it involves the N-terminus that is disordered and not detected in the crystallographic structure. The site does not overlap with the binding sites of the receptors that are at the edges of the molecule [40]. The sequence is conserved also in BMP4, and the biological activity of both molecules is affected by exogenous heparins, although the effect seems to be variable stimulatory [41] or inhibitory [42]. This N-terminal sequence is substituted in BMP6 and BMP7, being longer and with a lower density of basic residues. More important in our study is that this segment is absent in the commercial preparations of BMP6 that are biologically active, possibly because the basic residues interfere with expression and purification. Our preliminary data indicate that this sequence is important for heparin binding, and suggest the presence of a second heparin binding site exposed on the opposite site of the molecule that has lower affinity. Moreover, the BMP receptors were found to bind heparin [42], and it was proposed that they may bind Type II receptor and facilitate its interaction with Type I [3], thus acting as a co-receptors, similar to what has been described for Neogenin, which also binds to Type II before Type I [40]. The binding of HJV to heparin has not been studied yet.

7. Conclusions

Heparin interferes with the BMP6/SMAD pathway of hepcidin regulation, acting as a strong suppressor. The activity is also evident in vivo in animal models, and non-anticoagulant heparins are promising heparin antagonists that can be used for treatments of conditions with an excess of hepcidin, such as the anemia of chronic disease, also known as anemia of inflammation, which is the most common form of anemia in hospitalized patients, and the iron-refractory iron-deficient anemia (IRIDA) mainly linked to genetic variations of the Tmprrs6 gene. An understanding of how heparin and heparan sulfates participate in the mechanism of BMP/SMAD pathways is emerging, but awaits clarification from further studies.

Acknowledgments: This work was partially supported by Telethon grant GGP15064 to PA, by Fondazione Cariplo 2012-0570 to PA and AN, and MIUR PRIN-10-11 to PA.

Conflicts of Interest: The authors declare non conflict of interest.

References

1. Turnbull, J.; Powell, A.; Guimond, S. Heparan sulfate: Decoding a dynamic multifunctional cell regulator. *Trends. Cell. Biol.* **2001**, *11*, 75–82. [CrossRef]
2. Rider, C.C. Heparin/heparan sulphate binding in the tgf-beta cytokine superfamily. *Biochem. Soc. Trans.* **2006**, *34*, 458–460. [CrossRef] [PubMed]
3. Kuo, W.J.; Digman, M.A.; Lander, A.D. Heparan sulfate acts as a bone morphogenetic protein coreceptor by facilitating ligand-induced receptor hetero-oligomerization. *Mol. Biol. Cell.* **2010**, *21*, 4028–4041. [CrossRef] [PubMed]
4. Capila, I.; Linhardt, R.J. Heparin-protein interactions. *Angew. Chem. Int. Ed. Engl.* **2002**, *41*, 391–412. [CrossRef]
5. Goldberg, R.; Meirovitz, A.; Hirshoren, N.; Bulvik, R.; Binder, A.; Rubinstein, A.M.; Elkin, M. Versatile role of heparanase in inflammation. *Matrix. Biol.* **2013**, *32*, 234–240. [CrossRef] [PubMed]
6. Nemeth, E.; Tuttle, M.S.; Powelson, J.; Vaughn, M.B.; Donovan, A.; Ward, D.M.; Ganz, T.; Kaplan, J. Hepcidin regulates cellular iron efflux by binding to ferroportin and inducing its internalization. *Science* **2004**, *306*, 2090–2093. [CrossRef] [PubMed]
7. Kuhn, L.C. Iron regulatory proteins and their role in controlling iron metabolism. *Metallomics* **2015**, *7*, 232–243. [CrossRef] [PubMed]
8. Rouault, T.; Klausner, R. Regulation of iron metabolism in eukaryotes. *Curr. Top. Cell. Regul.* **1997**, *35*, 1–19. [PubMed]
9. McKie, A.; Barrow, D.; Latunde-Dada, G.; Rolfs, A.; Sager, G.; Mudaly, E.; Mudaly, M.; Richardson, C.; Barlow, D.; Bomford, A.; et al. An iron-regulated ferric reductase associated with the absorption of dietary iron. *Science* **2001**, *291*, 1755–1759. [CrossRef] [PubMed]
10. Pantopoulos, K.; Porwal, S.K.; Tartakoff, A.; Devireddy, L. Mechanisms of mammalian iron homeostasis. *Biochemistry* **2012**, *51*, 5705–5724. [CrossRef] [PubMed]
11. Nemeth, E.; Ganz, T. The role of hepcidin in iron metabolism. *Acta. Haematol.* **2009**, *122*, 78–86. [CrossRef] [PubMed]
12. Camaschella, C.; Silvestri, L. Molecular mechanisms regulating hepcidin revealed by hepcidin disorders. *Scientific World J.* **2011**, *11*, 1357–1366. [CrossRef] [PubMed]
13. Ganz, T.; Nemeth, E. Hepcidin and disorders of iron metabolism. *Annu. Rev. Med.* **2011**, *62*, 347–360. [CrossRef] [PubMed]
14. Babitt, J.L.; Huang, F.W.; Xia, Y.; Sidis, Y.; Andrews, N.C.; Lin, H.Y. Modulation of bone morphogenetic protein signaling in vivo regulates systemic iron balance. *J. Clin. Investig.* **2007**, *117*, 1933–1939. [CrossRef] [PubMed]
15. Xia, Y.; Babitt, J.L.; Sidis, Y.; Chung, R.T.; Lin, H.Y. Hemojuvelin regulates hepcidin expression via a selective subset of bmp ligands and receptors independently of neogenin. *Blood* **2008**, *111*, 5195–5204. [CrossRef] [PubMed]
16. Poli, M.; Luscieti, S.; Gandini, V.; Maccarinelli, F.; Finazzi, D.; Silvestri, L.; Roetto, A.; Arosio, P. Transferrin receptor 2 and hfe regulate furin expression via mitogen-activated protein kinase/extracellular signal-regulated kinase (mapk/erk) signaling. Implications for transferrin-dependent hepcidin regulation. *Haematologica* **2010**, *95*, 1832–1840. [CrossRef] [PubMed]
17. Ganz, T.; Nemeth, E. Hepcidin and iron homeostasis. *Biochim. Biophys. Acta* **2012**, *1823*, 1434–1443. [CrossRef] [PubMed]
18. Verga Falzacappa, M.V.; Vujic Spasic, M.; Kessler, R.; Stolte, J.; Hentze, M.W.; Muckenthaler, M.U. Stat3 mediates hepatic hepcidin expression and its inflammatory stimulation. *Blood* **2007**, *109*, 353–358. [CrossRef] [PubMed]

19. Silvestri, L.; Pagani, A.; Nai, A.; De Domenico, I.; Kaplan, J.; Camaschella, C. The serine protease matriptase-2 (tmprss6) inhibits hepcidin activation by cleaving membrane hemojuvelin. *Cell. Metab.* **2008**, *8*, 502–511. [CrossRef] [PubMed]

20. Finberg, K.E.; Heeney, M.M.; Campagna, D.R.; Aydinok, Y.; Pearson, H.A.; Hartman, K.R.; Mayo, M.M.; Samuel, S.M.; Strouse, J.J.; Markianos, K.; et al. Mutations in tmprss6 cause iron-refractory iron deficiency anemia (irida). *Nat. Genet.* **2008**, *40*, 569–571. [CrossRef] [PubMed]

21. Meynard, D.; Kautz, L.; Darnaud, V.; Canonne-Hergaux, F.; Coppin, H.; Roth, M.P. Lack of the bone morphogenetic protein bmp6 induces massive iron overload. *Nat. Genet.* **2009**, *41*, 478–481. [CrossRef] [PubMed]

22. Drakesmith, H.; Nemeth, E.; Ganz, T. Ironing out ferroportin. *Cell. Metab.* **2015**, *22*, 777–787. [CrossRef] [PubMed]

23. Poli, M.; Asperti, M.; Ruzzenenti, P.; Regoni, M.; Arosio, P. Hepcidin antagonists for potential treatments of disorders with hepcidin excess. *Front. Pharmacol.* **2014**, *5*, 86. [CrossRef] [PubMed]

24. Sun, C.C.; Vaja, V.; Babitt, J.L.; Lin, H.Y. Targeting the hepcidin-ferroportin axis to develop new treatment strategies for anemia of chronic disease and anemia of inflammation. *Am. J. Hematol.* **2012**, *78*, 392–400. [CrossRef] [PubMed]

25. Poli, M.; Girelli, D.; Campostrini, N.; Maccarinelli, F.; Finazzi, D.; Luscieti, S.; Nai, A.; Arosio, P. Heparin: A potent inhibitor of hepcidin expression in vitro and in vivo. *Blood* **2011**, *117*, 997–1004. [CrossRef] [PubMed]

26. Casu, B.; Guerrini, M.; Guglieri, S.; Naggi, A.; Perez, M.; Torri, G.; Cassinelli, G.; Ribatti, D.; Carminati, P.; Giannini, G.; et al. Undersulfated and glycol-split heparins endowed with antiangiogenic activity. *J. Med. Chem.* **2004**, *47*, 838–848. [CrossRef] [PubMed]

27. Poli, M.; Asperti, M.; Naggi, A.; Campostrini, N.; Girelli, D.; Corbella, M.; Benzi, M.; Besson-Fournier, C.; Coppin, H.; Maccarinelli, F.; et al. Glycol-split nonanticoagulant heparins are inhibitors of hepcidin expression in vitro and in vivo. *Blood* **2014**, *123*, 1564–1573. [CrossRef] [PubMed]

28. Poli, M.; Asperti, M.; Ruzzenenti, P.; Mandelli, L.; Campostrini, N.; Martini, G.; Di Somma, M.; Maccarinelli, F.; Girelli, D.; Naggi, A.; et al. Oversulfated heparins with low anticoagulant activity are strong and fast inhibitors of hepcidin expression in vitro and in vivo. *Biochem. Pharmacol.* **2014**, *92*, 467–475. [CrossRef] [PubMed]

29. Asperti, M.; Naggi, A.; Esposito, E.; Ruzzenenti, P.; Di Somma, M.; Gryzik, M.; Arosio, P.; Poli, M. High sulfation and a high molecular weight are important for anti-hepcidin activity of heparin. *Front. Pharmacol.* **2015**, *6*, 316. [CrossRef] [PubMed]

30. Hirsh, J.; Warkentin, T.E.; Raschke, R.; Granger, C.; Ohman, E.M.; Dalen, J.E. Heparin and low-molecular-weight heparin: Mechanisms of action, pharmacokinetics, dosing considerations, monitoring, efficacy, and safety. *Chest* **1998**, *114*, 489S–510S. [CrossRef] [PubMed]

31. Ritchie, J.P.; Ramani, V.C.; Ren, Y.; Naggi, A.; Torri, G.; Casu, B.; Penco, S.; Pisano, C.; Carminati, P.; Tortoreto, M.; et al. SST0001, a chemically modified heparin, inhibits myeloma growth and angiogenesis via disruption of the heparanase/syndecan-1 axis. *Clin. Cancer. Res.* **2011**, *17*, 1382–1393. [CrossRef] [PubMed]

32. Yang, Y.; MacLeod, V.; Dai, Y.; Khotskaya-Sample, Y.; Shriver, Z.; Venkataraman, G.; Sasisekharan, R.; Naggi, A.; Torri, G.; Casu, B.; et al. The syndecan-1 heparan sulfate proteoglycan is a viable target for myeloma therapy. *Blood* **2007**, *110*, 2041–2048. [CrossRef] [PubMed]

33. Paliwal, R.; Paliwal, S.R.; Agrawal, G.P.; Vyas, S.P. Recent advances in search of oral heparin therapeutics. *Med. Res. Rev.* **2012**, *32*, 388–409. [CrossRef] [PubMed]

34. Vlodavsky, I.; Goldshmidt, O.; Zcharia, E.; Metzger, S.; Chajek-Shaul, T.; Atzmon, R.; Guatta-Rangini, Z.; Friedmann, Y. Molecular properties and involvement of heparanase in cancer progression and normal development. *Biochimie* **2001**, *83*, 831–839. [CrossRef]

35. Asperti, M.; Stuemler, T.; Poli, M.; Gryzik, M.; Lifshitz, L.; Meyron-Holtz, E.G.; Vlodavsky, I.; Arosio, P. Heparanase overexpression reduces hepcidin expression, affects iron homeostasis and alters the response to inflammation. *PLoS ONE* **2016**, *11*, e0164183. [CrossRef] [PubMed]

36. Wozney, J.M.; Rosen, V.; Celeste, A.J.; Mitsock, L.M.; Whitters, M.J.; Kriz, R.W.; Hewick, R.M.; Wang, E.A. Novel regulators of bone formation: Molecular clones and activities. *Science* **1988**, *242*, 1528–1534. [CrossRef] [PubMed]

37. Ruppert, R.; Hoffmann, E.; Sebald, W. Human bone morphogenetic protein 2 contains a heparin-binding site which modifies its biological activity. *Eur. J. Biochem.* **1996**, *237*, 295–302. [CrossRef] [PubMed]
38. Gandhi, N.S.; Mancera, R.L. Prediction of heparin binding sites in bone morphogenetic proteins (bmps). *Biochim. Biophys. Acta* **2012**, *1824*, 1374–1381. [CrossRef] [PubMed]
39. Choi, Y.J.; Lee, J.Y.; Park, J.H.; Park, J.B.; Suh, J.S.; Choi, Y.S.; Lee, S.J.; Chung, C.P.; Park, Y.J. The identification of a heparin binding domain peptide from bone morphogenetic protein-4 and its role on osteogenesis. *Biomaterials* **2010**, *31*, 7226–7238. [CrossRef] [PubMed]
40. Healey, E.G.; Bishop, B.; Elegheert, J.; Bell, C.H.; Padilla-Parra, S.; Siebold, C. Repulsive guidance molecule is a structural bridge between neogenin and bone morphogenetic protein. *Nat. Struct. Mol. Biol.* **2015**, *22*, 458–465. [CrossRef] [PubMed]
41. Zhao, B.; Katagiri, T.; Toyoda, H.; Takada, T.; Yanai, T.; Fukuda, T.; Chung, U.I.; Koike, T.; Takaoka, K.; Kamijo, R. Heparin potentiates the in vivo ectopic bone formation induced by bone morphogenetic protein-2. *J. Biol. Chem.* **2006**, *281*, 23246–23253. [CrossRef] [PubMed]
42. Kanzaki, S.; Takahashi, T.; Kanno, T.; Ariyoshi, W.; Shinmyouzu, K.; Tujisawa, T.; Nishihara, T. Heparin inhibits bmp-2 osteogenic bioactivity by binding to both bmp-2 and bmp receptor. *J. Cell. Physiol.* **2008**, *216*, 844–850. [CrossRef] [PubMed]

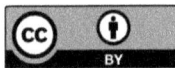

Review

Heparin, Heparan Sulphate and the TGF-β Cytokine Superfamily

Chris C. Rider * and Barbara Mulloy

Centre for Biomedical Sciences, School of Biological Sciences, Royal Holloway University of London, Egham, Surrey TW20 0EX, UK; b.mulloy@imperial.ac.uk
* Correspondence: c.rider@rhul.ac.uk

Academic Editors: Giangiacomo Torri and Jawed Fareed
Received: 29 March 2017; Accepted: 26 April 2017; Published: 29 April 2017

Abstract: Of the circa 40 cytokines of the TGF-β superfamily, around a third are currently known to bind to heparin and heparan sulphate. This includes TGF-β1, TGF-β2, certain bone morphogenetic proteins (BMPs) and growth and differentiation factors (GDFs), as well as GDNF and two of its close homologues. Experimental studies of their heparin/HS binding sites reveal a diversity of locations around the shared cystine-knot protein fold. The activities of the TGF-β cytokines in controlling proliferation, differentiation and survival in a range of cell types are in part regulated by a number of specific, secreted BMP antagonist proteins. These vary in structure but seven belong to the CAN or DAN family, which shares the TGF-β type cystine-knot domain. Other antagonists are more distant members of the TGF-β superfamily. It is emerging that the majority, but not all, of the antagonists are also heparin binding proteins. Any future exploitation of the TGF-β cytokines in the therapy of chronic diseases will need to fully consider their interactions with glycosaminoglycans and the implications of this in terms of their bioavailability and biological activity.

Keywords: heparin; heparan sulphate; TGF-β; bone morphogenetic protein (BMP); growth and differentiation factor (GDF); GDNF; BMP antagonists; noggin; sclerostin; gremlin

---

1. The TGF-β Cytokine Superfamily

The vertebrate TGF-β superfamily comprises some 40 cytokines, which regulate cellular activities encompassing proliferation, differentiation, and survival in diverse cell types (for reviews see [1–3]). They are thus important in tissue morphogenesis and development, as well as in regulating tissue homeostasis in the adult. Accordingly some members of the superfamily have come to the fore in the field of regenerative medicine, such as in the maintenance and subsequent differentiation of embryonic stem cells [1]. Moreover, aberrant signalling by TGF-β family cytokines occurs in a range of chronic diseases including tissue fibrosis and various cancers, and thus an understanding of their roles and modes of action is of relevance in effort to develop effective therapies for such diseases.

Within the superfamily, there are three TGF-βs [2], four activins [3], four neurotropic factors [4] and 21 bone morphogenetic proteins (BMPs)/growth and differentiation factors (GDFs) [5]. Across the superfamily a number of different receptors and signalling pathways are employed, but the canonical signalling pathway is via a complex of Type I and Type II serine/threonine kinases, cell surface receptors which activate cytoplasmic Smad transcription factors. The field of TGF-β family cytokine signalling and receptor usage has recently been reviewed elsewhere [6].

A further superfamily feature is a commonality of structure based on a cystine knot motif (Figure 1) Although variations occur, this typically contains within a sequence of some 110 residues, seven cysteines, of which six form intrachain disulphide bridges with the connectivity of CyS1-CyS5, CyS2-Cys6, and Cys3-CyS7. These covalent bridges give rise to a true knot structure, as CyS -2, -3, -6 and -7 together with neighbouring amino acids in the polypeptide chain, form an eight-membered circle of covalently linked residues, through which the CyS1-CyS5 linkage passes [7]. This covalent knot holds together a polypeptide fold in which two narrow β-strand finger loops project in near parallel from one face of a short α-helix [8,9]. A simply analogy of this structure is that of a hand (Figure 1A) bearing only two slightly curved fingers (the β-strand loops). The cystine knot region provides the palm, with the α-helix comprising the heel or wrist of the hand. Many but not all of the superfamily members exist as covalently linked dimers, held together by an interchain disulphide bridge between the two Cys4 residues which are un-partnered within the monomeric structure. This covalent bridge gives rise to an elongated, offset, face-to-face dimer in which the paired β-strand finger loops of each subunit extend away from the each other at opposite ends of the structure (Figure 1B).

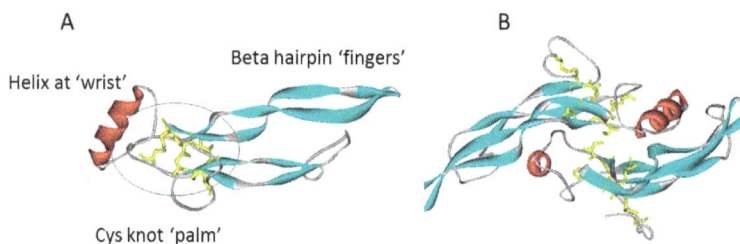

Figure 1. The TGF-β superfamily cystine knot fold, as typified by TGF-β1 (co-ordinates from 1KLC.pdb). Protein chains are shown in ribbon format: β-strands are blue, helices red, turns green; cystines are shown in yellow stick format. (**A**) TGF-β1 monomer showing the "hand" structures, with the cystine knot indicated by a green ellipse. (**B**) TGF-β1 dimer, the "wrist" of each hand is cupped in the other subunit. The view of the dimer is rotated by 90° with respect to the plane of 1A. The interchain disulphide bridge is visible in the centre of the structure.

2. Protein Antagonists of TGF-β Cytokines

The activities of a number of the TGF-β superfamily members are tightly regulated, in part through several secreted antagonist proteins which bind certain of these cytokines with high affinity, inhibiting cell surface receptor engagement, and thereby signalling. These antagonists include Noggin, Twisted Gastrulation (TSG), Chordin and Chordin-like proteins, and Follistatin (FST) and Follistatin like proteins (FSTLs). These antagonist proteins were initially recognised through their important roles in embryonic development [10]. A further family of seven antagonists is the Cerberus or Dan (CAN) family, which comprises Cerberus, Coco, Dan, Gremlin (also referred to as Gremlin-1), PRDC/gremlin-2, Sclerostin and USAG-1. Remarkably, the CAN family antagonists are also TGF-β superfamily members, by virtue of possessing the characteristic eight-membered cystine-knot domain [7]. The non-CAN antagonists, TSG, Chordin, and Noggin, but not Follistatin, possess more diverse variants of the cystine-knot motif within their larger structures, and therefore are distant members of the TGF-β superfamily [11].

3. Interactions of TGF-β Cytokines with Heparin and Heparan Sulphate

It has emerged that a number of the TGF-β superfamily cytokines bind to the sulphated polysaccharide heparin and heparan sulphate (HS) with interactions strong enough to be relevant at physiological ionic strength and pH. This was first established in the case of TGF-β1 by McCaffrey et al. [12]. Subsequently Lyon et al. [13] showed that heparin and highly sulphated liver HS bind both human TGF-β1 and TGF-β2, but not TGF-β3. On this basis, they proposed a discontinuous heparin/HS binding site based on basic residues located at the tips of the first finger loops (Figure 2A). The heparin binding affinity data for these two TGF-βs, and other superfamily members, are presented in Table 1.

Table 1. Heparin-binding affinity estimates of TGF-β superfamily cytokines.

Protein	Heparin Affinity		Reference
TGF-β1	HAC	$\geq$0.5 M	[13]
TGF-β2	HAC	$\geq$0.5 M	[13]
BMPs/GDFs			
BMP-2	SPR	K_d 20 nM	[14]
BMP-4	n.d.		-
BMP-6	n.d.		-
BMP-7	HAC	0.5 M	[15]
BMP-14/GDF-5	SPR	K_d 50 nM	[16]
BMP-15/GDF-9	HAC	$\approx$1.0 M	[17]
Neurotrophins			
GDNF	HAC	0.8 M	[18]
	SPR	K_d 23 nM	[19]
Artemin	HAC	23 nM	[18]
	SPR	K_d 45 nM	[19]
Neurturin	HAC	1.2 M	[18]
	SPR	K_d 115 nM	[19]
Can family antagonists			
Gremlin-1	HAC	0.8 M	[20]
	SPR	K_d 20 nM	[21]
Gremlin-2/PRDC	HAC	0.67 M	[22]
Sclerostin	n.d		-
Other antagonists			
Noggin	HAC	0.8 M	[23]
Chordin	HAC	1.0 M	[24]
Follistatin (288 isoform)	SPR	K_d 1.0 M	[25]

The techniques have been employed: heparin affinity chromatography, HAC, and surface plasmon resonance (SPR). HAC employs a NaCl gradient to elute the bound cytokine, and the concentration of salt required is given. This approach therefore investigates the ionic component of the binding interaction. For SPR, the estimated dissociation constant is presented. In comparing estimates from the different studies, it must be borne in mind that different laboratories will have used a variety of heparin immobilisation procedures and different batches of heparin.

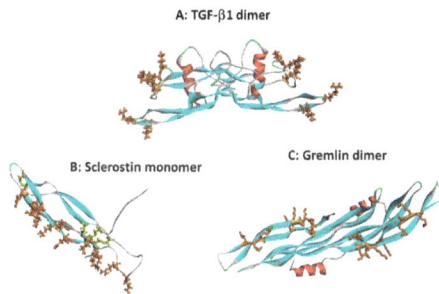

Figure 2. Heparin binding sites on TGF-β superfamily cytokines. Protein chains are shown as in Figure 1, and heparin binding site basic residues are shown in brown stick format. (**A**) The dimer of TGF-β1 (co-ordinates from 1KLC.pdb). Residues K25, R26, K31, K37, R94 and R97 form a discontinuous heparin binding site at the tips of the "fingers" [13]. (**B**) Sclerostin monomer (one of the NMR ensemble in 2K8P.pdb) with heparin-binding residues in brown. Cystine residues are shown in yellow stick format. Loop 3 (the second β-strand loop) and Loop 2 are both involved; residues K99, R102, R114, R116, R119, R131, R133, K134, R136, K142, K144 and R145 form a linear heparin binding site capable of accommodating a heparin dodecamer [26]. (**C**) The dimer of the CAN BMP antagonist gremlin (co-ordinates from 5AEJ.pdb). Here, the heparin binding residues are located largely along the second "finger", as for sclerostin; in the dimer both copies of the heparin binding site are on the concave face. Residues K145, K147, K148, K167, K168, K169, K174 and R177 have been identified as forming the heparin binding site [20]. The mode of dimerisation and the location of the heparin binding site both differ from those of TGF-β1.

The 21 TGF-β superfamily cytokines that are designated BMPs and GDFs can be grouped into subfamilies of between two and four members on the basis of sequence homology, and thereby presumably recent evolutionary divergence [5]. BMP-2 and -4 comprise one such subfamily. They possess amino terminal sequences, 13 and 15 residues in length, respectively, upstream of the first cysteine of their knot domains which are rich in the basic amino acids, Arg and Lys. In both cases, as previously reviewed [27], these contain heparin binding sites (see Figure 3). Mammalian BMP-2 and -4 show surprisingly high homology to the *Drosophila* morphogen decapentaplegic (Dpp). Dpp similarly binds to the cell surface HS proteoglycans Dally and dally-like, which are the *Drosophila* orthologs of mammalian glypicans [28].

```
Human BMP-2:                                QAKHKQRKRLKSSC
Human BMP-4:                             SPKHHSQRARKKKNKNC
Xenopus BMP-4:                            SPKQQRPRKKNKHC
Drosophila DPP:           DVSGGEGGGKGGRNKRQPRRPTRRKNHDDTC
Human GDNF:        SPDKQMAVLPRRERNRQAAAANPENSRGKGRRGQRGKNRGC
```

Figure 3. *N*-terminal sequences of some heparin binding BMPs. The sequences are shown ending with the first cysteine (shown in bold underlined font at the right hand side) of the knot domain. The basic residues lysine and arginine are highlighted in bold italics, and sequence regions experimentally implicated in heparin binding are boxed.

BMPs and GDFs of other subfamilies also bind to heparin and HS. Two highly homologous BMPs, BMP-6 [29] and BMP-7 [15,30,31], have both been shown to bind to heparin. The binding sites within these two BMPs are yet to be established, but their aminoterminal sequences are quite distinctive from those of BMP-2 and -4, being nearly three times longer. GDF-9 (BMP-15) [17] and most recently GDF-5 (BMP-14) [16], each representing a further subfamily, have also been shown to bind to heparin and HS. In neither case has the binding site been established. Predictive molecular docking calculations have indicated that a combination of unstructured *N*-terminal sequences and residues in the Cys knot region may combine to form heparin binding sites [32].

The four TGF-β superfamily neurotrophic factors are glial cell line-derived neurotrophic factor (GDNF), artemin, persephin and neurturin. All four regulate neuronal differentiation, share high sequence homology and signal at least in part through the cell surface tyrosine kinase Ret [33]. GDNF, artemin and neurturin have all been shown to bind to heparin [18] and to the HS proteoglycan syndecan-3 [19]. In the case of GDNF, the heparin binding site has been mapped to a 16-residue sequence containing 7 Arg and Lys residues immediately *N*-terminal to the first cysteine of the knot domain [18]. Although the *N*-terminal sequences of the other neurotrophins are considerably shorter than that of GDNF, those of artemin and neurturin, but not persephin are also enriched in basic residues. A notable feature of the binding of GDNF to heparin is its particular dependence on the presence of 2-*O*-sulphates [34].

4. Interactions of BMP Antagonist Proteins with Heparin and HS

Amongst the CAN family of antagonists, gremlin-1, gremlin-2, PRDC and sclerostin all bind to heparin and HS [20–22,26,35]. In each case the respective heparin binding sites lie within the cystine knot domain and involve exposed basic amino acid sidechains within the second β-strand finger loop [20,22,26,35]. For Dan and Cerberus, using molecular docking simulations we predicted a lack of affinity for heparin (see supplementary data, Rider and Mulloy, 2010 [5]), and for DAN this has since been confirmed experimentally [22]. We are unaware of any reports on the heparin/HS binding of Coco although on secretion it is retained on cell surfaces [36], a behaviour consistent with interaction with HS proteoglycans.

The more distantly related, non-CAN BMP antagonists are also heparin/HS binding proteins. This is well established for Noggin, which has a heparin binding site rich in basic residues aminoterminal to the cystine-knot domain [23] and lying within the "wrist" region of the polypeptide fold (Figure 4). Follistatin has been well characterised as a heparin binding protein that binds to cell surfaces through interaction with HS [37]. The heparin binding site has been identified as the sequence rich in basic amino acids between Lys75 and Arg6 [38]. The finding that follistatin complexed with myostatin (GDF-8) has much higher affinity for heparin than either of the two individual protein components [25] may be explained by the juxtaposition in the complex of the positively charged faces of myostatin and follistatin to form a single enhanced heparin binding site [39] (Figure 5). The follistatin–activin A complex also has enhanced affinity for heparin as measured by surface plasmon resonance, but is less stable to increased ionic strength than the follistatin-myostatin complex [25]. On the other hand, the follistatin related protein, follistatin-like 3, has no heparin binding site, and does not acquire heparin-binding properties when complexed with myostatin [40]. Chordin too binds heparin and HS, but the particular binding site involved has yet to be elucidated [24]. Thus, taken overall, current data reveal that the interaction with HS proteoglycans seems to be an important characteristic of the majority of the various BMP antagonist proteins. Moreover, at least in some instances, the complexes formed by BMPs and antagonists appear to have increased affinity for heparin, compared to the uncomplexed proteins.

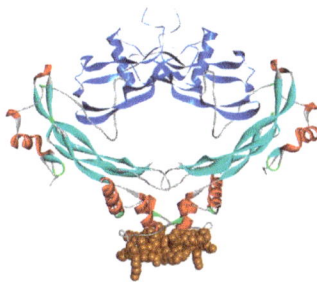

Figure 4. The heparin binding site of noggin in the noggin-BMP-7 complex (co-ordinates from 1M4U.pdb). Noggin is shown as described in Figure 1, with amino acids 133–144, encompassing a cluster of eight basic arginine and lysine residues, shown in brown CPK format; BMP-7 is shown in blue ribbon format.

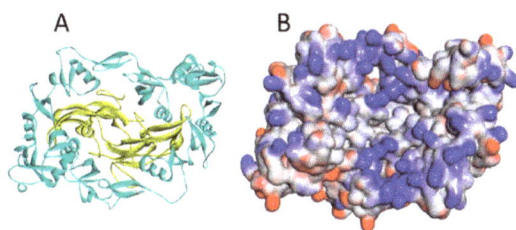

Figure 5. (**A**) The myostatin (yellow ribbon)/follistatin (turquoise ribbon) complex (3HH2.pdb); and (**B**) the same complex shown as a surface coloured according to interpolated charge (positive is blue, negative is red). Though myostatin does not have a heparin binding site, basic residues on its surface are located close to the follistatin binding site in the complex, increasing total affinity for heparin [40].

5. Heparin/HS Binding Sites of the TGF-β Cytokines

Returning to the more typical TGF-β superfamily members possessing the eight-residue circle cystine-knot, according to current knowledge, of the circa 40 mammalian proteins, two TGF-βs, six BMPs/GDFs, three out of four neurotrophins, and three of the CAN antagonists are known to bind to heparin/HS, around one third of the total number of proteins. With further study, this proportion is likely to rise, although given the paucity of clustered basic residues in some of the protein sequences, heparin/HS binding would appear to be far from a universal behaviour within this superfamily. Interestingly, within these proteins that do bind, their heparin/HS binding sites show considerable diversity. Thus, BMP-2, BMP-4, and GDNF have binding sites immediately aminoterminal to the cystine knot domain (Figure 3), whereas TGF-β1 and -β2 utilise the tips of their first β-strand finger loops (Figure 2A), and the CAN antagonists bind primarily via the surfaces of their second β-strand finger loops (Figure 2B,C). This leads to the conjecture that heparin/HS binding is a property acquired by certain members following the considerable divergence of this superfamily which occurred with the evolutionary emergence of the vertebrates. It would therefore appear to represent a fine-tuning mechanism for the biological activities of such proteins. It will be interesting to see whether future studies are able to determine whether or not each of the differing binding site locates can be associated with a different functional outcome of heparin/HS binding.

The Norrie disease protein, norrin, is an outlier of the cystine-knot family, possessing three β-strand loops per monomeric subunit. It activates the canonical Wnt/β-catenin pathway by binding to the the Frizzled4 cell surface receptor and the co-receptor low-density lipoprotein receptor related protein 5/6 (Lrp5/6). Like Wnt, it also interacts with cell surface HS proteoglycans. Mutational and structural studies of norrin have highlighted arginines 107, 109 and 115, which are located at the tip of the third β-strand loop as key residues in the GAG-binding site [41]. The triple substitution of these arginines with non-basic residues abolishes signalling activity and, interestingly, such a mutation occurs naturally, and is one causative of Norrie disease. These observations strongly implicate cell surface HS binding as critical for the normal functioning of norrin.

6. Effect of Heparin/HS Binding on TGF-β Cytokine Activity

Given that the TGF-β superfamily cytokines are relatively small, soluble glycoproteins, binding to HS proteoglycans of the extracellular matrix or on cell surfaces will have a major effect of restricting their diffusion away from sites of secretion within the tissues. This is well established for Dpp, the *Drosophila* homologue of BMP-2 and -4. Within the developing wing, a high concentration of Dpp defines the anterior-posterior axis, and a large body of work has established that the glypican HS proteoglycans dally and dally-like are not only responsible for maintaining this morphogenic gradient, but for transporting dpp across fields of cells to generate this gradient (reviewed by Nybakken and Perrimon [42]). Since there are close vertebrate homologues of all of the macromolecules involved in this mechanism it is reasonable to expect that BMP morphogenetic gradients are established and maintained by glypicans in higher organisms too.

Murine GDNF is another TGF-β cytokine for which there is clear evidence of the importance of HS in maintaining high localised concentrations of morphogens. In the initial stages of kidney formation, GDNF is expressed in the embryonic metanephric blastema and serves as a chemoattractant for cells of the ureteric bud which express the GDNF receptors. Contact between cells of these two embryonic structures results in the cellular condensation and proliferation events which lead to kidney formation [43]. The key role of GDNF in these events is revealed by the $GDNF^{-/-}$ mouse, in which there is a total absence of kidneys. Strikingly, this phenotype is recapitulated by homozygous knock-out of the gene encoding HS 2-*O*-sulphotransferase [44]. Since the binding of GDNF to heparin shows an unusually high dependence on the presence of 2-*O*-sulphate groups [34], these various studies support the paradigm that in the wild-type embryonic mouse, 2-*O*-sulphate replete HS is responsible for maintaining secreted GDNF within the metanephric blastema at concentrations sufficient to activate signalling in the arriving ureteric bud cells. In the absence of 2-*O*-sulphated HS, inadequate GDNF would be retained in this microenvironment. Further support for the role of HS proteoglycans in restricting the diffusion of GDNF within the tissues arises from studies of the administration of the recombinant cytokine into rat brain, whereupon a mutant lacking the heparin/HS binding domain was seen to diffuse more freely than the wild type cytokine [45].

Beyond the effect of HS binding restricting the diffusion of these cytokines, there is the issue of how binding to HS might affect their biological activities. Potentially the binding of small cytokine to bulky glycosaminoglycan chains might obscure their receptor binding sites, thereby inhibiting signalling activity. Alternatively, as is well established within the fibroblast growth factor (FGF) cytokine family, heparin and HS might serve as co-receptors, promoting signalling [46,47]. For FGF1, an initial step by which heparin promotes signalling activity is the formation of cytokine dimers through polypeptide-polysaccharide interactions. This dimerisation then facilitates receptor engagement [48]. Heparin-induced dimerisation is also a mechanism for promoting FGF2 signalling [49]. Since most TGF-β cytokines exist as disulphide-bridged dimers in circulation, a dimerisation function for GAG appears unnecessary with this superfamily. Moreover, as the locations of heparin/HS binding sites vary from one cytokine to another within the TGF-β family (see Figure 2), it may not necessarily be the case that GAG binding will affect TGF-β cytokine activity in a single, uniform way.

In one of the earliest studies of the effects of heparin/HS binding on BMP activity, a mutant of BMP-2 with abrogated heparin binding was found to be more active than the wild-type cytokine in chick limb bud assays [14]. This indicates that heparin binding is not obligatory for receptor activation, and thus that the co-receptor role for heparin/HS observed with FGFs does not apply for BMP-2. However the activity of wild type BMP-2 was increased by the addition of exogenous heparin [14]. Thus, interaction with extracellular matrix HS would appear to modulate the bioavailability of BMP-2. Essentially similar outcomes have been observed in subsequent studies [31,50–53]. Similar modulation of BMP-4 activity by heparin and HS has also been shown [54]. Of these studies, Jiao et al., have considered that the retention of a BMP on HS close to cell surfaces will not only retain the cytokine near its receptors facilitating signalling, but also in the vicinity of cellular internalisation mechanisms, promoting internalisation and turnover [50]. Thus, HS binding may facilitate both BMP signalling and turnover.

In embryonic stem cell differentiation exogenous heparin and highly sulphated HS have been shown to restore BMP-4 signalling to enable haematopoietic differentiation in HS-deficient cells [55]. Although this may appear to be consistent with a possible co-receptor function, a further study ascribed this effect to HS stabilising BMP-4 against degradation [56]. This indicates that the influence of HS on BMP signalling may well be dependent on cellular context. With BMP-7, biological activity in inhibiting cell proliferation in the subventricular zone of adult brain, a major site of neurogenesis, is also dependent on the presence of cell surface HS [57].

Beyond the BMPs, removal of heparin/HS binding for GDNF has no apparent effect on its receptor binding and cellular activity [18]. However the in vivo neuroprotective activity of GDNF in a rat model of Parkinson's disease of recombinant GDNF carrying this deletion was reduced compared to the wild-type protein, probably due to its lower retention at the site of administration [46] as previously mentioned. Overall, these studies show some similarity in the role of heparin and HS in BMP and GDNF signalling and bioavailability.

However, a major complication in attempting to assess the role of HS in BMP signalling within the tissues is the presence of the various BMP antagonist proteins, a high proportion of which themselves bind with high affinity to heparin and HS. Investigations in this area overall remain limited, but several instances provide some insight. Thus, as referred to above, the crystal structure of the follistatin isoform 288 complexed with myostatin (GDF-8) reveals a continuous electropositive surface generated at the interface between the two proteins. This accounts for the higher heparin binding affinity of the complex compared to the free follistatin [40,58]. Since there is no observation of the binding of myostatin to heparin/HS, binding to follistatin 288 would appear to be a mechanism for tethering the cytokine to cell surface HS. The antagonist Noggin, by binding to cell surface HS proteoglycans, is thought to reduce the diffusion of BMP-4 [23] thereby establishing morphogenetic gradients in the embryo. Interestingly, a mutation within the heparin binding site of Noggin which reduces its affinity underlies the congenital disorders of proximal subphalagism and conductive hearing loss [59], strongly implicating heparin-binding in the functioning of Noggin during development.

The high resolution crystal structure of gremlin-2 complexed with GDF-5 [60] shows a very different orientation of the two proteins in the complex compared to the noggin-BMP-7 structure

(Figure 4). In the former, the gremlin dimers are perpendicular to, and at the tips of the GDF-5 dimers, potentially allowing for the assembly of large repeat alternating "daisy chain" complexes of the two proteins, and formation of such multimers has been demonstrated in vitro [60]. Modelling the gremlin-2/BMP-2 complex on the gremlin-2/GDF-5 structure shows a large continuous basic surface patch at the interface of the antagonist and cytokine which may explain why the complex binds to heparin with higher affinity than either protein partner alone [22]. On the basis of these data, it may be suggested that HS chains in the tissues would promote the assembly of large gremlin-2/cytokine complexes with repeating heparin/HS binding sites would give rise to stable depots of the two proteins in the extracellular matrix and on cell surfaces close to their sites of secretion.

7. Heparin/HS Binding in the Therapeutic Applications of TGF-β Superfamily Cytokines

There has been widespread interest in exploiting the cellular regulatory activities of TGF-β cytokines in the therapy of a range of chronic diseases. A prominent instance of this is the clinical use of recombinant BMP-infused cements for non-unionising bone fractures and in the fusing of spinal vertebrae. Several groups are investigating whether the incorporation of heparin or HS into such biomaterials might provide for better bone growth outcomes by improving the bioavailability of BMP-2 through its slow release [61–63]. Heparin coatings for the titanium surfaces of skeletal implants are also under active consideration for the same reason [64]. Another area of interest is the potential therapeutic use of GDNF and related neurotrophins as neuroprotective and neuroregenerative agents in nervous system disease or injury. Although administration of recombinant GDNF has proved highly effective in rodent models of Parkinson's disease, a large clinical trial proved unsuccessful [65]. One major issue here is likely to be inadequate delivery of GDNF throughout the larger structures of human brain. This being the case, neurotrophin binding to HS may be disadvantageous in this application. Indeed, recently a variant of neurturin with reduced affinity for HS was found to diffuse further through brain and to be effective in regenerating dopaminergic nerve fibres a rat model of Parkinson's disease than GDNF [66]. In conclusion, where a TGF-β family cytokine binds heparin/HS, this property will be an important consideration in any potential therapeutic applications.

Conflicts of Interest: The authors declare no conflict of interest.

References

1. Watabe, T.; Miyazono, K. Roles of TGF-beta family signaling in stem cell renewal and differentiation. *Cell Res.* **2009**, *19*, 103–115. [CrossRef] [PubMed]
2. Fujio, K.; Komai, T.; Inoue, M.; Morita, K.; Okamura, T.; Yamamoto, K. Revisiting the regulatory roles of the TGF-beta family of cytokines. *Autoimmun. Rev.* **2016**, *15*, 917–922. [CrossRef] [PubMed]
3. Rodgarkia-Dara, C.; Vejda, S.; Erlach, N.; Losert, A.; Bursch, W.; Berger, W.; Schulte-Hermann, R.; Grusch, M. The activin axis in liver biology and disease. *Mutat. Res.* **2006**, *613*, 123–137. [CrossRef] [PubMed]
4. Saarma, M. GDNF—A stranger in the TGF-beta superfamily? *Eur. J. Biochem.* **2000**, *267*, 6968–6971. [CrossRef] [PubMed]
5. Rider, C.C.; Mulloy, B. Bone morphogenetic protein and growth differentiation factor cytokine families and their protein antagonists. *Biochem. J.* **2010**, *429*, 1–12. [CrossRef] [PubMed]
6. Yadin, D.; Knaus, P.; Mueller, T.D. Structural insights into BMP receptors: Specificity, activation and inhibition. *Cytokine Growth Factor Rev.* **2016**, *27*, 13–34. [CrossRef] [PubMed]
7. Avsian-Kretchmer, O.; Hsueh, A.J. Comparative genomic analysis of the eight-membered ring cystine knot-containing bone morphogenetic protein antagonists. *Mol. Endocrinol.* **2004**, *18*, 1–12. [CrossRef] [PubMed]
8. Daopin, S.; Piez, K.A.; Ogawa, Y.; Davies, D.R. Crystal structure of transforming growth factor-beta 2: An unusual fold for the superfamily. *Science* **1992**, *257*, 369–373. [CrossRef] [PubMed]
9. Scheufler, C.; Sebald, W.; Hulsmeyer, M. Crystal structure of human bone morphogenetic protein-2 at 2.7 A resolution. *J. Mol. Biol.* **1999**, *287*, 103–115. [CrossRef] [PubMed]

10. Mulloy, B.; Rider, C.C. The Bone Morphogenetic Proteins and Their Antagonists. *Vitam. Horm.* **2015**, *99*, 63–90. [PubMed]

11. Brazil, D.P.; Church, R.H.; Surae, S.; Godson, C.; Martin, F. BMP signalling: Agony and antagony in the family. *Trends Cell Biol.* **2015**, *25*, 249–264. [CrossRef] [PubMed]

12. McCaffrey, T.A.; Falcone, D.J.; Du, B. Transforming growth factor-beta 1 is a heparin-binding protein: identification of putative heparin-binding regions and isolation of heparins with varying affinity for TGF-beta 1. *J. Cell. Physiol.* **1992**, *152*, 430–440. [CrossRef] [PubMed]

13. Lyon, M.; Rushton, G.; Gallagher, J.T. The interaction of the transforming growth factor-betas with heparin/heparan sulfate is isoform-specific. *J. Biol. Chem.* **1997**, *272*, 18000–18006. [CrossRef] [PubMed]

14. Ruppert, R.; Hoffmann, E.; Sebald, W. Human bone morphogenetic protein 2 contains a heparin-binding site which modifies its biological activity. *Eur. J. Biochem.* **1996**, *237*, 295–302. [CrossRef] [PubMed]

15. McClarence, D. An Investigation into the Location of the Heparan Sulphate/Heparin-Binding Site of Human Bone Morphogenetic Protein-7. Ph.D. Thesis, Royal Holloway University of London, London, UK, 2011.

16. Ayerst, B.I.; Smith, R.A.; Nurcombe, V.; Day, A.J.; Merry, C.L.; Cool, S.M. Growth Differentiation Factor 5-Mediated Enhancement of Chondrocyte Phenotype Is Inhibited by Heparin: Implications for the Use of Heparin in the Clinic and in Tissue Engineering Applications. *Tissue Eng. Part. A* **2017**. [CrossRef]

17. Watson, L.N.; Mottershead, D.G.; Dunning, K.R.; Robker, R.L.; Gilchrist, R.B.; Russell, D.L. Heparan sulfate proteoglycans regulate responses to oocyte paracrine signals in ovarian follicle morphogenesis. *Endocrinology* **2012**, *153*, 4544–4555. [CrossRef] [PubMed]

18. Alfano, I.; Vora, P.; Mummery, R.S.; Mulloy, B.; Rider, C.C. The major determinant of the heparin binding of glial cell-line-derived neurotrophic factor is near the N-terminus and is dispensable for receptor binding. *Biochem. J.* **2007**, *404*, 131–140. [CrossRef] [PubMed]

19. Bespalov, M.M.; Sidorova, Y.A.; Tumova, S.; Ahonen-Bishopp, A.; Magalhaes, A.C.; Kulesskiy, E.; Paveliev, M.; Rivera, C.; Rauvala, H.; Saarma, M. Heparan sulfate proteoglycan syndecan-3 is a novel receptor for GDNF, neurturin, and artemin. *J. Cell. Biol.* **2011**, *192*, 153–169. [CrossRef] [PubMed]

20. Tatsinkam, A.J.; Mulloy, B.; Rider, C.C. Mapping the heparin-binding site of the BMP antagonist gremlin by site-directed mutagenesis based on predictive modelling. *Biochem. J.* **2015**, *470*, 53–64. [CrossRef] [PubMed]

21. Chiodelli, P.; Mitola, S.; Ravelli, C.; Oreste, P.; Rusnati, M.; Presta, M. Heparan sulfate proteoglycans mediate the angiogenic activity of the vascular endothelial growth factor receptor-2 agonist gremlin. *Arterioscler. Thromb. Vasc. Biol.* **2011**, *31*, e116–e127. [CrossRef] [PubMed]

22. Kattamuri, C.; Nolan, K.; Thompson, T.B. Analysis and identification of the Grem2 heparin/heparan-sulfate binding motif. *Biochem. J.* **2017**, *474*, 1093–1107. [CrossRef] [PubMed]

23. Paine-Saunders, S.; Viviano, B.L.; Economides, A.N.; Saunders, S. Heparan sulfate proteoglycans retain Noggin at the cell surface: A potential mechanism for shaping bone morphogenetic protein gradients. *J. Biol. Chem.* **2002**, *277*, 2089–2096. [CrossRef] [PubMed]

24. Jasuja, R.; Allen, B.L.; Pappano, W.N.; Rapraeger, A.C.; Greenspan, D.S. Cell-surface heparan sulfate proteoglycans potentiate chordin antagonism of bone morphogenetic protein signaling and are necessary for cellular uptake of chordin. *J. Biol. Chem.* **2004**, *279*, 51289–51297. [CrossRef] [PubMed]

25. Zhang, F.; Beaudet, J.M.; Luedeke, D.M.; Walker, R.G.; Thompson, T.B.; Linhardt, R.J. Analysis of the interaction between heparin and follistatin and heparin and follistatin-ligand complexes using surface plasmon resonance. *Biochemistry* **2012**, *51*, 6797–6803. [CrossRef] [PubMed]

26. Veverka, V.; Henry, A.J.; Slocombe, P.M.; Ventom, A.; Mulloy, B.; Muskett, F.W.; Muzylak, M.; Greenslade, K.; Moore, A.; Zhang, L.; et al. Characterization of the structural features and interactions of sclerostin: molecular insight into a key regulator of Wnt-mediated bone formation. *J. Biol. Chem.* **2009**, *284*, 10890–10900. [CrossRef] [PubMed]

27. Rider, C.C. Heparin/heparan sulphate binding in the TGF-beta cytokine superfamily. *Biochem. Soc. Trans.* **2006**, *34*, 458–460. [CrossRef] [PubMed]

28. Akiyama, T.; Kamimura, K.; Firkus, C.; Takeo, S.; Shimmi, O.; Nakato, H. Dally regulates Dpp morphogen gradient formation by stabilizing Dpp on the cell surface. *Dev. Biol.* **2008**, *313*, 408–419. [CrossRef] [PubMed]

29. Brkljacic, J.; Pauk, M.; Erjavec, I.; Cipcic, A.; Grgurevic, L.; Zadro, R.; Inman, G.J.; Vukicevic, S. Exogenous heparin binds and inhibits bone morphogenetic protein 6 biological activity. *Int. Orthop.* **2013**, *37*, 529–541. [CrossRef] [PubMed]

30. Irie, A.; Habuchi, H.; Kimata, K.; Sanai, Y. Heparan sulfate is required for bone morphogenetic protein-7 signaling. *Biochem. Biophys. Res. Commun.* **2003**, *308*, 858–865. [CrossRef]

31. Takada, T.; Katagiri, T.; Ifuku, M.; Morimura, N.; Kobayashi, M.; Hasegawa, K.; Ogamo, A.; Kamijo, R. Sulfated polysaccharides enhance the biological activities of bone morphogenetic proteins. *J. Biol. Chem.* **2003**, *278*, 43229–43235. [CrossRef] [PubMed]

32. Gandhi, N.S.; Mancera, R.L. Prediction of heparin binding sites in bone morphogenetic proteins (BMPs). *Biochim. Biophys. Acta* **2012**, *1824*, 1374–1381. [CrossRef] [PubMed]

33. Bespalov, M.M.; Saarma, M. GDNF family receptor complexes are emerging drug targets. *Trends Pharmacol. Sci.* **2007**, *28*, 68–74. [CrossRef] [PubMed]

34. Rickard, S.M.; Mummery, R.S.; Mulloy, B.; Rider, C.C. The binding of human glial cell line-derived neurotrophic factor to heparin and heparan sulfate: importance of 2-O-sulfate groups and effect on its interaction with its receptor, GFRalpha1. *Glycobiology.* **2003**, *13*, 419–426. [CrossRef] [PubMed]

35. Nolan, K.; Kattamuri, C.; Luedeke, D.M.; Deng, X.; Jagpal, A.; Zhang, F.; Linhardt, R.J.; Kenny, A.P.; Zorn, A.M.; Thompson, T.B. Structure of protein related to Dan and Cerberus: Insights into the mechanism of 368 bone morphogenetic protein antagonism. *Structure* **2013**, *21*, 1417–1429. [CrossRef] [PubMed]

36. Gao, H.; Chakraborty, G.; Lee-Lim, A.P.; Mo, Q.; Decker, M.; Vonica, A.; Shen, R.; Brogi, E.; Brivanlou, A.H.; Giancotti, F.G. The BMP inhibitor Coco reactivates breast cancer cells at lung metastatic sites. *Cell.* **2012**, *150*, 764–779. [CrossRef] [PubMed]

37. Sidis, Y.; Mukherjee, A.; Keutmann, H.; Delbaere, A.; Sadatsuki, M.; Schneyer, A. Biological activity of follistatin isoforms and follistatin-like-3 is dependent on differential cell surface binding and specificity for activin, myostatin, and bone morphogenetic proteins. *Endocrinology* **2006**, *147*, 3586–3597. [CrossRef] [PubMed]

38. Inouye, S.; Ling, N.; Shimasaki, S. Localization of the heparin binding site of follistatin. *Mol. Cell. Endocrinol.* **1992**, *90*, 1–6. [CrossRef]

39. Cash, J.N.; Rejon, C.A.; McPherron, A.C.; Bernard, D.J.; Thompson, T.B. The structure of myostatin:follistatin 288: insights into receptor utilization and heparin binding. *Embo. J.* **2009**, *28*, 2662–2676. [CrossRef] [PubMed]

40. Cash, J.N.; Angerman, E.B.; Kattamuri, C.; Nolan, K.; Zhao, H.; Sidis, Y.; Keutmann, H.T.; Thompson, T.B. Structure of myostatin.follistatin-like 3: N-terminal domains of follistatin-type molecules exhibit alternate modes of binding. *J. Biol. Chem.* **2012**, *287*, 1043–1053. [CrossRef] [PubMed]

41. Chang, T.H.; Hsieh, F.L.; Zebisch, M.; Harlos, K.; Elegheert, J.; Jones, E.Y. Structure and functional properties of Norrin mimic Wnt for signalling with Frizzled4, Lrp5/6, and proteoglycan. *Elife.* **2015**, *4*. [CrossRef] [PubMed]

42. Nybakken, K.; Perrimon, N. Heparan sulfate proteoglycan modulation of developmental signaling in Drosophila. *Biochim. Biophys. Acta.* **2002**, *1573*, 280–291. [CrossRef]

43. Schedl, A.; Hastie, N.D. Cross-talk in kidney development. *Curr. Opin. Genet. Dev.* **2000**, *10*, 543–549. [CrossRef]

44. Bullock, S.L.; Fletcher, J.M.; Beddington, R.S.; Wilson, V.A. Renal agenesis in mice homozygous for a gene trap mutation in the gene encoding heparan sulfate 2-sulfotransferase. *Genes Dev.* **1998**, *12*, 1894–1906. [CrossRef] [PubMed]

45. Piltonen, M.; Bespalov, M.M.; Ervasti, D.; Matilainen, T.; Sidorova, Y.A.; Rauvala, H.; Saarma, M.; Mannisto, P.T. Heparin-binding determinants of GDNF reduce its tissue distribution but are beneficial for the protection of nigral dopaminergic neurons. *Exp. Neurol.* **2009**, *219*, 499–506. [CrossRef] [PubMed]

46. Pellegrini, L. Role of heparan sulfate in fibroblast growth factor signalling: A structural view. *Curr. Opin. Struct. Biol.* **2001**, *11*, 629–634. [CrossRef]

47. Mohammadi, M.; Olsen, S.K.; Goetz, R. A protein canyon in the FGF-FGF receptor dimer selects from an a la carte menu of heparan sulfate motifs. *Curr. Opin. Struct. Biol.* **2005**, *15*, 506–516. [CrossRef] [PubMed]

48. Brown, A.; Robinson, C.J.; Gallagher, J.T.; Blundell, T.L. Cooperative heparin-mediated oligomerization of fibroblast growth factor-1 (FGF1) precedes recruitment of FGFR2 to ternary complexes. *Biophys. J.* **2013**, *104*, 1720–1730. [CrossRef] [PubMed]

49. Goodger, S.J.; Robinson, C.J.; Murphy, K.J.; Gasiunas, N.; Harmer, N.J.; Blundell, T.L.; Pye, D.A.; Gallagher, J.T. Evidence that heparin saccharides promote FGF2 mitogenesis through two distinct mechanisms. *J. Biol. Chem.* **2008**, *283*, 13001–13008. [CrossRef] [PubMed]

50. Jiao, X.; Billings, P.C.; O'Connell, M.P.; Kaplan, F.S.; Shore, E.M.; Glaser, D.L. Heparan sulfate proteoglycans (HSPGs) modulate BMP2 osteogenic bioactivity in C2C12 cells. *J. Biol. Chem.* **2007**, *282*, 1080–1086. [CrossRef] [PubMed]

51. Kanzaki, S.; Takahashi, T.; Kanno, T.; Ariyoshi, W.; Shinmyouzu, K.; Tujisawa, T.; Nishihara, T. Heparin inhibits BMP-2 osteogenic bioactivity by binding to both BMP-2 and BMP receptor. *J. Cell. Physiol.* **2008**, *216*, 844–850. [CrossRef] [PubMed]

52. Zhao, B.; Katagiri, T.; Toyoda, H.; Takada, T.; Yanai, T.; Fukuda, T.; Chung, U.I.; Koike, T.; Takaoka, K.; Kamijo, R. Heparin potentiates the In Vivo ectopic bone formation induced by bone morphogenetic protein-2. *J. Biol. Chem* **2006**, *281*, 23246–23253. [CrossRef] [PubMed]

53. Kanzaki, S.; Ariyoshi, W.; Takahashi, T.; Okinaga, T.; Kaneuji, T.; Mitsugi, S.; Nakashima, K.; Tsujisawa, T.; Nishihara, T. Dual effects of heparin on BMP-2-induced osteogenic activity in MC3T3-E1 cells. *Pharmacol. Rep.* **2011**, *63*, 1222–1230. [CrossRef]

54. Khan, S.A.; Nelson, M.S.; Pan, C.; Gaffney, P.M.; Gupta, P. Endogenous heparan sulfate and heparin modulate bone morphogenetic protein-4 signaling and activity. *Am. J. Physiol. Cell. Physiol.* **2008**, *294*, C1387–C1397. [CrossRef] [PubMed]

55. Holley, R.J.; Pickford, C.E.; Rushton, G.; Lacaud, G.; Gallagher, J.T.; Kouskoff, V.; Merry, C.L. Influencing hematopoietic differentiation of mouse embryonic stem cells using soluble heparin and heparan sulfate saccharides. *J. Biol. Chem.* **2011**, *286*, 6241–6252. [CrossRef] [PubMed]

56. Kraushaar, D.C.; Rai, S.; Condac, E.; Nairn, A.; Zhang, S.; Yamaguchi, Y.; Moremen, K.; Dalton, S.; Wang, L. Heparan sulfate facilitates FGF and BMP signaling to drive mesoderm differentiation of mouse embryonic stem cells. *J. Biol. Chem.* **2012**, *287*, 22691–22700. [CrossRef] [PubMed]

57. Douet, V.; Arikawa-Hirasawa, E.; Mercier, F. Fractone-heparan sulfates mediate BMP-7 inhibition of cell proliferation in the adult subventricular zone. *Neurosci. Lett* **2012**, *528*, 120–125. [CrossRef] [PubMed]

58. Cash, J.N.; Angerman, E.B.; Keutmann, H.T.; Thompson, T.B. Characterization of follistatin-type domains and their contribution to myostatin and activin A antagonism. *Mol. Endocrinol.* **2012**, *26*, 1167–1178. [CrossRef] [PubMed]

59. Masuda, S.; Namba, K.; Mutai, H.; Usui, S.; Miyanaga, Y.; Kaneko, H.; Matsunaga, T. A mutation in the heparin-binding site of noggin as a novel mechanism of proximal symphalangism and conductive hearing loss. *Biochem. Biophys. Res. Commun.* **2014**, *447*, 496–502. [CrossRef] [PubMed]

60. Nolan, K.; Kattamuri, C.; Rankin, S.A.; Read, R.J.; Zorn, A.M.; Thompson, T.B. Structure of Gremlin-2 in Complex with GDF5 Gives Insight into DAN-Family-Mediated BMP Antagonism. *Cell. Rep.* **2016**, *16*, 2077–2086. [CrossRef] [PubMed]

61. Bramono, D.S.; Murali, S.; Rai, B.; Ling, L.; Poh, W.T.; Lim, Z.X.; Stein, G.S.; Nurcombe, V.; van Wijnen, A.J.; Cool, S.M. Bone marrow-derived heparan sulfate potentiates the osteogenic activity of bone morphogenetic protein-2 (BMP-2). *Bone* **2012**, *50*, 954–964. [CrossRef] [PubMed]

62. Hettiaratchi, M.H.; Miller, T.; Temenoff, J.S.; Guldberg, R.E.; McDevitt, T.C. Heparin microparticle effects on presentation and bioactivity of bone morphogenetic protein-2. *Biomaterials* **2014**, *35*, 7228–7238. [CrossRef] [PubMed]

63. Kim, R.Y.; Lee, B.; Park, S.N.; Ko, J.H.; Kim, I.S.; Hwang, S.J. Is Heparin Effective for the Controlled Delivery of High-Dose Bone Morphogenetic Protein-2? *Tissue Eng. Part. A* **2016**, *22*, 801–817. [CrossRef] [PubMed]

64. Kim, S.E.; Kim, C.S.; Yun, Y.P.; Yang, D.H.; Park, K.; Kim, S.E.; Jeong, C.M.; Huh, J.B. Improving osteoblast functions and bone formation upon BMP-2 immobilization on titanium modified with heparin. *Carbohydr. Polym.* **2014**, *114*, 123–132. [CrossRef]

65. Hegarty, S.V.; O'Keeffe, G.W.; Sullivan, A.M. Neurotrophic factors: From neurodevelopmental regulators to novel therapies for Parkinson's disease. *Neural Regen Res.* **2014**, *9*, 1708–1711. [PubMed]

66. Runeberg-Roos, P.; Piccinini, E.; Penttinen, A.M.; Matlik, K.; Heikkinen, H.; Kuure, S.; Bespalov, M.M.; Peranen, J.; Garea-Rodriguez, E.; Fuchs, E.; et al. Developing therapeutically more efficient Neurturin variants for treatment of Parkinson's disease. *Neurobiol. Dis* **2016**, *96*, 335–345. [CrossRef] [PubMed]

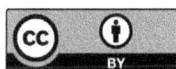

Review

Heparin and Heparin-Derivatives in Post-Subarachnoid Hemorrhage Brain Injury: A Multimodal Therapy for a Multimodal Disease

Erik G. Hayman [1], Akil P. Patel [1], Robert F. James [2] and J. Marc Simard [1,*]

[1] Department of Neurosurgery, University of Maryland School of Medicine, Baltimore, MD 21201, USA; ehayman@som.umaryland.edu (E.G.H.); appatel@som.umaryland.edu (A.P.P.)

[2] Department of Neurosurgery, University of Louisville, Louisville, KY 40208, USA; robert.james@louisville.edu

* Correspondence: msimard@som.umaryland.edu; Tel.: +1-410-328-0850; Fax: +1-410-328-0124

Academic Editors: Giangiacomo Torri and Jawed Fareed
Received: 29 March 2017; Accepted: 26 April 2017; Published: 2 May 2017

Abstract: Pharmacologic efforts to improve outcomes following aneurysmal subarachnoid hemorrhage (aSAH) remain disappointing, likely owing to the complex nature of post-hemorrhage brain injury. Previous work suggests that heparin, due to the multimodal nature of its actions, reduces the incidence of clinical vasospasm and delayed cerebral ischemia that accompany the disease. This narrative review examines how heparin may mitigate the non-vasospastic pathological aspects of aSAH, particularly those related to neuroinflammation. Following a brief review of early brain injury in aSAH and heparin's general pharmacology, we discuss potential mechanistic roles of heparin therapy in treating post-aSAH inflammatory injury. These roles include reducing ischemia-reperfusion injury, preventing leukocyte extravasation, modulating phagocyte activation, countering oxidative stress, and correcting blood-brain barrier dysfunction. Following a discussion of evidence to support these mechanistic roles, we provide a brief discussion of potential complications of heparin usage in aSAH. Our review suggests that heparin's use in aSAH is not only safe, but effectively addresses a number of pathologies initiated by aSAH.

Keywords: heparin; enoxaparin; subarachnoid hemorrhage; edema; brain injury; inflammation

1. Introduction

Despite decades of research, aneurysmal subarachnoid hemorrhage (aSAH) significantly compromises quality of life in those patients who survive their initial hemorrhage. Half of all surviving patients demonstrate some significant deficit of language, memory, or executive function [1–4], with only a third of survivors ultimately returning to work [5]. Consistent with these clinical findings, radiographic evaluation of survivors of aSAH demonstrates significant degrees of brain atrophy and other signs of global brain injury [6,7]. Although infarction due to vasospasm undoubtedly explains the acquisition of new focal deficits following aSAH, vasospasm-centered theories do not compellingly account for this global brain injury, especially given that effective pharmacologic prevention of vasospasm fails to improve outcomes following aSAH [8].

Modern understandings of post-SAH brain injury recognize the importance of other pathophysiological processes [9,10] emphasizing inflammation in particular as a central component of post-SAH brain injury [11]. SAH generates a wide variety of hemoglobin breakdown products capable of wide dissemination via the CSF, leading to global inflammation via activation of receptors such as toll-like receptor 4 [12,13], attraction of inflammatory phagocytes [14], and creation of a pro-oxidative environment via depletion of anti-oxidants [15]. Several clinical studies link this systemic inflammatory response to brain injury and poor outcome following aSAH [7,16–19]. Therefore, mitigating this inflammatory response presents an attractive therapeutic approach to improving outcomes following aSAH. Although specific inhibition of pro-inflammatory regulators, such as cytokines, represents a valid therapeutic strategy [20], aSAH activates multiple inflammatory pathways, suggesting that blockade of any single upstream inflammatory initiator may not adequately curb the downstream inflammatory response.

Multiple lines of clinical and pre-clinical evidence suggest that the endogenous anti-coagulant heparin effectively reduces inflammation and improves outcomes following aSAH [21–24]. Perhaps because of its clinical use as an anti-coagulant and its widely studied interactions with the coagulation cascade, clinicians remain relatively ignorant heparin's promiscuous interaction with a number of biological processes, especially those involved with inflammation. Although this absence of specificity typically hinders the application of drugs like heparin as therapeutic agents, these pleiotropic effects may prove advantageous in the complex inflammatory milieu accompanying aSAH. This review seeks to summarize the potential benefits of heparin therapy in the context of aSAH, with a particular emphasis on its anti-inflammatory properties.

2. Early Brain Injury, Inflammation, and Blood-Brain Barrier Failure in Aneurysmal Subarachnoid Hemorrhage

Aneurysm rupture initiates two separate pathologic events that contribute to global brain injury. The initial rupture rapidly raises intracranial pressure, leading to cerebral hypoperfusion, possible cerebral circulatory arrest, and global brain injury analogous to that of cardiac arrest [25]. The second occurs gradually in the days following hemorrhage as the subarachnoid blood clot breaks down, releasing a variety of hemoglobin and coagulation by-products into the CSF, where they undergo global distribution. Although these events negatively affect nearly every aspect of the CNS, they have a number of specific consequences for the brain, of which vasospasm represents only a single component.

SAH induces a significant degree of CNS inflammation, both from activation of the brain's endogenous microglia as well as influx of circulating leukocytes [26–30]. Inflammatory activation of these cells has a number of deleterious effects. Activated microglia mediate the significant neuronal apoptosis observed following experimental SAH [26]. Brain invasion by circulating neutrophils induces microvascular dysfunction [31], endothelial injury [32], and memory deficits via NMDA receptor dysfunction [29]. Perivascular invasion by leukocytes plays a role in vasospasm, as blockade of invasion via monoclonal antibody prevents vasospasm in both rabbits [33] and monkeys [34]. Generation of reactive species such as peroxynitrite via phagocyte-derived inducible nitric oxide synthase contributes to oxidative brain injury following aSAH [35]. This inflammatory state following aSAH mediates brain injury over several weeks [36]. Despite its clear role in brain injury following aSAH, this inflammatory response is not entirely detrimental. Both endogenous and circulating phagocytes mediate hemoglobin clearance following hemorrhage [37,38]. Activated microglia and their inflammatory cytokines also promote neurogenesis in non-aSAH models via activation of the brain's stem cell compartment [39,40], a relevant finding given evidence of increased neurogenesis following human aSAH [41]. However, despite these potentially beneficial effects, the excess inflammation that follows aSAH causes more harm than benefit, especially in the early post-ictal period.

Besides directly modulating the CNS microenvironment, aSAH induces failure of the blood brain barrier with consequent vasogenic edema formation. Diverse mechanisms underlie this phenomenon, as ischemia-hypoperfusion injury and hemorrhagic products within the subarachnoid space both contribute to blood-brain barrier (BBB) dysfunction following aSAH [42–44]. Besides brain swelling due to vasogenic edema [45], BBB dysfunction contributes to several other pathologic processes. Perfusion studies in patients with delayed cerebral ischemia following aSAH demonstrate abnormal permeability of the BBB prior to actual infarction [46]. Experimental studies link the loss of white matter integrity to BBB disruption following SAH [47]. Finally, the BBB represents a crucial gateway for inflammatory cell infiltration of the brain [48]; loss of barrier integrity could augment this already significant neuroinflammatory response to aSAH.

3. Heparin—Physiologic and Pharmacologic Roles

The heparins refer to a class of endogenous glycosaminoglycans originally isolated from canine liver cells during investigations of endogenous coagulants (hence, the Greek root *hepar* meaning "liver") [49]. Heparin molecules consist of linear polymeric chains of heavily sulfated polysaccharide chains. This high degree of sulfation imparts the highest negative charge density of any known biological macromolecule, allowing heparin to interact with a large number of proteins [50]. Given its context of discovery as well as its utility as an anticoagulant, traditional understandings of heparin's pharmacologic actions situate it within the clotting cascade. Within this understanding, heparin's primary role is to bind antithrombin III, inducing an allosteric activation of the latter that allows antithrombin III to inhibit the clotting Factor Xa, a phenomenon relatively independent of the size of the heparin molecule [51]. By virtue of heparin's large size and high negative charge, the heparin-antithrombin III complex may also bind thrombin and inactivate thrombin, although this action crucially depends on sufficient chain length to bind both antithrombin III and thrombin. Low molecular weight heparins exploit this latter property to inhibit Factor Xa without appreciable anti-thrombin activity. Of note, the anti-coagulant properties of heparin depend on its negative charge to allow for both thrombin binding and allosteric activation of antithrombin III; stripping heparin molecules of their negatively charged sulfate moieties reduces heparin's function as an anticoagulant [52].

Despite the prominence of anti-coagulation in heparin's clinical applications, several lines of evidence suggest that anti-coagulation is not heparin's primary physiologic role. Despite its initial discovery in mammals, heparin-like molecules exist in a wide variety of species lacking a formal hematologic system, including arthropods and echinoderms [53]. Furthermore, within mammals, mast cells and basophils represent the most abundant histologic source of heparin [54]; the importance of these cells in allergic and anti-helminthic response would seem to situate heparin within the broader schema of type 2 immune responses [55]. Finally, besides well-characterized interactions with antithrombin III, heparin promiscuously interacts with a variety of inflammatory proteins and chemokines [56]. While heparin's anticoagulant properties undoubtedly play a role in inflammatory physiology, a simple understanding of heparin as anticoagulant neglects heparin's broader role as a modulator of inflammatory function.

Heparin and its derivative molecules possess significant anti-inflammatory activity [57]. Heparin and heparinoids exert their anti-inflammatory effects through a wide variety of mechanisms. At the level of signal transduction, they reduce LPS-induced nuclear translocation of NF-κβ and the associated inflammatory response both in vitro and in vivo, although mechanistic explanations of this phenomenon are lacking [58,59]. Heparin molecules bind and inhibit cellular adhesion molecules such as the selectins [60,61], thereby preventing lymphocyte homing and extravasation. Heparin binds with high affinity to a number of inflammatory cytokines including IL-12 [62] and IL-2 [63], potentially sequestering them. Heparin prevents activation of the effector cells of inflammation, such as neutrophils and macrophages [64,65]. Finally, heparin directly inhibits molecular mediators of inflammation, such as elastase [66] and major basic protein [67]. Compellingly, the anti-inflammatory actions of heparin may be independent of its anti-coagulant activity [68]. Given its potent role as an anti-inflammatory agent, several clinical trials have evaluated heparin and its derivatives in diseases of inappropriate inflammation, including sepsis [69,70], and asthma [71].

Heparin's main clinical roles in the management of aSAH, prevention of VTE and systemic heparinization during endovascular treatment of aneurysms, exploit its anticoagulant properties. However, the broader role of heparin outside the coagulation cascade argues for a broader utility in aneurysmal SAH. Several clinical studies already suggest that heparin and its low molecular weight derivative enoxaparin reduce the incidence of clinical vasospasm and delayed cerebral infarction following aneurysmal SAH [21,24,72], although the literature is not entirely consistent in this result [73];

a previous review already discussed the role of heparin in the prevention of delayed cerebral ischemia following aneurysmal SAH [74]. Beyond vasospasm, however, heparin may improve outcomes in aSAH by preventing inflammation and restoring blood-brain barrier integrity. Given the increasing recognition of inflammation, edema, and blood-brain barrier dysfunction as mediators of poor outcome following aSAH, these extravascular effects of heparin represent an even more important aspect of its therapeutic efficacy than the prevention of vasospasm.

4. Heparin in Post-SAH Brain Injury

4.1. Ischemia-Reperfusion Injury

A hallmark of aneurysm rupture is a transient period of hypoperfusion or even frank intracranial circulatory arrest secondary to the acute rise in intracranial pressure at ictus. Although other factors, such as CSF dissemination of blood products, undoubtedly play a role in secondary brain injury, the ischemia-reperfusion injury at ictus is arguably the predominant injury following aSAH, as its clinical correlate, loss of consciousness at ictus, remains one of the best predictors of outcome following aSAH [75,76]. Multiple studies demonstrate the efficacy of heparin and its derivatives in ischemia-reperfusion injury. Several studies in rats demonstrate reduced infarct volume following heparin and heparin-derivative administration following transient cerebral arterial occlusion [77–81]. Both the efficacy of non-anticoagulating 2,3-*O*-desulfated heparin derivative in vivo [79] as well as the neuroprotection low molecular weight heparin affords against ischemia-reperfusion injury in vitro [82] suggest that heparin and its derivatives exert these effects independently of their actions on the coagulation cascade. Proposed modes of action include neutralization of oxidative species [83] and inhibition of neuronal apoptosis [84], although neither of these studies provide definitive evidence of these modes of action.

4.2. Leukocyte Extravasation

Mobilization of leukocytes from the periphery into inflamed tissue (leukocyte extravasation) is a crucial component of inflammation generally and post-SAH neuroinflammation specifically [85]. Administration of low dose heparin following experimental SAH reduces the number of inflammatory cells within the CNS [22]. Although studies of heparin in SAH do not address leukocyte extravasation explicitly, several animal models of neuroinflammatory injury suggest that heparins directly inhibit this process. Administration of unfractionated heparin following murine TBI reduces leukocyte extravasation as demonstrated by in vivo microscopy [86]. Administration of low molecular weight heparin yields similar results [87]. Compellingly, an in vivo microscopy study of experimental meningitis also demonstrates a reduction in leukocyte extravasation with heparin administration, a phenomenon attributable to both a reduction in leukocyte sticking and leukocyte rolling to the endothelium [88]. These findings of reduced leukocyte adhesion and leukocyte extravasation following heparin administration in disparate neuroinflammatory conditions suggests a common mechanism of action. Although the movement of leukocytes from the vascular to the parenchymal compartment is a complex process, adhesion of leukocytes to the vessel wall critically depends on interactions between cell surface glycoproteins and selectins, surface lectins expressed by both leukocytes (L-selectin) and endothelial cells (E-selectin) [89]. Given current knowledge of heparin's effects on endothelium-leukocyte interactions, inhibition of leukocyte expressed selectin [90] provides a plausible candidate mechanism to explain its effects on leukocyte extravasation. Several studies demonstrate that heparin-mediated inhibition of selectins occurs independently of anti-coagulation [60,91]. Consistent with these observations, studies of heparin in experimental TBI [86] note equivalent efficacy of low, non-anticoagulating heparin doses compared to higher doses with regard to leukocyte extravasation.

4.3. Inflammatory Activation

Although heparin's effects on leukocyte extravasation mediate some aspects of its anti-inflammatory processes, heparin may also reduce injury by modulating inflammatory cell activation. A key effector mechanism in the pathological neuroinflammatory response following SAH is phagocyte activation, resulting in production of direct mediators of pathology such as peroxynitrite [35] and matrix metalloproteinase-9 [47]. Given that heparin's effects on leukocyte extravasation do not readily account for the reduction in endogenous microglial activation observed with heparinization following SAH [22], heparin's effects on activation of inflammatory cells appear relevant to SAH. Given heparin's wide array of interactions with inflammatory mediators, no single mechanism of heparin induced immunoquiescence likely accounts for its full pleiotropic effects. Nevertheless, several interesting candidate mechanisms bear further discussion.

The receptor for advanced glycation end-products (RAGE) expressed on phagocytes mediates a number of inflammatory effects via activation of NF-κB [92]; SAH induces RAGE expression throughout the cortex by both neurons and microglia [93]. Furthermore, SAH induces the expression and release of a number of RAGE ligands, including HMGB1 [93–98] and S100B [99–102], within the CNS. Consistent with its inflammatory role, inhibition of RAGE signaling reduces inflammation and improves functional outcomes following experimental SAH [103–105]. Heparins, including low molecular weight heparins and non-anticoagulating derivatives such as 2,3-O-desulfated heparin, inhibit interactions between RAGE and its ligands with a high degree of specificity [65,106–110]. Although not well studied in SAH, pharmacologic blockade of HMGB1 duplicates some of the beneficial effects of enoxaparin following experimental TBI, including reduction of leukocyte extravasation, suggesting that heparin mediates some of its effects via modulating RAGE's interactions with its ligands [111]. Blockade of RAGE inhibition may account for some of heparin's effects on inflammatory cell activation.

Another potential mechanism of inflammatory modulation focuses on macrophage polarization. Although overly simplistic, macrophages and microglia roughly partition into two distinct phenotypes [112]. The M1 phenotype promotes anti-cellular immune responses important to viral and tumor defense. Consistent with this function, M1 phagocytes mediate a variety of biological effects relevant to post-SAH brain injury including peroxynitrite production via upregulation of inducible nitric oxide synthase and production of inflammatory cytokines including IL-1β, processes that contribute to early brain injury following SAH [35,113]. M2 phagocytes, in contrast, have opposite effects, reducing nitric oxide via arginine consumption and producing anti-inflammatory cytokines. Modulation of phagocyte polarization from a M1 to a M2 phenotype appears protective in SAH [114]. As mentioned previously, mast cells and basophils are the predominant sources of physiologic heparin [115]. This association strongly suggests that heparin plays a role in allergic and anti-helminthic responses. A common murine marker of M2 phenotype, the Ym1 receptor appears necessary for generation of a Type II immune response [116,117]. Compellingly, heparin appears to be a physiologic ligand of Ym1 [118]. Although direct evaluations of heparin's physiologic effects on phagocyte polarization are lacking, a study of oral enoxaparin in experimental ulcerative colitis demonstrates modulation of colonic macrophages from an M1 to an M2 phenotype with enoxaparin administration [119], a finding consistent with this hypothesized physiologic role. Further studies are required, however, to establish whether heparin modulates phagocyte polarization in aSAH.

4.4. Oxidative Stress

Production of reactive oxidative species (ROS) by activated phagocytes mediates significant injury following SAH [35]. Strategies to reduce oxidative stress following experimental SAH demonstrate numerous beneficial effects [120–123]. Heparin demonstrates a number of anti-oxidant effects. Extracellular superoxide dismutase (EC-SOD), a powerful anti-oxidant enzyme, demonstrates specific heparin binding [124,125]. From a physiologic standpoint, binding of EC-SOD to cell surface heparan sulfate sequesters EC-SOD to the cell surface, as mutations in the heparin-binding domain of SOD or administration of IV heparin results in release of EC-SOD into circulating fluids [126,127]. Aside from increasing circulating levels of EC-SOD, heparin also appears to induce its synthesis [128]. This release of EC-SOD into circulating fluids increases its activity, as heparin administration into the CSF of rabbits overexpressing EC-SOD results in a 27-fold increase in SOD activity within the CSF [129]. Although not studied in subarachnoid hemorrhage, systemic administration of enoxaparin enhances brain SOD activity in experimental cerebral ischemia-reperfusion injury [83], confirming the relevance of this phenomenon to intracranial pathology. Thioredoxin reductase, another enzyme thought protective in oxidative brain injury [130,131], also demonstrates high affinity binding to heparin [132], although the significance of this interaction is unclear. Several in vitro studies demonstrate direct antioxidant actions of the heparin molecule itself independent of any associated co-enzyme [133,134]. Taken together, these findings suggest that heparin may ameliorate the oxidative injury generated following aSAH.

4.5. Blood-Brain Barrier Dysfunction and Vasogenic Edema

Edema formation following SAH portends a poor prognosis [42]. Blood-brain barrier dysfunction and its associated vasogenic edema therefore present highly plausible therapeutic targets in aSAH. Multiple lines of evidence, in both aSAH and other injuries, suggest that heparin reduces blood-brain barrier dysfunction and its associated vasogenic edema. In a murine endovascular perforation model of SAH, pretreatment with low dose heparin reduced edema formation at 24 h following injury, with improved early behavioral outcome [23]. Heparin administration in other forms of experimental brain injury reduces blood-brain barrier dysfunction and edema formation in models as diverse as TBI [86,87,111,135], ischemic stroke [78,136], intracerebral hemorrhage [137,138], and meningitis [88]. A human study of TBI patients corroborates these findings, demonstrating more rapid resolution of pathologic CT imaging features, especially edema, with early enoxaparin administration [139].

Given the intimate association between inflammation and edema, heparin's anti-edema effects most likely derive from its anti-inflammatory properties. However, heparin demonstrates significant interaction with two molecules relevant to edema formation following aSAH, vascular endothelial growth factor (VEGF) and bradykinin (BK) [42]. VEGF, an angiogenic protein initially identified as a vascular permeability factor, binds heparin [140]. The effects of heparin on VEGF-endothelial cell interactions are complex. At low concentrations, heparin appears to enhance binding of VEGF to its receptor; however, at progressively higher concentrations heparin inhibits VEGF binding [141]. This inhibitory effect is sensitive to both the sulfation [141] and the size of heparin molecules employed [142]. Given the role of VEGF in SAH-mediated edema specifically and brain edema generally, heparin inhibition of VEGF presents a plausible albeit uninvestigated mode of edema reduction. Like VEGF, the interactions between heparin and bradykinin appear complex. While mast cell-derived heparin is crucial to both bradykinin formation and vascular permeability in allergic conditions [143], other studies suggest that intravenous heparin inhibits bradykinin induced vascular permeability [144]. Furthermore, bradykinin-mediated edema in aSAH occurs very early following hemorrhage [145]. Taken together, these findings suggests that heparin's interactions with bradykinin may not be relevant to its effects on edema.

5. Complications of Heparin Therapy in aSAH

5.1. Heparin Induced Thrombocytopenia (HIT)

Heparin-induced thrombocytopenia is arguably the most feared heparin related complication. An autoimmune phenomenon, HIT results from antibody formation to the heparin-platelet factor 4 complex, resulting in both platelet depletion and a paradoxical pro-thrombotic state with significant risk of both arterial and venous thromboembolic complications [146]. Although studies suggest that 3 to 5 percent of patients undergoing intravenous unfractionated heparin will develop HIT, the incidence of symptomatic HIT following SAH may be much higher, with a reported incidence between 5% and 15% [147,148]. Although general studies associate LMWH with a reduced risk of symptomatic HIT, the one comparison available to date finds no difference in rates of HIT between LMWH and UFH in SA [148]. Despite its associated thrombocytopenia, ischemic complications represent a particular concern with symptomatic HIT. Several large series identify increased risk of stroke, death, and poor outcome in SAH patients with HIT [147,149]. Risk factors identified for HIT in a multivariate analysis of patients with aSAH included female gender, clip treatment of aneurysm, and greater number of vasospasm treatments [149]. This last association may reflect either increased risk of HIT due to use of catheter heparinization in the treatment of vasospasm or, alternatively, an increased risk of cerebral ischemia due to a HIT-induced pro-thrombotic state. In our own reported series of low dose infusion for aneurysmal SAH, none of the forty-three treated patients developed symptomatic HIT [21], despite use of clip treatment and prolonged (fourteen day) heparin exposure. This lower than expected incidence could reflect the use of a low dose (12 U/kg/h), reduced auto-antibody production due to heparin's anti-inflammatory properties, a reduced incidence of vasospasm, or an inadequate number of subjects to assess HIT in this population. Since publication of this initial experience, two incidences of symptomatic HIT (2/150 patients) have developed in patients undergoing low dose heparin infusion, requiring cessation of their heparin infusion. Both patients required multiple interventions for vasospasm, with one experiencing a good recovery; the other died secondary to cerebral infarction. Although the low incidence of HIT in this population and excellent preliminary results of patients treated with low dose heparin outweigh this low risk of HIT, the apparently increased risk of cerebral ischemia from HIT in aSAH mandates vigilant screening for this condition.

5.2. Hemorrhagic Complications

Aside from HIT, fear of bleeding forms the other principal concern with heparin administration following aSAH. Patients with aSAH experience increased brain hemorrhage risk due to a variety of circumstances: aneurysm re-rupture prior to definitive treatment, periprocedural bleeding from surgery or a ventriculostomy, or hemorrhage into infarcted brain tissue. Although some experiences with systemic heparinization during endovascular treatment of ruptured aneurysms suggests that this practice does not increase the risk of hemorrhage or aneurysm re-bleeding [150,151], others suggest a significant risk of brain hemorrhage with this practice [152]. Ventriculostomy (EVD) placement followed by systemic heparinization for aSAH appears to be relatively safe, with multiple studies finding a low risk of significant EVD hemorrhage with systemic heparinization [151,153,154]. However, heparinization does appear to increase the risk of minor EVD hemorrhage [154]. In most reports of heparin or its derivatives as a therapeutic modality for vasospasm, hemorrhagic complications are either rare or non-existent [21,24,72], although one study noted an increased risk of non-significant bleeding in patients receiving enoxaparin compared to controls [73]. This low reported risk of hemorrhage is especially striking given the early (less than 12 h) post-operative initiation of heparin in at least one of these studies study [21]. The relatively low rate of hemorrhagic complications in these therapeutic studies of heparin most likely derive from a combination of low, non-anticoagulating doses of heparin as well as the relative safety of heparin use even following procedural interventions. Thus, the available evidence generally does not support the fears of hemorrhagic complications with heparinization following aneurysmal SAH.

6. Heparin Derivatives

Although unfractionated heparin is perhaps the best studied member of the heparin family in the context of aSAH, its theoretical associated risk of hemorrhagic complications might preclude its use in certain patients, such as those with difficult to secure aneurysms. However, as briefly discussed earlier, heparin's interactions with other molecular partners depends crucially on both the size and sulfation of the heparin molecule; modification of either of these parameters has significant effects on heparin's pharmacologic effects. As previously discussed, the unfractionated heparin used clinically consists of polysaccharide polymers of significantly variable length. Cleavage of these polymers using either chemical or enzymatic digestion yields the low-molecular weight heparins.

Low molecular weight heparins such as enoxaparin provide several advantages over standard unfractionated heparin, including more predictable clinical dosing and relatively specific anti-factor Xa activity [51]. Aside from digestion of unfractionated heparin, chemical synthesis of heparin's anti-thrombin binding pentasaccharide motif yields fondaparinux, a potent anti-coagulant with highly specific inhibition of factor Xa without significant risk of heparin induced thrombocytopenia [155]. Aside from modification of polymer length, several other strategies change heparin's pharmacological effects via chemical modification. Due to its high degree of sulfation, heparin possesses a significant high negative charge density, allowing for ionic interactions with a wide variety of molecular partners, including anti-thrombin III. Chemical desulfation reduces heparin's anticoagulant properties while retaining its interactions with other molecular pathways. 2,3-O-desulfated heparin, prepared via cold alkaline hydrolysis of native heparin, demonstrates markedly reduced anti-thrombin III binding with a concurrent reduction in anti-coagulant activity while still retaining native heparin's desirable anti-inflammatory effects such as selectin binding, RAGE blockade, and protease inhibition [108]. Replacement of the N-sulfate group with an acetyl side chain similarly reduces anticoagulant activity without compromising anti-inflammatory and anti-protease effects [156,157]. Although 6-O-desulfated heparin demonstrates reduced anti-coagulant activity with retained blockade of inflammatory receptors such as RAGE, loss of the 6-O-sulfate moiety also results in decreased selectin inhibition with compromised anti-inflammatory activity [158]. Finally, periodate cleavage of the 2,3 vicinal diols in uronate residues yield so-called glycol-split heparins, a class of heparin with reduced anticoagulant activity despite retained sulfate moieties. These glycol-split heparins demonstrate reduced anticoagulant activity while retaining useful features of native heparin, such as elastase inhibition and cytokine binding [157]. Although a full review of chemically modified heparinoids lies well-beyond the scope of this article, several of these molecules, especially 2,3-O-desulfated heparin, demonstrate a desirable blend of anti-inflammatory features with reduced anti-coagulant activity that might prove useful in aneurysmal SAH. Figure 1 depicts a summary of these modified heparin species along with salient characteristics.

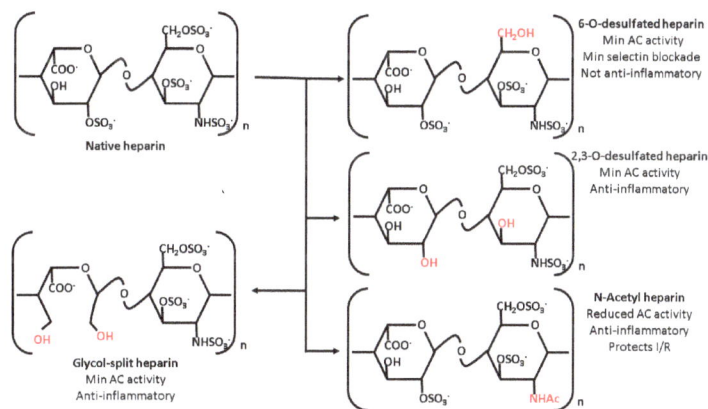

Figure 1. Summary of heparin chemical derivatives. Chemical modification of unfractionated heparin modulates its pharmacology. Although all derivatives discussed demonstrate reduced anticoagulant activity, chemical modification also affects heparin's other pharmacologic properties in a regiospecific manner. 2,3-O-desulfated heparin demonstrates nearly retained selecting and RAGE inhibition; 6-O-desulfated heparin, despite numerous sulfated residues, fails to bind selectins and does not demonstrate significant anti-inflammatory effects in vivo. Although less well studied in inflammation, N-acetyl heparin does demonstrate evidence of efficacy in ischemia-reperfusion (I/R) injury despite reduced anticoagulant activity. Finally, glycol split heparin retains the ability to inhibit proteases such as elastase despite reduced anti-coagulant activity.

7. Conclusions

Given the complexity of brain injury following aneurysmal subarachnoid hemorrhage, no single therapeutic modality is likely to address all aspects relevant to its treatment. Given the multimodal nature of heparin's interactions with mediators of post-SAH brain injury, as summarized in the accompanying figure (Figure 2), heparin and heparin derivatives may form a significantly better class of therapeutic for aSAH than more well-defined pharmacologic agents. Although initial clinical and experimental work suggests the efficacy of heparin in aSAH, these studies are relatively preliminary, with further clinical work required to confirm the utility of heparin. Furthermore, the absence of clear mechanistic insight into heparin's therapeutic effects mandates further experimental work, as a better understanding of heparin's mechanism of action could lead to improved and safer heparin derivatives. Nevertheless, heparin for aSAH represents a promising way forward in a disease much in need of effective therapy.

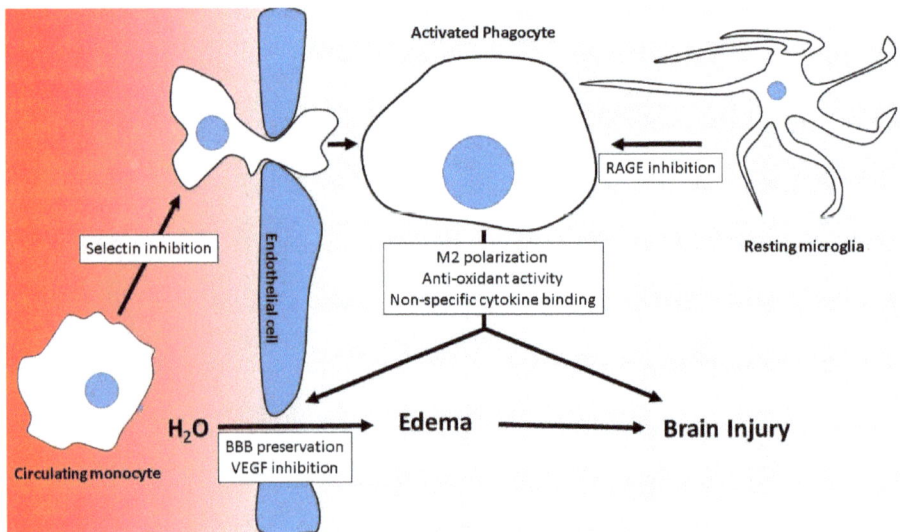

Figure 2. Summary of heparin's modes of action. Several confluent processes combine to injure the brain including extravasation of circulating cells into the brain parenchyma, activation of microglia, production of harmful molecules and cytokines by activated phagocytes, and blood-brain barrier breakdown with subsequent vasogenic edema formation. Heparin antagonizes these processes, with heparin's mechanisms of action indicated in the white boxes.

Acknowledgments: This work was supported by grants to JMS from the National Institute of Neurological Disorders and Stroke (NS060801; NS061808) and the National Heart, Lung and Blood Institute (HL082517).

Conflicts of Interest: The authors declare no conflicts of interest.

References

1. Ogden, J.A.; Utley, T.; Mee, E.W. Neurological and psychosocial outcome 4 to 7 years after subarachnoid hemorrhage. *Neurosurgery* **1997**, *41*, 25–34. [PubMed]
2. Hackett, M.L.; Anderson, C.S. Health outcomes 1 year after subarachnoid hemorrhage: An international population-based study. The australian cooperative research on subarachnoid hemorrhage study group. *Neurology* **2000**, *55*, 658–662. [PubMed]

3. Kreiter, K.T.; Copeland, D.; Bernardini, G.L.; Bates, J.E.; Peery, S.; Claassen, J.; Du, Y.E.; Stern, Y.; Connolly, E.S.; Mayer, S.A. Predictors of cognitive dysfunction after subarachnoid hemorrhage. *Stroke* **2002**, *33*, 200–208. [PubMed]

4. Al-Khindi, T.; Macdonald, R.L.; Schweizer, T.A. Cognitive and functional outcome after aneurysmal subarachnoid hemorrhage. *Stroke* **2010**, *41*, e519–e536. [PubMed]

5. Haley, E.C., Jr. Measuring cognitive outcome after subarachnoid hemorrhage. *Ann. Neurol.* **2006**, *60*, 502–504. [PubMed]

6. Kivisaari, R.P.; Salonen, O.; Servo, A.; Autti, T.; Hernesniemi, J.; Ohman, J. Mr imaging after aneurysmal subarachnoid hemorrhage and surgery: A long-term follow-up study. *AJNR Am. J. Neuroradiol.* **2001**, *22*, 1143–1148. [PubMed]

7. Tam, A.K.; Kapadia, A.; Ilodigwe, D.; Li, Z.; Schweizer, T.A.; Macdonald, R.L. Impact of global cerebral atrophy on clinical outcome after subarachnoid hemorrhage. *J. Neurosurg.* **2013**, *119*, 198–206. [PubMed]

8. Macdonald, R.L.; Higashida, R.T.; Keller, E.; Mayer, S.A.; Molyneux, A.; Raabe, A.; Vajkoczy, P.; Wanke, I.; Bach, D.; Frey, A.; et al. Randomised trial of clazosentan, an endothelin receptor antagonist, in patients with aneurysmal subarachnoid hemorrhage undergoing surgical clipping (conscious-2). *Acta Neurochir. Suppl.* **2013**, *115*, 27–31. [PubMed]

9. Cossu, G.; Messerer, M.; Oddo, M.; Daniel, R.T. To look beyond vasospasm in aneurysmal subarachnoid haemorrhage. *Biomed. Res. Int.* **2014**, *2014*, 628597. [PubMed]

10. Rowland, M.J.; Hadjipavlou, G.; Kelly, M.; Westbrook, J.; Pattinson, K.T. Delayed cerebral ischaemia after subarachnoid haemorrhage: Looking beyond vasospasm. *Br. J. Anaesth.* **2012**, *109*, 315–329. [PubMed]

11. Lucke-Wold, B.P.; Logsdon, A.F.; Manoranjan, B.; Turner, R.C.; McConnell, E.; Vates, G.E.; Huber, J.D.; Rosen, C.L.; Simard, J.M. Aneurysmal subarachnoid hemorrhage and neuroinflammation: A comprehensive review. *Int. J. Mol. Sci.* **2016**, *17*, 497. [CrossRef] [PubMed]

12. Lin, S.; Yin, Q.; Zhong, Q.; Lv, F.L.; Zhou, Y.; Li, J.Q.; Wang, J.Z.; Su, B.Y.; Yang, Q.W. Heme activates tlr4-mediated inflammatory injury via myd88/trif signaling pathway in intracerebral hemorrhage. *J. Neuroinflamm.* **2012**, *9*, 46. [CrossRef] [PubMed]

13. Kwon, M.S.; Woo, S.K.; Kurland, D.B.; Yoon, S.H.; Palmer, A.F.; Banerjee, U.; Iqbal, S.; Ivanova, S.; Gerzanich, V.; Simard, J.M. Methemoglobin is an endogenous toll-like receptor 4 ligand-relevance to subarachnoid hemorrhage. *Int. J. Mol. Sci.* **2015**, *16*, 5028–5046. [CrossRef] [PubMed]

14. Gallia, G.L.; Tamargo, R.J. Leukocyte-endothelial cell interactions in chronic vasospasm after subarachnoid hemorrhage. *Neurol. Res.* **2006**, *28*, 750–758. [CrossRef] [PubMed]

15. Ayer, R.E.; Zhang, J.H. Oxidative stress in subarachnoid haemorrhage: Significance in acute brain injury and vasospasm. *Acta Neurochir. Suppl.* **2008**, *104*, 33–41. [PubMed]

16. Chou, S.H.; Feske, S.K.; Atherton, J.; Konigsberg, R.G.; De Jager, P.L.; Du, R.; Ogilvy, C.S.; Lo, E.H.; Ning, M. Early elevation of serum tumor necrosis factor-alpha is associated with poor outcome in subarachnoid hemorrhage. *J. Investig. Med.* **2012**, *60*, 1054–1058. [CrossRef] [PubMed]

17. Hanafy, K.A.; Morgan Stuart, R.; Fernandez, L.; Schmidt, J.M.; Claassen, J.; Lee, K.; Sander Connolly, E.; Mayer, S.A.; Badjatia, N. Cerebral inflammatory response and predictors of admission clinical grade after aneurysmal subarachnoid hemorrhage. *J. Clin. Neurosci.* **2010**, *17*, 22–25. [CrossRef] [PubMed]

18. McMahon, C.J.; Hopkins, S.; Vail, A.; King, A.T.; Smith, D.; Illingworth, K.J.; Clark, S.; Rothwell, N.J.; Tyrrell, P.J. Inflammation as a predictor for delayed cerebral ischemia after aneurysmal subarachnoid haemorrhage. *J. Neurointerv. Surg.* **2013**, *5*, 512–517. [CrossRef] [PubMed]

19. Tam, A.K.; Ilodigwe, D.; Mocco, J.; Mayer, S.; Kassell, N.; Ruefenacht, D.; Schmiedek, P.; Weidauer, S.; Pasqualin, A.; Macdonald, R.L. Impact of systemic inflammatory response syndrome on vasospasm, cerebral infarction, and outcome after subarachnoid hemorrhage: Exploratory analysis of conscious-1 database. *Neurocrit. Care* **2010**, *13*, 182–189. [CrossRef] [PubMed]

20. Jedrzejowska-Szypulka, H.; Larysz-Brysz, M.; Kukla, M.; Snietura, M.; Lewin-Kowalik, J. Neutralization of interleukin-1beta reduces vasospasm and alters cerebral blood vessel density following experimental subarachnoid hemorrhage in rats. *Curr. Neurovasc. Res.* **2009**, *6*, 95–103. [CrossRef] [PubMed]

21. Simard, J.M.; Aldrich, E.F.; Schreibman, D.; James, R.F.; Polifka, A.; Beaty, N. Low-dose intravenous heparin infusion in patients with aneurysmal subarachnoid hemorrhage: A preliminary assessment. *J. Neurosurg.* **2013**, *119*, 1611–1619. [CrossRef] [PubMed]

22. Simard, J.M.; Tosun, C.; Ivanova, S.; Kurland, D.B.; Hong, C.; Radecki, L.; Gisriel, C.; Mehta, R.; Schreibman, D.; Gerzanich, V. Heparin reduces neuroinflammation and transsynaptic neuronal apoptosis in a model of subarachnoid hemorrhage. *Transl. Stroke Res.* **2012**, *3*, 155–165. [CrossRef] [PubMed]

23. Altay, O.; Suzuki, H.; Hasegawa, Y.; Sorar, M.; Chen, H.; Tang, J.; Zhang, J.H. Effects of low-dose unfractionated heparin pretreatment on early brain injury after subarachnoid hemorrhage in mice. *Acta Neurochir. Suppl.* **2016**, *121*, 127–130. [PubMed]

24. Bruder, M.; Won, S.Y.; Kashefiolasl, S.; Wagner, M.; Brawanski, N.; Dinc, N.; Seifert, V.; Konczalla, J. Effect of heparin on secondary brain injury in patients with subarachnoid hemorrhage: An additional "h" therapy in vasospasm treatment. *J. Neurointerv. Surg.* **2017**. neurintsurg–2016–012925. [CrossRef] [PubMed]

25. Grote, E.; Hassler, W. The critical first minutes after subarachnoid hemorrhage. *Neurosurgery* **1988**, *22*, 654–661. [CrossRef] [PubMed]

26. Hanafy, K.A. The role of microglia and the tlr4 pathway in neuronal apoptosis and vasospasm after subarachnoid hemorrhage. *J. Neuroinflamm.* **2013**, *10*, 83. [CrossRef] [PubMed]

27. Jackowski, A.; Crockard, A.; Burnstock, G.; Russell, R.R.; Kristek, F. The time course of intracranial pathophysiological changes following experimental subarachnoid haemorrhage in the rat. *J. Cereb. Blood Flow Metab.* **1990**, *10*, 835–849. [CrossRef] [PubMed]

28. Moraes, L.; Grille, S.; Morelli, P.; Mila, R.; Trias, N.; Brugnini, A.; Luberas, L.N.; Biestro, A.; Lens, D. Immune cells subpopulations in cerebrospinal fluid and peripheral blood of patients with aneurysmal subarachnoid hemorrhage. *Springerplus* **2015**, *4*, 195. [CrossRef] [PubMed]

29. Provencio, J.J.; Swank, V.; Lu, H.; Brunet, S.; Baltan, S.; Khapre, R.V.; Seerapu, H.; Kokiko-Cochran, O.N.; Lamb, B.T.; Ransohoff, R.M. Neutrophil depletion after subarachnoid hemorrhage improves memory via nmda receptors. *Brain Behav. Immun.* **2016**, *54*, 233–242. [CrossRef] [PubMed]

30. Provencio, J.J.; Fu, X.; Siu, A.; Rasmussen, P.A.; Hazen, S.L.; Ransohoff, R.M. Csf neutrophils are implicated in the development of vasospasm in subarachnoid hemorrhage. *Neurocrit. Care* **2010**, *12*, 244–251. [CrossRef] [PubMed]

31. Xu, H.; Testai, F.D.; Valyi-Nagy, T.; M, N.P.; Zhai, F.; Nanegrungsunk, D.; Paisansathan, C.; Pelligrino, D.A. vap-1 blockade prevents subarachnoid hemorrhage-associated cerebrovascular dilating dysfunction via repression of a neutrophil recruitment-related mechanism. *Brain Res.* **2015**, *1603*, 141–149. [CrossRef] [PubMed]

32. Satoh, S.; Yamamoto, Y.; Toshima, Y.; Ikegaki, I.I.; Asano, T.; Suzuki, Y.; Shibuya, M. Fasudil, a protein kinase inhibitor, prevents the development of endothelial injury and neutrophil infiltration in a two-haemorrhage canine subarachnoid model. *J. Clin. Neurosci.* **1999**, *6*, 394–399. [CrossRef]

33. Pradilla, G.; Wang, P.P.; Legnani, F.G.; Ogata, L.; Dietsch, G.N.; Tamargo, R.J. Prevention of vasospasm by anti-cd11/cd18 monoclonal antibody therapy following subarachnoid hemorrhage in rabbits. *J. Neurosurg.* **2004**, *101*, 88–92. [CrossRef] [PubMed]

34. Clatterbuck, R.E.; Gailloud, P.; Ogata, L.; Gebremariam, A.; Dietsch, G.N.; Murphy, K.J.; Tamargo, R.J. Prevention of cerebral vasospasm by a humanized anti-cd11/cd18 monoclonal antibody administered after experimental subarachnoid hemorrhage in nonhuman primates. *J. Neurosurg.* **2003**, *99*, 376–382. [CrossRef] [PubMed]

35. Iqbal, S.; Hayman, E.G.; Hong, C.; Stokum, J.A.; Kurland, D.B.; Gerzanich, V.; Simard, J.M. Inducible nitric oxide synthase (nos-2) in subarachnoid hemorrhage: Regulatory mechanisms and therapeutic implications. *Brain Circ.* **2016**, *2*, 8–19. [PubMed]

36. Kooijman, E.; Nijboer, C.H.; van Velthoven, C.T.; Mol, W.; Dijkhuizen, R.M.; Kesecioglu, J.; Heijnen, C.J. Long-term functional consequences and ongoing cerebral inflammation after subarachnoid hemorrhage in the rat. *PLoS ONE* **2014**, *9*, e90584. [CrossRef] [PubMed]

37. Schallner, N.; Pandit, R.; LeBlanc, R.; Thomas, A.J.; Ogilvy, C.S.; Zuckerbraun, B.S.; Gallo, D.; Otterbein, L.E.; Hanafy, K.A. Microglia regulate blood clearance in subarachnoid hemorrhage by heme oxygenase-1. *J. Clin. Investig.* **2015**, *125*, 2609–2625. [CrossRef] [PubMed]

38. Matz, P.; Turner, C.; Weinstein, P.R.; Massa, S.M.; Panter, S.S.; Sharp, F.R. Heme-oxygenase-1 induction in glia throughout rat brain following experimental subarachnoid hemorrhage. *Brain Res.* **1996**, *713*, 211–222. [CrossRef]

39. Bernardino, L.; Agasse, F.; Silva, B.; Ferreira, R.; Grade, S.; Malva, J.O. Tumor necrosis factor-alpha modulates survival, proliferation, and neuronal differentiation in neonatal subventricular zone cell cultures. *Stem Cells* **2008**, *26*, 2361–2371. [CrossRef] [PubMed]

40. Shigemoto-Mogami, Y.; Hoshikawa, K.; Goldman, J.E.; Sekino, Y.; Sato, K. Microglia enhance neurogenesis and oligodendrogenesis in the early postnatal subventricular zone. *J. Neurosci.* **2014**, *34*, 2231–2243. [CrossRef] [PubMed]

41. Sgubin, D.; Aztiria, E.; Perin, A.; Longatti, P.; Leanza, G. Activation of endogenous neural stem cells in the adult human brain following subarachnoid hemorrhage. *J. Neurosci. Res.* **2007**, *85*, 1647–1655. [CrossRef] [PubMed]

42. Hayman, E.G.; Wessell, A.; Gerzanich, V.; Sheth, K.N.; Simard, J.M. Mechanisms of global cerebral edema formation in aneurysmal subarachnoid hemorrhage. *Neurocrit. Care* **2017**, *26*, 301–310. [CrossRef] [PubMed]

43. Simard, J.M.; Geng, Z.; Woo, S.K.; Ivanova, S.; Tosun, C.; Melnichenko, L.; Gerzanich, V. Glibenclamide reduces inflammation, vasogenic edema, and caspase-3 activation after subarachnoid hemorrhage. *J. Cereb. Blood Flow Metab.* **2009**, *29*, 317–330. [CrossRef] [PubMed]

44. Germano, A.; Avella, D.; Imperatore, C.; Caruso, G.; Tomasello, F. Time-course of blood-brain barrier permeability changes after experimental subarachnoid haemorrhage. *Acta Neurochir. (Wien)* **2000**, *142*, 575–580; discussion 580–581. [CrossRef] [PubMed]

45. Claassen, J.; Carhuapoma, J.R.; Kreiter, K.T.; Du, E.Y.; Connolly, E.S.; Mayer, S.A. Global cerebral edema after subarachnoid hemorrhage: Frequency, predictors, and impact on outcome. *Stroke* **2002**, *33*, 1225–1232. [CrossRef] [PubMed]

46. Ivanidze, J.; Kesavabhotla, K.; Kallas, O.N.; Mir, D.; Baradaran, H.; Gupta, A.; Segal, A.Z.; Claassen, J.; Sanelli, P.C. Evaluating blood-brain barrier permeability in delayed cerebral infarction after aneurysmal subarachnoid hemorrhage. *AJNR Am. J. Neuroradiol.* **2015**, *36*, 850–854. [CrossRef] [PubMed]

47. Egashira, Y.; Zhao, H.; Hua, Y.; Keep, R.F.; Xi, G. White matter injury after subarachnoid hemorrhage: Role of blood-brain barrier disruption and matrix metalloproteinase-9. *Stroke* **2015**, *46*, 2909–2915. [CrossRef] [PubMed]

48. Carvey, P.M.; Hendey, B.; Monahan, A.J. The blood-brain barrier in neurodegenerative disease: A rhetorical perspective. *J. Neurochem.* **2009**, *111*, 291–314. [CrossRef] [PubMed]

49. Wardrop, D.; Keeling, D. The story of the discovery of heparin and warfarin. *Br. J. Haematol.* **2008**, *141*, 757–763. [CrossRef] [PubMed]

50. Capila, I.; Linhardt, R.J. Heparin-protein interactions. *Angew. Chem. Int. Ed. Engl.* **2002**, *41*, 391–412. [CrossRef]

51. Gray, E.; Mulloy, B.; Barrowcliffe, T.W. Heparin and low-molecular-weight heparin. *Thromb. Haemost.* **2008**, *99*, 807–818. [CrossRef] [PubMed]

52. Wei, M.; Gao, Y.; Tian, M.; Li, N.; Hao, S.; Zeng, X. Selectively desulfated heparin inhibits p-selectin-mediated adhesion of human melanoma cells. *Cancer Lett.* **2005**, *229*, 123–126. [CrossRef] [PubMed]

53. Medeiros, G.F.; Mendes, A.; Castro, R.A.; Bau, E.C.; Nader, H.B.; Dietrich, C.P. Distribution of sulfated glycosaminoglycans in the animal kingdom: Widespread occurrence of heparin-like compounds in invertebrates. *Biochim. Biophys. Acta* **2000**, *1475*, 287–294. [CrossRef]

54. Ronnberg, E.; Melo, F.R.; Pejler, G. Mast cell proteoglycans. *J. Histochem. Cytochem.* **2012**, *60*, 950–962. [CrossRef] [PubMed]

55. Pulendran, B.; Artis, D. New paradigms in type 2 immunity. *Science* **2012**, *337*, 431–435. [CrossRef] [PubMed]

56. Pomin, V.H.; Mulloy, B. Current structural biology of the heparin interactome. *Curr. Opin. Struct. Biol.* **2015**, *34*, 17–25. [CrossRef] [PubMed]

57. Lever, R.; Page, C.P. Non-anticoagulant effects of heparin: An overview. *Handb. Exp. Pharmacol.* **2012**, 281–305.

58. Li, X.; Li, Z.; Zheng, Z.; Liu, Y.; Ma, X. Unfractionated heparin ameliorates lipopolysaccharide-induced lung inflammation by downregulating nuclear factor-kappab signaling pathway. *Inflammation* **2013**, *36*, 1201–1208. [CrossRef] [PubMed]

59. Li, X.; Zheng, Z.; Li, X.; Ma, X. Unfractionated heparin inhibits lipopolysaccharide-induced inflammatory response through blocking p38 mapk and nf-kappab activation on endothelial cell. *Cytokine* **2012**, *60*, 114–121. [CrossRef] [PubMed]

60. Koenig, A.; Norgard-Sumnicht, K.; Linhardt, R.; Varki, A. Differential interactions of heparin and heparan sulfate glycosaminoglycans with the selectins. Implications for the use of unfractionated and low molecular weight heparins as therapeutic agents. *J. Clin. Investig.* **1998**, *101*, 877–889. [CrossRef] [PubMed]

61. Stevenson, J.L.; Choi, S.H.; Varki, A. Differential metastasis inhibition by clinically relevant levels of heparins—Correlation with selectin inhibition, not antithrombotic activity. *Clin. Cancer Res.* **2005**, *11*, 7003–7011. [CrossRef] [PubMed]

62. Hasan, M.; Najjam, S.; Gordon, M.Y.; Gibbs, R.V.; Rider, C.C. Il-12 is a heparin-binding cytokine. *J. Immunol.* **1999**, *162*, 1064–1070. [PubMed]

63. Najjam, S.; Gibbs, R.V.; Gordon, M.Y.; Rider, C.C. Characterization of human recombinant interleukin 2 binding to heparin and heparan sulfate using an elisa approach. *Cytokine* **1997**, *9*, 1013–1022. [CrossRef] [PubMed]

64. Cohen-Mazor, M.; Mazor, R.; Kristal, B.; Kistler, E.B.; Ziv, I.; Chezar, J.; Sela, S. Heparin interaction with the primed polymorphonuclear leukocyte cd11b induces apoptosis and prevents cell activation. *J. Immunol. Res.* **2015**, *2015*, 751014. [CrossRef] [PubMed]

65. Li, L.; Ling, Y.; Huang, M.; Yin, T.; Gou, S.M.; Zhan, N.Y.; Xiong, J.X.; Wu, H.S.; Yang, Z.Y.; Wang, C.Y. Heparin inhibits the inflammatory response induced by lps and hmgb1 by blocking the binding of hmgb1 to the surface of macrophages. *Cytokine* **2015**, *72*, 36–42. [CrossRef] [PubMed]

66. Spencer, J.L.; Stone, P.J.; Nugent, M.A. New insights into the inhibition of human neutrophil elastase by heparin. *Biochemistry* **2006**, *45*, 9104–9120. [CrossRef] [PubMed]

67. Swaminathan, G.J.; Myszka, D.G.; Katsamba, P.S.; Ohnuki, L.E.; Gleich, G.J.; Acharya, K.R. Eosinophil-granule major basic protein, a c-type lectin, binds heparin. *Biochemistry* **2005**, *44*, 14152–14158. [CrossRef] [PubMed]

68. Shastri, M.D.; Stewart, N.; Horne, J.; Zaidi, S.T.; Sohal, S.S.; Peterson, G.M.; Korner, H.; Gueven, N.; Patel, R.P. Non-anticoagulant fractions of enoxaparin suppress inflammatory cytokine release from peripheral blood mononuclear cells of allergic asthmatic individuals. *PLoS ONE* **2015**, *10*, e0128803. [CrossRef] [PubMed]

69. Wang, C.; Chi, C.; Guo, L.; Wang, X.; Guo, L.; Sun, J.; Sun, B.; Liu, S.; Chang, X.; Li, E. Heparin therapy reduces 28-day mortality in adult severe sepsis patients: A systematic review and meta-analysis. *Crit. Care* **2014**, *18*, 563. [CrossRef] [PubMed]

70. Chande, N.; MacDonald, J.K.; Wang, J.J.; McDonald, J.W. Unfractionated or low molecular weight heparin for induction of remission in ulcerative colitis: A cochrane inflammatory bowel disease and functional bowel disorders systematic review of randomized trials. *Inflamm. Bowel Dis.* **2011**, *17*, 1979–1986. [CrossRef] [PubMed]

71. Duong, M.; Cockcroft, D.; Boulet, L.P.; Ahmed, T.; Iverson, H.; Atkinson, D.C.; Stahl, E.G.; Watson, R.; Davis, B.; Milot, J.; et al. The effect of ivx-0142, a heparin-derived hypersulfated disaccharide, on the allergic airway responses in asthma. *Allergy* **2008**, *63*, 1195–1201. [CrossRef] [PubMed]

72. Wurm, G.; Tomancok, B.; Nussbaumer, K.; Adelwohrer, C.; Holl, K. Reduction of ischemic sequelae following spontaneous subarachnoid hemorrhage: A double-blind, randomized comparison of enoxaparin versus placebo. *Clin. Neurol. Neurosurg.* **2004**, *106*, 97–103. [CrossRef] [PubMed]

73. Siironen, J.; Juvela, S.; Varis, J.; Porras, M.; Poussa, K.; Ilveskero, S.; Hernesniemi, J.; Lassila, R. No effect of enoxaparin on outcome of aneurysmal subarachnoid hemorrhage: A randomized, double-blind, placebo-controlled clinical trial. *J. Neurosurg.* **2003**, *99*, 953–959. [CrossRef] [PubMed]

74. Simard, J.M.; Schreibman, D.; Aldrich, E.F.; Stallmeyer, B.; Le, B.; James, R.F.; Beaty, N. Unfractionated heparin: Multitargeted therapy for delayed neurological deficits induced by subarachnoid hemorrhage. *Neurocrit. Care* **2010**, *13*, 439–449. [CrossRef] [PubMed]

75. Wang, J.; Alotaibi, N.M.; Akbar, M.A.; Ayling, O.G.; Ibrahim, G.M.; Macdonald, R.L.; Noble, A.; Molyneux, A.; Quinn, A.; Schatlo, B.; et al. Loss of consciousness at onset of aneurysmal subarachnoid hemorrhage is associated with functional outcomes in good-grade patients. *World Neurosurg.* **2017**, *98*, 308–313. [CrossRef] [PubMed]

76. Suwatcharangkoon, S.; Meyers, E.; Falo, C.; Schmidt, J.M.; Agarwal, S.; Claassen, J.; Mayer, S.A. Loss of consciousness at onset of subarachnoid hemorrhage as an important marker of early brain injury. *JAMA Neurol.* **2016**, *73*, 28–35. [CrossRef] [PubMed]

77. Quartermain, D.; Li, Y.S.; Jonas, S. The low molecular weight heparin enoxaparin reduces infarct size in a rat model of temporary focal ischemia. *Cerebrovasc. Dis.* **2003**, *16*, 346–355. [CrossRef] [PubMed]

78. Li, P.A.; He, Q.P.; Siddiqui, M.M.; Shuaib, A. Posttreatment with low molecular weight heparin reduces brain edema and infarct volume in rats subjected to thrombotic middle cerebral artery occlusion. *Brain Res.* **1998**, *801*, 220–223. [CrossRef]

79. Mocco, J.; Shelton, C.E.; Sergot, P.; Ducruet, A.F.; Komotar, R.J.; Otten, M.L.; Sosunov, S.A.; Macarthur, R.B.; Kennedy, T.P.; Connolly, E.S., Jr. O-desulfated heparin improves outcome after rat cerebral ischemia/reperfusion injury. *Neurosurgery* **2007**, *61*, 1297–1303; discussion 1303–1304. [CrossRef] [PubMed]

80. Smith, D.R.; Ducker, T.B.; Kempe, L.G. Temporary experimental intracranial vascular occlusion. Effect of massive doses of heparin on brain survival. *J. Neurosurg.* **1969**, *30*, 537–544. [CrossRef] [PubMed]

81. Yanaka, K.; Spellman, S.R.; McCarthy, J.B.; Oegema, T.R., Jr.; Low, W.C.; Camarata, P.J. Reduction of brain injury using heparin to inhibit leukocyte accumulation in a rat model of transient focal cerebral ischemia. I. Protective mechanism. *J. Neurosurg.* **1996**, *85*, 1102–1107. [CrossRef] [PubMed]

82. Zhang, Z.G.; Lu, T.S.; Yuan, H.Y. Neuroprotective effects of ultra-low-molecular-weight heparin in vitro and vivo models of ischemic injury. *Fundam. Clin. Pharmacol.* **2011**, *25*, 300–303. [CrossRef] [PubMed]

83. Zhang, Z.G.; Zhang, Q.Z.; Cheng, Y.N.; Ji, S.L.; Du, G.H. Antagonistic effects of ultra-low-molecular-weight heparin against cerebral ischemia/reperfusion injury in rats. *Pharmacol. Res.* **2007**, *56*, 350–355. [CrossRef] [PubMed]

84. Zhang, Z.G.; Sun, X.; Zhang, Q.Z.; Yang, H. Neuroprotective effects of ultra-low-molecular-weight heparin on cerebral ischemia/reperfusion injury in rats: Involvement of apoptosis, inflammatory reaction and energy metabolism. *Int. J. Mol. Sci.* **2013**, *14*, 1932–1939. [CrossRef] [PubMed]

85. Xu, H.L.; Garcia, M.; Testai, F.; Vetri, F.; Barabanova, A.; Pelligrino, D.A.; Paisansathan, C. Pharmacologic blockade of vascular adhesion protein-1 lessens neurologic dysfunction in rats subjected to subarachnoid hemorrhage. *Brain Res.* **2014**, *1586*, 83–89. [CrossRef] [PubMed]

86. Nagata, K.; Kumasaka, K.; Browne, K.D.; Li, S.; St-Pierre, J.; Cognetti, J.; Marks, J.; Johnson, V.E.; Smith, D.H.; Pascual, J.L. Unfractionated heparin after tbi reduces in vivo cerebrovascular inflammation, brain edema and accelerates cognitive recovery. *J. Trauma Acute Care Surg.* **2016**, *81*, 1088–1094. [CrossRef] [PubMed]

87. Li, S.; Marks, J.A.; Eisenstadt, R.; Kumasaka, K.; Samadi, D.; Johnson, V.E.; Holena, D.N.; Allen, S.R.; Browne, K.D.; Smith, D.H.; et al. Enoxaparin ameliorates post-traumatic brain injury edema and neurologic recovery, reducing cerebral leukocyte endothelial interactions and vessel permeability in vivo. *J. Trauma Acute Care Surg.* **2015**, *79*, 78–84. [CrossRef] [PubMed]

88. Weber, J.R.; Angstwurm, K.; Rosenkranz, T.; Lindauer, U.; Freyer, D.; Burger, W.; Busch, C.; Einhaupl, K.M.; Dirnagl, U. Heparin inhibits leukocyte rolling in pial vessels and attenuates inflammatory changes in a rat model of experimental bacterial meningitis. *J. Cereb. Blood Flow Metab.* **1997**, *17*, 1221–1229. [CrossRef] [PubMed]

89. McEver, R.P. Selectins: Initiators of leucocyte adhesion and signalling at the vascular wall. *Cardiovasc. Res.* **2015**, *107*, 331–339. [CrossRef] [PubMed]

90. Nelson, R.M.; Cecconi, O.; Roberts, W.G.; Aruffo, A.; Linhardt, R.J.; Bevilacqua, M.P. Heparin oligosaccharides bind L- and P-selectin and inhibit acute inflammation. *Blood* **1993**, *82*, 3253–3258. [PubMed]

91. Sudha, T.; Phillips, P.; Kanaan, C.; Linhardt, R.J.; Borsig, L.; Mousa, S.A. Inhibitory effect of non-anticoagulant heparin (s-nach) on pancreatic cancer cell adhesion and metastasis in human umbilical cord vessel segment and in mouse model. *Clin. Exp. Metastasis* **2012**, *29*, 431–439. [CrossRef] [PubMed]

92. Byun, K.; Yoo, Y.; Son, M.; Lee, J.; Jeong, G.B.; Park, Y.M.; Salekdeh, G.H.; Lee, B. Advanced glycation end-products produced systemically and by macrophages: A common contributor to inflammation and degenerative diseases. *Pharmacol. Ther.* **2017**. [CrossRef] [PubMed]

93. Li, H.; Wu, W.; Sun, Q.; Liu, M.; Li, W.; Zhang, X.S.; Zhou, M.L.; Hang, C.H. Expression and cell distribution of receptor for advanced glycation end-products in the rat cortex following experimental subarachnoid hemorrhage. *Brain Res.* **2014**, *1543*, 315–323. [CrossRef] [PubMed]

94. Zhao, X.D.; Mao, H.Y.; Lv, J.; Lu, X.J. Expression of high-mobility group box-1 (hmgb1) in the basilar artery after experimental subarachnoid hemorrhage. *J. Clin. Neurosci.* **2016**, *27*, 161–165. [CrossRef] [PubMed]

95. Chang, C.Z.; Wu, S.C.; Kwan, A.L.; Lin, C.L. 4'-O-beta-d-glucosyl-5-O-methylvisamminol, an active ingredient of saposhnikovia divaricata, attenuates high-mobility group box 1 and subarachnoid hemorrhage-induced vasospasm in a rat model. *Behav. Brain Funct.* **2015**, *11*, 28. [CrossRef] [PubMed]

96. Sokol, B.; Wozniak, A.; Jankowski, R.; Jurga, S.; Wasik, N.; Shahid, H.; Grzeskowiak, B. Hmgb1 level in cerebrospinal fluid as a marker of treatment outcome in patients with acute hydrocephalus following aneurysmal subarachnoid hemorrhage. *J. Stroke Cerebrovasc. Dis.* **2015**, *24*, 1897–1904. [CrossRef] [PubMed]

97. Sun, Q.; Wu, W.; Hu, Y.C.; Li, H.; Zhang, D.; Li, S.; Li, W.; Li, W.D.; Ma, B.; Zhu, J.H.; et al. Early release of high-mobility group box 1 (hmgb1) from neurons in experimental subarachnoid hemorrhage in vivo and in vitro. *J. Neuroinflamm.* **2014**, *11*, 106. [CrossRef] [PubMed]

98. Nakahara, T.; Tsuruta, R.; Kaneko, T.; Yamashita, S.; Fujita, M.; Kasaoka, S.; Hashiguchi, T.; Suzuki, M.; Maruyama, I.; Maekawa, T. High-mobility group box 1 protein in csf of patients with subarachnoid hemorrhage. *Neurocrit. Care* **2009**, *11*, 362–368. [CrossRef] [PubMed]

99. Murakami, K.; Koide, M.; Dumont, T.M.; Russell, S.R.; Tranmer, B.I.; Wellman, G.C. Subarachnoid hemorrhage induces gliosis and increased expression of the pro-inflammatory cytokine high mobility group box 1 protein. *Transl. Stroke Res.* **2011**, *2*, 72–79. [CrossRef] [PubMed]

100. Kellermann, I.; Kleindienst, A.; Hore, N.; Buchfelder, M.; Brandner, S. Early csf and serum s100b concentrations for outcome prediction in traumatic brain injury and subarachnoid hemorrhage. *Clin. Neurol. Neurosurg.* **2016**, *145*, 79–83. [CrossRef] [PubMed]

101. Brandner, S.; Xu, Y.; Schmidt, C.; Emtmann, I.; Buchfelder, M.; Kleindienst, A. Shunt-dependent hydrocephalus following subarachnoid hemorrhage correlates with increased S100B levels in cerebrospinal fluid and serum. *Acta Neurochir. Suppl.* **2012**, *114*, 217–220. [PubMed]

102. Stranjalis, G.; Korfias, S.; Psachoulia, C.; Kouyialis, A.; Sakas, D.E.; Mendelow, A.D. The prognostic value of serum S-100B protein in spontaneous subarachnoid haemorrhage. *Acta Neurochir. (Wien)* **2007**, *149*, 231–237; discussion 237–238. [CrossRef] [PubMed]

103. Haruma, J.; Teshigawara, K.; Hishikawa, T.; Wang, D.; Liu, K.; Wake, H.; Mori, S.; Takahashi, H.K.; Sugiu, K.; Date, I.; et al. Anti-high mobility group box-1 (hmgb1) antibody attenuates delayed cerebral vasospasm and brain injury after subarachnoid hemorrhage in rats. *Sci. Rep.* **2016**, *6*, 37755. [CrossRef] [PubMed]

104. Hao, G.; Dong, Y.; Huo, R.; Wen, K.; Zhang, Y.; Liang, G. Rutin inhibits neuroinflammation and provides neuroprotection in an experimental rat model of subarachnoid hemorrhage, possibly through suppressing the rage-nf-kappab inflammatory signaling pathway. *Neurochem. Res.* **2016**, *41*, 1496–1504. [CrossRef] [PubMed]

105. Li, H.; Yu, J.S.; Zhang, D.D.; Yang, Y.Q.; Huang, L.T.; Yu, Z.; Chen, R.D.; Yang, H.K.; Hang, C.H. Inhibition of the receptor for advanced glycation end-products (rage) attenuates neuroinflammation while sensitizing cortical neurons towards death in experimental subarachnoid hemorrhage. *Mol. Neurobiol.* **2017**, *54*, 755–767. [CrossRef] [PubMed]

106. Myint, K.M.; Yamamoto, Y.; Doi, T.; Kato, I.; Harashima, A.; Yonekura, H.; Watanabe, T.; Shinohara, H.; Takeuchi, M.; Tsuneyama, K.; et al. Rage control of diabetic nephropathy in a mouse model: Effects of rage gene disruption and administration of low-molecular weight heparin. *Diabetes* **2006**, *55*, 2510–2522. [CrossRef] [PubMed]

107. Liu, R.; Mori, S.; Wake, H.; Zhang, J.; Liu, K.; Izushi, Y.; Takahashi, H.K.; Peng, B.; Nishibori, M. Establishment of in vitro binding assay of high mobility group box-1 and s100a12 to receptor for advanced glycation endproducts: Heparin's effect on binding. *Acta Med. Okayama* **2009**, *63*, 203–211. [PubMed]

108. Rao, N.V.; Argyle, B.; Xu, X.; Reynolds, P.R.; Walenga, J.M.; Prechel, M.; Prestwich, G.D.; MacArthur, R.B.; Walters, B.B.; Hoidal, J.R.; et al. Low anticoagulant heparin targets multiple sites of inflammation, suppresses heparin-induced thrombocytopenia, and inhibits interaction of rage with its ligands. *Am. J. Physiol. Cell Physiol.* **2010**, *299*, C97–C110. [CrossRef] [PubMed]

109. Ling, Y.; Yang, Z.Y.; Yin, T.; Li, L.; Yuan, W.W.; Wu, H.S.; Wang, C.Y. Heparin changes the conformation of high-mobility group protein 1 and decreases its affinity toward receptor for advanced glycation endproducts in vitro. *Int. Immunopharmacol.* **2011**, *11*, 187–193. [CrossRef] [PubMed]

110. Takeuchi, A.; Yamamoto, Y.; Munesue, S.; Harashima, A.; Watanabe, T.; Yonekura, H.; Yamamoto, H.; Tsuchiya, H. Low molecular weight heparin suppresses receptor for advanced glycation end products-mediated expression of malignant phenotype in human fibrosarcoma cells. *Cancer Sci.* **2013**, *104*, 740–749. [CrossRef] [PubMed]

111. Li, S.; Eisenstadt, R.; Kumasaka, K.; Johnson, V.E.; Marks, J.; Nagata, K.; Browne, K.D.; Smith, D.H.; Pascual, J.L. Does enoxaparin interfere with hmgb1 signaling after tbi? A potential mechanism for reduced cerebral edema and neurologic recovery. *J. Trauma Acute Care Surg.* **2016**, *80*, 381–387; discussion 387–389. [CrossRef] [PubMed]

112. Loane, D.J.; Kumar, A. Microglia in the tbi brain: The good, the bad, and the dysregulated. *Exp. Neurol.* **2016**, *275 Pt 3*, 316–327. [CrossRef] [PubMed]

113. Sozen, T.; Tsuchiyama, R.; Hasegawa, Y.; Suzuki, H.; Jadhav, V.; Nishizawa, S.; Zhang, J.H. Role of interleukin-1beta in early brain injury after subarachnoid hemorrhage in mice. *Stroke* **2009**, *40*, 2519–2525. [CrossRef] [PubMed]

114. You, W.; Wang, Z.; Li, H.; Shen, H.; Xu, X.; Jia, G.; Chen, G. Inhibition of mammalian target of rapamycin attenuates early brain injury through modulating microglial polarization after experimental subarachnoid hemorrhage in rats. *J. Neurol. Sci.* **2016**, *367*, 224–231. [CrossRef] [PubMed]

115. Farrugia, B.L.; Lord, M.S.; Melrose, J.; Whitelock, J.M. Can we produce heparin/heparan sulfate biomimetics using "mother-nature" as the gold standard? *Molecules* **2015**, *20*, 4254–4276. [CrossRef] [PubMed]

116. Arora, M.; Chen, L.; Paglia, M.; Gallagher, I.; Allen, J.E.; Vyas, Y.M.; Ray, A.; Ray, P. Simvastatin promotes th2-type responses through the induction of the chitinase family member ym1 in dendritic cells. *Proc. Natl. Acad. Sci. USA* **2006**, *103*, 7777–7782. [CrossRef] [PubMed]

117. Cai, Y.; Kumar, R.K.; Zhou, J.; Foster, P.S.; Webb, D.C. ym1/2 promotes th2 cytokine expression by inhibiting 12/15(s)-lipoxygenase: Identification of a novel pathway for regulating allergic inflammation. *J. Immunol.* **2009**, *182*, 5393–5399. [CrossRef] [PubMed]

118. Chang, N.C.; Hung, S.I.; Hwa, K.Y.; Kato, I.; Chen, J.E.; Liu, C.H.; Chang, A.C. A macrophage protein, Ym1, transiently expressed during inflammation is a novel mammalian lectin. *J. Biol. Chem.* **2001**, *276*, 17497–17506. [CrossRef] [PubMed]

119. Lean, Q.Y.; Eri, R.D.; Randall-Demllo, S.; Sohal, S.S.; Stewart, N.; Peterson, G.M.; Gueven, N.; Patel, R.P. Orally administered enoxaparin ameliorates acute colitis by reducing macrophage-associated inflammatory responses. *PLoS ONE* **2015**, *10*, e0134259. [CrossRef] [PubMed]

120. Lu, H.; Zhang, D.M.; Chen, H.L.; Lin, Y.X.; Hang, C.H.; Yin, H.X.; Shi, J.X. *N*-acetylcysteine suppresses oxidative stress in experimental rats with subarachnoid hemorrhage. *J. Clin. Neurosci.* **2009**, *16*, 684–688. [CrossRef] [PubMed]

121. Endo, H.; Nito, C.; Kamada, H.; Yu, F.; Chan, P.H. Reduction in oxidative stress by superoxide dismutase overexpression attenuates acute brain injury after subarachnoid hemorrhage via activation of akt/glycogen synthase kinase-3beta survival signaling. *J. Cereb. Blood Flow Metab.* **2007**, *27*, 975–982. [CrossRef] [PubMed]

122. Yamaguchi, M.; Zhou, C.; Heistad, D.D.; Watanabe, Y.; Zhang, J.H. Gene transfer of extracellular superoxide dismutase failed to prevent cerebral vasospasm after experimental subarachnoid hemorrhage. *Stroke* **2004**, *35*, 2512–2517. [CrossRef] [PubMed]

123. Froehler, M.T.; Kooshkabadi, A.; Miller-Lotan, R.; Blum, S.; Sher, S.; Levy, A.; Tamargo, R.J. Vasospasm after subarachnoid hemorrhage in haptoglobin 2-2 mice can be prevented with a glutathione peroxidase mimetic. *J. Clin. Neurosci.* **2010**, *17*, 1169–1172. [CrossRef] [PubMed]

124. Sandstrom, J.; Carlsson, L.; Marklund, S.L.; Edlund, T. The heparin-binding domain of extracellular superoxide dismutase c and formation of variants with reduced heparin affinity. *J. Biol. Chem.* **1992**, *267*, 18205–18209. [PubMed]

125. Adachi, T.; Yamnamoto, M.; Hara, H. Heparin-affinity of human extracellular-superoxide dismutase in the brain. *Biol. Pharm. Bull.* **2001**, *24*, 191–193. [CrossRef] [PubMed]

126. Sandstrom, J.; Nilsson, P.; Karlsson, K.; Marklund, S.L. 10-fold increase in human plasma extracellular superoxide dismutase content caused by a mutation in heparin-binding domain. *J. Biol. Chem.* **1994**, *269*, 19163–19166. [PubMed]

127. Adachi, T.; Yamada, H.; Futenma, A.; Kato, K.; Hirano, K. Heparin-induced release of extracellular-superoxide dismutase form (V) to plasma. *J. Biochem.* **1995**, *117*, 586–590. [CrossRef] [PubMed]

128. Adachi, T.; Hara, H.; Yamada, H.; Yamazaki, N.; Yamamoto, M.; Sugiyama, T.; Futenma, A.; Katagiri, Y. Heparin-stimulated expression of extracellular-superoxide dismutase in human fibroblasts. *Atherosclerosis* **2001**, *159*, 307–312. [CrossRef]

129. Nakane, H.; Chu, Y.; Faraci, F.M.; Oberley, L.W.; Heistad, D.D. Gene transfer of extracellular superoxide dismutase increases superoxide dismutase activity in cerebrospinal fluid. *Stroke* **2001**, *32*, 184–189. [CrossRef] [PubMed]

130. Chen, T.Y.; Tsai, K.L.; Lee, T.Y.; Chiueh, C.C.; Lee, W.S.; Hsu, C. Sex-specific role of thioredoxin in neuroprotection against iron-induced brain injury conferred by estradiol. *Stroke* **2010**, *41*, 160–165. [CrossRef] [PubMed]

131. Baratz-Goldstein, R.; Deselms, H.; Heim, L.R.; Khomski, L.; Hoffer, B.J.; Atlas, D.; Pick, C.G. Thioredoxin-mimetic-peptides protect cognitive function after mild traumatic brain injury (mtbi). *PLoS ONE* **2016**, *11*, e0157064. [CrossRef] [PubMed]

132. Liu, S.Y.; Stadtman, T.C. Heparin-binding properties of selenium-containing thioredoxin reductase from hela cells and human lung adenocarcinoma cells. *Proc. Natl. Acad. Sci. USA* **1997**, *94*, 6138–6141. [CrossRef] [PubMed]

133. Ross, M.A.; Long, W.F.; Williamson, F.B. Inhibition by heparin of fe(II)-catalysed free-radical peroxidation of linolenic acid. *Biochem. J.* **1992**, *286 (Pt 3)*, 717–720. [CrossRef] [PubMed]

134. Albertini, R.; Rindi, S.; Passi, A.; Pallavicini, G.; De Luca, G. Heparin protection against Fe2+ -and Cu2+ -mediated oxidation of liposomes. *FEBS Lett.* **1996**, *383*, 155–158. [CrossRef]

135. Wahl, F.; Grosjean-Piot, O.; Bareyre, F.; Uzan, A.; Stutzmann, J.M. Enoxaparin reduces brain edema, cerebral lesions, and improves motor and cognitive impairments induced by a traumatic brain injury in rats. *J. Neurotrauma* **2000**, *17*, 1055–1065. [CrossRef] [PubMed]

136. Pratt, J.; Boudeau, P.; Uzan, A.; Imperato, A.; Stutzmann, J. Enoxaparin reduces cerebral edemaafter photothrombotic injury in the rat. *Haemostasis* **1998**, *28*, 78–85. [CrossRef] [PubMed]

137. Xi, G.; Wagner, K.R.; Keep, R.F.; Hua, Y.; de Courten-Myers, G.M.; Broderick, J P.; Brott, T.G.; Hoff, J.T. Role of blood clot formation on early edema development after experimental intracerebral hemorrhage. *Stroke* **1998**, *29*, 2580–2586. [CrossRef] [PubMed]

138. Gong, Y.; Xi, G.H.; Keep, R.F.; Hoff, J.T.; Hua, Y. Complement inhibition attenuates brain edema and neurological deficits induced by thrombin. *Acta Neurochir. Suppl.* **2005**, *95*, 389–392. [PubMed]

139. Kim, L.; Schuster, J.; Holena, D.N.; Sims, C.A.; Levine, J.; Pascual, J.L. Early initiation of prophylactic heparin in severe traumatic brain injury is associated with accelerated improvement on brain imaging. *J. Emerg. Trauma Shock* **2014**, *7*, 141–148. [PubMed]

140. Bruce, J.N.; Criscuolo, G.R.; Merrill, M.J.; Moquin, R.R.; Blacklock, J.B.; Oldfield, E.H. Vascular permeability induced by protein product of malignant brain tumors: Inhibition by dexamethasone. *J. Neurosurg.* **1987**, *67*, 880–884. [CrossRef] [PubMed]

141. Tessler, S.; Rockwell, P.; Hicklin, D.; Cohen, T.; Levi, B.Z.; Witte, L.; Lemischka, I.R.; Neufeld, G. Heparin modulates the interaction of vegf165 with soluble and cell associated flk-1 receptors. *J. Biol. Chem.* **1994**, *269*, 12456–12461. [PubMed]

142. Marchetti, M.; Vignoli, A.; Russo, L.; Balducci, D.; Pagnoncelli, M.; Barbui, T.; Falanga, A. Endothelial capillary tube formation and cell proliferation induced by tumor cells are affected by low molecular weight heparins and unfractionated heparin. *Thromb. Res.* **2008**, *121*, 637–645. [CrossRef] [PubMed]

143. Oschatz, C.; Maas, C.; Lecher, B.; Jansen, T.; Bjorkqvist, J.; Tradler, T.; Sedlmeier, R.; Burfeind, P.; Cichon, S.; Hammerschmidt, S.; et al. Mast cells increase vascular permeability by heparin-initiated bradykinin formation in vivo. *Immunity* **2011**, *34*, 258–268. [CrossRef] [PubMed]

144. Carr, J. The anti-inflammatory action of heparin: Heparin as an antagonist to histamine, bradykinin and prostaglandin e1. *Thromb. Res.* **1979**, *16*, 507–516. [CrossRef]

145. Thal, S.C.; Sporer, S.; Schmid-Elsaesser, R.; Plesnila, N.; Zausinger, S. Inhibition of bradykinin b2 receptors before, not after onset of experimental subarachnoid hemorrhage prevents brain edema formation and improves functional outcome. *Crit. Care Med.* **2009**, *37*, 2228–2234. [CrossRef] [PubMed]

146. Gupta, S.; Tiruvoipati, R.; Green, C.; Botha, J.; Tran, H. Heparin induced thrombocytopenia in critically ill: Diagnostic dilemmas and management conundrums. *World J. Crit. Care Med.* **2015**, *4*, 202–212. [CrossRef] [PubMed]

147. Hoh, B.L.; Aghi, M.; Pryor, J.C.; Ogilvy, C.S. Heparin-induced thrombocytopenia type II in subarachnoid hemorrhage patients: Incidence and complications. *Neurosurgery* **2005**, *57*, 243–248; discussion 243–248. [CrossRef] [PubMed]

148. Kim, G.H.; Hahn, D.K.; Kellner, C.P.; Komotar, R.J.; Starke, R.; Garrett, M.C.; Yao, J.; Cleveland, J.; Mayer, S.A.; Connolly, E.S. The incidence of heparin-induced thrombocytopenia type II in patients with subarachnoid hemorrhage treated with heparin versus enoxaparin. *J. Neurosurg.* **2009**, *110*, 50–57. [CrossRef] [PubMed]

149. Mehta, B.P.; Sims, J.R.; Baccin, C.E.; Leslie-Mazwi, T.M.; Ogilvy, C.S.; Nogueira, R.G. Predictors and outcomes of suspected heparin-induced thrombocytopenia in subarachnoid hemorrhage patients. *Interv. Neurol.* **2014**, *2*, 160–168. [CrossRef] [PubMed]

150. Shimamura, N.; Naraoka, M.; Matsuda, N.; Ohkuma, H. Safety of preprocedural antiplatelet medication in coil embolization of ruptured cerebral aneurysms at the acute stage. *Interv. Neuroradiol.* **2014**, *20*, 413–417. [CrossRef] [PubMed]

151. Hoh, B.L.; Nogueira, R.G.; Ledezma, C.J.; Pryor, J.C.; Ogilvy, C.S. Safety of heparinization for cerebral aneurysm coiling soon after external ventriculostomy drain placement. *Neurosurgery* **2005**, *57*, 845–849; discussion 845–849. [CrossRef] [PubMed]

152. Egashira, Y.; Yoshimura, S.; Enomoto, Y.; Ishiguro, M.; Asano, T.; Iwama, T. Ultra-early endovascular embolization of ruptured cerebral aneurysm and the increased risk of hematoma growth unrelated to aneurysmal rebleeding. *J. Neurosurg.* **2013**, *118*, 1003–1008. [CrossRef] [PubMed]

153. Zachariah, J.; Snyder, K.A.; Graffeo, C.S.; Khanal, D.R.; Lanzino, G.; Wijdicks, E.F.; Rabinstein, A.A. Risk of ventriculostomy-associated hemorrhage in patients with aneurysmal subarachnoid hemorrhage treated with anticoagulant thromboprophylaxis. *Neurocrit. Care* **2016**, *25*, 224–229. [CrossRef] [PubMed]

154. Bruder, M.; Schuss, P.; Konczalla, J.; El-Fiki, A.; Lescher, S.; Vatter, H.; Seifert, V.; Guresir, E. Ventriculostomy-related hemorrhage after treatment of acutely ruptured aneurysms: The influence of anticoagulation and antiplatelet treatment. *World Neurosurg.* **2015**, *84*, 1653–1659. [CrossRef] [PubMed]

155. Bauer, K.A. Fondaparinux: Basic properties and efficacy and safety in venous thromboembolism prophylaxis. *Am. J. Orthop. (Belle Mead NJ)* **2002**, *31*, 4–10. [PubMed]

156. Zhang, Y.; Zhao, Z.; Guan, L.; Mao, L.; Li, S.; Guan, X.; Chen, M.; Guo, L.; Ding, L.; Cong, C.; et al. *N*-acetyl-heparin attenuates acute lung injury caused by acid aspiration mainly by antagonizing histones in mice. *PLoS ONE* **2014**, *9*, e97074. [CrossRef] [PubMed]

157. Veraldi, N.; Hughes, A.J.; Rudd, T.R.; Thomas, H.B.; Edwards, S.W.; Hadfield, L.; Skidmore, M.A.; Siligardi, G.; Cosentino, C.; Shute, J.K.; et al. Heparin derivatives for the targeting of multiple activities in the inflammatory response. *Carbohydr. Polym.* **2015**, *117*, 400–407. [CrossRef] [PubMed]

158. Wang, L.; Brown, J.R.; Varki, A.; Esko, J.D. Heparin's anti-inflammatory effects require glucosamine 6-*O*-sulfation and are mediated by blockade of l- and p-selectins. *J. Clin. Investig.* **2002**, *110*, 127–136. [CrossRef] [PubMed]

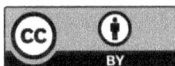

molecules

MDPI

Article

The Impact of the Low Molecular Weight Heparin Tinzaparin on the Sensitization of Cisplatin-Resistant Ovarian Cancers—Preclinical In Vivo Evaluation in Xenograft Tumor Models

Thomas Mueller [1], Daniel Bastian Pfankuchen [2], Kathleen Wantoch von Rekowski [2], Martin Schlesinger [2], Franziska Reipsch [1] and Gerd Bendas [2,*]

[1] Department of Internal Medicine IV, Oncology/Hematology, Martin-Luther-University Halle-Wittenberg, Ernst-Grube-Straße 40, 06120 Halle (Saale), Germany; thomas.mueller@medizin.uni-halle.de (T.M.); freipsch@gmail.com (F.R.)
[2] Department of Pharmacy, University Bonn, An der Immenburg 4, 53121 Bonn, Germany; danielpfankuchen@uni-bonn.de (D.B.P.); Kathleen.Wantoch@uni-bonn.de (K.W.v.R.); martin.schlesinger@uni-bonn.de (M.S.)
* Correspondence: gbendas@uni-bonn.de; Tel.: +49-228-735-250

Academic Editor: Giangiacomo Torri
Received: 28 March 2017; Accepted: 28 April 2017; Published: 3 May 2017

Abstract: Resistance formation of tumors against chemotherapeutics is the major obstacle in clinical cancer therapy. Although low molecular weight heparin (LMWH) is an important component in oncology referring to guideline-based antithrombotic prophylaxis of tumor patients, a potential interference of LMWH with chemoresistance is unknown. We have recently shown that LMWH reverses the cisplatin resistance of A2780cis human ovarian cancer cells in vitro. Here we address the question whether this LMWH effect is also valid under in vivo conditions. Therefore, we established tumor xenografts of A2780 and cisplatin resistant A2780cis cells in nude mice and investigated the impact of daily tinzaparin applications (10 mg/kg BW) on anti-tumor activity of cisplatin (6 mg/kg BW, weekly) considering the tumor growth kinetics. Intratumoral platinum accumulation was detected by GF-AAS. Xenografts of A2780 and A2780cis cells strongly differed in cisplatin sensitivity. As an overall consideration, tinzaparin co-treatment affected the response to cisplatin of A2780cis, but not A2780 tumors in the later experimental time range. A subgroup analysis confirmed that initially smaller A2780cis tumors benefit from tinzaparin, but also small A2780 xenografts. Tinzaparin did not affect cisplatin accumulation in A2780cis xenografts, but strongly increased the platinum content in A2780, obviously related to morphological differences in both xenografts. Although we cannot directly confirm a return of A2780cis cisplatin resistance by tinzaparin, as shown in vitro, the present findings give reason to discuss heparin effects on cytostatic drug efficiency for small tumors and warrants further investigation.

Keywords: cisplatin; low molecular weight heparin (LMWH); ovarian cancer; resistance

---

1. Introduction

Cancer-associated thrombosis is an important mortality factor in malignant tumor diseases [1]. Therefore, antithrombotic prophylaxis or treatment is a common component in the therapeutic regimes of patients with malignancies. Based on the current clinical guidelines for antithrombotic treatment of cancer patients, low molecular weight heparin (LMWH) is the drug of choice [2,3]. Consequently, tremendous amounts of clinical data exist concerning the clinical treatment of cancer patients with LMWH. The retrospective analysis of those clinical data implies that anticoagulation by LMWH could possess a survival benefit for certain cancer patients, which probably goes beyond solely an antithrombotic efficiency [4]. This postulate has been addressed by a high number of preclinical investigations during the last two decades to figure out the potential mode of action. LMWH was shown to affect the metastatic capacities of various carcinomas by interfering with different functional axes, such as cell adhesion [5], migration [6], chemokine and growth factor signaling [7] or the enzymatic activity of heparanase [8].

However, little is known whether and how LMWH affects the classical chemotherapeutic treatment of cancer. One can presume that attenuation of thrombosis formation close to the solid tumors increases the accessibility for chemotherapeutics and decreases the interstitial pressure, both leading to higher drug efficiency. A number of studies refer to those mechanisms and display a therapeutic effect for the combination of LMWH and chemotherapy [9–11]. A retrospective consideration of the combination of LMWH with chemotherapy in patients with small cell lung cancer suggest a protective effect of heparin [12].

Nevertheless, acquired tumor cell resistance against single or series of chemotherapeutics is the major obstacle in clinical treatment of cancer, such as ovarian carcinomas [13]. The molecular mechanisms of those chemoresistance phenomena are manifold and often less understood. Cisplatin, the standard drug for clinical treatment of ovarian cancer and several other tumor entities is also often restricted in its efficiency by resistance formation of tumors [14]. Consequently, chemoresistance appears as attractive target to overcome restrictions in chemotherapeutic treatment. However, findings for a potential interference of heparin application and chemoresistance are hardly known [15].

We have recently shown that cisplatin-resistant A2780cis ovarian cancer cells were "resensitized" for cisplatin cytotoxicity to the level of non-resistant A2780 cells by a therapeutic LMWH (tinzaparin) concentration in a preclinical in vitro setting [16]. Considering the outstanding role of LMWH in cancer treatment, this surprising and novel finding linking LMWH application in cancer treatment with a potential circumvention of chemoresistance could have a high clinical relevance. However, the molecular mechanisms are not fully elucidated. It was shown that tinzaparin has no effect on the intracellular drug levels thus the higher efficiency in the resistant cells is not simply related to transport mechanisms. A whole genome analysis of tinzaparin pretreated resistant A2780cis cells confirmed that tinzaparin possesses a complex impact on signaling and gene regulatory mechanisms reversing the resistance phenomenon. Obviously, this LMWH efficiency is related to the cellular proteoglycans.

In a further step to evaluate the value of this finding here we address the question whether the chemoresistance overcoming capacity of tinzaparin is potentially valid and detectable under in vivo conditions. Considering the strong differences between in vitro 2D-cytotoxicity assays and in vivo tumor growth models we aimed to draw a parallel by establishing A2780 and A2780cis tumor xenografts in mice and investigated their cisplatin treatment in response to tinzaparin.

2. Results

To investigate the efficiency of cisplatin treatment and the impact of tinzaparin co-treatment for tumor growth under in vivo conditions, xenograft tumors in nude mice were established using the A2780 and cisplatin-resistant A2780cis cell line. In both trials, tumor bearing mice were divided into four groups with a similar mean tumor volume ($n = 8$) at start of treatment. Furthermore, the groups were set up to contain small, middle and larger tumors at the start of treatment with similar distribution between the groups. Mice were treated with saline, tinzaparin, cisplatin or a combination of tinzaparin with cisplatin, respectively.

2.1. Comparison of the Xenograft Tumor Models

First, for a direct comparison of both tumor models regarding growth rate and response to cisplatin, the respective data of the saline- and cisplatin-groups were combined in one graph, which is shown in Figure 1. Overall, the A2780 tumors showed a higher growth rate compared to A2780cis tumors. A2780 tumors of the saline treated control group reached the maximal acceptable tumor volume much earlier than A2780cis tumors. Cisplatin treatment led to a clear growth inhibition effect compared to saline control in the A2780 model with a reduction of tumor growth of more than 50% when analyzed on days 7 and 9 (Figure 1). A much lower impact of cisplatin on tumor growth was observed in the A2780cis model with a growth inhibition of less than 30% (Figure 1). Thus, the in vitro cisplatin resistance of A2780cis cells was reproduced in vivo as xenograft tumors, although the relative difference in cisplatin sensitivity between both models turned out to be of lesser extent as compared to in vitro conditions.

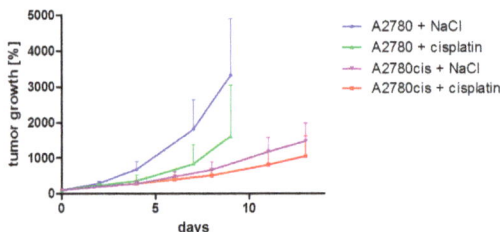

Figure 1. Comparison of A2780 and A2780cis tumor models regarding growth rate and response to cisplatin. Shown is the increase of mean tumor volumes of each group ($n = 8$) ± standard deviation normalized to day 0 (start of treatment). In the A2780 model, the treatment and monitoring of the saline control group was discontinued on day 9 after four mice had reached the maximal acceptable tumor volume. Mice of cisplatin group were monitored for a prolonged time, which is not depicted here. In the A2780cis model, monitoring of the control group was discontinued on day 15 when six mice had reached the maximal acceptable tumor volume whereas the cisplatin group was monitored for a prolonged time. The data depicted here are derived from the complete data sets shown in Figures 3 and 4.

To investigate whether the differences in growth rate of both tumor models were reflected by morphological differences, we investigated the structural peculiarities of both tumor models. Histological examination after HE staining revealed differences predominantly with regard to the vascularization. A2780cis tumors are highly vascularized and contain well-structured vessels of different shapes and diameters. A2780 tumors are even more vascularized, show structured vessels, but are also characterized by particular high occurrence of hemorrhages. This correlates with the red-blue colored appearance of A2780 tumors when subcutaneously grown in nude mice. For further characterization and comparison of both tumor models, we performed Azan-staining, which is useful to visualize extracellular matrix material and fibrous structures. This revealed an additional difference between both models. As shown in Figure 2, a typical feature of the A2780cis tumor tissue is a characteristic composition of tumor cells together with septal structures. Such tissue pattern is scarcely found in A2780 tumors.

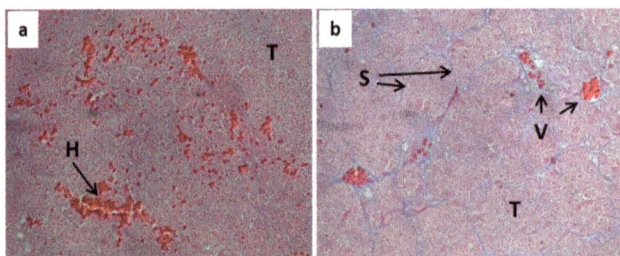

Figure 2. Histological analysis of tumor tissue of A2780 (**a**) and A2780cis tumors (**b**) after Azan-staining. A2780cis tumors show a characteristic composition of tumor cells together with septal structures. Particular high occurrence of hemorrhages is a typical feature of A2780 tumors. (T—tumor tissue, H—hemorrhage, S—septum, V—vessel; 400 × magnification).

2.2. Impact of Tinzaparin on Tumor Growth and Response to Cisplatin Treatment

Tinzaparin was given as daily injections of 10 mg/kg body weight which was well tolerated; no weight loss or bleeding complications were observed. However, considering the combined graphs, treatment with tinzaparin alone resulted in a tumor growth inhibition effect in the A2780 model (Figure 3). In contrast, no tumor growth inhibition by tinzaparin alone was observed in the A2780cis model (Figure 4).

This obvious difference in tinzaparin effects in the two tumor models can be explained with a more detailed view on the individual mice data. Analyses of individual mice revealed a more heterogeneous tumor growth under tinzaparin treatment compared to treatment with saline, preferentially in the A2780 model. A2780 tumors with small initial volume seemed to be inhibited which explains the shift of the mean graph of the tinzaparin group (Figure 3). Interestingly, one of the tumors with smaller initial volume within the tinzaparin groups of both models did not grow or showed regression with no further growth. This was exclusively observed for the solely tinzaparin treated groups.

The combination of cisplatin as a once weekly application of 6 mg/kg body weight and tinzaparin did not result in an additional growth inhibition effect in both models, at least in an observation frame up to day 15. At this time point, part of the mice of each group had reached the maximal acceptable tumor volume and had to be removed from the study. Mice, which had not reached the maximal acceptable tumor volume at this time point, were maintained for the experiment. Therefore, a smaller number of mice (4 vs. 4 in A2780 and 3 vs. 3 in A2780cis) were monitored for an additional time period. This subgroup analysis revealed a difference between the two tumor models. An improved tumor growth inhibition effect of the combination treatment with cisplatin and tinzaparin became evident in the A2780cis model (Figure 4) but not in the A2780 tumor model (Figure 3).

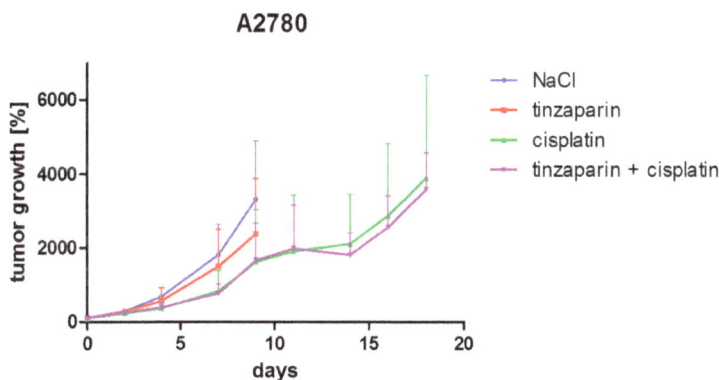

Figure 3. Analysis of tumor growth inhibition in the A2780 model. The increase of mean tumor volumes of each group ($n = 8$) $\pm$ standard deviation is illustrated normalized to day 0 (start of treatment). Tinzaparin was administered as daily injections of 10 mg/kg body weight. Cisplatin (6 mg/kg body weight) was given once weekly for two weeks. A third cisplatin injection was omitted due to incomplete recovery of mouse body weight after the second injection. Control group received saline. The treatment and monitoring of both the control group and the tinzaparin group was discontinued on day 9 after four mice had reached the maximal acceptable tumor volume, respectively. On day 11, two tumors in the cisplatin group and two tumors in the cisplatin/tinzaparin group had reached the maximal acceptable tumor volume and the mice were removed from the study. On day 14, further two mice of each group were removed. The remaining four mice of both groups were monitored until day 18.

The tumor growth inhibition in the later stages of experiment (Figure 4) refers to a preferential effect of the combined tinzaparin and cisplatin treatment on initially smaller tumors. To strengthen this postulation, a comparison of combination treatment vs. cisplatin alone was performed by separately analyzing the three tumors with the smallest initial volume from each group, respectively. This revealed a more evident effect of tinzaparin co-treatment on cisplatin induced growth inhibition in A2780cis model than in Figure 4 (Figure 5a), but A2780 xenografts (Figure 5b) also appear to benefit from tinzaparin when considering the smallest tumors, which was not expected from Figure 3.

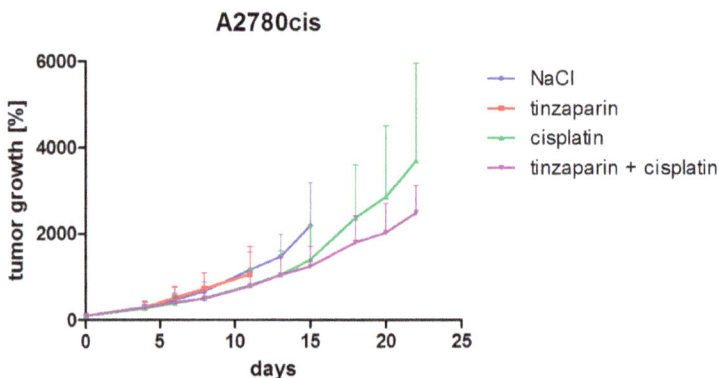

Figure 4. Analysis of tumor growth inhibition in the A2780cis model. Shown is the increase of mean tumor volumes of each group ($n = 8$) $\perp$ standard deviation normalized to day 0 (start of treatment). Tinzaparin was administered as daily injections of 10 mg/kg body weight. Cisplatin (6 mg/kg) was given once weekly for three weeks. Control group received saline. The treatment and monitoring of the tinzaparin group was discontinued on day 11 after four mice had reached the maximal acceptable tumor volume. Monitoring of control group was continued until day 15 when six mice had reached the maximal acceptable tumor volume. In addition, five tumors in the cisplatin group and five tumors in the cisplatin/tinzaparin group had reached the maximal acceptable tumor volume and the mice were removed from the study on day 15. The remaining three mice of both groups were monitored until day 22.

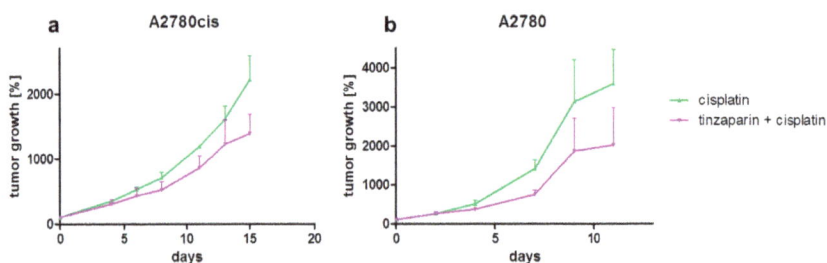

Figure 5. Impact of tinzaparin on cisplatin treatment of tumors with small initial volume. Shown is the increase of mean tumor volumes of each group ($n = 3$) $\pm$ standard deviation normalized to day 0 (start of treatment), (**a**) A2780cis and (**b**) A2780 xenografts. Tinzaparin and cisplatin treatment was as mentioned before.

2.3. The Impact of Tinzaparin On Tumor Platination

In order to elucidate whether the tinzaparin treatment of mice had an impact on the cisplatin accumulation in the tumor tissue and thus higher cisplatin levels could explain the attenuated tumor growth kinetics in the A2780cis xenografts at the later time points, platinum concentrations were detected in the tumor tissue by the GF-AAS technique. Therefore, A2780 and A2780cis tumors were taken from tinzaparin-treated and -untreated mice at two different time points after the last cisplatin application. For each time point, the non-LMWH treated platinum concentration was set as 100% to individually illustrate changes in the platinum levels induced by heparin. It becomes evident that in A2780 tumors both, at day 3 and 10 post cisplatin injection the daily tinzaparin dosis affects drastically the platinum content (Figure 6a) showing four- to fivefold higher platinum concentrations. This is in contrast to our in vitro findings that displayed no effect of tinzaparin on cisplatin uptake by A2780 cells [16]. However, we cannot directly compare these findings since we have no information on the intratumor localization of the drug. Nevertheless, the higher platinum concentrations induced by tinzaparin is obviously not reflected by a higher overall cytotoxicity, as indicated in Figure 3.

In strict contrast, tinzaparin treatment had no or only a negligible impact on platinum accumulation in the cisplatin resistant tumor xenografts (Figure 6b). This is a clear indication that the slower tumor growth kinetics in the combined cisplatin and tinzaparin treatment compared to the cisplatin group at the later experimental time points is not related to higher drug concentrations within the tumor tissue.

One can assume that the strong differences in platinum accumulation reflect the morphological differences between both tumor xenografts, shown in Figure 2. In the A2780 model, which is characterized by a lesser organized tissue structure as compared to the A2780cis model, tinzaparin treatment could have impacted the intratumoral cisplatin distribution thereby resulting in improved accumulation.

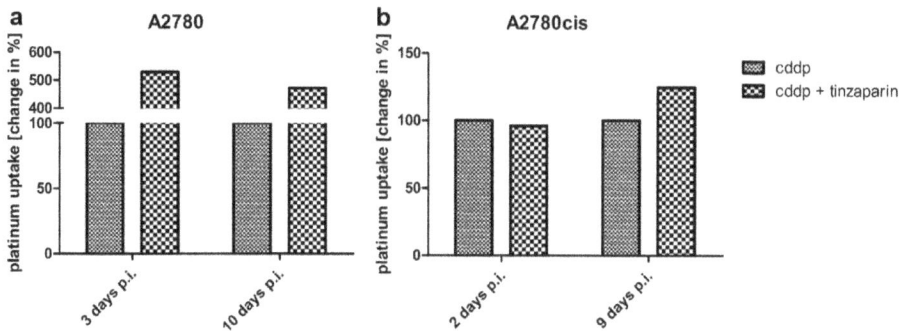

Figure 6. Detection of intratumoral platinum accumulation in A2780 (**a**) and A2780cis (**b**) tumor xenografts. Tumor samples were taken after 3 and 10 (A2780) or after 2 and 9 days (A2780cis) following the last cisplatin injection. The platinum concentration of tinzaparin treated tumors was normalized to only cisplatin treated tumors which were set to 100%, heparin induced changes were displayed in %.

3. Discussion

Considerable progress in elucidating beneficial effects of heparin treatment of cancer has been documented during the last two decades, which goes beyond the guideline-based application of LMWH to circumvent or treat venous thrombotic events [17,18]. Most attention has been given to the meanwhile experimentally confirmed fact that heparin impacts the metastatic spread of carcinomas [5]. In doing this, heparin possesses multiple "pleiotropic" effects to interfere with the tumor cell communication and the support, given by host or stroma components [19,20]. Consequently, heparin blocks tumors at an early development stage. However, little is known whether heparin can additionally affect tumors in an early stage of development or existing solid tumors, i.e., by assisting cytostatics. The cytostatic treatment of cancer patients is often hampered by the rapid development of cancer cell resistance against single or whole classes of cytostatic agents [21]. Despite heparin is a common constituent in clinical cancer therapy, a certain link between chemoresistance and heparin does not exist.

We could recently show in an in vitro approach that the LMWH tinzaparin reverses the cisplatin resistance in human A2780 ovarian cancer cells by a genetic reprogramming and a deregulation of more than 3700 genes, although cytotoxic or apoptotic effects of the LMWH doses used could be excluded [16]. The molecular mechanisms are still not elucidated and a matter of ongoing research.

Here we performed a first adaptation of this finding to in vivo relevant conditions and compare for the first time the cytostatic activity in a wild-type and cisplatin resistant subtype of a tumor cell line in relation to a LMWH therapeutic application. We provide evidence that the cisplatin resistance of A2780cis cells is maintained in the mice xenograft model, when compared to A2780 cell xenografts. However, the resistant cell xenografts display an overall slower growth kinetic than the wild-type ones and both tumor models show morphological differences, which requires a selective interpretation of cisplatin cytotoxicity response. This emphasizes impressively that the in vitro conditions of a plain 2D cultivation of pure tumor cell cultures are severely limited when transferred to experimental in vivo conditions, where the tumor cells are embedded and impacted by connective tissues, stroma cells. Furthermore, their access to the drugs is thus not a simple diffusion process but mediated and restricted by the blood vasculature.

Based on these differences in growth rate and morphology between the xenografts of A2780 and A2780cis we could not simply expect a sensitization of A2780cis cells for cisplatin by tinzaparin resulting in a similar behavior like the A2780 cells, as the cells adapted in vitro. Nevertheless, the overall consideration of tumor growth kinetics referred to a slightly diminished growth rate for A2780cis after day 15 in the tinzaparin and cisplatin combination group (Figure 4). This is a clear, but not a significant indication for improved cytotoxic activity in presence of tinzaparin. It turns out that the initially smallest A2780cis tumors are mostly influenced by the tinzaparin application and display the most evident growth retardation. Since tinzaparin hardly affected the cisplatin accumulation in the A2780cis xenografts (Figure 6) and did not display an intrinsic effect on growth inhibition (Figure 4) this could point to a higher sensitivity for cisplatin as reason for growth reduction.

The smallest A2780 tumors also displayed a slower growth rate co-treated with cisplatin and tinzaparin when compared to the solely cisplatin treated groups. However, the background of this type of "sensitization" seems different from A2780cis, since A2780 xenografts accumulated massively higher amounts of cisplatin in the tumor tissue by tinzaparin activity, obviously enforced by the leaky tissue structure. We can presently not explain completely the reason for this difference in cisplatin vascular leakage triggered by tinzaparin between A2780 and A2780cis. Since both xenografts are highly vascularized, the much higher leakage in A2780 xenografts seems to be related to the hemorrhagic regions and thus an even higher intratumoral bleeding when heparinized, and not a functional effect of tinzaparin on intact vasculature. However, the up to fivefold higher cisplatin concentrations in A2780 tumor tissue in presence of tinzaparin appear as the primary reason for slower growth, although intrinsic effects of tinzaparin alone might also play a role, as indicated in Figure 3.

Despite these obvious differences in A2780 and A2780cis concerning morphology and uptake characteristics and the different background of the term "sensitization" in both models, it is interesting to point out that only the tumors in early stages are susceptible for LMWH effects, as indicated for the anti-metastatic approaches with heparin.

Our postulations on a sensitization of tumors for chemotherapy do hardly find clear reflections by existing clinical data, since the classical data for clinical outcomes like progression free survival or overall survival probably also cover a potential better response to cytostatics. However, our postulations might be in line with those studies which explicitly focus on cytostatic efficiency [9,10,12] that proposed a beneficial effect of LMWH. These findings warrant further investigations to probably open new aspects for heparin applications in oncology.

4. Materials and Methods

4.1. Cell Lines

A2780 and cisplatin-resistant A2780cis human ovarian carcinoma cell lines were from the ECACC (Salisbury, UK); No. 93112519 (A2780) and No. 93112517 (A2780cis) and cultivated (37 °C, 5% CO_2)

in RPMI1640 medium containing 10% FCS, 1.5% L-glutamine and 1% penicillin/streptomycin (PAN Biotech, Aidenbach, Germany). After purchase, cells were frozen in aliquots (master cell bank) from which they were cultivated for a maximum of ten passages for the present study. Cell authentication was confirmed by short tandem repeat (STR) profiling.

4.2. Animal Studies

The investigations of this study were approved by the Laboratory Animal Care Committee of Sachsen-Anhalt, Germany. Xenograft tumors were generated in athymic nude mice (Charles River, Sulzfeld, Germany) using the ovarian carcinoma cell lines A2780 and A2780cis. Eight million cells of either cell line were resuspended in PBS and injected subcutaneously into the flank of mice. After establishment of tumors, mice were divided into four groups with a similar mean tumor volume ($n = 8$) at start of treatment and with similar distribution of tumor volumes between the groups. Tinzaparin was given as daily i.p. injections of 10 mg/kg body weight. Cisplatin (6 mg/kg BW) was administered i.p. once weekly. The control group received normal saline. Tumor growth and response to therapy was monitored by caliper measurements and tumor volume calculation using the formula $a^2 \times b \times 0.5$ with a being the short and b the long dimension.

4.3. Tumor Lysis and Measurement of Intratumoral Platinum Accumulation

The kinetic of cisplatin uptake by A2780 and A2780cis tumors was analyzed by graphite furnace atomic absorption spectrometry (GF-AAS). Tumor samples were taken at the indicated time points and snap frozen. At time of detection, tumors were dissected with a scalpel, lysed with 65% nitric acid suprapur® (Merck Chemicals, Schwalbach, Germany) for one hour at 80 °C followed by GF-AAS investigation, as indicated before [16]. Measured platinum concentrations were related to the tumor weights.

4.4. Histological Analyses

For hematoxylin and eosin (HE) staining, necropsied tumors were cross-sectioned, fixed in 4% formalin, embedded in paraffin, sliced with a RM 2245 microtome (4–5 µm, Leica, Wetzlar, Germany), dewaxed and rehydrated by decreasing alcohol series from xylene up to bi-distilled water. The slices were stained with hematoxylin (Dako, Hamburg, Germany), followed by several washing steps with tap water and bi-distilled water. Subsequently, the slices were stained with eosin (Merck Chemicals GmbH, Darmstadt, Germany). After staining, the slices were dehydrated by ascending alcohol series and fixed with Roti®-Histokit (Carl Roth GmbH & Co. KG, Karlsruhe, Germany).

For Azan staining, the dewaxed and rehydrated tissue slices were initially stained with an azocarmine (Morphisto®, Frankfurt a.M., Germany) solution. After some washing steps with bi-distilled water and the nuclei differentiation with aniline (Baacklab®, Schwerin, Germany) in 95% ethanol, the slices were treated with 5% phosphomolybdic acid (Baacklab®). Subsequently they were rinsed with bi-distilled water and stained with a solution of aniline blue and Orange G (Baacklab®). Afterwards the slices were washed with bi-distilled water, dehydrated by ascending alcohol series and fixed with Roti®-Histokitt (Carl Roth GmbH & Co. KG).

Acknowledgments: This work has partly been supported by LEO Pharma GmbH. The authors would like to thank for this support. DBP was supported by Hilmer Stiftung by a Ph.D. student scholarship.

Author Contributions: T.M. and G.B. conceived and designed the study; T.M. and F.R. performed the animal studies; D.B.P. and K.W.v.R. analyzed the platinum content, M.S. analyzed the data and contributed to writing the ms.; T.M. and G.B. wrote the paper.

Conflicts of Interest: The authors declare no conflict of interest. The founding sponsors had no role in the design of the study; in the collection, analyses, or interpretation of data; in the writing of the manuscript, and in the decision to publish the results.

References

1. Ay, C.; Pabinger, I.; Cohen, A.T. Cancer-associated venous thromboembolism: Burden, mechanisms, and management. *Thromb. Haemost.* **2017**, *117*, 219–230. [CrossRef] [PubMed]
2. Mandalà, M.; Falanga, A.; Roila, F. ESMO Guidelines Working Group Venous thromboembolism in cancer patients: ESMO Clinical Practice Guidelines for the management. *Ann. Oncol. Off. J. Eur. Soc. Med. Oncol.* **2010**, *21* (Suppl. 5), v274–v276. [CrossRef] [PubMed]
3. Lyman, G.H.; Bohlke, K.; Khorana, A.A.; Kuderer, N.M.; Lee, A.Y.; Arcelus, J.I.; Balaban, E.P.; Clarke, J.M.; Flowers, C.R.; Francis, C.W.; et al. Venous thromboembolism prophylaxis and treatment in patients with cancer: American society of clinical oncology clinical practice guideline update 2014. *J. Clin. Oncol. Off. J. Am. Soc. Clin. Oncol.* **2015**, *33*, 654–656. [CrossRef] [PubMed]
4. Schünemann, H.J.; Ventresca, M.; Crowther, M.; Briel, M.; Zhou, Q.; Garcia, D.; Lyman, G.; Noble, S.; Macbeth, F.; Griffiths, G.; et al. Use of heparins in patients with cancer: Individual participant data meta-analysis of randomised trials study protocol. *BMJ Open* **2016**, *6*, e010569. [CrossRef] [PubMed]
5. Bendas, G.; Borsig, L. Cancer cell adhesion and metastasis: Selectins, integrins, and the inhibitory potential of heparins. *Int. J. Cell Biol.* **2012**, *2012*, 676731. [CrossRef] [PubMed]
6. Zhong, G.; Gong, Y.; Yu, C.; Wu, S.; Ma, Q.; Wang, Y.; Ren, J.; Zhang, X.; Yang, W.; Zhu, W. Significantly inhibitory effects of low molecular weight heparin (Fraxiparine) on the motility of lung cancer cells and its related mechanism. *Tumour Biol. J. Int. Soc. Oncodev. Biol. Med.* **2015**, *36*, 4689–4697. [CrossRef] [PubMed]
7. Knelson, E.H.; Nee, J.C.; Blobe, G.C. Heparan sulfate signaling in cancer. *Trends Biochem. Sci.* **2014**, *39*, 277–288. [CrossRef] [PubMed]
8. Vlodavsky, I.; Singh, P.; Boyango, I.; Gutter-Kapon, L.; Elkin, M.; Sanderson, R.D.; Ilan, N. Heparanase: From basic research to therapeutic applications in cancer and inflammation. *Drug Resist. Updat. Rev. Comment. Antimicrob. Anticancer Chemother.* **2016**, *29*, 54–75. [CrossRef] [PubMed]
9. Altinbas, M.; Coskun, H.S.; Er, O.; Ozkan, M.; Eser, B.; Unal, A.; Cetin, M.; Soyuer, S. A randomized clinical trial of combination chemotherapy with and without low-molecular-weight heparin in small cell lung cancer. *J. Thromb. Haemost. JTH* **2004**, *2*, 1266–1271. [CrossRef] [PubMed]
10. Lebeau, B.; Baud, M.; Masanes, M.-J.; Febvre, M.; Mokhtari, T.; Chouaïd, C. Optimization of small-cell lung cancer chemotherapy with heparin: A comprehensive retrospective study of 239 patients treated in a single specialized center. *Chemotherapy* **2011**, *57*, 253–258. [CrossRef] [PubMed]
11. Icli, F.; Akbulut, H.; Utkan, G.; Yalcin, B.; Dincol, D.; Isikdogan, A.; Demirkazik, A.; Onur, H.; Cay, F.; Büyükcelik, A. Low molecular weight heparin (LMWH) increases the efficacy of cisplatinum plus gemcitabine combination in advanced pancreatic cancer. *J. Surg. Oncol.* **2007**, *95*, 507–512. [CrossRef] [PubMed]
12. Altinbas, M.; Dikilitas, M.; Ozkan, M.; Dogu, G.G.; Er, O.; Coskun, H.S. The effect of small-molecular-weight heparin added to chemotherapy on survival in small-cell lung cancer—A retrospective analysis. *Indian J. Cancer* **2014**, *51*, 324–329. [CrossRef] [PubMed]
13. Ali, A.Y.; Farrand, L.; Kim, J.Y.; Byun, S.; Suh, J.-Y.; Lee, H.J.; Tsang, B.K. Molecular determinants of ovarian cancer chemoresistance: New insights into an old conundrum. *Ann. N. Y. Acad. Sci.* **2012**, *1271*, 58–67. [CrossRef] [PubMed]
14. Ferreira, J.A.; Peixoto, A.; Neves, M.; Gaiteiro, C.; Reis, C.A.; Assaraf, Y.G.; Santos, L.L. Mechanisms of cisplatin resistance and targeting of cancer stem cells: Adding glycosylation to the equation. *Drug Resist. Updat. Rev. Comment. Antimicrob. Anticancer Chemother.* **2016**, *24*, 34–54. [CrossRef] [PubMed]
15. Niu, Q.; Wang, W.; Li, Y.; Ruden, D.M.; Wang, F.; Li, Y.; Wang, F.; Song, J.; Zheng, K. Low molecular weight heparin ablates lung cancer cisplatin-resistance by inducing proteasome-mediated ABCG2 protein degradation. *PLoS ONE* **2012**, *7*, e41035. [CrossRef] [PubMed]
16. Pfankuchen, D.B.; Stölting, D.P.; Schlesinger, M.; Royer, H.-D.; Bendas, G. Low molecular weight heparin tinzaparin antagonizes cisplatin resistance of ovarian cancer cells. *Biochem. Pharmacol.* **2015**, *97*, 147–157. [CrossRef] [PubMed]
17. Zacharski, L.R.; Ornstein, D.L. Heparin and cancer. *Thromb. Haemost.* **1998**, *80*, 10–23. [CrossRef] [PubMed]
18. Ornstein, D.L.; Zacharski, L.R. The use of heparin for treating human malignancies. *Haemostasis* **1999**, *29* (Suppl. S1), 48–60. [CrossRef] [PubMed]

19. Stevenson, J.L.; Choi, S.H.; Varki, A. Differential metastasis inhibition by clinically relevant levels of heparins—Correlation with selectin inhibition, not antithrombotic activity. *Clin. Cancer Res. Off. J. Am. Assoc. Cancer Res.* **2005**, *11*, 7003–7011. [CrossRef] [PubMed]
20. Stevenson, J.L.; Varki, A.; Borsig, L. Heparin attenuates metastasis mainly due to inhibition of P- and L-selectin, but non-anticoagulant heparins can have additional effects. *Thromb. Res.* **2007**, *120* (Suppl. 2), S107–S111. [CrossRef]
21. Pattabiraman, D.R.; Weinberg, R.A. Tackling the cancer stem cells—What challenges do they pose? *Nat. Rev. Drug Discov.* **2014**, *13*, 497–512. [CrossRef] [PubMed]

Sample Availability: Samples of the compounds are not available from the authors.

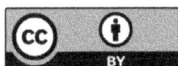

molecules

MDPI

Review

Functional Assays in the Diagnosis of Heparin-Induced Thrombocytopenia: A Review

Valentine Minet [1,*], Jean-Michel Dogné [1] and François Mullier [2]

[1]   Department of Pharmacy, Namur Thrombosis and Hemostasis Center (NTHC), Namur Research Institute for LIfe Sciences (NARILIS), University of Namur, Namur 5000, Belgium; jean-michel.dogne@unamur.be
[2]   CHU UCL Namur, Namur Thrombosis and Hemostasis Center (NTHC), Hematology Laboratory, Université catholique de Louvain, Yvoir 5530, Belgium; mullierfrançois@gmail.com
*   Correspondence: valentine.minet@unamur.be; Tel.: +32-81-72-42-92

Academic Editors: Giangiacomo Torri and Jawed Fareed
Received: 15 March 2017; Accepted: 8 April 2017; Published: 11 April 2017

Abstract: A rapid and accurate diagnosis in patients with suspected heparin-induced thrombocytopenia (HIT) is essential for patient management but remains challenging. Current HIT diagnosis ideally relies on a combination of clinical information, immunoassay and functional assay results. Platelet activation assays or functional assays detect HIT antibodies that are more clinically significant. Several functional assays have been developed and evaluated in the literature. They differ in the activation endpoint studied; the technique or technology used; the platelet donor selection; the platelet suspension (washed platelets, platelet rich plasma or whole blood); the patient sample (serum or plasma); and the heparin used (type and concentrations). Inconsistencies in controls performed and associated results interpretation are common. Thresholds and performances are determined differently among papers. Functional assays suffer from interlaboratory variability. This lack of standardization limits the evaluation and the accessibility of functional assays in laboratories. In the present article, we review all the current activation endpoints, techniques and methodologies of functional assays developed for HIT diagnosis.

Keywords: heparin-induced thrombocytopenia; diagnosis; functional assay; platelets

---

1. Introduction

Accurate and rapid diagnosis of heparin-induced thrombocytopenia (HIT) is essential to improve clinical management of patients. Because thrombocytopenia is rather frequent in hospitalized patients receiving heparin, clinicians must distinguish the uncommon patient with HIT among the many without [1]. Accurate diagnosis is crucial as overdiagnosis may expose the patient to alternative anticoagulant treatment conferring a significant risk for major bleeding complications. Moreover, physicians are very reluctant to reintroduce heparin in such patients [2,3]. Misdiagnosis will delay the initiation of the alternative treatment, increasing thrombotic risk and mortality [4]. Clinical scoring systems, such as the 4Ts score or the HEP score, are helpful in estimating the probability of HIT [5,6]. A low probability 4Ts score appears to be a robust means of excluding HIT [7,8] but does not rule out HIT in all cases [9,10] and may be difficult to apply [11]. Patients with intermediate and high probability scores require further evaluation [7]. HIT is often difficult to exclude or to confirm based on clinical information alone [1]. HIT diagnosis requires laboratory testing. Two types of assays are available: immunoassays and functional assays [1]. Immunoassays detect binding of anti-PF4/heparin antibodies (Ab). Functional assays or platelet activation assays investigate if these antibodies are able to activate platelets in the presence of heparin. Depending on the clinical setting, only 10%–50% of patients with positive immunoassays have platelet-activating antibodies [12]. HIT cannot be confirmed by immunoassays alone because of low positive predictive value [13]. A recent systematic review and meta-analysis concluded that only five immunoassays evaluated have a high sensitivity (>95%) and a high specificity (>90%) [14]. Moreover, optical density (OD) values of immunoassays vary among laboratories and need standardization of the OD ranges [15]. Performing a functional assay in the case of positive immunoassay is highly needed to reduce overdiagnosis and subsequent mistreatment of patients without HIT [16]. An integrated diagnostic approach combining clinical information with immunoassays and functional assays is recommended and provides a guide to decision making facing a patient suspected of HIT [5,14,17]. Making a timely and accurate diagnosis of HIT remains an important challenge because of limitations of current diagnostic tests. Functional assays considered as gold standards, i.e., ^{14}C-serotonin release assay (^{14}C-SRA) and heparin-induced platelet activation (HIPA)), require a highly specialized laboratory and are not widely available [18]. Several platelet activation assays avoiding limitations of previous assays have been developed. We provide an overview of all current laboratory endpoints, techniques, assay variations and results interpretation in functional assays for HIT diagnosis.

2. Principles of Functional Assays

In functional tests, donor platelets are incubated with patient serum/plasma and heparin. If clinically significant patient's HIT antibodies are present with an optimal heparin–PF4 stoichiometric ratio, this leads to the formation of a heparin–antibody–PF4 complex that will bind to FcγRIIa receptors on the platelet and induce donor platelets activation. This in vitro reaction results in platelet changes including release of α-granules and dense bodies, generation of platelet microparticles (PMPs), upregulation of various membrane glycoproteins (GP) and ultimately platelet aggregation. These platelet changes may be used as endpoints in functional assays (Figure 1) [19].

3. Activation Endpoints

3.1. Release of Dense Granules Content

3.1.1. Release of Serotonin

Almost all circulating serotonin is accumulated and stored in the dense granules of platelets [20,21]. When platelets are activated by HIT antibodies, they release serotonin in the supernatant. The measurement of the serotonin release can be used to detect HIT antibody-induced platelet activation within patient serum or plasma [22]. The first assay proposed to measure this release of serotonin as a platelet activation point in the diagnosis of HIT was the ^{14}C-serotonin release assay (^{14}C-SRA) [23]. To perform this assay, donor platelet-rich plasma (PRP) is pre-incubated with radioactive ^{14}C-serotonin. Radiolabeled serotonin enters dense granules of platelets. After a washing procedure, washed platelets are incubated with patient serum/plasma and heparin followed by a centrifugation step where supernatants are collected and radioactivity is measured using a β-counter [22].

Alternatives to study platelet serotonin release have been described in the literature. These techniques avoid the use of a radioactive agent and measure the release of intraplatelet endogenous serotonin. The first technique is the enzyme linked immunosorbent assay (ELISA) [24]. During the incubation step, endogenous serotonin is released from dense granules to the supernatant. After a centrifugation step, the serotonin contained in the supernatant is quantified with an ELISA [24–26]. The second technique to quantify serotonin released in the supernatant from platelets is the high-pressure liquid chromatography (HPLC) [25–27] coupled to a fluorescent detector [27] or to an electrochemical detector [25]. The third technology analyses intraplatelet serotonin content using flow cytometry [28]. After the incubation step, platelets were identified using an antiCD41a monoclonal antibody that recognizes a calcium-dependent complex of GPIIb/IIIa expressed on normal platelets. Intraplatelet serotonin content was detected with an antiserotonin antibody labelling after fixation and permeabilization of platelets. Platelets activation was independently shown by annexin V binding [28].

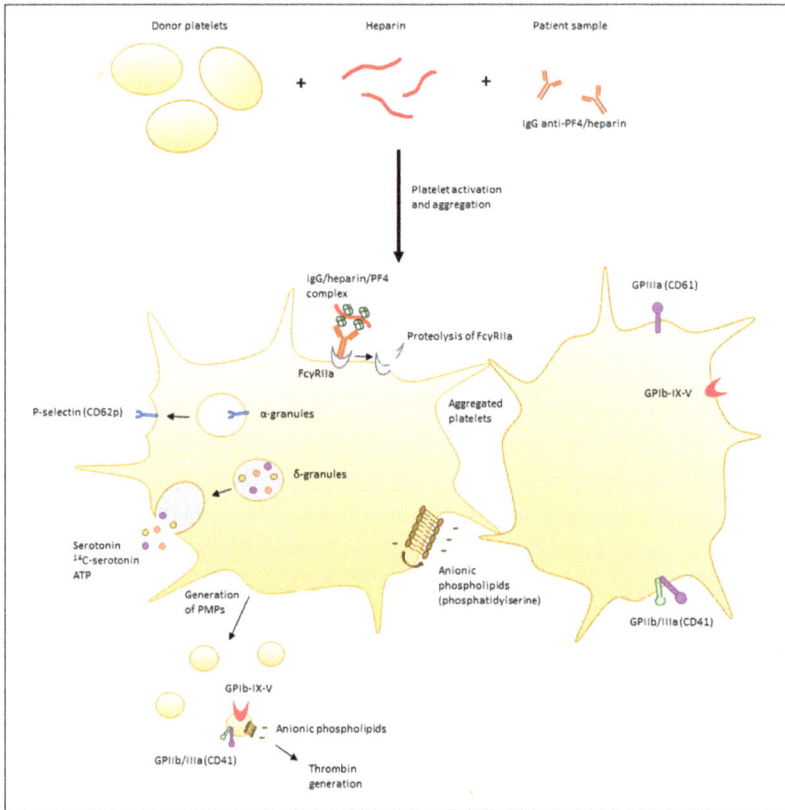

Figure 1. Platelet changes induced by heparin-induced thrombocytopenia (HIT) antibodies and detected in HIT functional assays. Donor platelets, heparin and the patient sample are incubated in vitro. Clinically significant antibodies lead to the formation of an antibody/heparin/PF4 complex that binds to FcγRIIa receptors on the platelet and induces donor platelets activation and aggregation. The following platelet changes are induced and may be used as endpoints in functional assays: proteolysis of the FcγRIIa receptor; translocation of p-selectin (CD62p) from α-granules to the platelet surface; release of δ-granules (dense granules) content containing serotonin; ATP and preincubated radiolabeled serotonin; generation of PMPs; procoagulant activity of PMPs with thrombin generation; translocation of anionic phospholipids such as phosphatidylserine to the outer surface by a flip-flop mechanism; and aggregation of platelets. GPIIIa (CD61) and GPIIb/IIIa (CD41) are two platelet and PMP surface glycoproteins (GP) expressed on normal platelets. GPIb–IX–V is a subunit of the von Willebrand factor receptor complex expressed on the surface of platelets and PMPs. (IgG: immunoglobulin G, PF4: platelet factor 4, ATP: adenosine triphosphate, PMPs: platelet microparticles.)

3.1.2. Release of Adenosine Triphosphate (ATP)

The platelet dense granules contain large stores of ATP [29]. ATP release from platelets during platelet activation induced by HIT antibodies can be measured using a lumiaggregometer [29]. Luciferase–luciferin reagent is added to the platelet samples, it reacts with released ATP to generate adenyl–luciferon. A chemiluminescent reaction occurs when adenyl–luciferin oxides. The light emitted is proportional to the quantity of ATP present in the aggregometer cuvette [19]. Another group reported the use of a standard scintillation counter to quantify the released ATP [30].

3.1.3. Platelet Aggregation

The platelet aggregation endpoint can be measured in three different ways.

Visual Assessment

HIPA test is based on visual assessment of platelet aggregation in U-bottomed polystyrene microtiter wells with rotating steel balls used to agitate the platelets [31–35]. Donor platelets, patient serum and heparin are stirred using a magnetic stirrer. The wells are examined visually against an indirect light source at 5-min intervals. A change in appearance of the reaction mixture from turbidity (nonaggregated platelets) to transparency (aggregated platelets) is considered a positive result [36].

Optical Aggregometry

The heparin-induced platelet aggregation test (PAT) evaluates platelet aggregation using conventional light transmission aggregometry (LTA) [33,37]. The test principle is similar to HIPA, except that the platelet aggregation endpoint is not evaluated visually but with the use of an optical aggregometer. The reaction mixture is stirred in a cuvette at 37 °C between a light source and a photocell and the light transmission is recorded over time. Aggregation is detected by an increase in light transmission through the platelet suspension [38].

Impedance Aggregometry

Platelet aggregation can be detected with the heparin-induced multiple electrode aggregometry (HIMEA) [39–44]. The reaction mixture is incubated and stirred in a cuvette containing two pairs of sensor electrodes. When platelet aggregation occurs, platelets stick on the electrodes inducing an enhancement of the electrical resistance between them. This change in impedance is recorded over time in the whole blood impedance analyzer (Multiplate® analyzer, Dynabyte Medical, Munich, Germany).

3.1.4. Expression of Platelet Membrane Glycoproteins

During platelet activation, changes are induced in the platelet membranes with expression of surface markers. These platelet activation markers can be studied in flow cytometry with the use of fluorescent-labeled ligand [38]. Expression of anionic phospholipids and P-selectin have been proposed in the literature as identification markers of platelet activation [45–50]. During platelet activation, a membrane flip-flop mechanism translocates anionic phospholipids such as phosphatidylserine to the outer surface. Annexin V is a protein that binds with high affinity and specificity to anionic phospholipids expressed on the surface of activated platelets [19]. P-selectin is a protein stored in the membranes of the α-granules of resting platelets. Upon platelet activation, P-selectin (CD62P) is translocated to the platelet surface [19,38] and can be measured using a labelled anti-P-selectin antibody. Platelet marker antibodies are also used to identify the platelet population. Anti-CD61 and anti-CD41 recognize two platelet surface GP: platelet GPIIIa (CD61) [50] and platelet complex GPIIb/IIIa (CD41), respectively [45,46,48,51]. After the in vitro platelet activation by HIT antibodies, the platelet mixture is incubated with two fluorescent-labelled ligands: one to identify platelets and the other to detect activated platelets. The proportion of activated platelets is obtained by two-color flow cytometry.

3.1.5. Generation of Platelets Microparticles

Platelets activated by HIT sera generate platelet-derived microparticles [52–54]. PMPs are quantified using flow cytometry. After the incubation step, platelet mixture is incubated with a fluorescent-labelled antibody to identify platelets and PMPs such as anti-CD41 [51,55–57] or anti-GPIbα [58], the latter monoclonal antibody links a subunit of the von Willebrand factor receptor complex (GPIb–IX–V) expressed on the surface of platelets and PMPs [19]. Annexin-V may be added to bind anionic phospholipids as a platelet activation marker [51,55–57]. PMPs are distinguished from platelets by their size and scatter parameters.

3.1.6. Procoagulant Activity

Platelet-derived microparticles generated by HIT antibodies are procoagulant and lead to thrombin generation [53]. The procoagulant activity of HIT IgG antibodies can be measured with the thrombin generation assay (TGA) using a fluorometer [59,60]. At the end of the incubation with HIT antibodies, recombinant human tissue factor is added and coagulation is triggered with the addition of a fluorogenic substrate and calcium chloride. The peptidic fluorogenic substrate is hydrolysed by thrombin and releases a product which emits fluorescence. The fluorescence intensity is recorded over time and converted into a peak of active thrombin concentration against time [61].

3.1.7. FcγRIIa Proteolysis

FcγRIIa agonists lead to cleavage of the receptor and the retention of a 32-kDa membrane bound component [62,63]. Identification of the proteolytic fragment of FcγRIIa with a Western blot analysis could serve as a surrogate marker for HIT [64]. After the incubation time, platelet activation is stopped with EDTA in the presence of protease inhibitors. Platelets are centrifuged and solubilized in lysis buffer. To measure proteolysis, lysates are separated by SDS-PAGE and detected by Western blot analysis using goat anti-human FcγRIIa with avidin–horseradish peroxidase and chemiluminescence [64]. The percentage proteolysis is determined using scanning densitometry.

3.1.8. Intracellular Luciferase Cell Activity

Cuker and collaborators recently developed a new functional assay to identify cell-activating anti-PF4/heparin antibodies without need for donor platelets but using a cell-line that can be stored at -80 °C [65]. DT40 chicken B lymphocyte cells were transiently transfected to express human FcγRIIA and a luciferase reporter. The PF4/heparin/plasma mixtures are added to the resultant transgenic B-cell line. HIT immune complexes bind to B cells and cross-link the FcγRIIA which induces an intracellular signaling cascade, ultimately leading to luciferase activation, resulting in a luminescence signal. Luciferase activity is measured with a luminometer using Luciferase Assay Reagent. Data are reported as the signal induced by patient plasma relative to the absence of plasma (fold-basal) [65].

4. Platelets

4.1. Whole Blood, PRP or Washed Platelets

Donor platelets can be used in three different ways: either as washed platelets, as PRP or as whole blood.

Whole blood does not require platelet preparation after the blood drawn and is therefore more rapid to obtain than PRP or washed platelets.

To obtain PRP, a simple centrifugation of whole blood at a low speed (150 to 180 g for 10 to 15 min at room temperature) is needed [32]. PRP is sometimes adjusted to 250,000–300,000 platelets/μL [29,42,48,66]. PRP is technically less demanding than washed platelets and can be performed in a non-specialist clinical laboratory [19].

To prepare washed platelets, blood is collected into acid–citrate–dextrose (ACD) solution. ACD reduces the pH in order to prevent platelet aggregation that would occur during platelet pelleting [36]. ACD also chelates the calcium in blood preventing coagulation. A low speed centrifugation is performed to obtain PRP. Platelets are isolated from PRP by successive centrifugation steps and re-suspended in calcium- and magnesium-free Tyrode's buffer at pH 6.3 with glucose and apyrase. The absence of calcium and magnesium allows the activation of coagulation factors and platelets to be avoided [36]. Apyrase is an enzyme that prevents adenosine diphosphate (ADP) accumulation from the platelets by degrading adenine nucleotides. It maintains platelet sensitivity to subsequent ADP stimulation that occurs during the second phase of HIT antibody-induced platelet activation [32,67]. Platelets are resuspended into calcium- and magnesium-containing Tyrode's buffer at physiological pH (pH 7.4) without apyrase or hirudin to allow HIT-induced platelet activation [36].

Platelet washing is a time-consuming procedure requiring experience and care to avoid excessive platelet activation [19,51]. Although, the mild background platelet activation generated during the washing procedure can be advantageous in HIT assays, excessive platelet activation can occur in inexperienced hands and lead to erroneous results [19]. Washed platelets are best suited for specialist or referral laboratories assessing many HIT sera/plasma as this facilitates acquisition of sufficient technical experience to perform the assay successfully on a consistent basis [36]. In the nonspecialist clinical laboratories, the technicians may not have the experience or training to perform platelet washing properly and a PRP-based assay may be more appropriate [19].

Washed platelet-based assays are considered more sensitive and possibly more specific than PRP or whole blood-based assay tests for some biological reasons [19,36,68]: (i) the wash step eliminates possible interfering substances potentially causing heparin independent aggregation such as IgG or acute-phase proteins (e.g., fibrinogen) [69]; (ii) the high centrifugation during washing may induce platelet granule release of PF4 with greater formation of PF4/heparin antigen complexes [19]; (iii) the use of apyrase prevents platelets from becoming refractory to subsequent ADP-mediated potentiation of HIT-antibody-induced activation; (iv) the physiological calcium concentrations induce optimal IgG-mediated platelet activation [36,69].

Previous studies have compared PAT, a PRP aggregation test to SRA, a washed platelets activation assay. They suggested that PAT has lower sensitivity than SRA and may miss cases of true HIT [33,35,70,71]. In contrast, another study reported a similarly high sensitivity for PAT in comparison to SRA but with a lower specificity for PAT [72]. It is believed that when performed under controlled conditions with highly responsive platelets and with a two-point system, the sensitivity and specificity of PRP-based assay can approach or be similar to washed platelet-based assays [19,33]. More recent studies compared the performances of SRA to newer PRP or whole-blood-based tests and showed close or similar sensitivity and specificity [27,42,44,56,73]. No direct comparison of functional assays using the same patient samples with the same platelet donors using PRP and washed platelets has been described in the literature.

4.2. Platelet Donor Selection

It was reported that serum/plasma of a patient with HIT highly activates autologous platelets [74,75]. It has been potentially explained by a persisting high expression of FcγRIIa on platelets [75], baseline platelet activation and higher availability of PF4 in patients with acute HIT [76]. However, use of autologous PRP can be limited by the patient thrombocytopenia, hence the use of donor platelets to perform the functional assay [36,77].

Platelets from different donors vary considerably in their reactivity to HIT antibodies [19]. A potential explanation is the genetic polymorphism of the FcγRIIa receptor [78]. Two polymorphisms have been identified: Arg/His131 [79–84] and Gln/Lys127 [85]. It is of utmost importance to select platelets from responsive donors as it was shown that using a high responder donor for HIT investigation improves the sensitivity of the functional assay [86,87]. Indeed, platelets with poor reactivity may give false negative results with weak HIT antibodies [44,88]. Selection of platelets from a high responder donor seems to be the most important factor affecting the sensitivity of the HIT antibody functional assay [19]. In order to select responsive donors, different approaches have been adopted. Some laboratories use platelets from four different donors to minimize the variability of platelets. Some laboratories identify a number of "good responders" among the laboratory staff [19]. These known reactive donors are potential platelet donors when a HIT functional assay is needed. The identification can be realized in two ways. First, platelet donors may be tested individually against strong and weak positive control sera/plasma using a functional assay [27]. Platelet donors inducing a high platelet response with strong and with the weak positive control will be selected. Weak positive control sera/plasma are obtained from dilution of a well-characterized strong HIT sera/plasma [22]. The anti-CD9 monoclonal antibody ALB6 cross-links the FcγRIIa receptor and can be used as a platelet activator to select good donors [41,89,90]. The 5B9 is a chimeric IgG1 antibody to PF4/H complexes that mimics human HIT antibodies [91] which can potentially be used to select responsive donors.

Platelets should be obtained from donors that did not take medications impairing platelet function such as acetylsalicylic acid or non-steroid anti-inflammatory drugs (NSAIDs) [19,32]. Garlic, antihistamines, and naturopathic medications should also be avoided because of their effect on platelets [19,32,41].

For the use of HIMEA- and LTA-evaluating donor platelets aggregation, Morel-Kopp et al suggest to collect blood following ISTH-SSC recommendations [92]. These SSC/ISTH guidelines have been established for the standardization of LTA and recommend that treatment with drugs known to reversibly (e.g., NSAIDs except aspirin) or irreversibly (e.g., aspirin, thienopyridines) inhibit platelet function should be stopped at least 3 days and 10 days, respectively, before sampling [92]. Although, it is recognized in the literature that antiplatelet compounds should be avoided in donor blood, this is not systematically mentioned and minimum time between the last drug intake and the blood drawn may differ among papers [32,40,41,49,93]. Sono-Koree et al. evaluated the effects of aspirin and ibuprofen on donor platelets in responsive platelet donors to HIT antibodies using HPLC-SRA [27]. They concluded that the effects of these NSAIDs were donor specific and markedly decreased responses to HIT antibodies in several donors. They observed a return to normal platelet function in all donors by 1 week following drug ingestion and implemented a conservative approach, restricting SRA platelet donation in subjects who have ingested NSAIDs in the past 10–14 days [27].

Healthy donors with no platelet dysfunction should be selected to prevent false negatives. To ensure the good reactivity of platelets, donor platelets may be tested with common platelet activators such as collagen, ADP, arachidonic acid or thrombin receptor activating peptide (TRAP) during a pre-screening test [33,40]. Moreover, working with healthy donor blood decreases the risk of potential interfering substances that may cause false positives.

The number of donor(s) to perform a functional assay for the diagnosis of one suspected HIT patient varies from one to four among studies [18,27,41]. In general, studies using a high number of donors to minimize the variability of platelets selected them randomly [15,18]. This is less recommended as platelet donors are not easily available, therefore it may not be possible to obtain platelets from four donors to perform the assay on a regular basis [19]. Previous identification of highly responsive donors among the laboratory staff allows only one or two donors to be tested when a HIT functional assay is needed [18,19,41]. Some studies that worked with two or three donors known to be reactive to HIT antibodies did not test them separately but mixed their platelets to perform the HIT functional assay [15,27,58,94,95].

When performing the HIT assay with donor whole blood, blood group O or the same group as the patient should be used to avoid an ABO incompatibility reaction [40,56]. When working with PRP or washed platelets, ABO blood group discrepancies are inconsequential and may be ignored [22,31,36].

No international standardized guidelines for the appropriate selection of platelet donors to perform HIT functional assays currently exist. This may lead to interlaboratory variability [96].

5. Patient Sample

Functional assays may be performed with either patient serum or plasma [22,23,41]. An exception is the TGA requiring preferably plasma because it contains coagulation proteins that are needed for thrombin generation [61]. Testing should be performed using acute serum or plasma because HIT antibodies are transient [32]. Residual thrombin may contaminate patient serum or plasma and cause platelet activation leading to false positive results (e.g., patient with disseminated intravascular coagulation) [19,36]. The patient sample could be first heated at 56 °C for 30–45 min to inactivate thrombin [22,27]. Then, a high-speed centrifugation is performed (8000–12,000 g for 5–10 min) to remove fibrin(ogen)gel and other precipitates [23,32,36]. Complement proteins are also destroyed by heat inactivation but they are not required for IgG-dependent platelet activation in HIT [32]. However, overheating the patient sample can generate aggregated IgG causing platelet activation [19,23,36].

This heat-inactivation is not systematically performed for HIT functional assays in the literature. Morel-Kopp et al. do not recommend the heat inactivation of the patient sample before HIMEA testing because it may decrease antibody titers and affect platelet aggregation results [41].

6. Heparin

In vivo, unfractionated heparin (UFH) caused the HIT syndrome more frequently than low molecular weight heparin (LMWH) [16]. In vitro, studies demonstrated greater capacity of UFH to form highly immunogenic ultra large PF4/heparin/IgG complexes than LMWH [97]. In functional assays, UFH is commonly used [26,28,40–42], LMWH may be tested in parallel [18,25,58,98]. LMWH exhibits nearly 100% in vitro cross-reactivity to HIT antibodies using functional assays [27,48,99,100]. In others studies, LMWH showed less cross-reactivity compared with UFH, varying from low [101] to very high [102–104] cross-reactivity. These inconsistencies may be explained by a lack of standardization of test conditions such as source of donor platelets or optimal tested concentrations [102]. Two studies demonstrated that using reviparin, a LMWH, enhanced the sensitivity of the functional assay in comparison to UFH, because of the formation of more stable PF4/heparin complexes due to the narrow range in the molecular weight [98,105]. In the literature, reviparin or enoxaparin are used as LMWH in functional assays [18].

The concentration of heparin in the assay is critically important to induce maximal platelet activation/aggregation, maximizing the sensitivity of the assay [19]. Indeed, heparin and PF4 form heparin–antibody–PF4 complexes that activate platelets only over a narrow molar range [106,107]. Variable heparin concentrations are used in platelet activation assays for HIT diagnosis [18,88]. Pharmacologic heparin concentrations of 0.1 to 0.3 IU/mL are optimal for the formation of the heparin/PF4 complex in washed platelet-based assays [23]. For PRP-based assays, the optimal heparin concentrations are between 0.5 and 1.0 IU/mL [19,102]. Whole blood assays commonly use 1.0 IU/mL as low heparin concentration [39–43,56]. The rationale for using higher concentrations of heparin in whole blood and PRP-based assays compared to washed platelet-based assays is the presence of heparin binding proteins in plasma [88]. Multiple low heparin concentrations comprised in the optimal range may be tested in parallel during the same functional assay [18,22]. A high heparin concentration condition is recommended to enhance the specificity of the assay [19]. Indeed, high dose heparin disrupts the PF4/heparin complex [108] by saturating the heparin binding sites of all PF4 molecules. It suppresses platelet activation induced by HIT antibodies [19]. The high heparin concentration commonly used for washed platelet-based assays is 100 IU/mL [18,22,27]. In PRP-based assays and in whole blood-based assays, heparin at 100 IU/mL may not always completely suppress the HIT antibody-induced platelet activation because of the presence of heparin-binding proteins [19]. This partial inhibition may be acceptable or a higher concentration of heparin (i.e., 200 to 500 IU/mL) may be used to obtain a higher inhibition of the HIT-mediated platelet reaction [19,41,56].

Contaminating heparin in the patient sample can interfere with assay performances by inducing inappropriate final heparin concentrations in the assay [109,110]. Heparinase [110,111], resin for anions [58,112] or thiophilic adsorption chromatography [113] have been used to remove heparin contamination in the patient sample. Elimination of residual heparin in patient samples before performing a HIT functional assay is not a common practice in HIT diagnosis. In order to prevent an erroneous result caused by contaminating heparin, Morel-Kopp et al. recommend, whenever possible, to collect blood at least 4 h after cessation of an unfractionated heparin infusion and at least 12 h after a dose of LMWH [41].

7. Controls

Functional assays require strict quality controls [68]. Several controls have been described in the literature but they are not systematically performed [88]. There is a high variability of controls tested between laboratories.

7.1. Negative Controls

An appropriate negative control is needed to ensure the absence of platelet activation/aggregation of donor platelets in the presence of heparin with a negative sample [68]. To perform this negative control, the test sample may be replaced by a healthy control sample, a previously tested negative patient sample or a commercially available negative control sample [88].

The buffer control is a test condition performed in the absence of added heparin to prove the absence of donor platelets response with the patient sample without heparin [114].

7.2. Heparin Dependency

To verify that platelet activation/aggregation is FcγRIIa receptor-dependent and to prove the heparin dependency, two test conditions may be performed as a confirmation step [18]. First, the high heparin concentration condition disrupts PF4/heparin complexes and prevents the antibody-induced platelet activation response [18]. Second, the monoclonal antibody IV.3 blocks the FcγRIIa receptor and inhibits HIT-antibody-mediated platelet activation [18,19]. Heparin at high concentration or monoclonal antibody IV.3 should be added before donor platelets [18]. IV.3 is tested in the presence of a low heparin concentration [22], proving that the heparin dependency enhances the specificity of the assay [19,36].

7.3. Positive Controls

An appropriate positive control is required to verify that the platelets are sufficiently reactive and to ensure that the assay can adequately detect platelet-activating antibodies [68,88,115]. A known HIT-positive serum/plasma sample should be tested in parallel as standard control response [19]. HIT-positive serum/plasma of well-documented HIT are stored frozen and remain stable for many years [68]. Studies revealed that HIT sera stored at −70 °C continue to react well when used in the SRA or enzyme-immunoassay (EIA) more than two decades later [32,116,117]. The use of one or more "strong positive" and one or more "weak positive" HIT sera/plasma have been recommended [22,32,88,118]. "Strong positive" HIT controls are diluted to obtain "weak positive" HIT sera/plasma [22]. Weak-positive controls ensure the assay is sensitive enough to detect patients with HIT and assess variability in assay performance over time [22,118].

In theory, a HIT-mimicking monoclonal antibody may be used as a positive control [32]. For example, KKO, an IgG2bκ antibody [119] or 5B9, an IgG1 antibody (5B9) [91] are two monoclonal antibodies that activate human platelets through a heparin- and PF4-dependent mechanism that is mediated through FcγRIIA [91,119]. However, the correlation between the human platelets responsiveness and the reactivity to HIT antibodies needs to be evaluated to determine if a HIT-mimicking monoclonal antibody could be valuable in HIT diagnosis.

Platelet activating agonist controls may be used to ensure the good platelet responsiveness [88]. Heat-aggregated human IgG is sometimes used as an immune complex control added with and without IV.3 to ensure that the platelets respond to an "IgG agonist" and also to validate the FcγRIIa inhibition step as IV.3 inhibits platelet activation by heat-aggregated IgG [19,22,32,58]. Heat-aggregated IgG may be prepared from pooled normal sera by heat treatment at 63 °C for 20 min, followed by a 10-min centrifugation at 12,000 g [120]. Donor platelet reactivity may be tested in platelet aggregation assay with common platelet activators such as ADP, collagen, arachidonic acid or TRAP [33,40,41,77].

Some laboratories proposed a positive IgG-specific anti-PF4/heparin EIA as a quality control to avoid a false-positive SRA report as incongruous results may occur (i.e., positive SRA in combination with negative EIA and an atypical clinical presentation) [12,14,22,94,121,122].

8. Other Variations

Donor platelets are incubated with patient serum/plasma and heparin in all functional assays. This preanalytical step may differ for the agitation force, the incubation time and the incubation temperature among different functional assays or for the same functional assay. The incubation temperature may vary from room temperature [24,27,34,45] to 25–28 °C [48,51] to 37 °C [45,55]. To agitate, occasional gentle mixing [24,48], low speed [27], agitation of 1000 rpm [29,34,42] or 1200 rpm [55] are used. The incubation period may vary from 15 min [41,42] to 20 min [55,56] to 30 min [45,48,51] to 45 min [34] for up to 60 min [22,27,45]. The ratio of donor platelets to the patient sample is usually 3.75:1 for washed platelet-based assays [22,27] and usually between 1:0.5 and 1:1 for PRP and whole blood-based assays [36,39,40,55]. To collect donor platelets, ACD, citrate or hirudin tubes are often used. ACD tubes are used for washed platelet-based assays [22,27,58]. Citrate tubes are commonly used for PRP or whole blood-based assays [19,39,42,44,55]. Hirudin tubes are often used preferably for HIMEA as it improves assay sensitivity [39,89] by avoiding issues of calcium concentrations affecting platelet response (and also the problem of calcium depletion in under-filled citrate tubes [41]). Heparin tubes are avoided in order to prevent increase of final heparin concentration in the test.

9. Results Expression

Results expression is specific to the endpoint and the technology used. Functional assays using the release of radiolabeled or unradiolabeled serotonin as an endpoint (^{14}C-SRA, EIA-SRA, HPLC-SRA) often express the results as a percentage of serotonin release to account for inter- and intra-individual variability in platelet serotonin content [25,27]. Expression of raw serotonin values may be used [24,25,28]. Platelet activation assays measuring ATP release reported luminescence results in moles of ATP per amount of platelets [29]. HIPA results are expressed as the presence or absence of a visual platelet aggregation [34]. PAT results are expressed as the area under the aggregation curve [44] or as percentage of aggregation [40,123]. HIMEA results are most commonly expressed as the area under the aggregation curve [39,40,42,43]. The aggregation velocity and the lag-time may be also used [41,89]. Flow cytometry experiments measuring the expression of platelet activation markers express results as a percentage of activated platelets [46,48–50,124]. Flow cytometry assays that detect generated PMPs may express results as the amount or the percentage of PMPs [51,58]. For the FcγRIIa proteolysis assay, results are determined as the percentage of proteolysis [64]. Some studies express the final results as a ratio between results at the low heparin concentration and at the high heparin concentration [51,55,56,95] or as a ratio between results at the low heparin concentration and in the absence of heparin [61]. The ratio low/high heparin concentration takes into account the heparin dependency confirmation step in the final result expression but is not applicable to each functional assay as the result at the high heparin concentration may be zero in HIMEA for instance [41].

10. Results Interpretation

According to the results of the test condition and controls, several situations are possible (Table 1).

In the first situation, the results of the functional assay are negative in the absence of added heparin (buffer control), at the low heparin concentration(s), at the high heparin concentration and with the monoclonal antibody IV.3. This is observed in the case of a true negative, i.e., the patient has really no HIT or in the case of a false negative. The latter may occur if the donor platelets were not sufficiently reactive because the donor is not a good responder to HIT antibodies or because he/she took antiplatelet agents. Another potential cause is a problem that occurred during the experiment. To avoid a false negative, it is highly important to obtain platelets from one or more good platelet responder that has been selected previously. Positive controls performed in parallel are essential to verify that donor platelets are optimally reactive and that the donor did not fail to mention antiplatelet compounds intake in the previous days [22]. Positive controls ensure that no technical problem occurs during the experiment and that the assay can adequately detect platelet activation or aggregation [22,68,88,115].

The second situation occurs in the case of a true HIT because of a positive reaction that occurs only with the low heparin concentration(s). Absence of platelet reaction with the high heparin concentration and the monoclonal antibody IV.3 conditions prove that the platelet reaction is heparin-dependent. The negative response in the absence of added heparin demonstrates that heparin is needed to activate/aggregate platelets.

Table 1. Different patterns with a combination of functional assay results (platelet response) at four test conditions (i.e., absence of added heparin, low concentration(s) and high concentration of heparin and monoclonal antibody IV.3). Potential causes of each pattern are provided. Negative and positive controls are not represented in the table. Neg: negative, Pos: positive, Ab: antibody, IgG: immunoglobulin G, HLA: human leukocyte antigen.

Pattern	Absence of Added Heparin	Low Concentration(s) of Heparin	High Concentration of Heparin	Monoclonal Ab IV.3	Potential Causes
1	Neg	Neg	Neg	Neg	No HIT HIT and low platelet reactivity Technical problem
2	Neg	Pos	Neg	Neg	HIT
3	Pos	Pos	Neg	Neg	HIT with residual heparin Syndromes of autoimmune HIT: Delayed-onset HIT Persisting HIT Spontaneous HIT syndrome Fondaparinux-associated HIT
4	Pos	Pos	Neg	Pos	Residual thrombin Very strong HIT
5	Pos	Pos	Pos	Neg	Heat-aggregated IgG High-titer HLA class I alloantibodies Systemic lupus erythematosus Other platelet-activating factor
6	Pos	Pos	Pos	Pos	Very strong HIT

In the third situation, the difference with the HIT laboratory profile is a positive response occurring in the buffer control. There are at least two potential explanations for strong platelet activation/aggregation in the absence of added heparin along with an inhibition at high heparin concentration and by FcγRIIa blocking antibody [36,113,125–131]. First, residual heparin may be present in the patient sample [109,110]. Second, HIT antibodies that activate platelets even in the absence of heparin may exist in the patient sample [96,113]. These antibodies are generated in four syndromes of autoimmune HIT: delayed-onset HIT, persisting HIT, spontaneous HIT syndrome and fondaparinux-associated HIT [125]. Platelet activation occurs in the absence of heparin because the HIT antibodies recognize PF4 bound to platelet-associated chondroitin sulfate [125,132]. Delayed-onset HIT indicates HIT that begins or worsens despite stopping heparin [125,133–135]. Persisting HIT is a HIT syndrome that takes several weeks to recover [125,128]. Spontaneous HIT syndrome is a disorder clinically and serologically resembling HIT but without proximate heparin exposure [125–127,136,137]. Fondaparinux-associated HIT is a HIT syndrome that occurs during fondaparinux treatment, the causal association of fondaparinux and HIT is controversial [138]. These disorders highlight the need of the buffer control to diagnose them from a typical HIT [114].

In the fourth situation, we observe a platelet activation/aggregation with each condition except at the high heparin concentration. The platelet response is not inhibited by monoclonal antibody IV.3 but only by a high heparin concentration. This may be mediated by residual thrombin [58,94]. Indeed, thrombin is a potent platelet activator [64]. This activation progressively decreases from buffer control to low heparin concentration to high heparin concentration [36]. To prevent this false positive, heat-inactivation of the patient sample at 56 °C before performing the assay is performed [22,27]. Another laboratory practice to inactivate thrombin is to add hirudin to the patient sample [18,34,36,94]. These results may also be obtained with strongly-reacting HIT sera/plasma [94]. Some very strong HIT samples may induce platelet activation/aggregation that is not inhibited by monoclonal antibody IV.3 but with a high heparin concentration [36,94]. These strongly-reacting HIT antibodies are able to activate platelets without heparin [122].

In the fifth situation, a platelet response is observed in each condition except with the monoclonal antibody IV.3. A potential explanation is the presence of immune complexes in the patient sample such as heat-aggregated human IgG [22,77,98]. Heat-aggregated IgG may be produced during an inappropriate heat-inactivation of the patient sample [19,23,36]. They induce FcγRIIa-dependent platelet activation even in the presence of high heparin concentration but which is inhibited by the monoclonal antibody IV.3 [98,139]. The reaction profile may also occur in the presence of high-titer HLA class I alloantibodies as they react with HLA class I antigens present in high density on platelets [36]. Systemic lupus erythematosus or other platelet-activating factors may also be responsible for this situation [36,78,140]. Inhibition by IV.3 is not entirely specific for the HIT antibody-induced platelet activation [19].

The sixth reaction pattern presents a positive platelet reaction at each condition. This may be caused by very strong HIT antibodies that activate platelets in the presence of monoclonal antibody IV.3 but even with a high concentration of heparin [36,68,141].

Thrombotic thrombocytopenic purpura may lead to variable activation in the presence of heparin that is not inhibited by FcγRIIa-blocking monoclonal antibody [32,63,78]. It has been mentioned that elevated acute-phase reactant proteins such as fibrinogen, commonly present in plasma from critically ill patients, may cause heparin-dependent platelet aggregation in PAT [69,142,143].

The result of a functional assay is considered positive if a positive reaction occurs with the low heparin concentration(s) and is inhibited by the high heparin concentration and by monoclonal antibody IV.3 (pattern 2 and 3) [19]. The result is considered negative if no platelet activation occurs with no, low and high heparin concentration and with monoclonal antibody IV.3 (pattern 1) along with an appropriate reaction of the positive controls. When samples cannot be classified as either positive or negative, they are designated as "indeterminate results" (patterns 4, 5 and 6) [22]. In these indeterminate reactions, platelet activation/aggregation occurs with low heparin concentration but is not inhibited by high heparin concentration and/or IV.3 [64]. Facing an indeterminate result, strategies have been proposed in the literature. The first solution is to repeat the experiment with another properly heat-inactivated sample [19]. On the one hand, a sample not sufficiently heated may still be contaminated by residual thrombin and induce pattern 4. On the other hand, an overheated sample may contain heat-aggregated IgG and be responsible of pattern 5 [27]. An interpretable result may be obtained when the assay is repeated using another heat-inactivated aliquot [94]. The second solution (that may be coupled with the first solution) is to repeat the assay using different platelet donors; the subsequent test may yield a clear negative or positive result [32,94]. An explanation is that platelet activation by immune antibodies such as HLA or thrombotic thrombocytopenic purpura antibodies may be dependent on donor platelet phenotype [27]. The third solution is to take into account the result of an anti-PF4/heparin EIA to assess for the presence or absence of anti-PF4/heparin antibodies in indeterminate samples [12,36,94]. EIA assays have a high sensitivity and a negative result essentially rules out HIT [68]. They are often performed before functional assays as recommended in diagnosis algorithms [5,14]. In case of a positive EIA, the fourth solution is to retest dilutions of patient samples. A clear HIT pattern of reactivity may be obtained and indicates that very strong HIT antibodies are present [22,94].

The possible different reaction pattern, caused by other factors than HIT antibodies able to activate platelets, highlights the importance of running appropriate controls when performing a functional assay for the diagnosis of HIT.

11. Threshold and Performances

Different ways to determine a threshold in the literature are used to separate positive and negative platelet reactions. A cut-off may be defined in the laboratory because of its traditional use in the literature [22,27,144,145]. This is often the case with SRA whose threshold of 20% was historically defined by Sheridan et al. [23]. However, some authors favor the use of a higher cut-off of 50% [3,22,32,146] as this better discriminates between HIT and non-HIT thrombocytopenia [3,36]. The mean negative control value + 2 SD [47,112,147] or + 3 SD [24,42] may be used as the threshold. Some papers suggest that each laboratory should determine its own cut-off based on negative control using local donors [41,56]. A receiver operating characteristic (ROC) curve analysis is sometimes performed to determine the threshold value that gives maximal sensitivity and specificity [24,40,95]. Because functional tests are not used as screening tests but as confirmatory tests, a better specificity should be preferred over a better sensitivity [26,42]. The ROC curve of a functional assay is obtained against a reference standard. Functional assays, SRA [24,26,42,44,48] or HIPA [95] are sometimes used as reference in the literature to calculate the performances of the studied functional assay. More recently, the diagnosis of HIT based on the opinion of two or three independent experts was used as the reference standard [40,43,56,115,121,124,148]. Experts use all available clinical information, including follow-up data on each patient with HIT suspicion to make the diagnosis blinded to the results of the laboratory tests [115]. This expert consensus diagnosis has been questioned in the literature [115,149]. The combination of SRA with EIA has been proposed as a reference standard [68,149]. Clinico-biological conclusion combining a biological result, such as SRA or HIPA, with clinical parameters has also been used or proposed as a reference standard [65,115,150]. No universally accepted reference standards to measure performances of functional assay currently exist [7,151]. Since the studies do not use the same reference standard, clear-cut definitions of the specificities and sensitivities of the available functional assays are not given [69]. Moreover, even for the same functional assay, interlaboratory differences in methodology exist and performances reported by one laboratory do not necessarily apply to others [22].

12. Existing Functional Assays and Their Characteristics

SRA and HIPA are two washed platelet-based assays, often considered as reference standards for diagnosing HIT [14,18] although no universally accepted gold standard for HIT exists [65]. The reported sensitivity and specificity of SRA and HIPA are over 95% [115,151,152]. HIPA requires no special equipment and a moderate level of expertise but its activation endpoint is evaluated subjectively with possible visual interferences (Table 2) [14,36,69].

Table 2. Functional assays described in the literature for the diagnosis of HIT and associated technique/technology, studied endpoint, platelet suspension, advantages and limitations. SRA: serotonin-release assay, [14]C: carbon-14, EIA: enzyme-immunoassay, HPLC: high-pressure liquid chromatography, FCA: flow cytometry assay, HIPA: heparin-induced platelet activation, PAT: platelet aggregation assay, HIMEA: heparin-induced multiple electrode aggregometry, ATP: adenosine triphosphate, PMPGA: platelet microparticle generation assay, TGA: thrombin generation assay, PRP: platelet rich plasma, GP: glycoproteins, PMPs: platelet microparticles.

Assay	Technique/Technology	Endpoint	Platelets Used	Advantages	Limitations
[14]C-SRA	β-counter	^{14}C-radiolabeled serotonin release from dense granules of activated platelets	Washed platelets (PRP)	High sensitivity; High specificity	Time-consuming; High technical expertise; Radioactivity and specific license; Expensive equipment; Limited availability
EIA-SRA	ELISA	Serotonin release from dense granules of activated platelets	Washed platelets	Endogenous serotonin; No radioactive serotonin preloading; No special equipment needed; Quantitative determination of serotonin	Time-consuming
HPLC-SRA	HPLC	Serotonin release from dense granules of activated platelets	Washed platelets	Endogenous serotonin; No radioactive serotonin preloading; Rapid; Quantitative determination of serotonin	High technical expertise; Expensive equipment; Not widely available
FCA-intraplatelet serotonin	Flow cytometer	Loss of intraplatelet content of serotonin from activated platelets	PRP	Rapid; Reproducible	High technical expertise; Expensive equipment; Not widely available
HIPA	Visual observation	Visual assessment of platelet aggregation	Washed platelets	High sensitivity; High specificity; No special equipment needed; Repeated evaluation of platelet activation over time; Moderate level of expertise required; Moderate time consumption	Subjective visual assessment; Possible interference with visual interpretation
PAT	Aggregometer	Change of light transmittance caused by platelet aggregation	PRP	Largely available equipment in laboratory; Easy-to-perform; Objective assessment of platelet aggregation; Record over time	Low sensitivity; Moderate specificity
HIMEA	Multiple electrode platelet aggregometry	Changes in impedance caused by platelet aggregation on electrodes	Whole blood	Easy-to-perform; Semi-automated; No platelet handling and preparation; Moderate level of expertise required; Rapid; Largely available equipment in laboratory	Compatible blood group donor
ATP release assay	Lumiaggregometer/Standard scintillation counter	Detection of ATP release from activated platelets	Washed platelets; PRP	Easy-to-perform; Rapid	Not widely available
FCA-membrane GP	Flow cytometer	Expression of platelet activation markers (anionic phospholipids or P-selectin) in platelet population (CD61 or CD41)	PRP	Rapid; Cost-effective	Expensive equipment; High technical expertise; Not widely available
PMPGA	Flow cytometer	Generation of PMPs	Washed platelets; Whole blood; PRP	Rapid; Cost-effective	Expensive equipment; High technical expertise; Not widely available
TGA	Fluorometer	Generation of thrombin	PRP		
FcγRIIa proteolysis assay	Western blot/densitometer	Proteolysis of FcγRIIa	Washed platelets	Specific for FcγRIIa-mediated platelet activation	Not widely available
DT40-luciferase	Luminometer	Luciferase activity induced by cell activation	Platelet substitutes: chicken B lymphocytes	No need of donor platelets; Cell line stored at −80 °C and retrieved as needed/Easy-to-perform	Not widely available

SRA is not available in most routine hospital laboratories because it requires the use of radioactive material with expensive special equipment and a specific license [36,38]. This assay needs a high level of expertise and is time-consuming [22]. SRA is available to most clinicians only as send-outs to highly specialized laboratories and it does not provide results in real time necessary to guide initial management [14,148,152]. Moreover, even if SRA is available in the laboratory, the result may be obtained with a delay of several days [2]. SRA is not applicable for immediate patient management but rather for an ultimate HIT diagnosis [22]. Moreover, it has been reported that 10% of samples tested for HIT with SRA are initially classified as indeterminate which further delays accurate diagnosis [64,94]. SRA may also be performed with PRP [65,153] but this is a less common practice [22,112]. Because most of the laboratories try to avoid radioactivity for regulatory and safety issues [1] and because a rapid assay is very desirable in HIT diagnosis, researchers developed and evaluated new techniques. Alternative "non-radioactive serotonin-release assays" have been proposed in the literature using ELISA [24–26], HPLC [25–27] or flow cytometry [28]. A common advantage of these techniques is that they measure endogenous serotonin, avoiding the ^{14}C-serotonin platelet preloading step of SRA which simplifies the preanalytical procedure. ELISA does not require special equipment except a microplate spectrophotometer but it is a time-consuming assay procedure [24,25]. HPLC and flow cytometry are special equipment, with a high initial capital cost, that require technical expertise but these technologies offer a larger availability compared to a radioactive assay [26]. Studies that compared non-radioactive serotonin-release assay to SRA demonstrated similar performances [24,27] but further evaluation is needed. PAT was the first HIT assay described in the literature [37]. PAT has the advantage of easy handling but its sensitivity and specificity were demonstrated to be inferior to SRA/HIPA even when good platelet donors were selected [1,14,33,42,69]. HIMEA performed with whole blood proved to be a more sensitive and specific assay than PAT [40,42,89] and showed similar performances to SRA [40,42,44,89]. This semi-automated assay has the advantage of being easy-to-perform, requiring a moderate level of expertise. The equipment needed is a multiple electrode platelet aggregometer, widely used for antiplatelet treatment monitoring [154] and largely available in laboratories [39]. Its rapid turnaround time [41,42] and large availability reduce the time taken to confirm a HIT diagnosis and should have a positive impact on patient management [41]. Working with whole blood does not require platelet handling and preparation but has the limitation of needing a compatible blood group donor to avoid an ABO response [40]. More studies are needed to confirm the equivalence of HIMEA to SRA/HIPA [41]. A standard HIMEA protocol has been proposed by the SSC of the ISTH to serve as a standard for multicenter studies [41]. ATP release assay is a rapid and easy-to-perform assay that has been evaluated in one paper for HIT diagnosis [29]. Concordance with SRA was very good but needs further evaluation [29]. Flow cytometry assays (FCA) measuring platelet activation markers have been proposed in HIT diagnosis [45–51,95,124]. Studies showed good correlation between FCA and SRA [48,49], HIPA [50,95] or final clinical HIT diagnosis [124]. Flow cytometry measuring PMPs was evaluated as a functional assay [51,55–58]. Washed platelets [58], whole blood [55–57] or PRP [51] were used. Studies showed that PMPs as a platelet activation endpoint gave comparable results with SRA [55,56,58]. Further studies evaluating flow cytometry in the diagnosis of HIT are needed [14]. FCA requires high technical expertise and a high initial outlay on expensive equipment; however, this is cost-effective [48,51,95] and rapid [48,50,51,95,124]. TGA was investigated in the research setting in one study [61]. Results of the TGA correlated well with the results of PAT. They concluded that generation of thrombin could potentially be used for the diagnosis of HIT but needs further evaluation [14]. FcγRIIa proteolysis was shown to be at least as specific as the SRA for the diagnosis of HIT [64]. This endpoint has the advantage of being specific for FcγRIIa-mediated platelet activation [64]. For example, thrombin is a potent platelet activator that will not cause proteolysis of FcγRIIa [64]. DT40-luciferase was proposed as a functional cell-based assay not requiring donor platelets [65]. The cell line may be stored at $-80\ ^\circ$C and retrieved as needed. This assay showed better discrimination than two commercial immunoassays. It is easy-to-perform but not widely available. Stability of the transfected cell line and larger prospective validation are needed.

Specialized laboratories use mainly ^{14}C-SRA, HIPA, PAT or HIMEA as a functional assay to diagnose HIT. Other methods presented in Table 2 are more used in a research perspective but they may become more available for routine use. Indeed, the evolution of technology and the reduction of the equipment cost can render some sophisticated techniques more accessible, such as HPLC (HPLC-SRA) or flow cytometry (FCA-membrane GP, PMPGA, FCA-intraplatelet serotonin).

13. Conclusions

An ideal functional assay would be easy-to-perform, rapid, widely available in real-time, standardized and would have excellent performance. On-demand HIT testing has the potential to have a positive clinical and economic impact [155]. In confirmed HIT patients, it improves clinical outcomes by enabling earlier appropriate treatment and reduce costs by preventing expensive complications. In non-HIT patients, it could reduce overdiagnosis, unnecessary treatment and replacement anticoagulant drug costs [65,155]. Practically, few laboratories are currently able to perform a functional assay [2,42]. Among laboratories performing functional assays, there is currently a high variability in pre-analytical sample preparation and handling [22], platelet donors selection, controls performed, heparin concentrations used, testing methodologies and results interpretation [88]. The variability in HIT functional assays among laboratories reflects the lack of consensus recommendations on HIT testing and indicates a need for proficiency testing to assess assay performances [88]. Functional assays with few technical limitations facilitate their standardization and increase their accessibility in laboratories. Further standardization and evaluation of functional assays based on consensus guidelines would be valuable for a rapid and accurate diagnosis of HIT.

Author Contributions: V.M. wrote the paper. F.M., J.M.D. and V.M. revised the manuscript and approved the final version.

Conflicts of Interest: The authors declare no conflict of interest.

References

1. Bakchoul, T. An update on heparin-induced thrombocytopenia: Diagnosis and management. *Expert Opin. Drug Saf.* **2016**, *15*, 787–797. [CrossRef] [PubMed]
2. Greinacher, A. Too many hits in HIT? *Am. J. Hematol.* **2007**, *82*, 1035–1036. [CrossRef] [PubMed]
3. Lo, G.K.; Sigouin, C.S.; Warkentin, T.E. What is the potential for overdiagnosis of heparin-induced thrombocytopenia? *Am. J. Hematol.* **2007**, *82*, 1037–1043. [CrossRef] [PubMed]
4. Elalamy, I.; Tardy-Poncet, B.; Mulot, A.; de Maistre, E.; Pouplard, C.; Nguyen, P.; Cleret, B.; Gruel, Y.; Lecompte, T.; Tardy, B.; et al. Risk factors for unfavorable clinical outcome in patients with documented heparin-induced thrombocytopenia. *Thromb. Res.* **2009**, *124*, 554–559. [CrossRef] [PubMed]
5. Greinacher, A. Heparin-induced thrombocytopenia. *N. Engl. J. Med.* **2015**, *373*, 1883–1884. [PubMed]
6. Joseph, L.; Gomes, M.P.; Al Solaiman, F.; St John, J.; Ozaki, A.; Raju, M.; Dhariwal, M.; Kim, E.S. External validation of the HIT Expert Probability (HEP) score. *Thromb. Haemost.* **2015**, *113*, 633–640. [CrossRef] [PubMed]
7. Cuker, A.; Gimotty, P.A.; Crowther, M.A.; Warkentin, T.E. Predictive value of the 4Ts scoring system for heparin-induced thrombocytopenia: A systematic review and meta-analysis. *Blood* **2012**, *120*, 4160–4167. [CrossRef] [PubMed]
8. Lo, G.K.; Juhl, D.; Warkentin, T.E.; Sigouin, C.S.; Eichler, P.; Greinacher, A. Evaluation of pretest clinical score (4 T's) for the diagnosis of heparin-induced thrombocytopenia in two clinical settings. *J. Thromb. Haemost.* **2006**, *4*, 759–765. [CrossRef] [PubMed]
9. Favaloro, E.J. Toward improved diagnosis of HIT. *Blood* **2015**, *126*, 563–564. [CrossRef] [PubMed]
10. Linkins, L.A.; Bates, S.M.; Lee, A.Y.; Heddle, N.M.; Wang, G.; Warkentin, T.E. Combination of 4Ts score and PF4/H-PaGIA for diagnosis and management of heparin-induced thrombocytopenia: Prospective cohort study. *Blood* **2015**, *126*, 597–603. [CrossRef] [PubMed]

11. Nagler, M.; Fabbro, T.; Wuillemin, W.A. Prospective evaluation of the interobserver reliability of the 4Ts score in patients with suspected heparin-induced thrombocytopenia. *J. Thromb. Haemost.* **2012**, *10*, 151–152. [CrossRef] [PubMed]

12. Warkentin, T.E. How I diagnose and manage HIT. *ASH Educ. Program Book* **2011**, *1*, 143–149. [CrossRef] [PubMed]

13. Nagler, M.; Bachmann, L.M.; Ten Cate, H.; Ten Cate-Hoek, A. Diagnostic value of immunoassays for heparin-induced thrombocytopenia: A systematic review and meta-analysis. *Blood* **2015**, *127*, 546–557. [CrossRef] [PubMed]

14. Nagler, M.; Bakchoul, T. Clinical and laboratory tests for the diagnosis of heparin-induced thrombocytopenia. *Thromb. Haemost.* **2016**, *116*, 823–834. [CrossRef] [PubMed]

15. Greinacher, A.; Ittermann, T.; Bagemuhl, J.; Althaus, K.; Furll, B.; Selleng, S.; Lubenow, N.; Schellong, S.; Sheppard, J.I.; Warkentin, T.E. Heparin-induced thrombocytopenia: Towards standardization of platelet factor 4/heparin antigen tests. *J. Thromb. Haemost.* **2010**, *8*, 2025–2031. [CrossRef] [PubMed]

16. Linkins, L.A.; Dans, A.L.; Moores, L.K.; Bona, R.; Davidson, B.L.; Schulman, S.; Crowther, M. Treatment and prevention of heparin-induced thrombocytopenia: Antithrombotic therapy and prevention of thrombosis: American College of Chest Physicians evidence-based clinical practice guidelines. *Chest J.* **2012**, *141*, e495S–e530S. [CrossRef] [PubMed]

17. Farm, M.; Bakchoul, T.; Frisk, T.; Althaus, K.; Odenrick, A.; Norberg, E.M.; Berndtsson, M.; Antovic, J.P. Evaluation of a diagnostic algorithm for Heparin-Induced Thrombocytopenia. *Thromb. Res.* **2017**, *152*, 77–81. [CrossRef] [PubMed]

18. Bakchoul, T.; Zollner, H.; Greinacher, A. Current insights into the laboratory diagnosis of HIT. *Int. J. Lab. Hematol.* **2014**, *36*, 296–305. [CrossRef] [PubMed]

19. Michelson, A.D. *Platelets*, 2nd ed.; Elsevier Academic Press: Amsterdam, The Netherlands, 2011; pp. 861–886.

20. De Jong, W.H.; Wilkens, M.H.; de Vries, E.G.; Kema, I.P. Automated mass spectrometric analysis of urinary and plasma serotonin. *Anal. Bioanal. Chem.* **2010**, *396*, 2609–2616. [CrossRef] [PubMed]

21. Brand, T.; Anderson, G.M. The measurement of platelet-poor plasma serotonin: A systematic review of prior reports and recommendations for improved analysis. *Clin. Chem.* **2011**, *57*, 1376–1386. [CrossRef] [PubMed]

22. Warkentin, T.E.; Arnold, D.M.; Nazi, I.; Kelton, J.G. The platelet serotonin-release assay. *Am. J. Hematol.* **2015**, *90*, 564–572. [CrossRef] [PubMed]

23. Sheridan, D.; Carter, C.; Kelton, J.G. A diagnostic test for heparin-induced thrombocytopenia. *Blood* **1986**, *67*, 27–30. [PubMed]

24. Harenberg, J.; Huhle, G.; Giese, C.; Wang, L.C.; Feuring, M.; Song, X.H.; Hoffmann, U. Determination of serotonin release from platelets by enzyme immunoassay in the diagnosis of heparin-induced thrombocytopenia. *Br. J. Haematol.* **2000**, *109*, 182–186. [CrossRef] [PubMed]

25. Koch, S.; Odel, M.; Schmidt-Gayk, H.; Walch, S.; Budde, U.; Harenberg, J. Development of an HPLC method for the diagnosis of heparin-induced thrombocytopenia. *Anastesiol. Intensivmed. Notfallmed. Schmerzther.* **2002**, *37* (Suppl. S1), S12. [CrossRef]

26. Fouassier, M.; Bourgerette, E.; Libert, F.; Pouplard, C.; Marques-Verdier, A. Determination of serotonin release from platelets by HPLC and ELISA in the diagnosis of heparin-induced thrombocytopenia: Comparison with reference method by [C]-serotonin release assay. *J. Thromb. Haemost.* **2006**, *4*, 1136–1139. [CrossRef] [PubMed]

27. Sono-Koree, N.K.; Crist, R.A.; Frank, E.L.; Rodgers, G.M.; Smock, K.J. A high-performance liquid chromatography method for the serotonin release assay is equivalent to the radioactive method. *Int. J. Lab. Hematol.* **2016**, *38*, 72–80. [CrossRef] [PubMed]

28. Gobbi, G.; Mirandola, P.; Tazzari, P.L.; Ricci, F.; Caimi, L.; Cacchioli, A.; Papa, S.; Conte, R.; Vitale, M. Flow cytometry detection of serotonin content and release in resting and activated platelets. *Br. J. Haematol.* **2003**, *121*, 892–896. [CrossRef] [PubMed]

29. Stewart, M.W.; Etches, W.S.; Boshkov, L.K.; Gordon, P.A. Heparin-induced thrombocytopenia: An improved method of detection based on lumi-aggregometry. *Br. J. Haematol.* **1995**, *91*, 173–177. [CrossRef] [PubMed]

30. Teitel, J.M.; Gross, P.; Blake, P.; Garvey, M.B. A bioluminescent adenosine nucleotide release assay for the diagnosis of heparin-induced thrombocytopenia. *Thromb. Haemost.* **1996**, *76*, 479. [PubMed]

31. Greinacher, A.; Michels, I.; Kiefel, V.; Mueller-Eckhardt, C. A rapid and sensitive test for diagnosing heparin-associated thrombocytopenia. *Thromb. Haemost.* **1991**, *66*, 734–736. [PubMed]

32. Warkentin, T.E.; Moore, J.C. Laboratory evaluation of heparin-induced thrombocytopenia. In *Quality in Laboratory Hemostasis and Thrombosis*, 2nd ed.; Kitchen, S., Olson, J.D., Preston, F.E., Eds.; Wiley-Blackwell: Chichester, West Sussex, UK; Hoboken, NJ, USA, 2009.

33. Chong, B.H.; Burgess, J.; Ismail, F. The clinical usefulness of the platelet aggregation test for the diagnosis of heparin-induced thrombocytopenia. *Thromb. Haemost.* **1993**, *69*, 344–350. [PubMed]

34. Eichler, P.; Budde, U.; Haas, S.; Kroll, H.; Loreth, R.M.; Meyer, O.; Pachmann, U.; Potzsch, B.; Schabel, A.; Albrecht, D.; et al. First workshop for detection of heparin-induced antibodies: Validation of the heparin-induced platelet-activation test (HIPA) in comparison with a PF4/heparin ELISA. *Thromb. Haemost.* **1999**, *81*, 625–629. [PubMed]

35. Greinacher, A.; Amiral, J.; Dummel, V.; Vissac, A.; Kiefel, V.; Mueller-Eckhardt, C. Laboratory diagnosis of heparin-associated thrombocytopenia and comparison of platelet aggregation test, heparin-induced platelet activation test, and platelet factor 4/heparin enzyme-linked immunosorbent assay. *Transfusion* **1994**, *34*, 381–385. [CrossRef] [PubMed]

36. Warkentin, T.; Greinacher, A. *Heparin-Induced Thrombocytopenia*, 5th ed.; CRC Press: Boca Raton, FL, USA, 2012.

37. Fratantoni, J.C.; Pollet, R.; Gralnick, H.R. Heparin-induced thrombocytopenia: Confirmation of diagnosis with in vitro methods. *Blood* **1975**, *45*, 395–401. [PubMed]

38. Prechel, M.; Jeske, W.P.; Walenga, J.M. Anticoagulants, Antiplatelets, and Thrombolytics. In *Anticoagulants, Antiplatelets, and Thrombolytics*; Mousa, S.A., Ed.; Humana Press Inc.: Totowa, NJ, USA, 2004; Volume 93, pp. 83–94.

39. Elalamy, I.; Galea, V.; Hatmi, M.; Gerotziafas, G.T. Heparin-induced multiple electrode aggregometry: A potential tool for improvement of heparin-induced thrombocytopenia diagnosis. *J. Thromb. Haemost.* **2009**, *7*, 1932–1934. [CrossRef] [PubMed]

40. Minet, V.; Bailly, N.; Douxfils, J.; Osselaer, J.C.; Laloy, J.; Chatelain, C.; Elalamy, I.; Chatelain, B.; Dogne, J.M.; Mullier, F. Assessment of the performances of AcuStar HIT and the combination with heparin-induced multiple electrode aggregometry: A retrospective study. *Thromb. Res.* **2013**, *132*, 352–359. [CrossRef] [PubMed]

41. Morel-Kopp, M.C.; Mullier, F.; Gkalea, V.; Bakchoul, T.; Minet, V.; Elalamy, I.; Ward, C.M. Heparin-induced multi-electrode aggregometry method for heparin-induced thrombocytopenia testing: Communication from the SSC of the ISTH. *J. Thromb. Haemost.* **2016**, *14*, 2548–2552. [CrossRef] [PubMed]

42. Galea, V.; Khaterchi, A.; Robert, F.; Gerotziafas, G.; Hatmi, M.; Elalamy, I. Heparin-induced multiple electrode aggregometry is a promising and useful functional tool for heparin-induced thrombocytopenia diagnosis: Confirmation in a prospective study. *Platelets* **2013**, *24*, 441–447. [CrossRef] [PubMed]

43. Minet, V.; Baudar, J.; Bailly, N.; Douxfils, J.; Laloy, J.; Lessire, S.; Gourdin, M.; Devalet, B.; Chatelain, B.; Dogne, J.M.; et al. Rapid exclusion of the diagnosis of immune HIT by AcuStar HIT and heparin-induced multiple electrode aggregometry. *Thromb. Res.* **2014**, *133*, 1074–1078. [CrossRef] [PubMed]

44. Morel-Kopp, M.C.; Aboud, M.; Tan, C.W.; Kulathilake, C.; Ward, C. Whole blood impedance aggregometry detects heparin-induced thrombocytopenia antibodies. *Thromb. Res.* **2010**, *125*, e234–e239. [CrossRef] [PubMed]

45. Gobbi, G.; Mirandola, P.; Tazzari, P.L.; Talarico, E.; Caimi, L.; Martini, G.; Papa, S.; Conte, R.; Manzoli, F.A.; Vitale, M. New laboratory test in flow cytometry for the combined analysis of serologic and cellular parameters in the diagnosis of heparin-induced thrombocytopenia. *Cytom. Part B Clin. Cytom.* **2004**, *58*, 32–38. [CrossRef] [PubMed]

46. Tomer, A.; Masalunga, C.; Abshire, T.C. Determination of heparin-induced thrombocytopenia: A rapid flow cytometric assay for direct demonstration of antibody-mediated platelet activation. *Am. J. Hematol.* **1999**, *61*, 53–61. [CrossRef]

47. Vitale, M.; Tazzari, P.; Ricci, F.; Mazza, M.A.; Zauli, G.; Martini, G.; Caimi, L.; Manzoli, F.A.; Conte, R. Comparison between different laboratory tests for the detection and prevention of heparin-induced thrombocytopenia. *Cytometry* **2001**, *46*, 290–295. [CrossRef] [PubMed]

48. Tomer, A. A sensitive and specific functional flow cytometric assay for the diagnosis of heparin-induced thrombocytopenia. *Br. J. Haematol.* **1997**, *98*, 648–656. [CrossRef] [PubMed]

49. Solano, C.; Mutsando, H.; Self, M.; Morel-Kopp, M.C.; Mollee, P. Using HitAlert flow cytometry to detect heparin-induced thrombocytopenia antibodies in a tertiary care hospital. *Blood Coagul. Fibrinolysis* **2013**, *24*, 365–370. [CrossRef] [PubMed]

50. Malicev, E.; Kozak, M.; Rozman, P. Evaluation of a flow cytometric assay for the confirmation of heparin-induced thrombocytopenia. *Int. J. Lab. Hematol.* **2016**, *38*, 240–245. [CrossRef] [PubMed]

51. Kerenyi, A.; Debreceni, I.B.; Olah, Z.; Ilonczai, P.; Bereczky, Z.; Nagy, B., Jr.; Muszbek, L.; Kappelmayer, J. Evaluation of flow cytometric HIT assays in relation to an IgG-specific immunoassay and clinical outcome. *Cytom. Part B Clin. Cytom.* **2016**. [CrossRef] [PubMed]

52. Campello, E.; Radu, C.M.; Duner, E.; Lombardi, A.M.; Spiezia, L.; Bendo, R.; Ferrari, S.; Simioni, P.; Fabris, F. Activated platelet-derived and leukocyte-derived circulating microparticles and the risk of thrombosis in heparin-induced thrombocytopenia: A role for PF4-bearing microparticles? *Cytom. Part B Clin. Cytom.* **2017**. [CrossRef] [PubMed]

53. Warkentin, T.E.; Hayward, C.P.; Boshkov, L.K.; Santos, A.V.; Sheppard, J.A.; Bode, A.P.; Kelton, J.G. Sera from patients with heparin-induced thrombocytopenia generate platelet-derived microparticles with procoagulant activity: An explanation for the thrombotic complications of heparin-induced thrombocytopenia. *Blood* **1994**, *84*, 3691–3699. [PubMed]

54. Hughes, M.; Hayward, C.P.; Warkentin, T.E.; Horsewood, P.; Chorneyko, K.A.; Kelton, J.G. Morphological analysis of microparticle generation in heparin-induced thrombocytopenia. *Blood* **2000**, *96*, 188–194. [PubMed]

55. Mullier, F.; Bailly, N.; Cornet, Y.; Dubuc, E.; Robert, S.; Osselaer, J.C.; Chatelain, C.; Dogne, J.M.; Chatelain, B. Contribution of platelet microparticles generation assay to the diagnosis of type II heparin-induced thrombocytopenia. *Thromb. Haemost.* **2010**, *103*, 1277–1281. [CrossRef] [PubMed]

56. Mullier, F.; Minet, V.; Bailly, N.; Devalet, B.; Douxfils, J.; Chatelain, C.; Elalamy, I.; Dogne, J.M.; Chatelain, B. Platelet microparticle generation assay: A valuable test for immune heparin-induced thrombocytopenia diagnosis. *Thromb. Res.* **2014**, *133*, 1068–1073. [CrossRef] [PubMed]

57. Minet, V.; Bailly, N.; Dogne, J.M.; Mullier, F. Platelet microparticle generation assay for heparin-induced thrombocytopenia diagnosis: How should we express the results? *Thromb. Res.* **2015**, *136*, 175–177. [CrossRef] [PubMed]

58. Lee, D.H.; Warkentin, T.E.; Denomme, G.A.; Hayward, C.P.; Kelton, J.G. A diagnostic test for heparin-induced thrombocytopenia: Detection of platelet microparticles using flow cytometry. *Br. J. Haematol.* **1996**, *95*, 724–731. [CrossRef] [PubMed]

59. Hemker, H.C.; Giesen, P.; Al Dieri, R.; Regnault, V.; de Smedt, E.; Wagenvoord, R.; Lecompte, T.; Beguin, S. Calibrated automated thrombin generation measurement in clotting plasma. *Pathophysiol. Haemost. Thromb.* **2003**, *33*, 4–15. [CrossRef] [PubMed]

60. Hemker, H.C.; Giesen, P.; AlDieri, R.; Regnault, V.; de Smed, E.; Wagenvoord, R.; Lecompte, T.; Beguin, S. The calibrated automated thrombogram (CAT): A universal routine test for hyper- and hypocoagulability. *Pathophysiol. Haemost. Thromb.* **2002**, *32*, 249–253. [CrossRef] [PubMed]

61. Tardy-Poncet, B.; Piot, M.; Chapelle, C.; France, G.; Campos, L.; Garraud, O.; Decousus, H.; Mismetti, P.; Tardy, B. Thrombin generation and heparin-induced thrombocytopenia. *J. Thromb. Haemost.* **2009**, *7*, 1474–1481. [CrossRef] [PubMed]

62. Gardiner, E.E.; Karunakaran, D.; Arthur, J.F.; Mu, F.T.; Powell, M.S.; Baker, R.I.; Hogarth, P.M.; Kahn, M.L.; Andrews, R.K.; Berndt, M.C. Dual ITAM-mediated proteolytic pathways for irreversible inactivation of platelet receptors: De-ITAM-izing FcgammaRIIa. *Blood* **2008**, *111*, 165–174. [CrossRef] [PubMed]

63. Gardiner, E.E.; Al-Tamimi, M.; Mu, F.T.; Karunakaran, D.; Thom, J.Y.; Moroi, M.; Andrews, R.K.; Berndt, M.C.; Baker, R.I. Compromised ITAM-based platelet receptor function in a patient with immune thrombocytopenic purpura. *J. Thromb. Haemost.* **2008**, *6*, 1175–1182. [CrossRef] [PubMed]

64. Nazi, I.; Arnold, D.M.; Smith, J.W.; Horsewood, P.; Moore, J.C.; Warkentin, T.E.; Crowther, M.A.; Kelton, J.G. FcgammaRIIa proteolysis as a diagnostic biomarker for heparin-induced thrombocytopenia. *J. Thromb. Haemost.* **2013**, *11*, 1146–1153. [CrossRef] [PubMed]

65. Cuker, A.; Rux, A.H.; Hinds, J.L.; Dela Cruz, M.; Yarovoi, S.V.; Brown, I.A.; Yang, W.; Konkle, B.A.; Arepally, G.M.; Watson, S.P.; et al. Novel diagnostic assays for heparin-induced thrombocytopenia. *Blood* **2013**, *121*, 3727–3732. [CrossRef] [PubMed]

66. Lewis, S.M.; Bain, B.J.; Bates, I.; Dacie, J.V.; Dacie, J.V. *Dacie and Lewis Practical Haematology*, 10th ed.; Churchill Livingstone: Philadelphia, PA, USA, 2006; pp. 475–478.

67. Polgar, J.; Eichler, P.; Greinacher, A.; Clemetson, K.J. Adenosine diphosphate (ADP) and ADP receptor play a major role in platelet activation/aggregation induced by sera from heparin-induced thrombocytopenia patients. *Blood* **1998**, *91*, 549–554. [PubMed]

68. Warkentin, T.E.; Greinacher, A.; Gruel, Y.; Aster, R.H.; Chong, B.H. Laboratory testing for heparin-induced thrombocytopenia: A conceptual framework and implications for diagnosis. *J. Thromb. Haemost.* **2011**, *9*, 2498–2500. [CrossRef] [PubMed]

69. Leo, A.; Winteroll, S. Laboratory diagnosis of heparin-induced thrombocytopenia and monitoring of alternative anticoagulants. *Clin. Diagn. Lab. Immunol.* **2003**, *10*, 731–740. [CrossRef] [PubMed]

70. Favaloro, E.J.; Bernal-Hoyos, E.; Exner, T.; Koutts, J. Heparin-induced thrombocytopenia: Laboratory investigation and confirmation of diagnosis. *Pathology* **1992**, *24*, 177–183. [CrossRef] [PubMed]

71. Walenga, J.M.; Jeske, W.P.; Fasanella, A.R.; Wood, J.J.; Ahmad, S.; Bakhos, M. Laboratory diagnosis of heparin-induced thrombocytopenia. *Clin. Appl. Thromb. Hemost.* **1999**, *5*, S21–S27. [CrossRef] [PubMed]

72. Pouplard, C.; Amiral, J.; Borg, J.Y.; Laporte-Simitsidis, S.; Delahousse, B.; Gruel, Y. Decision analysis for use of platelet aggregation test, carbon 14-serotonin release assay, and heparin-platelet factor 4 enzyme-linked immunosorbent assay for diagnosis of heparin-induced thrombocytopenia. *Am. J. Clin. Pathol.* **1999**, *111*, 700–706. [CrossRef] [PubMed]

73. Morel-Kopp, M.C.; Aboud, M.; Tan, C.W.; Kulathilake, C.; Ward, C. Heparin-induced thrombocytopenia: Evaluation of IgG and IgGAM ELISA assays. *Int. J. Lab. Hematol.* **2011**, *33*, 245–250. [CrossRef] [PubMed]

74. Kappa, J.R.; Fisher, C.A.; Berkowitz, H.D.; Cottrell, E.D.; Addonizio, V.P. Heparin-induced platelet activation in sixteen surgical patients: Diagnosis and management. *J. Vasc. Surg.* **1987**, *5*, 101–109. [CrossRef]

75. Chong, B.H.; Pilgrim, R.L.; Cooley, M.A.; Chesterman, C.N. Increased expression of platelet IgG Fc receptors in immune heparin-induced thrombocytopenia. *Blood* **1993**, *81*, 988–993. [PubMed]

76. Chong, B.H.; Murray, B.; Berndt, M.C.; Dunlop, L.C.; Brighton, T.; Chesterman, C.N. Plasma P-selectin is increased in thrombotic consumptive platelet disorders. *Blood* **1994**, *83*, 1535–1541. [PubMed]

77. Griffiths, E.; Dzik, W.H. Assays for heparin-induced thrombocytopenia. *Transfus. Med.* **1997**, *7*, 1–11. [CrossRef] [PubMed]

78. Arman, M.; Krauel, K. Human platelet IgG Fc receptor FcgammaRIIA in immunity and thrombosis. *J. Thromb. Haemost.* **2015**, *13*, 893–908. [CrossRef] [PubMed]

79. Warmerdam, P.A.; van de Winkel, J.G.; Gosselin, E.J.; Capel, P.J. Molecular basis for a polymorphism of human Fc gamma receptor II (CD32). *J. Exp. Med.* **1990**, *172*, 19–25. [CrossRef] [PubMed]

80. Clark, M.R.; Stuart, S.G.; Kimberly, R.P.; Ory, P.A.; Goldstein, I.M. A single amino acid distinguishes the high-responder from the low-responder form of Fc receptor II on human monocytes. *Eur. J. Immunol.* **1991**, *21*, 1911–1916. [CrossRef] [PubMed]

81. Tomiyama, Y.; Kunicki, T.J.; Zipf, T.F.; Ford, S.B.; Aster, R.H. Response of human platelets to activating monoclonal antibodies: Importance of Fc gamma RII (CD32) phenotype and level of expression. *Blood* **1992**, *80*, 2261–2268. [PubMed]

82. Burgess, J.K.; Lindeman, R.; Chesterman, C.N.; Chong, B.H. Single amino acid mutation of Fc gamma receptor is associated with the development of heparin-induced thrombocytopenia. *Br. J. Haematol.* **1995**, *91*, 761–766. [CrossRef] [PubMed]

83. Brandt, J.T.; Isenhart, C.E.; Osborne, J.M.; Ahmed, A.; Anderson, C.L. On the role of platelet Fc gamma RIIa phenotype in heparin-induced thrombocytopenia. *Thromb. Haemost.* **1995**, *74*, 1564–1572. [PubMed]

84. Denomme, G.A.; Warkentin, T.E.; Horsewood, P.; Sheppard, J.A.; Warner, M.N.; Kelton, J.G. Activation of platelets by sera containing IgG1 heparin-dependent antibodies: An explanation for the predominance of the Fc gammaRIIa "low responder" (his131) gene in patients with heparin-induced thrombocytopenia. *J. Lab. Clin. Med.* **1997**, *130*, 278–284. [CrossRef]

85. Norris, C.F.; Pricop, L.; Millard, S.S.; Taylor, S.M.; Surrey, S.; Schwartz, E.; Salmon, J.E.; McKenzie, S.E. A naturally occurring mutation in Fc gamma RIIA: A Q to K127 change confers unique IgG binding properties to the R131 allelic form of the receptor. *Blood* **1998**, *91*, 656–662. [PubMed]

86. Bachelot-Loza, C.; Saffroy, R.; Lasne, D.; Chatellier, G.; Aiach, M.; Rendu, F. Importance of the FcgammaRIIa-Arg/His-131 polymorphism in heparin-induced thrombocytopenia diagnosis. *Thromb. Haemost.* **1998**, *79*, 523–528. [PubMed]

87. Francis, J.L. A critical evaluation of assays for detecting antibodies to the heparin-PF4 complex. *Semin. Thromb. Hemost.* **2004**, *30*, 359–368. [CrossRef] [PubMed]

88. Price, E.A.; Hayward, C.P.M.; Moffat, K.A.; Moore, J.C.; Warkentin, T.E.; Zehnder, J.L. Laboratory testing for heparin-induced thrombocytopenia is inconsistent in North America: A survey of North American specialized coagulation laboratories. *Thromb. Haemost.* **2007**, *98*, 1357–1361. [CrossRef] [PubMed]

89. Morel-Kopp, M.C.; Tan, C.W.; Brighton, T.A.; McRae, S.; Baker, R.; Tran, H.; Mollee, P.; Kershaw, G.; Joseph, J.; Ward, C.; et al. Validation of whole blood impedance aggregometry as a new diagnostic tool for HIT: Results of a large Australian study. *Thromb. Haemost.* **2012**, *107*, 575–583. [CrossRef] [PubMed]

90. Rollin, J.; Pouplard, C.; Gratacap, M.P.; Leroux, D.; May, M.A.; Aupart, M.; Gouilleux-Gruart, V.; Payrastre, B.; Gruel, Y. Polymorphisms of protein tyrosine phosphatase CD148 influence FcgammaRIIA-dependent platelet activation and the risk of heparin-induced thrombocytopenia. *Blood* **2012**, *120*, 1309–1316. [CrossRef] [PubMed]

91. Rollin, J.; Pouplard, C.; Sung, H.C.; Leroux, D.; Saada, A.; Gouilleux-Gruart, V.; Thibault, G.; Gruel, Y. Increased risk of thrombosis in FcgammaRIIA 131RR patients with HIT due to defective control of platelet activation by plasma IgG2. *Blood* **2015**, *125*, 2397–2404. [CrossRef] [PubMed]

92. Cattaneo, M.; Cerletti, C.; Harrison, P.; Hayward, C.P.; Kenny, D.; Nugent, D.; Nurden, P.; Rao, A.K.; Schmaier, A.H.; Watson, S.P.; et al. Recommendations for the standardization of light transmission aggregometry: A consensus of the working party from the platelet physiology subcommittee of SSC/ISTH. *J. Thromb. Haemost.* **2013**, *11*, 1183–1189. [CrossRef] [PubMed]

93. Legnani, C.; Cini, M.; Pili, C.; Boggian, O.; Frascaro, M.; Palareti, G. Evaluation of a new automated panel of assays for the detection of anti-PF4/heparin antibodies in patients suspected of having heparin-induced thrombocytopenia. *Thromb. Haemost.* **2010**, *104*, 402–409. [CrossRef] [PubMed]

94. Moore, J.C.; Arnold, D.M.; Warkentin, T.E.; Warkentin, A.E.; Kelton, J.G. An algorithm for resolving 'indeterminate' test results in the platelet serotonin release assay for investigation of heparin-induced thrombocytopenia. *J. Thromb. Haemost.* **2008**, *6*, 1595–1597. [CrossRef] [PubMed]

95. Poley, S.; Mempel, W. Laboratory diagnosis of heparin-induced thrombocytopenia: Advantages of a functional flow cytometric test in comparison to the heparin-induced platelet-activation test. *Eur. J. Haematol.* **2001**, *66*, 253–262. [CrossRef] [PubMed]

96. Tan, C.W.; Ward, C.M.; Morel-Kopp, M.C. Evaluating heparin-induced thrombocytopenia: The old and the new. *Semin. Thromb. Hemost.* **2012**, *38*, 135–143. [CrossRef] [PubMed]

97. Greinacher, A.; Gopinadhan, M.; Gunther, J.U.; Omer-Adam, M.A.; Strobel, U.; Warkentin, T.E.; Papastavrou, G.; Weitschies, W.; Helm, C.A. Close approximation of two platelet factor 4 tetramers by charge neutralization forms the antigens recognized by HIT antibodies. *Arterioscler. Thrombo. Vasc. Biol.* **2006**, *26*, 2386–2393. [CrossRef] [PubMed]

98. Krauel, K.; Hackbarth, C.; Furll, B.; Greinacher, A. Heparin-induced thrombocytopenia: In vitro studies on the interaction of dabigatran, rivaroxaban, and low-sulfated heparin, with platelet factor 4 and anti-PF4/heparin antibodies. *Blood* **2012**, *119*, 1248–1255. [CrossRef] [PubMed]

99. Warkentin, T.E.; Levine, M.N.; Hirsh, J.; Horsewood, P.; Roberts, R.S.; Gent, M.; Kelton, J.G. Heparin-induced thrombocytopenia in patients treated with low-molecular-weight heparin or unfractionated heparin. *N. Engl. J. Med.* **1995**, *332*, 1330–1335. [CrossRef] [PubMed]

100. Greinacher, A.; Michels, I.; Mueller-Eckhardt, C. Heparin-associated thrombocytopenia: The antibody is not heparin specific. *Thromb. Haemost.* **1992**, *67*, 545–549. [PubMed]

101. Kikta, M.J.; Keller, M.P.; Humphrey, P.W.; Silver, D. Can low molecular weight heparins and heparinoids be safely given to patients with heparin-induced thrombocytopenia syndrome? *Surgery* **1993**, *114*, 705–710. [PubMed]

102. Vun, C.M.; Evans, S.; Chong, B.H. Cross-reactivity study of low molecular weight heparins and heparinoid in heparin-induced thrombocytopenia. *Thromb. Res.* **1996**, *81*, 525–532. [CrossRef]

103. Makhoul, R.G.; Greenberg, C.S.; McCann, R.L. Heparin-associated thrombocytopenia and thrombosis: A serious clinical problem and potential solution. *J. Vasc. SurG.* **1986**, *4*, 522–528. [CrossRef]

104. Chong, B.H.; Ismail, F.; Cade, J.; Gallus, A.S.; Gordon, S.; Chesterman, C.N. Heparin-induced thrombocytopenia: Studies with a new low molecular weight heparinoid, Org 10172. *Blood* **1989**, *73*, 1592–1596. [CrossRef] [PubMed]

105. Greinacher, A.; Feigl, M.; Mueller-Eckhardt, C. Crossreactivity studies between sera of patients with heparin associated thrombocytopenia and a new low molecular weight heparin, reviparin. *Thromb. Haemost.* **1994**, *72*, 644–645. [PubMed]

106. Greinacher, A.; Alban, S.; Omer-Adam, M.A.; Weitschies, W.; Warkentin, T.E. Heparin-induced thrombocytopenia: A stoichiometry-based model to explain the differing immunogenicities of unfractionated heparin, low-molecular-weight heparin, and fondaparinux in different clinical settings. *Thromb. Res.* **2008**, *122*, 211–220. [CrossRef] [PubMed]

107. Rauova, L.; Poncz, M.; McKenzie, S.E.; Reilly, M.P.; Arepally, G.; Weisel, J.W.; Nagaswami, C.; Cines, D.B.; Sachais, B.S. Ultralarge complexes of PF4 and heparin are central to the pathogenesis of heparin-induced thrombocytopenia. *Blood* **2005**, *105*, 131–138. [CrossRef] [PubMed]

108. Greinacher, A.; Potzsch, B.; Amiral, J.; Dummel, V.; Eichner, A.; Mueller-Eckhardt, C. Heparin-associated thrombocytopenia: Isolation of the antibody and characterization of a multimolecular PF4-heparin complex as the major antigen. *Thromb. Haemost.* **1994**, *71*, 247–251. [PubMed]

109. White, M.M.; Siders, L.; Jennings, L.K.; White, F.L. The effect of residual heparin on the interpretation of heparin-induced platelet aggregation in the diagnosis of heparin-associated thrombocytopenia. *Thromb. Haemost.* **1992**, *68*, 88. [PubMed]

110. Potzsch, B.; Keller, M.; Madlener, K.; Muller-Berghaus, G. The use of heparinase improves the specificity of crossreactivity testing in heparin-induced thrombocytopenia. *Thromb. Haemost.* **1996**, *76*, 1121. [PubMed]

111. Socher, I.; Kroll, H.; Jorks, S.; Santoso, S.; Sachs, U.J. Heparin-independent activation of platelets by heparin-induced thrombocytopenia antibodies: A common occurrence. *J. Thromb. Haemost.* **2008**, *6*, 197–200. [CrossRef] [PubMed]

112. Arepally, G.; Reynolds, C.; Tomaski, A.; Amiral, J.; Jawad, A.; Poncz, M.; Cines, D.B. Comparison of PF4/heparin ELISA assay with the 14C-serotonin release assay in the diagnosis of heparin-induced thrombocytopenia. *Am. J. Clin. Pathol.* **1995**, *104*, 648–654. [CrossRef] [PubMed]

113. Prechel, M.M.; McDonald, M.K.; Jeske, W.P.; Messmore, H.L.; Walenga, J.M. Activation of platelets by heparin-induced thrombocytopenia antibodies in the serotonin release assay is not dependent on the presence of heparin. *J. Thromb. Haemost.* **2005**, *3*, 2168–2175. [CrossRef] [PubMed]

114. Horlait, G.; Minet, V.; Mullier, F.; Michaux, I. Persistent heparin-induced thrombocytopenia: Danaparoid cross-reactivity or delayed-onset heparin-induced thrombocytopenia? A case report. *Blood Coagul. Fibrinolysis* **2017**, *28*, 193–197. [CrossRef] [PubMed]

115. Tardy, B.; Presles, E.; Akrour, M.; de Maistre, E.; Lecompte, T.; Tardy-Poncet, B. Experts' opinion or the serotonin release assay as a gold standard for the diagnosis of heparin-induced thrombocytopenia (HIT)? *J. Thromb. Haemost.* **2011**, *9*, 1667–1669. [CrossRef] [PubMed]

116. Warkentin, T.E.; Sheppard, J.A.; Moore, J.C.; Cook, R.J.; Kelton, J.G. Studies of the immune response in heparin-induced thrombocytopenia. *Blood* **2009**, *113*, 4963–4969. [CrossRef] [PubMed]

117. Warkentin, T.E.; Sheppard, J.I.; Moore, J.C.; Kelton, J.G. The use of well-characterized sera for the assessment of new diagnostic enzyme-immunoassays for the diagnosis of heparin-induced thrombocytopenia. *J. Thromb. Haemost.* **2010**, *8*, 216–218. [CrossRef] [PubMed]

118. Warkentin, T.E.; Hayward, C.P.; Smith, C.A.; Kelly, P.M.; Kelton, J.G. Determinants of donor platelet variability when testing for heparin-induced thrombocytopenia. *J. Lab. Clin. Med.* **1992**, *120*, 371–379. [PubMed]

119. Arepally, G.M.; Kamei, S.; Park, K.S.; Kamei, K.; Li, Z.Q.; Liu, W.; Siegel, D.L.; Kisiel, W.; Cines, D.B.; Poncz, M. Characterization of a murine monoclonal antibody that mimics heparin-induced thrombocytopenia antibodies. *Blood* **2000**, *95*, 1533–1540. [PubMed]

120. Warkentin, T.E.; Sheppard, J.I. Generation of platelet-derived microparticles and procoagulant activity by heparin-induced thrombocytopenia IgG/serum and other IgG platelet agonists: A comparison with standard platelet agonists. *Platelets* **1999**, *10*, 319–326. [PubMed]

121. Warkentin, T.E.; Sheppard, J.A.; Moore, J.C.; Moore, K.M.; Sigouin, C.S.; Kelton, J.G. Laboratory testing for the antibodies that cause heparin-induced thrombocytopenia: How much class do we need? *J. Lab. Clin. Med.* **2005**, *146*, 341–346. [CrossRef] [PubMed]

122. Pauzner, R.; Greinacher, A.; Selleng, K.; Althaus, K.; Shenkman, B.; Seligsohn, U. False-positive tests for heparin-induced thrombocytopenia in patients with antiphospholipid syndrome and systemic lupus erythematosus. *J. Thromb. Haemost.* **2009**, *7*, 1070–1074. [CrossRef] [PubMed]

123. Isenhart, C.E.; Brandt, J.T. Platelet aggregation studies for the diagnosis of heparin-induced thrombocytopenia. *Am. J. Clin. Pathol.* **1993**, *99*, 324–330. [CrossRef] [PubMed]

124. Garritsen, H.S.; Probst-Kepper, M.; Legath, N.; Eberl, W.; Samaniego, S.; Woudenberg, J.; Schuitemaker, J.H.; Kroll, H.; Gurney, D.A.; Moore, G.W.; et al. High sensitivity and specificity of a new functional flow cytometry assay for clinically significant heparin-induced thrombocytopenia antibodies. *Int. J. Lab. Hematol.* **2014**, *36*, 135–143. [CrossRef] [PubMed]

125. Warkentin, T.E. Clinical picture of heparin-induced thrombocytopenia (HIT) and its differentiation from non-HIT thrombocytopenia. *Thromb. Haemost.* **2016**, *116*, 813–822. [CrossRef] [PubMed]

126. Warkentin, T.E.; Basciano, P.A.; Knopman, J.; Bernstein, R.A. Spontaneous heparin-induced thrombocytopenia syndrome: 2 new cases and a proposal for defining this disorder. *Blood* **2014**, *123*, 3651–3654. [CrossRef] [PubMed]

127. Warkentin, T.E.; Makris, M.; Jay, R.M.; Kelton, J.G. A spontaneous prothrombotic disorder resembling heparin-induced thrombocytopenia. *Am. J. Med.* **2008**, *121*, 632–636. [CrossRef] [PubMed]

128. Kopolovic, I.; Warkentin, T.E. Progressive thrombocytopenia after cardiac surgery in a 67-year-old man. *Can. Med. Assoc. J.* **2014**, *186*, 929–933. [CrossRef] [PubMed]

129. Tvito, A.; Bakchoul, T.; Rowe, J.M.; Greinacher, A.; Ganzel, C. Severe and persistent heparin-induced thrombocytopenia despite fondaparinux treatment. *Am. J. Hematol.* **2015**, *90*, 675–678. [CrossRef] [PubMed]

130. Alsaleh, K.A.; Al-Nasser, S.M.; Bates, S.M.; Patel, A.; Warkentin, T.E.; Arnold, D.M. Delayed-onset HIT caused by low-molecular-weight heparin manifesting during fondaparinux prophylaxis. *Am. J. Hematol.* **2008**, *83*, 876–878. [CrossRef] [PubMed]

131. Pruthi, R.K.; Daniels, P.R.; Nambudiri, G.S.; Warkentin, T.E. Heparin-induced thrombocytopenia (HIT) during postoperative warfarin thromboprophylaxis. A second example of postorthopedic surgery 'spontaneous' HIT. *J. Thromb. Haemost.* **2009**, *7*, 499–501. [CrossRef] [PubMed]

132. Padmanabhan, A.; Jones, C.G.; Bougie, D.W.; Curtis, B.R.; McFarland, J.G.; Wang, D.; Aster, R.H. Heparin-independent, PF4-dependent binding of HIT antibodies to platelets: Implications for HIT pathogenesis. *Blood* **2015**, *125*, 155–161. [CrossRef] [PubMed]

133. Warkentin, T.E.; Kelton, J.G. Delayed-onset heparin-induced thrombocytopenia and thrombosis. *Ann. Intern. Med.* **2001**, *135*, 502–506. [CrossRef] [PubMed]

134. Rice, L.; Attisha, W.K.; Drexler, A.; Francis, J.L. Delayed-onset heparin-induced thrombocytopenia. *Ann. Intern. Med.* **2002**, *136*, 210–215. [CrossRef] [PubMed]

135. Warkentin, T.E.; Bernstein, R.A. Delayed-onset heparin-induced thrombocytopenia and cerebral thrombosis after a single administration of unfractionated heparin. *N. Engl. J. Med.* **2003**, *348*, 1067–1069. [CrossRef] [PubMed]

136. Mallik, A.; Carlson, K.B.; DeSancho, M.T. A patient with 'spontaneous' heparin-induced thrombocytopenia and thrombosis after undergoing knee replacement. *Blood Coagul. Fibrinolysis* **2011**, *22*, 73–75. [CrossRef] [PubMed]

137. Greinacher, A. Me or not me? The danger of spontaneity. *Blood* **2014**, *123*, 3536–3538. [CrossRef] [PubMed]

138. Warkentin, T.E. Fondaparinux: Does it cause HIT? Can it treat HIT? *Expert Rev. Hematol.* **2010**, *3*, 567–581. [CrossRef] [PubMed]

139. Greinacher, A.; Michels, I.; Liebenhoff, U.; Presek, P.; Mueller-Eckhardt, C. Heparin-associated thrombocytopenia: Immune complexes are attached to the platelet membrane by the negative charge of highly sulphated oligosaccharides. *Br. J. Haematol.* **1993**, *84*, 711–716. [CrossRef] [PubMed]

140. Duffau, P.; Seneschal, J.; Nicco, C.; Richez, C.; Lazaro, E.; Douchet, I.; Bordes, C.; Viallard, J.F.; Goulvestre, C.; Pellegrin, J.L.; et al. Platelet CD154 potentiates interferon-alpha secretion by plasmacytoid dendritic cells in systemic lupus erythematosus. *Sci. Transl. Med.* **2010**, *2*, 47ra63. [CrossRef] [PubMed]

141. Bakchoul, T.; Giptner, A.; Bein, G.; Santoso, S.; Sachs, U.J. Performance characteristics of two commercially available IgG-specific immunoassays in the assessment of heparin-induced thrombocytopenia (HIT). *Thromb. Res.* **2011**, *127*, 345–348. [CrossRef] [PubMed]

142. Warkentin, T.E. Heparin-induced thrombocytopenia in the ICU: A transatlantic perspective. *Chest J.* **2012**, *142*, 815–816. [CrossRef] [PubMed]

143. Warkentin, T.E. Heparin-induced thrombocytopenia: Pathogenesis and management. *Br. J. Haematol.* **2003**, *121*, 535–555. [CrossRef] [PubMed]

144. Berry, C.; Tcherniantchouk, O.; Ley, E.J.; Salim, A.; Mirocha, J.; Martin-Stone, S.; Stolpner, D.; Margulies, D.R. Overdiagnosis of heparin-induced thrombocytopenia in surgical ICU patients. *J. Am. Coll. Surg.* **2011**, *213*, 10–17. [CrossRef] [PubMed]

145. Demma, L.J.; Winkler, A.M.; Levy, J.H. A diagnosis of heparin-induced thrombocytopenia with combined clinical and laboratory methods in cardiothoracic surgical intensive care unit patients. *Anesthesia Analg.* **2011**, *113*, 697–702. [CrossRef] [PubMed]

146. Crowther, M.A.; Cook, D.J.; Albert, M.; Williamson, D.; Meade, M.; Granton, J.; Skrobik, Y.; Langevin, S.; Mehta, S.; Hebert, P.; et al. The 4Ts scoring system for heparin-induced thrombocytopenia in medical-surgical intensive care unit patients. *J. Crit. Care* **2010**, *25*, 287–293. [CrossRef] [PubMed]

147. Tawfik, N.M.; Hegazy, M.A.; Hassan, E.A.; Ramadan, Y.K.; Nasr, A.S. Egyptian experience of reliability of 4T's score in diagnosis of heparin induced thrombocytopenia syndrome. *Blood Coagul. Fibrinolysis* **2011**, *22*, 701–705. [CrossRef] [PubMed]

148. Cuker, A.; Arepally, G.; Crowther, M.A.; Rice, L.; Datko, F.; Hook, K.; Propert, K.J.; Kuter, D.J.; Ortel, T.L.; Konkle, B.A.; et al. The HIT Expert Probability (HEP) Score: A novel pre-test probability model for heparin-induced thrombocytopenia based on broad expert opinion. *J. Thromb. Haemost.* **2010**, *8*, 2642–2650. [CrossRef] [PubMed]

149. Warkentin, T.E. Platelet microparticle generation assay for detection of HIT antibodies: Advance, retreat, or too soon to tell? *Thromb. Res.* **2014**, *133*, 957–958. [CrossRef] [PubMed]

150. Sachs, U.J.; von Hesberg, J.; Santoso, S.; Bein, G.; Bakchoul, T. Evaluation of a new nanoparticle-based lateral-flow immunoassay for the exclusion of heparin-induced thrombocytopenia (HIT). *Thromb. Haemost.* **2011**, *106*, 1197–1202. [CrossRef] [PubMed]

151. Cuker, A. Clinical and laboratory diagnosis of heparin-induced thrombocytopenia: An integrated approach. *Semin. Thromb. Hemost.* **2014**, *40*, 106–114. [CrossRef] [PubMed]

152. Cuker, A.; Cines, D.B. How I treat heparin-induced thrombocytopenia. *Blood* **2012**, *119*, 2209–2218. [CrossRef] [PubMed]

153. Cines, D.B.; Kaywin, P.; Bina, M.; Tomaski, A.; Schreiber, A.D. Heparin associated thrombocytopenia. *N. Engl. J. Med.* **1980**, *303*, 788–795. [CrossRef] [PubMed]

154. Sibbing, D.; Braun, S.; Morath, T.; Mehilli, J.; Vogt, W.; Schomig, A.; Kastrati, A.; von Beckerath, N. Platelet reactivity after clopidogrel treatment assessed with point-of-care analysis and early drug-eluting stent thrombosis. *J. Am. Coll. Cardiol.* **2009**, *53*, 849–856. [CrossRef] [PubMed]

155. Caton, S.; O'Brien, E.; 'annelay, A.J.; Cook, R.G. Assessing the clinical and cost impact of on-demand immunoassay testing for the diagnosis of heparin induced thrombocytopenia. *Thromb. Res.* **2016**, *140*, 155–162. [CrossRef] [PubMed]

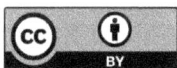

logo

Editorial

Advances in Heparins and Related Research. An Epilogue

Jawed Fareed *, Peter Bacher and Walter Jeske

Loyola University Medical Center, Maywood, IL 60153, USA; h.peter.bacher@gmail.com (P.B.); wjeske@luc.edu (W.J.)
* Correspondence: jfareed@luc.edu; Tel.: +1-708-216-3262

Received: 7 February 2018; Accepted: 8 February 2018; Published: 12 February 2018

The discovery of heparin in 1916 by Jay McLean, a medical student at Johns Hopkins University, not only provided a universal anticoagulant, but also laid the foundation for the discipline of hemostasis and thrombosis. Much of what is known today regarding bleeding and thrombotic disorders is based on the observations and scientific research on heparin and related drugs. The surgical, interventional, and medical usage of heparin has revolutionized medicine. For over one hundred years, new discoveries and innovative findings have continued to contribute to the expansion of our knowledge. The collection of manuscripts in this special issue of Molecules is a testimony of the continual progress in heparin sciences.

While heparin represents an old drug, the development of newer anticoagulants is primarily based on the knowledge of the mechanisms of the anticoagulant effects of heparin and related drugs. The newly developed non-vitamin K oral anticoagulants, including the anti-Xa and anti-IIa agents, along with the other mono-specific coagulation factor inhibitors, have been conceived based on the understanding of heparins's interactions with endogenous inhibitors in plasma. These single targeting agents, which include rivaroxaban, apixaban, edoxaban, betrixaban and dabigatran are agents with specific enzyme inhibitory profiles and do not exhibit the polypharmacologic profile of heparin. The multiple pharmacologic actions of heparin have been addressed for some years, and will continue to emerge as our knowledge of vascular pathology advances.

Over the last 25 years, several major developments have occurred that have revolutionized the scientific approaches and the clinical use of heparin and related drugs. The role of some of the contributors to this volume is demonstrated by the comprehensive manuscripts written by these leading scientists.

The introduction of fractionated heparins and the subsequent development of low molecular weight heparins (LMWHs) in the 1980s has added a new dimension to the management of surgical and medical thrombosis. Eventually, with knowledge of the composition and structure of LMWHs, synthetic heparins such as the pentasaccharide were developed by French investigators. Currently, biotechnology-based methods are being employed to design and develop heparin-related drugs. The identification of the antithrombin region and subsequent synthesis of heparin-related oligosaccharides such as the pentasaccharide laid the foundation for current research programs on the development of synthetic heparin mimetics and glycomimetics with broad clinical applications.

The step-wise clinical development of heparin and related drugs from their initial indication for surgical anticoagulation onwards to medical usage and prophylactic use for post-surgical thrombosis management played a key role in the expansion of the clinical indications of heparins and LMWHs. As pleiotropic agents, heparins target multiple sites, and accordingly are relevant in the management of diverse thrombotic and vascular disorders. Additional indications are established in the areas of cardiovascular disease, cancer, autoimmune diseases, neurodegenerative diseases and sepsis-associated coagulopathy. Much of the pharmacology of heparin remains to be explored.

Heparin is the only parenteral anticoagulant that has a clinically available antagonist, protamine sulfate. Progress in identifying additional heparin neutralizing agents has been met with limited success. Approaches such as heparin digesting enzymes including heparinase, recombinant platelet factor 4, polybrene, synthetic orgamomimetics and chromatographic methods have not provided clinically favorable results. Thus, protamine sulfate is the only antagonist that is clinically used for heparin and low molecular weight heparin neutralization.

The global contaminant crisis in 2008 was a wake-up call to all of the scientists, clinicians and regulatory bodies who use and study heparin. It prompted the establishment of defined guidelines and quality assurance procedures to confirm the structural integrity and activity of these biological compounds. With the introduction of methods such as nuclear magnetic resonance (NMR) and mass spectrometry (MS), the pioneering work of Italian scientists, in particular the Ronzoni Institute (Milan, Italy), led to the establishment of analytical methods to investigate the structure and corresponding functional relevance of the components of heparins. Such methods have since been applied to the quality assurance of heparins and the detection of impurities and contaminants. Through this effort, the heparins available globally have improved purity and are safer to use. Application of chemometric techniques and holistic approaches promises to make these analytical methods even more powerful. Several of the investigators who advanced and validated these methods have contributed to this special issue.

Heparin has provided a challenging opportunity to both clinicians and scientists for innovative research that has steadily advanced the therapeutic value of this poly-therapeutic agent. Scientists from various disciplines have initially focused on improving the isolation, purification and characterization of heparin and related glycosaminoglycans. The discovery of heparin also laid the foundation for the recognition of glycosaminoglycans as being of a broad group of biologically active polymers with functional and structural heterogeneity. This dedicated issue of Molecules is a testimony to these advances.

The contributions compiled in this special issue of Molecules describe a diverse array of basic science and clinical developments. Heparins have facilitated global scientific and clinical collaborations, which are also evident in this book. Through the efforts of the scientific group at the Ronzoni Institute, under the leadership of Professor Casu, the structural and functional relationships of heparins is being established. Many of the manuscripts in this issue represent collaborative and network-based scientific work.

Advances in technology and innovations in molecular and cellular biology coupled with integrated approaches have greatly amplified research in heparin related disciplines. Our understanding of the structure and biology of heparin is far from complete, and will continue to benefit from recent advances in structural analysis, where NMR methods have played a pivotal role. One of the major areas of ongoing research relates to the correlation of structure and function, which was perceived by Professor Casu and his group to be a crucial element in the understanding of heparins.

There have been concerns regarding the supply of unfractionated heparin, which is the only anticoagulant for surgical and interventional usage. The global porcine mucosal heparin supply is primarily controlled by Chinese manufacturers. Because of the biological nature of heparin, the US Congress has expressed concern about the potential shortage of this anticoagulant and its impact on healthcare https://energycommerce.house.gov/wp-content/uploads/2018/02/20180202FDA.pdf. The need to find alternate sources for heparin has been emphasized, and the option of reintroducing bovine heparin has been underscored. Bovine heparin had been used clinically in the initial stages of the development of this drug; however, because of the concerns over BSE and potential side effects, it was withdrawn from European and US markets. However, in light of the improved manufacturing processes and South American origin of the bovine tissue, these concerns may no longer relevant. Thus, the call for bovine heparin introduction is timely and will provide a reasonable alternate for porcine heparin. Additionally through further improvement of manufacturing, the potency of bovine heparin can be enhanced to equal the porcine potency and thus can be regarded as a biosimilar product. It should be underscored that despite minor structural differences bovine heparin is clinically comparable to porcine heparin.

Molecules **2018**, *23*, 390

Sheep provide another viable source of this anticoagulant. The sheep heparin is very similar to porcine heparin and can be manufactured to exhibit a comparable biochemical and pharmacological profile. Sheep heparins have also been used in the past for clinical usage. Currently sheep heparin is being developed for clinical purposes. Pre-clinical studies have shown that sheep heparin and low molecular weight heparins are comparable to their porcine counter-parts. Thus the development of sheep heparin is also timely and will be complimentary to the development of bovine heparin.

Some of the lead initiatives in heparin research are listed below, and will potentially be the topics of future manuscripts in Molecules:

1. Improved manufacturing and quality programs for heparins and related drugs. With the advancement in purification methods and improvements in quality assurance, the heparins available today are much purer and can be defined in terms of chemical nature and biologic activities.
2. Diversification of the sources for the manufacturing of heparin. Although the currently available heparin is primarily of porcine origin, additional sources including mamallian tissues and marine sources are also being used to obtain heparin and LMWHs with comparable biologic properties to the porcine material.
3. Re-introduction of bovine heparin for clinical use is now being considered by various regulatory agencies. A dedicated monograph to detail the specifications for bovine heparin has been introduced by Brazilian regulatory agencies. The USP and other agencies are also working on specific monographs dedicated to bovine heparin.
4. Molecular and structural analyses of heparin using advanced analytical approaches have provided additional tools to understand the structural characteristics of this complex polysaccharide. Biophysical methods have been used to characterize the solution structure and molecular interaction of heparin related drugs.
5. Therapeutic profiling of non-anticoagulant heparins has been a focus of intense pre-clinical and clinical research. Novel applications of heparin and non-anticoagulant heparins include neuromodulation, immunomodulation, and cytoprotection, as well as the treatment of inflammation and cancer.
6. Biosynthetic and recombinant heparins have been developed. Utilizing hybrid chemo-enzymatic methods, heparin analogues have been synthesized by various groups. The recombinant approaches have been of limited value, but may provide enzymes and other resources to develop bioheparins.
7. Enriched heparins with higher potency have recently been developed utilizingimproved purification and site-specific sulfation approaches.
8. Development of scientific guidelines to facilitate regulatory compliance and the introduction of improved and safer products. These guidelines have primarily been developed by clinicians and scientists with working experience with heparin. Product specifications, potency designation, biosimilarity and standardization are some of the considerations that will contribute to the development of safer therapeutic products.

The contributors to this special issue of Molecules represent some of the pioneers and leaders in their area of expertise. It is hoped that this compilation will also provide an integrated forum to initiate networking and international collaboration. This collection of articles in the form of a special issue was developed under the auspices of Ronzoni Institute and Loyola University Chicago. Both of these institutions are committed to increasing the awareness of heparin and related anticoagulants for the management of thrombosis and related disorders.

Conflicts of Interest: The authors declare no conflict of interest.

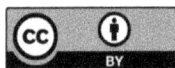

MDPI

St. Alban-Anlage 66

4052 Basel

Switzerland

Tel. +41 61 683 77 34

Fax +41 61 302 89 18

www.mdpi.com

Molecules Editorial Office

E-mail: molecules@mdpi.com

www.mdpi.com/journal/molecules

www.ingramcontent.com/pod-product-compliance
Lightning Source LLC
Chambersburg PA
CBHW051720210326
41597CB00032B/5543